TREATMENT OF CHILD ABUSE

Treatment of CHILD ABUSE

COMMON GROUND for MENTAL HEALTH, MEDICAL, and LEGAL PRACTITIONERS

2nd edition

Edited by
ROBERT M. REECE, M.D.
ROCHELLE F. HANSON, PH.D.
AND JOHN SARGENT, M.D.

FOREWORD BY WALTER F. MONDALE

JOHNS HOPKINS UNIVERSITY PRESS | BALTIMORE

Note to the Reader: This book discusses the treatment of child abuse *in general*. It is not intended to provide medical or legal advice regarding specific cases.

Drugs: The authors and publisher have made reasonable efforts to determine that the selection of drugs discussed in this text conforms to the practices of the general medical community. The medications described do not necessarily have specific approval by the U.S. Food and Drug Administration for the use in the diseases for which they are recommended. In view of ongoing research, changes in governmental regulations, and the constant flow of information relating to drug therapy and drug reactions, the reader is urged to check the package insert of each drug for any change in indications and dosage and for warnings and precautions. This is particularly important when the recommended agent is a new and/or infrequently used drug.

© 2000, 2014 Johns Hopkins University Press
All rights reserved. Published 2014
Printed in the United States of America on acid-free paper
9 8 7 6 5 4 3 2 1

Johns Hopkins University Press
2715 North Charles Street
Baltimore, Maryland 21218-4363
www.press.jhu.edu

Library of Congress Cataloging-in-Publication Data

Treatment of child abuse : common ground for mental health, medical, and legal practitioners / edited by Robert M. Reece, M.D., Rochelle F. Hanson, Ph.D., and John Sargent, M.D. ; foreword by Walter F. Mondale. — Second edition.
        pages cm
    Includes bibliographical references and index.
    ISBN-13: 978-1-4214-1272-6 (hardcover : alk. paper)
    ISBN-13: 978-1-4214-1273-3 (pbk. : alk. paper)
    ISBN-13: 978-1-4214-1274-0 (electronic)
    ISBN-10: 1-4214-1272-1 (hardcover : alk. paper)
    ISBN-10: 1-4214-1273-X (pbk. : alk. paper)
    ISBN-10: 1-4214-1274-8 (electronic)
    1. Child abuse—Treatment.   2. Abused children—Rehabilitation.
I. Reece, Robert M., editor of compilation.   II. Hanson, Rochelle F., 1962– editor of compilation.   III. Sargent, John, 1947– editor of compilation.
    RJ375.T74 2014
    616.85'8223—dc23   2013025012

A catalog record for this book is available from the British Library.

Special discounts are available for bulk purchases of this book.
For more information, please contact Special Sales at 410-516-6936
or specialsales@press.jhu.edu.

Johns Hopkins University Press uses environmentally friendly book materials, including recycled text paper that is composed of at least 30 percent post-consumer waste, whenever possible.

CONTENTS

CONTRIBUTORS

Ananda B. Amstadter, Ph.D.
Assistant Professor
Virginia Institute for Psychiatric and
    Behavioral Genetics
Virginia Commonwealth University
Richmond, VA

Christine Barron, M.D.
Assistant Professor of Pediatrics
    (Clinical)
The Warren Alpert Medical School of
    Brown University
Fellowship Director, Child Abuse
    Pediatrics
Child Protection Program
Hasbro Children's Hospital
Providence, RI

Judith V. Becker, Ph.D.
Professor, Department of Psychology
University of Arizona
Tucson, AZ

Leah E. Behl, Ph.D.
Child Abuse Research, Education, and
    Services Institute
Stratford, NJ

David S. Bennett, Ph.D.
Psychologist, Grow Clinic
St. Christopher's Hospital for Children
Professor, Department of Psychiatry
Drexel University College of Medicine
Philadelphia, PA

Erin C. Berenz, Ph.D.
Postdoctoral Fellow
Virginia Institute for Psychiatric and
    Behavioral Genetics
Virginia Commonwealth University
Richmond, VA

Lucy Berliner, M.S.W.
Director, Harborview Center for
    Sexual Assault and Traumatic
    Stress
University of Washington
Seattle, WA

Sandra L. Bloom, M.D.
Associate Professor
Drexel University School of Public
    Health
Philadelphia, PA
President, CommunityWorks
Distinguished Fellow, Andrus
    Children's Center
Yonkers, NY

Jeff Q. Bostic, M.D., Ed.D.
Associate Clinical Professor,
    Department of Psychiatry
Harvard Medical School
Director, School Psychiatry
Massachusetts General Hospital
Medical Director, Massachusetts Child
    Psychiatry Access Project Site at
    MGH
Boston, MA

Ernestine C. Briggs-King, Ph.D.
Assistant Professor of Psychiatry and
    Behavioral Sciences
Department of Psychiatry / Child
    and Family Mental Health and
    Developmental Neurology
Duke University School of
    Medicine
Durham, NC

Donald C. Bross, Ph.D., J.D.
Professor of Pediatrics
The Kempe Center
University of Colorado School of
    Medicine
Denver, CO

Adam Brown, Psy.D.
Clinical Assistant Professor of
    Psychiatry
Department of Child and Adolescent
    Psychiatry
New York University School of
    Medicine
New York, NY

Ruth C. Brown, Ph.D.
Postdoctoral Fellow
Virginia Commonwealth
    University
Virginia Institute for Psychiatric and
    Behavioral Genetics
Richmond, VA

Christopher Campbell, Ph.D.
Postdoctoral Psychology Fellow
University of Oklahoma Health
    Science Center
Oklahoma City, OK

Marianne Celano, Ph.D.
Professor of Psychiatry and Behavioral
    Sciences
Emory University
Associate Editor, *Journal of Family
    Psychology*
President, Society for Family
    Psychology
Atlanta, GA

Mark Chaffin, Ph.D.
Professor of Pediatrics
University of Oklahoma Health
    Sciences Center
Oklahoma City, OK

Kathleen M. Chard, Ph.D.
Veterans Administration CPT
    Implementation Director
Director, PTSD and Anxiety Disorders
    Division
Cincinnati Veterans Administration
    Medical Center
Associate Professor of Clinical
    Psychiatry
University of Cincinnati College of
    Medicine
Cincinnati, OH

Carla Kmett Danielson, Ph.D.
Associate Professor
National Crime Victims Research and
    Treatment Center
Medical University of South Carolina
Charleston, SC

Tatiana Davidson, Ph.D.
Mental Health Disparities and
    Diversity Program
Institute of Psychiatry and Behavioral
    Sciences
Medical University of South Carolina
Charleston, SC

Michael de Arellano, Ph.D.
Professor
National Crime Victims Research and
    Treatment Center
Medical University of South Carolina
Charleston, SC

Esther Deblinger, Ph.D.
Professor of Psychiatry
Rowan University—School of
    Osteopathic Medicine
Co-Director, Child Abuse
    Research Education Services
    (CARES) Institute
Stratford, NJ

Diane DePanfilis, Ph.D., M.S.W.
Director, Ruth Young Center for
    Families and Children
Professor, University of Maryland
    School of Social Work
Baltimore, MD

Erin C. Dunn, Sc.D., M.P.H.
Psychiatric and Neurodevelopmental
    Genetics Unit, Center for Human
    Genetic Research Massachusetts
    General Hospital
Department of Psychiatry, Harvard
    Medical School
Stanley Center for Psychiatric
    Research, The Broad Institute of
    Harvard and MIT
Boston, MA

Anna Edwards-Gaura, Ph.D.
National SafeCare Training and
    Research Center
Georgia State University
Atlanta, GA

Amanda M. Fanniff, Ph.D.
Assistant Professor
Pacific Graduate School
    of Psychology
Palo Alto University
Palo Alto, CA

Amanda K. Fingarson, D.O.
Instructor in Pediatrics
Northwestern University Feinberg
    School of Medicine
Chicago, IL

Martin A. Finkel, D.O., FAAP
Professor of Pediatrics
Medical Director, Rowan
    University—School of
    Osteopathic Medicine
Child Abuse Research
    Education Services (CARES)
    Institute
Stratford, NJ

Monica M. Fitzgerald, Ph.D.
Assistant Professor, Department of
    Pediatrics
University of Colorado–Denver
The Kempe Center for the Prevention
    and Treatment of Child Abuse and
    Neglect
The Gary Pavilion at Children's
    Hospital Colorado
Aurora, CO

Emalee G. Flaherty, M.D.
Professor of Pediatrics
Northwestern University Feinberg
    School of Medicine
Head, Division of Child Abuse Pediatrics
Ann & Robert H. Lurie Children's
    Hospital of Chicago
Chicago, IL

Robert P. Franks, Ph.D.
Director, Connecticut Center for
    Effective Practice
Vice President, Child Health and
    Development Institute
Farmington, CT

Beverly W. Funderburk, Ph.D.
Associate Professor of Research
Center on Child Abuse and Neglect
University of the Oklahoma Health
    Sciences Center's Department of
    Pediatrics
Oklahoma City, OK

Amy L. Gambow, M.S.
Palo Alto University
Palo Alto, CA

Rich Gilman, Ph.D.
Coordinator, Psychology and Special
    Education Programs
Division of Developmental and
    Behavioral Pediatrics
Cincinnati Children's Hospital Medical
    Center
Associate Professor, General Pediatrics
University of Cincinnati Medical
    School
Cincinnati, OH

Jordan Greenbaum, M.D.
Medical Director, Child Protection
    Team
Children's Healthcare of Atlanta
Atlanta GA

Rochelle F. Hanson, Ph.D.
Professor
National Crime Victims Research and
    Treatment Center
Medical University of South Carolina
Charleston, SC

Nicholas C. Heck, Ph.D.
Medical University of South Carolina
Charleston, SC

Sigalit Hoffman, M.D.
Assistant Professor in Psychiatry
Tufts University School of Medicine
Psychiatrist, Tufts Medical Center
Boston, MA

Soonjo Hwang, M.D.
Clinical/Research Fellow
National Institutes of Health, National
    Institute of Mental Health
Department of Psychiatry,
    Massachusetts General Hospital
Boston, MA

Sigrid James, Ph.D., LCSW
Associate Professor, Department of
    Social Work and Social Ecology
Loma Linda University School of
    Behavioral Health
Loma Linda, CA

Lisa H. Jaycox, Ph.D.
Senior Behavioral Scientist
RAND Corporation
Washington, DC

Sheryl H. Kataoka-Endo, M.D., M.S.H.S.
Assistant Professor of Psychiatry and
    Behavioral Health
University of California, Los Angeles,
    Health Services Research Center
Los Angeles, CA

Susan J. Kelley, RN, Ph.D., FAAN
Professor
Byrdine F. Lewis School of Nursing
    and Health Professions
Director, Project Healthy
    Grandparents
Georgia State University
Atlanta, GA

Hans B. Kersten, M.D.
Medical Director, Grow Clinic
St. Christopher's Hospital for
    Children

Associate Professor of Pediatrics
Drexel University College of Medicine
Philadelphia, PA

David J. Kolko, Ph.D., ABPP
Professor of Psychiatry, Psychology,
    and Pediatrics
University of Pittsburgh School of
    Medicine
Director, Special Services Unit
Western Psychiatric Institute and Clinic
Pittsburgh, PA

Jason M. Lang, Ph.D.
Associate Director, Connecticut Center
    for Effective Practice
Child Health and Development
    Institute of Connecticut
Assistant Professor, Department of
    Psychiatry
UCONN Health Center
Farmington, CT

Audra K. Langley, Ph.D.
Assistant Professor, Division of Child
    and Adolescent Psychiatry
University of California, Los Angeles,
    Semel Institute for Neuroscience
    and Human Behavior
Director of Training, Center for
    Resiliency, Hope, and Wellness in
    Schools
Chair, National Child Traumatic Stress
    Network School Committee
Los Angeles, CA

Jessica L. Laubach, B.S.
Department of Psychology
Carnegie Mellon University
Pittsburgh, PA

John Lutzker, Ph.D.
National SafeCare Training and
    Research Center
Georgia State University
Atlanta, GA

Kathi Makoroff, M.D., M.Ed.
Mayerson Center for Safe and Healthy
    Children
Cincinnati Children's Hospital Medical
    Center
Associate Professor of Pediatrics
University of Cincinnati College of
    Medicine
Cincinnati, OH

Erin McFry, M.P.H.
National SafeCare Training and
    Research Center
Georgia State University
Atlanta, GA

Colette McLean, LCSW
Rowan University—School
    of Osteopathic Medicine
Child Abuse Research Education
    Services (CARES) Institute
Stratford, NJ

Melissa McLean, LPC
Clinician
Rowan University—School of
    Osteopathic Medicine
CARES (Child Abuse Research
    Education and Service) Institute
Stratford, NJ

Walter F. Mondale
United States Senator, 1964–1976
42nd Vice President of the United
    States, 1977–1981
Senior Counsel, Dorsey Law Firm,
    Minneapolis, MN

Angela Montesanti, M.P.H.
National SafeCare Training and
    Research Center
Georgia State University
Atlanta, GA

Carryl P. Navalta, Ph.D.
Associate Professor, Department of
    Psychiatry
Boston University School of
    Medicine
Boston, MA

Michael W. Naylor, M.D.
Associate Professor of Psychiatry
University of Illinois at Chicago School
    of Medicine
Chicago, IL

Nicole R. Nugent, Ph.D.
Assistant Professor
Warren Alpert Medical School, Brown
    University
Providence, RI

Elisabeth Pollio, Ph.D.
Rowan University—School of
    Osteopathic Medicine

Child Abuse Research Education
    Services (CARES) Institute
Stratford, NJ

Mona Patel Potter, M.D.
Child and Adolescent Psychiatry,
    McLean Hospital
Instructor, Department of Psychiatry
Harvard Medical School
Boston, MA

Genevieve Preer, M.D.
Assistant Professor
Boston University School of Medicine
Boston, MA

Robert M. Reece, M.D.
Clinical Professor of Pediatrics
Tufts University School of Medicine
Editor, *The Quarterly Update*
North Falmouth, MA

Leslie Anne Ross, Psy.D.
Vice President, Leadership Center
Children's Institute Inc.
Los Angeles, CA

Melissa K. Runyon, Ph.D.
Professor of Psychiatry
Treatment Services Director, Rowan
    University—School of Osteopathic
    Medicine
Child Abuse Research Education
    Services (CARES) Institute
Stratford, NJ

John Sargent, M.D.
Director, Division of Child and
    Adolescent Psychiatry
Professor of Psychiatry and
    Pediatrics
Tufts University School of Medicine
Boston, MA

Benjamin E. Saunders, Ph.D.
Professor and Associate Director
National Crime Victims Research and
    Treatment Center
Department of Psychiatry and
    Behavioral Sciences
Medical University of South Carolina
Charleston, SC

Ronald C. Savage, Ed.D.
Chairman, International Pediatric
    Brain Injury Association
Philadelphia, PA

Glenn Saxe, M.D.
Arnold Simon Professor of Child and
    Adolescent Psychiatry
Chair, Department of Child and
    Adolescent Psychiatry
Director, New York University Child
    Study Center
New York, NY

Kimberly A. Schwartz, M.D., FAAP
Child Abuse Pediatrician
Boston Medical Center Child
    Protection Team
Boston, MA

Robert D. Sege, M.D., Ph.D.
Director, Division of Child and Family
    Advocacy
Medical Director, Child Protection
    Team, Boston Medical Center
Professor of Pediatrics
Boston University School of
    Medicine
Boston, MA

Shannon Self-Brown, Ph.D.
Associate Director, National SafeCare
    Training and Research Center
Associate Professor, Institute of Public
    Health
Georgia State University
Atlanta, GA

Jenelle Shanley, Ph.D.
National SafeCare Training and
    Research Center
Georgia State University
Atlanta, GA

Kimberly L. Shipman, Ph.D.
Assistant Professor, Department of
    Pediatrics
Program Director, Kempe Child
    Trauma Program
Kempe Center for the Prevention and
    Treatment of Child Abuse and
    Neglect
The Gary Pavilion at Children's
    Hospital Colorado
Aurora, CO

Shannon W. Simmons, M.D., M.P.H.
Acting Assistant Professor of
    Psychiatry
Department of Psychiatry and
    Behavioral Sciences

University of Washington School of
    Medicine
Seattle, WA

Brett Slingsby, M.D.
Assistant Professor of Pediatrics
University of South Dakota, Sanford
    School of Medicine
Child Abuse Pediatrician
Child's Voice
Sioux Falls, SD

Daniel W. Smith, Ph.D.
Professor of Psychiatry and Behavioral
    Sciences
Associate Dean for Faculty Affairs and
    Faculty Development
College of Medicine
Medical University of South Carolina
Charleston, SC

Bradley D. Stein, M.D., Ph.D.
Senior Natural Scientist, RAND
    Corporation
Associate Professor of Psychiatry
University of Pittsburgh
Pittsburgh, PA

Naomi Sugar, M.D. (deceased)
Clinical Professor of Pediatrics
General Pediatrics Division
University of Washington School of
    Medicine
Seattle, WA

Marcela M. Torres, Ph.D.
Instructor, Department of Pediatrics
University of Colorado School of
    Medicine
Child Trauma Program
Kempe Center for the Prevention and
    Treatment of Child Abuse and
    Neglect
Aurora, CO

Erika Tullberg, M.P.A., M.P.H.
Research Assistant Professor
Departments of Child and Adolescent
    Psychiatry and Psychiatry
New York University School of
    Medicine
New York, NY

Michael Ungar, Ph.D.
Killam Professor of Social Work
Dalhousie University

Network Director, Children and
    Youth in Challenging Contexts
    Network
Founder and Co-Director, Resilience
    Research Centre
Halifax, NS

Jeffrey N. Wherry, Ph.D., ABPP
Rockwell Professor of Human
    Development and Family Studies
    Director
Institute for Child and Family Studies
Texas Tech University
Lubbock, TX

Daniel Whitaker, Ph.D.
Professor, Georgia State University
Director, National SafeCare Training
    and Research Center
Director, Division of Health
    Promotion and Behavior
Atlanta, GA

Deborah M. Whitley, M.P.H., Ph.D.
Associate Professor, School of Social
    Work
Director, National Center on
    Grandparents Raising
    Grandchildren

Andrew Young School of Policy
    Studies
Georgia State University
Atlanta, GA

Marleen Wong, Ph.D.
Associate Dean and Clinical
    Professor
University of Southern
    California
Director, Field Education
University of Southern California
    School of Social Work
Los Angeles, CA

FOREWORD

In the early 1970s, I was deeply saddened by numerous media reports on child abuse and neglect in the United States. As I did more research, gathering information from frontline care providers and legal systems, I learned that our social and health systems suffered serious deficiencies in their responses to these tragedies. Child maltreatment impacts not only the direct victims—the children—but also their families and larger communities. All require our help. At that time, what appeared to be missing were targeted efforts for prevention and treatment. It was apparent that these issues needed immediate attention, but that addressing them would not be easy. Some parties expressed concern that efforts to alleviate child abuse would constitute an invasion of family privacy.

In 1973, as chairman of the Senate Subcommittee on Children and Youth, I held hearings on child abuse and neglect. We learned a great deal through these hearings and incorporated our findings into legislation, which culminated in the Child Abuse Prevention and Treatment Act (CAPTA). The purpose of CAPTA was to coordinate the identification, prevention, and treatment of child abuse and neglect at a national level, as well as to help states improve their systems for identifying, reporting, treating, and preventing all forms of child abuse and neglect. After working with colleagues in Congress and the Executive Branch, we saw our bill signed into law in 1974.

Much has happened since then, as demonstrated by the contents of this book. Despite consistent efforts over the past four decades, confirmed reports of child maltreatment hover around one million per year. However, we have made significant progress. Awareness of child maltreatment has greatly expanded. We have taken huge strides in demonstrating the effectiveness of a wide array of treatment and prevention programs, and we have significantly improved the dissemination and implementation of evidence-based practices into communities across the country. I believe this book will provide assistance and inspiration to all those who have dedicated their professional careers to improving the lives of abused children. Most importantly, I hope that this book will encourage all of us to continue pursuing new ways to ameliorate and prevent the unnecessary tragedy of child abuse.

Walter F. Mondale

PREFACE

Despite increased awareness and a decline in reported rates (Finkelhor & Jones, 2012; Finkelhor et al., 2010), child abuse and neglect remain a major public health problem in the United States in the twenty-first century. Nearly one million allegations of abuse and neglect are reported annually (U.S. Department of Justice, 2010). These experiences are associated with increased risk for myriad psychological and physical health consequences, both acutely and across the lifespan. Psychological difficulties, including depression, posttraumatic stress disorder, and substance abuse (e.g., Cisler et al., 2012; Dube, Felitti, et al., 2003; Dube, Miller, et al., 2006; Kilpatrick, Ruggerio, et al., 2003; Kilpatrick, Saunders, & Smith, 2002; Walsh et al., 2012), can further affect academic performance and educational attainment, relationship stability, risk for early pregnancy, and engagement in aggressive behavior that can result in involvement with the legal system. Research has also indicated that child abuse and neglect can cause neurobiological changes (Cohen et al., 2002; De Bellis et al., 2010) and are associated with smoking, obesity, and other chronic physical health conditions (Edwards et al., 2005; Ford et al., 2011; Williamson et al., 2002). The American Academy of Pediatrics has recently described child abuse and neglect as a crisis warranting multidisciplinary attention and creative individual and community remedies.

In the 13 years since publication of the first edition of Reece's *Treatment of Child Abuse*, much has changed. The mental health treatment community has emphasized the importance of rigorous research to identify effective treatments for traumatized children and adolescents. Federal and state agencies—such as the Substance Abuse and Mental Health Services Administration's (2013) National Registry of Evidence-based Programs and Practices, the National Child Traumatic Stress Network (www.nctsn.org), the Office of Justice Programs' Crimesolutions.gov (U.S. Department of Justice, 2013), and the California Evidence-Based Clearinghouse (Chadwick Center for Children and Families, 2013), to name a few—have identified trauma-informed, evidence-based practices to facilitate their widespread use among mental health, child welfare, and other professionals involved in providing services for abused children and their families. Furthermore, there have been significant efforts to enhance training and promote the widespread use of effective treatments among a broad range of child mental health professionals. The establishment of child abuse pediatrics as a subspecialty of pediatrics ensures accurate diagnosis and treatment of abuse and neglect and provides consistent education for pediatricians and family physicians in their training on abuse and neglect. In addition, improvements in foster care, development of trauma-informed care in residential treatment, attention to the experience and impact of bullying among abused and neglected youths, and awareness of the need for standards in the appropriate use of psychopharmacology for abused and neglected foster children—all have occurred in the past decade. Specific training in child abuse, neglect, and trauma treatment has been developed and promoted nationally for all professionals who care for children. Finally, there has been increased recognition of the psychological impact of this work on professionals, resulting in an awareness of the importance of self-care.

All of these issues are addressed in this book. Our hope is that the book will help professionals recognize the importance of evidence-based practices and promote widespread adoption of these practices among those involved in the care of abused and neglected children. The book begins with a focus on the identification of abuse and neglect and the psychosocial assessment of these children. Part II includes descriptions of several evidence-based and evidence-supported treatments for traumatized children and adolescents, including information on the research and theory underlying the interventions, as well as details of the treatment protocols. Part III addresses special populations and treatment approaches, including the Sanctuary Model of trauma-informed care, cultural modifications of evidence-based treatments, interventions to address bullying, and the treatment of children and adolescents who have engaged in sexual offenses. In part IV, the chapters cover the short- and long-term medical care of abused youth. The chapters in part V focus on a variety of approaches to the training of mental health professionals and physicians in trauma-informed, evidence-based care for abused children and how current theories are broadcast to the child abuse treatment community. A chapter on self-care for professionals working in this field is also included. Part VI includes a discussion about the exciting advances in psychopharmacology, the issues surrounding the interplay between genes and the environment, and the importance of resilience and recovery for victims of child maltreatment. Part VII is devoted to the significant legal implications of reporting, interviewing, courtroom testimony, and legal consequences for therapists.

We encourage readers to select those chapters of most interest and most use to their individual practices, as well as sharing of the book among colleagues and students entering the child abuse field. Effective responses to the challenge of child abuse and neglect need to be collaborative and multidisciplinary. Our hope is that this compilation of work will help each of you in your personal efforts and also aid in your collaborative practice. Finally we want to thank the authors who have so generously contributed their ideas, knowledge, and time. We hope that the lives of abused and neglected children are better for this.

References

Chadwick Center for Children and Families. (2013). *California Evidence-Based Clearinghouse for Child Welfare.* San Diego, CA: Author. www.cebc4cw.org

Cisler, J. M., Begle, A. M., Amstadter, A. B., Resnick, H. S., Danielson, C. K., Saunders, B. E., & Kilpatrick, D. G. (2012). Exposure to interpersonal violence and risk for PTSD, depression, delinquency, and binge drinking among adolescents: Data from the NSA-R. *Journal of Traumatic Stress, 25,* 33–40.

Cohen, J. A., Perel, J. M., Debellis, M., Friedman, M. J., & Putnam, F. W. (2002). Treating traumatized children: Clinical implications of the psychobiology of posttraumatic stress disorder. *Trauma, Violence & Abuse, 3*(2), 91–108.

De Bellis, M. D., Hooper, S. R., Woolley, D. P., & Shenk, C. E. (2010). Demographic, maltreatment, and neurobiological correlates of PTSD symptoms in children and adolescents. *Journal of Pediatric Psychology, 35*(5), 570–577.

Dube, S. R., Felitti, V. J., Dong, M., Chapman, D. P., Giles, W. H., & Anda, R. F. (2003). Childhood abuse, neglect and household dysfunction and the risk of illicit drug use: The Adverse Childhood Experience Study. *Pediatrics, 111*(3), 564–572.

Dube, S. R., Miller, J. W., Brown, D. W., Giles, W. H., Felitti, V. J., Dong, M., & Anda, R. F. (2006). Adverse childhood experiences and the association with ever using alcohol and initiating alcohol use during adolescence. *Journal of Adolescent Health, 38*(4), 444.e1–10.

Edwards, V. J., Anda, R. F., Dube, S. R., Dong, M., Chapman, D. F., & Felitti, V. J. (2005). The wide-ranging health consequences of adverse childhood experiences. In K. Kendall-Tackett and S. Giacomoni (Eds.), *Child Victimization: Maltreatment, Bullying, and Dating Violence, Prevention and Intervention.* Kingston, NJ: Civic Research Institute.

Finkelhor, D., & Jones, L. (2012). *Have sexual abuse and physical abuse declined since the 1990s?* Durham, NH: Crimes against Children Research Center.

Finkelhor, D., Turner, H. A., Ormrod, R. K., & Hamby, S. L. (2010). Trends in childhood violence and abuse exposure: Evidence from two national surveys. *Archives of Pediatrics & Adolescent Medicine 164*(3), 238–242.

Ford, E. S., Anda, R. F., Edwards, V. J., Perry, G. S., Zhao, G., Tsai, J., et al. (2011). Adverse childhood experiences and smoking status in five states. *Preventive Medicine, 53,* 188–193.

Kilpatrick, D. G., Ruggiero, K. J., Acierno, R., Saunders, B. E., Resnick, H. S., & Best, C. L. (2003). Violence and risk of PTSD, major depression, substance abuse/dependence, and comorbidity: Results from the National Survey of Adolescents. *Journal of Consulting and Clinical Psychology, 71,* 692–700.

Kilpatrick, D. G., Saunders, B. E., & Smith, D. W. (2002). *Research in brief: Youth victimization—Prevalence and implications* (NCJ 194972). Washington, DC: U.S. Department of Justice, National Institute of Justice.

Substance Abuse and Mental Health Services Administration. (2013). *National Registry of Evidence-based Programs and Practices.* Washington, DC: U.S. Department of Health and Human Services. www.nrepp.samhsa.gov

U.S. Department of Justice, Office of Justice Programs. (2013). CrimeSolutions.gov. Washington, DC: Author. http://crimesolutions.gov/TopicDetails.aspx?ID=60

Walsh, K., Danielson, C. K., McCauley, J., Hanson, R. F., Smith, D. W., Resnick, H. S., et al. (2012). Longitudinal trajectories of PTSD symptoms and binge drinking among adolescent girls: The role of sexual victimization. *Journal of Adolescent Health, 50*(1), 54–59. doi:10.1016/j.jadohealth.2011.05.017

Williamson, D. F., Thompson, T. J., Anda, R. F., Dietz, W. H., & Felitti, V. J. (2002). Body weight, obesity, and self-reported abuse in childhood. *International Journal of Obesity, 26,* 1075–1082.

PART I Initial Contact with the Abused Child

JORDAN GREENBAUM, M.D.
MARIANNE CELANO, PH.D.

Identification, Mandated Reporting Requirements, and Referral for Mental Health Evaluation and Treatment

GENERAL CONSIDERATIONS

A medical provider may encounter a child victim of abuse or neglect under a variety of circumstances, whether routine pediatric visits with the primary care physician or nurse practitioner, or acute care in the emergency department or surgical suite for injuries related to abuse or neglect, or intake exams at a juvenile detention center. The allegations of maltreatment may or may not have been previously identified and known to the provider. The child may disclose abuse spontaneously to the clinician, surprising both professional and parent. In some cases, the parent seeks medical attention for the child specifically because of concerns about maltreatment. Rarely, a child may present for medical care unaccompanied by an adult, with an allegation of abuse and a request for treatment and protection. This chapter considers issues relevant to the clinician who is providing care to a possible victim of abuse or neglect, including mandated reporting, patient privacy rules, and confidentiality, and provides an overview of the medical evaluation in cases of suspected maltreatment. We discuss how to determine the type of mental health treatment appropriate for a child and the best "fit" between child and therapist.

MANDATORY REPORTING OF ABUSE AND NEGLECT

As a condition for receiving federal funding through the Child Abuse Prevention and Treatment Act (CAPTA; Pub. L. No. 93-273; 43 U.S.C. §§ 5101–5119), states are required to implement statutes mandating certain adults to report suspected child abuse and neglect to authorities (National Association of Counsel for Children, 2012). As of April 2010, 48 states and the District of Columbia defined specific types of professionals (typically including health care workers and mental health providers) as mandated reporters, while New Jersey and Wyoming required all persons to report suspicions, without specifying any particular professional group (Child Welfare Information Gateway, 2010). Typically, state statutes require some level of certainty akin to "reasonable suspicion" or simply require that the reporter should have "reason to believe" or "suspect" that maltreatment has occurred before mandating a report, but there is ample room for interpretation and the provider may struggle with the decision. The purpose of the law is to empower mandated reporters and others to serve as a "safety net" for victimized children. As such, the level of certainty required to report suspected abuse is intended to be considerably lower than that associated with child protective service "case substantiation" or criminal conviction. Providers need not be certain that abuse or neglect has occurred before making a report, and typically this level of certainty is not possible without investigation that goes beyond the actions of the medical provider. It is the provider's responsibility merely to report concerns about possible abuse and then allow authorities to assess the situation and determine whether maltreatment has occurred.

Nearly all states (47 and the District of Columbia, as of December 2009) define penalties for a mandated reporter who fails to report suspected child maltreatment (Child Welfare Information Gateway, 2009); in most states the act is considered a misdemeanor. On the other hand, all 50 states and the District of Columbia also provide immunity from civil and criminal liability for any mandated reporter who makes a report "in good faith." This immunity is effective even when abuse or neglect is not substantiated by investigation (Child Welfare Information Gateway, 2012). In addition, many states also provide immunity for actions taken by the mandated reporter after the initial report, including participation in judicial proceedings and assistance with the investigation.

Finally, some states provide immunity for health care professionals when they undertake specific activities associated with the report of suspected maltreatment. These activities may include performing a physical exam; obtaining relevant laboratory tests, radiographs, or photographs; disclosing medical records or other pertinent information to authorities; and taking a child into emergency protective custody (Child Welfare Information Gateway, 2012).

State statutes vary, but many require that the mandated reporter make contact with authorities within a given time after determining the suspicion for abuse. This is often defined as within a 24-hour period. It is important to remember that the mandated reporter is responsible for the report and should not rely on others to call social services. A provider who sends a child with injuries suspicious for physical abuse to the emergency department and relies on staff there to recognize the concern and make the report is jeopardizing the safety of the child, as well as leaving himself or herself open to criminal or civil liability for failure to report.

PATIENT PRIVACY RULES AND CONFIDENTIALITY

In 2002 the Department of Health and Human Services established the Privacy Rule—the Standards for Privacy of Individually Identifiable Health Information (U.S. Department of Health and Human Services, Office of Civil Rights, 2003)—to implement the privacy requirement of the Health Insurance Portability and Accountability Act (HIPAA) passed by Congress in 1996 (Pub. L. No. 104-191). The Privacy Rule ensures the protection of individually identifiable health information and applies to "covered entities," including physicians and psychologists who document and exchange patient information in electronic form. While this rule provides strict control of the circumstances under which patient information may be released, there are important exceptions for cases of suspected child abuse and neglect. Specifically, medical and mental health providers are permitted to release protected health information (PHI) without parental or patient consent when required by law (e.g., mandatory reporting law). They are allowed to release relevant PHI to law enforcement and child protective service agencies to help these authorities avert or reduce a serious threat to a child's health or safety. They may also release this information in response to a court order, warrant, subpoena, or summons issued by a judicial officer (Podrid, 2003). The HIPAA regulations do not preempt state laws that call for reporting of disease, injury, child abuse, or death or reporting for public health surveillance purposes. If a provider discloses PHI, he or she must inform the child or the child's representative immediately, unless doing so would place the child at risk of serious harm.

Other details of the Privacy Rule are also important. Unless the state designates law enforcement as an entity to receive and investigate reports of suspected child maltreatment, the health care professional may disclose only limited information without authorization of the legal guardian; such limitations do not apply to child protective service agencies. In some situations the health care provider may believe the child or someone else is in imminent danger, and the health professional is then allowed to provide PHI to law enforcement. Occasionally, health care providers are asked to provide PHI even when they themselves have not reported the suspected abuse or neglect. They are allowed to do so without guardian authorization under certain conditions, including when it is permissible by state law, when it is necessary to protect the child or others from serious harm, and if the PHI released is relevant to the alleged maltreatment. Further details of the HIPAA regulation, Privacy Rule, and exceptions to HIPAA may be found elsewhere (Committee on Child Abuse and Neglect, American Academy of Pediatrics, 2010; Podrid, 2003).

The HIPAA regulations also require that legal guardians receive information describing their rights to confidentiality and to protection of health information related to the child. The guardian is asked to sign a form indicating that he or she has received and understands the rights. While the guardian ordinarily has access to the child's medical record, it is the prerogative of the health care provider to decide whether to allow the guardian such access when there are concerns about abuse or neglect. Specifically, if concerned that access to this information will endanger the child (e.g., the parent is the suspected abuser), the provider may refuse the guardian access (American Academy of Pediatrics, 2010).

Because of mandatory reporting laws and HIPAA exceptions, it is critically important for medical and mental health providers to make certain that adolescents are aware of limits in patient confidentiality. Thus, providers should make it clear early in the discussion that the child's disclosures regarding abuse or neglect will necessitate notification of authorities. In most cases, this also means the child's parents will learn of the disclosure. Confidentiality must also be breached if the child discloses harm to, or plans to harm, himself or herself or others.

MEDICAL EVALUATION OF SUSPECTED CHILD ABUSE AND NEGLECT

Physical Abuse

According to the Department of Health and Human Services, approximately 695,000 children were victims of maltreatment in 2010. Physical abuse was the second most common form of maltreatment and was identified in 17.6% of the children (U.S. Department of Health and Human Services, Administration on Children, Youth and Families, 2010). This type of abuse occurs in all age groups, but the most severely injured tend to be the youngest children. In 2010, 79% of fatal child maltreatment involved children less than 4 years old, with nearly 48% occurring in children less than 12 months of age. Of fatal cases, 45% involved physical abuse, either alone or in combination with other forms of maltreatment (U.S. Department of Health and Human Services, Administration on Children, Youth and Families, 2010).

Physical abuse is often manifested by skin injuries such as bruises, abrasions, and burns but may also take the form of inflicted fractures, closed head injury, mucosal trauma, asphyxial injury, or blunt force trauma to the thorax. Distinguishing abusive injuries from accidental ones may be difficult, and medical providers must rely heavily on information from a detailed history of the trauma event, as well as a thorough physical exam, often with supplemental diagnostic testing (Kellogg & Committee on Child Abuse and Neglect, 2007; Maguire, 2010). The history obtained from the caregiver should include a timeline of events prior to the reported trauma, extending to the time when medical attention was obtained. It is helpful to begin the account at the time when the child was last known to be acting completely normally, without signs or symptoms of injury. Specific details of the injury event itself (when and where it occurred, activities of the child at the time of the event, presence of witnesses, position of the child before/after a fall, child's response to the event, physical characteristics of the environment in which the event occurred) will help the provider understand the circumstances, assess the feasibility, and determine the likely mechanism and degree of force involved in the reported event. Comparing the mechanism and degree of force implied by the caregiver's history with what would be required to cause the observed injury will help determine the likelihood that the reported scenario actually caused the injury to the child.

When a child presents with a clear injury and the caregiver denies any episodes of trauma, concerns about maltreatment should arise. In a study of children 0–3 years of age admitted for head injuries, Hettler and Greenes (2003) found that "no history of trauma" had a specificity of 97% for inflicted trauma and a positive predictive value of 92%. In addition, changes in the caregiver's explanation of the injury event were significantly more likely in cases of "definite abuse" than in cases of "not definite abuse." Flaherty (2006) found that caregivers' initial explanation of the trauma event in children hospitalized for physical abuse contained elements of truth in over 90% of cases, particularly explanations involving the trigger for the abuse (e.g., crying, vomiting, toilet training) and the circumstances surrounding the trauma event (e.g., family conflict).

In evaluating a child for possible physical abuse, it is critical to consider underlying medical conditions that may mimic abuse, such as coagulopathies, osteogenesis imperfecta, glutaric aciduria, and vitamin D–deficient rickets. The medical provider needs to obtain detailed information on the child's past medical history, current and recent medications, and developmental and family history, as well as a review of systems, as such information can help rule out inherited and acquired diseases. A thorough developmental history may also aid in determining whether the child has the motor and cognitive skills implied in the trauma history.

A thorough physical exam is necessary in cases of suspected physical abuse, both to document injuries and to assess for possible medical conditions that may influence the interpretation of injuries. Bruising in nonmobile infants and children and bruising in ordinarily protected areas of the body (genitals, inner thighs, torso, ears, neck, and soft portion of the cheeks) have been shown to be associated with inflicted trauma (Labbe & Caouette, 2001; Pierce et al., 2010; Sugar et al., 1999). Any bruises, abrasions, or lacerations of the skin or mucosal surfaces should be measured and, if possible, photographed. Documentation should include the size, shape, color, and location of the injury and a description of associated findings such as swelling and tenderness. Photographs should contain a measurement tool or small object of known size (e.g., a nickel) and should include close-up views of the injury, as well as mid-range and more distant perspectives that show an anatomical landmark. All photographs should be identified and should be stored securely (Ricci, 2011).

Supplemental diagnostic testing to assess for occult inflicted trauma and possible organic disease depends on the nature and severity of the presenting injury, the child's age, any concerns about specific medical conditions raised by the history or physical findings, and the degree of suspicion for abuse. As infants and very young children tend to experience the most severe forms of abuse (National Association of Counsel for Children, 2012) and are at increased risk of inflicted fractures and abusive head injury (Pandya et al., 2009; Piteau et al., 2012), comprehensive testing for these children may include skeletal survey; noncontrast head CT; MRI of the brain and/or cervical spine; laboratory testing for hematologic disorders, occult abdominal trauma, and bone disease; formal ophthalmologic consultation; and in some circumstances, abdominal CT and tests for specific medical conditions (e.g., osteogenesis imperfecta) (Kellogg & Committee on Child Abuse and Neglect, 2007). Full skeletal surveys (using standards published in American College of Radiology, 1997, p. 23) have been shown to identify occult fractures in a substantial number of cases of suspected inflicted trauma (Belfer, Klein, & Orr, 2001; Hansen & Campbell, 2009; Hicks & Stolfe, 2007). In Belfer et al.'s (2001) study of children hospitalized for alleged abuse, 26% of the patients undergoing a skeletal survey had occult fractures. In its guidelines on diagnostic imaging of child abuse, the American Academy of Pediatrics, Section on Radiology (2000) recommends a complete skeletal survey in children under 2 years old for whom there are suspicions of abuse. Other specific recommendations for diagnostic imaging in cases of possible physical abuse are described elsewhere (Meyer et al., 2011).

In summary, the medical evaluation of suspected physical abuse involves careful analysis of information from a wide variety of sources, including history, thorough physical exam, and in many cases, ancillary testing and consultations by pediatric subspecialists. No single finding is pathognomonic for abuse, and a complete differential diagnosis must be considered.

Sexual Abuse

Sexual abuse is common in the United States. Results of one study employing a telephone survey indicated that 9.6% of girls and 6.7% of boys aged 2–17 years had been abused in the past year (Finkelhor et al., 2005). Medical providers are often asked to assess child victims for possible abuse, typically because a child has made concerning statements about possible molestation or a caregiver has noted unusual or sexualized behavior by the child or has observed signs and/or symptoms that suggest anogenital trauma or infection. The medical evaluation includes a thorough history (from the child and/or caregiver, depending on the child's age, developmental abilities, and circumstances), a comprehensive physical exam with detailed anogenital exam, and potentially, collection of trace evidence, sexually transmitted infection (STI) testing, and/or pregnancy and STI prophylaxis (Adams et al., 2007; Kellogg & Committee on Child Abuse and Neglect, 2005). The examiner should interview the child alone, if feasible, and use developmentally appropriate, nonleading questions to guide the exam and to gain information relevant to making the decision to report to authorities. If the child is over 2 years old, the parent should be interviewed outside the child's presence. It is important for the provider to document statements made by the child and the caregiver accurately, using direct quotations whenever possible.

The physical exam is important for documentation of any injuries, assessment and treatment of medical conditions (related or unrelated to sexual abuse), and screening for emotional and behavioral issues or developmental delays. It may also play a critical role in reassuring the child that his or her body is normal (or that injuries will heal and infections will be treated), in allaying fears of long-term catastrophic consequences (genitals will be permanently disfigured and everyone will "know" the child has been abused), and dispelling other misperceptions (a 5-year-old fearing she is pregnant). Careful documentation of exam findings includes detailed descriptions of injuries, discharges, focal lesions, normal variants, and nonspecific changes; diagrams are helpful, and photo or video documentation is ideal. Baseline testing for STIs is guided by the type of sexual contact alleged and by the history of symptoms, as well as by exam findings. The Centers for Disease Control and Prevention (2010) has published guidelines on STI testing and treatment.

The medical provider conducting the exam should have a thorough knowledge of prepubertal and adolescent anatomy, as well as normal variations in hymenal appearance. The provider should be proficient in the use of the various techniques that provide the most optimal views of the genitalia and anus. Many providers lack such training and experience (Adams et al., 2012), and often it is more appropriate to delay the exam 1–2 days if this will allow the child to be evaluated by an experienced provider. Not all children need an immediate exam; such urgency is typically necessary only if the alleged abuse may have occurred within the past 72 hours and trace evidence and/or biological material may be present, if the child is symptomatic (pain, bleeding, discharge, fever, etc.), if there are concerns about the child's emotional state (depression, psychosis, agitation, suicidal or homicidal ideation), or if the child may be in danger (possible harm by perpetrator or caregiver).

After the interview and exam, the medical professional provides recommendations and referrals to the child and family, as appropriate. This may include mental health assessment and treatment for the child and family, a developmental evaluation for the child, follow-up STI testing, and/or referrals to pediatric subspecialists for further evaluation of possible medical conditions. When abuse is suspected, child welfare and law enforcement should be notified and information gleaned from the assessment clearly communicated to investigators.

Child Neglect

Neglect is the most common form of maltreatment reported to authorities. According to data from the Department of Health and Human Services, more than 75% of maltreated child victims experienced neglect in 2010 (National Association of Counsel for Children, 2012). Medical evaluations of suspected neglect typically include a comprehensive physical exam to assess hygiene, growth and development, and general health and to check for untreated medical conditions. In cases of failure to thrive, laboratory testing may be done and is guided by history, exam findings, and results of prior medical evaluations. In assessments of possible physical neglect, photographs are often helpful, and documentation should include a description of the child's clothing, general appearance, affect, and behavior. A developmental screen is necessary because many neglected children have demonstrable delays and require referrals for comprehensive testing. Toxicology testing of urine or hair samples may be indicated if there is concern about exposure to drugs or other toxins.

MENTAL HEALTH ASSESSMENT

Some children exposed to abuse and other traumatic events have no evidence of mental health problems or experience only transient symptoms before returning to their previous level of functioning (Bonanno & Mancini, 2008; Kendall-Tackett, Williams, & Finkelhor, 1993). However, substantial proportions of abused children develop serious emotional and behavioral difficulties and health risks in adolescence (Boney-McCoy & Finkelhor, 1995; Hussey, Chang, & Kotch, 2006) or develop risky behaviors and health problems in adulthood (Schilling, Aseltine, & Gore, 2007). Therefore, a comprehensive assessment of the child victim's mental health needs is strongly recommended during the initial evaluation of the abuse.

A burgeoning literature documents the family processes (e.g., coercive parent-child interactions) contributing to the risk of abuse (Silber et al., 1993), as well as those (e.g., support from a nonoffending caregiver) that contribute to children's recovery from abuse (Conte & Schuerman, 1987). Abuse and its sequelae (e.g., separation from family members) can lead to adverse outcomes for all family members, including strained or conflictual family relationships, which can in turn place children at risk for developing mental health disorders. Furthermore, many victimized children bear the burden of cumulative trauma exposure; for these children, maltreatment is better conceptualized as a childrearing condition or context than as a discrete event (Finkelhor, Ormrod, & Turner, 2007). As a result, the mental health evaluation should be guided by an ecological systemic perspective in which the child victim's functioning and development are shaped by complex, transactional processes at the levels of the individual child, the family, and the community.

Given the documented impact of child maltreatment on a range of developmental outcomes, there is a broad consensus that mental health assessment should address the child's functioning across all key domains (e.g., emotional, cognitive, behavioral, social, and psychobiological) of his or her life (Margolin & Vickerman, 2007). Indeed, the ways in which abuse affects children's mental health are heterogeneous, depending on many factors, including the child's age and pre-morbid functioning, the timing of abuse onset, the child's exposure to other traumatic and adverse events, and the relationship of the abuser to the child. Symptoms in one domain (e.g., intrusive thoughts or images) may trigger symptoms in other domains (e.g., poor academic achievement or peer adjustment) by derailing the child from normal developmental tasks and acquisition of related competencies.

Assessment of the child's functioning across domains typically includes administering standardized measures of child behavior through the parent. As child physical abuse often occurs in the context of parental attributional bias, such as hypervigilance to child noncompliance or negative interpretation of child behaviors (Milner, 2003), abusive parents may report a higher level of negative child behaviors than nonabusive parents or teachers. Therefore, it is important to obtain data about the child's behavior from other adults in the child's life in addition to the parent. If appropriate, the mental health evaluation should include standardized measures of emotional and behavioral functioning designed to be completed by the child; child-report versions of most standardized assessment instruments are available for children over the age of 6 years.

In recent years, the concept of posttraumatic stress has emerged as a unifying framework for understanding and treating the problems of children who have experienced abuse and exposure to domestic violence (Vickerman & Margolin, 2007). As a substantial minority of child victims meet some or all of the criteria for posttraumatic stress disorder (PTSD) in the aftermath of abuse (Saunders, Berliner, & Hanson, 2004), clinicians should use assessment tools developed specifically to evaluate exposure to traumatic events and trauma-related symptoms for victims of child maltreatment. Many maltreated children have been exposed to other

traumatic events in addition to their abuse (Dong et al., 2004). Trauma screening should therefore include questions about exposure to an array of specific traumatic events, including rape, intimate partner violence, community violence, natural disasters, and invasive medical procedures (Margolin et al., 2009). After identification of a trauma history, the clinician should evaluate the impact of the traumatic event(s) on the child, using standardized measures of trauma-related symptoms. These semi-structured interviews or behavior checklists are valid tools for assessing PTSD symptoms among children over the age of 6 years; there are comparatively few valid and reliable instruments for assessing PTSD among children during the first five years of life.

Mental health evaluations of maltreated children should be developmentally informed. A developmental perspective is needed because the psychological sequelae of maltreatment depend in part on the child's developmental capacities. For example, children under the age of 5 years are often not able to communicate thoughts and feelings relevant to PTSD symptoms (e.g., fear, intrusive reminders of trauma, or the sense of a foreshortened future) and may manifest trauma symptoms in different ways than older children (e.g., posttraumatic play, regression of developmental skills, inappropriate sexual behaviors). Indeed, the DSM-IV diagnostic criteria for PTSD have been challenged on the grounds that they are developmentally inappropriate for very young children (Chu & Lieberman, 2010).

Assessment of the child's family context is needed to develop an appropriate case formulation and to identify and prioritize treatment targets. At a minimum, the evaluation should include information on the following: (1) family constellation and structure; (2) current parent-child relationship; (3) parental stress; (4) family health problems, including mental health and developmental disabilities; (5) parental substance abuse; (6) family support and resources; and (7) parenting practices, including the use of physical discipline strategies. An additional consideration is the parents' own trauma histories. Many parents involved in the child welfare system were abused or neglected as children or have experienced traumatic events in adulthood. Past or present experiences of traumatic stress can interfere in parents' ability to regulate their emotions, parent effectively, and maintain a safe and stable home environment for their children. Thus, it is important to gather information from the parent about his or her own trauma history as a part of the child's mental health assessment.

Some parts of the family assessment may be conducted in a different service setting or by a different evaluator than the setting or evaluator used in the mental health assessment of the maltreated child. Separate assessments may be indicated when one family member is the alleged perpetrator or when evaluation of the family member requires competencies that the child's evaluator does not have (e.g., substance abuse evaluation). If a child has been sexually victimized by an older child or adolescent in the family, the alleged perpetrator should also receive a mental health assessment. Although it is now known that youth who commit sexual offenses are more like other adolescent offenders than like adult sex offenders, evaluation using empirically supported risk assessment instruments is indicated (Ryan, Leversee, & Lane, 2010) to ascertain pedophilic interest, extent of denial or minimization of harm, and risk for reoffending, and in setting treatment goals. The timing and nature of the assessment of the adult perpetrator(s) in the family depend on the forensic investigation and the case plan developed by the statutory child protection agency; however, in most cases, a psychological or psychiatric evaluation of the perpetrator is needed to guide treatment, reduce the risk of recidivism, and determine the viability of family reunification. Assessment of sexual offenders is considered an area of specialty practice that requires specialized knowledge and training.

Culturally influenced values, beliefs, and practices must be taken into account when evaluating the child and family in child maltreatment cases. Values and beliefs informed by a family's or community's cultural, religious, and racial/ethnic identification include those related to sexuality, nudity, discipline practices, family boundaries, respect for elders, personal and familial privacy, gender roles, and help-seeking attitudes (Saunders, Berliner, & Hanson, 2004). There is well-documented variability across cultural groups in perceptions about the helpfulness and purpose of mental health services (U.S. Department of Health and Human Services, 2001), and different cultures define child maltreatment differently, depending on how these cultures have developed in response to social, economic, and political contexts (Fontes, 2005). To maximize the accuracy of mental health assessment in child maltreatment cases, clinicians should build rapport, overcome language barriers, respect families' values and beliefs while ensuring children's safety, include clergy and extended family members, as appropriate, and create a welcoming and respectful agency environment.

Two additional considerations must be addressed early in the assessment process in child maltreatment cases. The first is the safety of the child's current living environment. As many abused children continue to live with the family member who has hurt them or in families where intimate partner violence occurs, the clinician's first task is to assess the level of risk for harm in the child's environment and to engage in direct safety planning, in collaboration with other involved systems of care (Saunders, Berliner, & Hanson, 2004). Evaluation of risk also aids in identifying initial treatment targets for the family (e.g., treatment for substance abuse or behavior management skills for the parent) and contraindications for beginning trauma-informed therapy at a particular time. Targeted treatment of fear and anxiety symptoms might be ineffective or even harmful in situations in which it is appropriate for a child to be afraid and vigilant to danger.

A second important consideration in child maltreatment cases is the parents' perspective on the maltreatment charges (Saunders, Berliner, & Hanson, 2004). Parents exhibit a range of emotional reactions to children's abuse disclosures, including anger, disbelief, fear, shock, worry, and numbness. They may dispute the abuse allegations or minimize the harmful impact of the abuse on the child. It is important to remember that a parent's first reaction to the abuse disclosure is not always his or her best reaction, and many parents adopt a more supportive stance toward the child over time and with treatment. For some parents with a trauma history, their children's disclosure of traumatic experiences may trigger trauma-related symptoms such as numbness (i.e., appearing to be disengaged) or disabling anxiety. Identification of parents' perceptions, attitudes, and feelings about the alleged abuse is critical to the development of a meaningful and realistic treatment plan, particularly because a successful therapy outcome for maltreated children usually requires a high degree of parental investment and participation in the treatment process.

REFERRAL TO MENTAL HEALTH TREATMENT

Children with Symptoms

There is considerable consensus in the clinical and research literature on the important intervention objectives and strategies for maltreated children presenting with trauma-related symptoms. These children benefit from evidence-based, trauma-focused psychotherapy delivered to the child victim and his or her nonoffending caregiver(s). Based primarily on cognitive behavioral therapy (CBT) models, these interventions feature a combination of the following treatment components: (1) education about abuse and trauma, (2) regulation of emotions and coping, (3) parent training or parent-child relationship building, (4) trauma reexposure, (5) cognitive processing and restructuring of trauma, and (6) safety planning. Evidence-based interventions for children's PTSD symptoms related to abuse have been extensively reviewed (Dong et al., 2004; Saunders Berliner, & Hanson, 2004), and many of these models are discussed in this volume. Similarly, evidence-based family interventions have been developed and tested to help parents at risk for physically abusing their children and to help children who are affected by physical abuse. These interventions, based on behavioral therapy or CBT, work with the parent and child together to teach parents developmentally appropriate, nonviolent parenting skills and to improve parent-child interactions. A growing literature supports the efficacy of evidence-based family interventions in improving parenting skills and child behavior problems and in reducing physical abuse reports (Runyon & Urquiza, 2011).

Although clinical trials have established the efficacy of specific interventions in treating abuse-related symptoms or family processes for various populations, this research is only one factor to consider in treatment planning in a given case. The process of identifying the best mental health treatment for a given child and family requires consideration of multiple factors, consistent with evidence-based practice in professional psychology. Evidence-based practice is defined as the integration of research with clinical expertise in the context of patient characteristics, culture, and preferences (Levant et al., 2006). Clinical expertise includes the clinician's competency and confidence in a given intervention model, experience and comfort in treating a specific mental health problem or patient population, clinical formulation of the case, and access to appropriate professional supervision and support. In the case of child maltreatment, patient characteristics include the child's presenting problems (including co-morbidities), current risk and protective factors for mental health problems and revictimization, family structure and processes, culturally influenced beliefs and values, preferences for a given type of treatment, and access to mental health services. Evidence-based practice is the clinical decision-making process of tying together these three components—research, clinical expertise, and patient characteristics—on behalf of a particular child and family. The following case examples illustrate evidence-based practice in cases of child maltreatment.

Case 1. On forensic interview, a 24-year-old Caucasian mother reports that her 5-year-old son has witnessed her boyfriend's threats and physical aggression toward her on multiple occasions and that her boyfriend has also used corporal punishment to "discipline" her son. The boy presents with nightmares, frequent tantrums, oppositional behavior, and aggression toward siblings, with increased problems since the boyfriend left the home. The mother states that while she feels safer with her boyfriend out of the home, he was the only one who could control her son. The clinician refers the family to a colleague who is trained in Parent-Child Interaction Therapy (McNeil & Hembree-Kigin, 2010), with the goal of strengthening the parent-child bond and reducing behavioral problems before implementing a trauma-focused intervention.

Case 2. A 9-year-old African American boy with autism was sexually abused by an adolescent male cousin; the mother learned about the abuse when she "walked in" on the cousin attempting to penetrate her son. The child presents with cognitive delay (consistent with autism) and mild symptoms of anxiety, but the mother endorses symptoms of PTSD, in part related to her own sexual victimization in childhood. In addition, the parents report marital tension related to their different ways of coping with the abuse and their different relationships with the adolescent perpetrator (the father's nephew). According to the clinician's formulation, the child's anxiety is attributable mostly to his mother's emotional reaction to the abuse and to the ensuing marital tension. The clinician elects to do an adapted version of Trauma-Focused Cognitive Behavioral Therapy (TF-CBT) (Cohen, Mannarino, & Deblinger, 2006) for the couple and child, and she refers the mother to individual therapy. TF-CBT

is adapted such that the child and parents receive psychoeducation about abuse and safety planning, with the rest of the modules (including the mother's narrative about learning of her son's abuse) completed by the parents only.

Case 3. A 7-year-old Caucasian boy with a history of physical abuse and neglect is placed into his second foster home in two years. The earlier placement failed due to the boy's aggressive, hyperactive behavior, stealing, and chronic bedwetting. A previous mental health provider diagnosed attention-deficit/hyperactivity disorder and prescribed stimulant medication, which led to improved behavior and concentration. However, the boy continues to wet the bed nightly, and he now "sneaks" food and drink into his bedroom. The caseworker is worried that this placement may fail, because the foster mother has complained to her about the bedwetting. The child doesn't remember the physical abuse, which occurred when he was a toddler, or the neglect he experienced when he lived with his mother. He denies nightmares, sleep disturbance, or other symptoms of traumatic stress. His father is deceased, and the caseworker is seeking termination of parental rights for the mother. The clinician, in consultation with the caseworker and pediatrician, recommends behavioral treatment for nocturnal enuresis, with a plan to review the case for other treatment targets once the bedwetting is reduced.

Case 4. A 10-year-old daughter of parents who emigrated from Pakistan presents for treatment of PTSD symptoms following her substantiated allegation of sexual victimization by a Caucasian man in the neighborhood. The female clinician recommends TF-CBT to reduce the PTSD symptoms and refers the family to a male colleague at her agency. The parents do not keep the first TF-CBT appointment or return the male clinician's calls. The female clinician calls the family and learns that their cultural beliefs proscribe girls' discussion of sexual material with any males, including male doctors, particularly if the mother is not present. The mother also states that she and her husband do not want their daughter to write a narrative about the sexual abuse experience (a key feature of TF-CBT), as it is not proper for 10-year-old girls to talk or think about sex. The female clinician consults with her male colleague and agrees to begin supportive psychotherapy with the girl, hoping to build stronger rapport with the family over several sessions while she completes Web-based training in TF-CBT. She then implements TF-CBT without the narrative, a form of TF-CBT that has been shown to be efficacious (Deblinger et al., 2011), with supervision and support from her male colleague.

Case 5. A 16-year-old Caucasian girl with a history of multiple traumas, including chronic sexual abuse by her paternal grandfather (now deceased), presents with her mother for treatment of depression. The girl has had two previous psychiatric hospitalizations for suicidal ideation or threats, and she regularly engages in nonlethal cutting on her arms and legs. A trial of antidepressant medication has alleviated some of her depressive symptoms but has not reduced her self-destructive behavior or suicidal ideation. The clinician determines that the girl is not at imminent risk for harming herself or others but feels she is not stable enough to participate in a trauma-focused intervention at this time. The clinician refers the girl to a colleague who does Dialectical Behavioral Therapy, an evidence-based intervention that reduces suicidal and self-destructive behavior among adolescents (Miller, Rathus, & Linehan, 2006).

Some children or parents may be too psychiatrically unstable or cognitively limited to benefit from any of the evidence-based, trauma-focused interventions; in these cases, mental health interventions are oriented toward crisis stabilization, resource utilization, and safety planning. For example, a parent or child with a current substance abuse problem is unlikely to benefit from trauma-focused therapy until he or she has stopped using substances to avoid trauma symptoms. In this case, the patient may need substance abuse treatment before beginning a trauma-focused intervention.

In conclusion, acceptable interventions for symptoms and behaviors related to child maltreatment are developmentally informed, culturally sensitive, driven by a clinical case formulation, conducted by a qualified therapist, and accepted by the family and community. Given the current knowledge base on interventions for maltreated children, these interventions should be evidence-based and/or theoretically sound. Above all, they should do no harm.

Children without Symptoms

Not all children exposed to sexual or physical abuse develop detectable adverse outcomes (Kendall-Tackett, Williams, & Finkelhor, 1993), and some may exhibit delayed negative reactions (Bonanno & Mancini, 2008) as they develop or as they accumulate additional traumatic experiences and adversities. Even in the absence of presenting symptoms, the abuse has an effect on children because it is developmentally inappropriate (in the case of sexual abuse), it changes the relationship within which it is embedded, and it leads to changes in how the child views others and the world. There is currently no consensus on the recommended treatment for maltreated children without detectable psychological difficulties; however, at a minimum, the child and family may need some education about the nature of trauma and the effects of abuse on children. Some children without symptoms have families characterized by social isolation, coercive or authoritarian

parenting, and/or marital conflict. These family processes may constitute risk factors for maltreatment and adverse developmental outcomes for the child. For this reason, marital and family relationships and processes are appropriate targets for clinical intervention (Saunders, Berliner, & Hanson, 2004), even in the absence of symptoms in the child.

References

Adams, J. A., Kaplan, R. A., Starling, S. P., Mehta, N. H., Finkel, M. A., Botash, A. S., et al. (2007). Guidelines for medical care of children who may have been sexually abused. *Journal of Pediatric and Adolescent Gynecology, 20*, 163–172.

Adams, J. A., Starling, S. P., Frasier, L. D., Palusci, V. J., Shapiro, R. A., Finkel, M. A., & Botash, A. S. (2012). Diagnostic accuracy in child sexual abuse medical evaluation: Role of experience, training, and expert case review. *Child Abuse & Neglect, 36*(5), 383–392.

American Academy of Pediatrics, Section on Radiology. (2000). Diagnostic imaging of child abuse. *Pediatrics, 105*(6), 1345–1348.

American College of Radiology. (1997). *ACR standards for skeletal surveys in children*. Resolution 22. Reston, VA: Author.

Belfer, R. A., Klein, B. L., & Orr, L. (2001). Use of the skeletal survey in the evaluation of child maltreatment. *American Journal of Emergency Medicine, 19*, 122–124.

Bonanno, G. A., & Mancini, A. D. (2008). The human capacity to thrive in the face of potential trauma. *Pediatrics, 121*(2), 369–375.

Boney-McCoy, S., & Finkelhor, D. (1995). Psychosocial sequelae of violent victimization in a national youth sample. *Journal of Consulting and Clinical Psychology, 63*(5), 726–736.

Centers for Disease Control and Prevention. (2010). Sexually transmitted diseases treatment guidelines, 2010. *MMWR Recommendations and Reports, 59*(RR-12), 1–110.

Child Welfare Information Gateway. (2009). *Penalties for failure to report and false reporting of child abuse and neglect: summary of state laws*. Washington, DC: U.S. Department of Health and Human Services, Administration for Children and Families, Administration on Children, Youth and Families, Children's Bureau. www.childwelfare.gov/systemwide/laws_policies /statutes/report.cfm

Child Welfare Information Gateway. (2010). *Mandatory reporters of child abuse and neglect: Summary of state laws*. Washington, DC: U.S. Department of Health and Human Services, Administration for Children and Families, Administration on Children, Youth and Families, Children's Bureau. www.childwelfare.gov/systemwide/laws_policies/statutes /manda.cfm

Child Welfare Information Gateway. (2012). *Immunity for reporters of child abuse and neglect*. Washington, DC: U.S. Department of Health and Human Services, Administration for Children and Families, Administration on Children, Youth and Families, Children's Bureau. www.childwelfare.gov /systemwide/laws_policies/statutes/immunity.pdf

Chu, A. T., & Lieberman, A. F. (2010). Clinical implications of traumatic stress from birth to age five. *Annual Review of Clinical Psychology, 6*, 469–494.

Cohen, J. A., Mannarino, A. P., & Deblinger, E. (2006). *Treating trauma and traumatic grief in children and adolescents*. New York, NY: Guilford Press.

Committee on Child Abuse and Neglect, American Academy of Pediatrics. (2010). Policy statement—Child abuse, confidentiality, and the Health Insurance Portability and Accountability Act. *Pediatrics, 125*(1), 197–201.

Conte, J. R., & Schuerman, J. R. (1987). Factors associated with an increased impact of child sexual abuse. *Child Abuse & Neglect, 11*(2), 201–211.

Deblinger, E., Mannarino, A. P., Cohen, J. A., Runyon, M. K., & Steer, R. A. (2011). Trauma-focused cognitive behavioral therapy for children: Impact of the trauma narrative and treatment length. *Depression and Anxiety, 28*(1), 67–75.

Dong, M., Anda, R. F., Felitti, V. J., Dube, S. R., Williamson, D. F., Thompson, T. J., et al. (2004). The interrelatedness of multiple forms of childhood abuse, neglect, and household dysfunction. *Child Abuse & Neglect, 28*(7), 771–784.

Finkelhor, D., Ormrod, R. K., & Turner, H. A. (2007). Poly-victimization: A neglected component in child victimization. *Child Abuse & Neglect, 31*(1), 7–26.

Finkelhor, D., Ormond, R., Turner, H., & Hamby, S. L. (2005). The victimization of children and youth: A comprehensive national survey. *Child Maltreatment, 10*, 5–25.

Flaherty, E. G. (2006). Analysis of caretaker histories in abuse: Comparing initial histories with subsequent confessions. *Child Abuse & Neglect, 30*(7), 789–798.

Fontes, L. A. (2005). *Child abuse and culture: Working with diverse families*. New York, NY: Guilford Press.

Hansen, K. K., & Campbell, K. A. (2009). How useful are skeletal surveys in the second year of life? *Child Abuse & Neglect, 33*, 278–281.

Hettler, J., & Greenes, D. S. (2003). Can the initial history predict whether a child with a head injury has been abused? *Pediatrics, 111*(3), 602–607.

Hicks, R., & Stolfe, A. (2007). Skeletal surveys in children with burns caused by child abuse. *Pediatric Emergency Care, 23*(5), 308–313.

Hussey, J. M., Chang, J. J., & Kotch, J. B. (2006). Child maltreatment in the United States: Prevalence, risk factors, and adolescent health consequences. *Pediatrics, 118*(3), 933–942.

Kellogg, N., & Committee on Child Abuse and Neglect, American Academy of Pediatrics. (2005). The evaluation of sexual abuse in children. *Pediatrics, 116*(2), 506–512.

Kellogg, N. D., & Committee on Child Abuse and Neglect, American Academy of Pediatrics. (2007). Clinical report: Evaluation of suspected child physical abuse. *Pediatrics, 119*(6), 1232–1241. Updated May 2012.

Kendall-Tackett, K. A., Williams, L. M., & Finkelhor, D. (1993). Impact of sexual abuse on children: A review and synthesis of recent empirical studies. *Psychological Bulletin, 113*(1), 164–180.

Labbe, J., & Caouette, G. (2001). Recent skin injuries in normal children. *Pediatrics, 108*(2), 271–276.

Levant, R. F., Barlow, D. H., David, K. W., Hagglund, K. J., Hollon, S. D., Johnson, J. D., et al. (2006). Evidence-based practice in psychology. *American Psychologist, 61*(4), 271–285.

Maguire, S. (2010). Which injuries may indicate child abuse? *Archives of Diseases in Childhood: Education and Practice Edition, 95*, 170–177.

Margolin, G., & Vickerman, K. A. (2007). Posttraumatic stress in children and adolescents exposed to family violence: I. Overview and issues. *Professional Psychology: Research and Practice, 38*(6), 613–619.

Margolin, G., Vickerman, K. A., Ramos, M. C., Serrano, S. D., Gordis, E. B., Iturralde, E., et al. (2009). Youth exposed to violence: Stability, co-occurrence, and context. *Clinical Child and Family Psychology Review, 12*(1), 39–54.

McNeil, C., & Hembree-Kigin, T. L. (2010). *Parent-Child Interaction Therapy*. New York, NY: Springer.

Meyer, J. S., Gunderman, R., Coley, B. D., Bulas, D., Garber, M., Karmazyn, B., et al., Expert Panel on Pediatric Imaging. (2011). ACR appropriateness criteria: Suspected physical abuse—child. *Journal of the American College of Radiology, 8*, 87–94.

Miller, A. L., Rathus, J. H., & Linehan, M. M. (2006). *Dialectical behavior therapy with suicidal adolescents*. New York, NY: Guilford Press.

Milner, J. S. (2003). Social information processing in high-risk and physically abusive parents. *Child Abuse & Neglect, 27*(1), 7–20.

National Association of Counsel for Children. (2012). *Child maltreatment*. www.naccchildlaw.org/?page=child maltreatment

Pandya, N. K., Baldwin, K., Wolfgruber, H., Hayley, B. A., Christian, C. W., Drummond, D. S., et al. (2009). Child abuse and orthopaedic injury patterns: Analysis at a level 1 pediatric trauma center. *Journal of Pediatric Orthopedics, 29*, 618–625.

Pierce, M. C., Kaczor, K., Aldridge, S., O'Flynn, J., & Lorenz, D. J. (2010). Bruising characteristics discriminating physical child abuse from accidental trauma. *Pediatrics, 125*(1), 67–74.

Piteau, S. J., Ward, M. G. K., Barrowman, N. J., & Plint, A. C. (2012). Clinical and radiographic characteristics associated with abusive and nonabusive head trauma: A systematic review. *Pediatrics, 130*(2), 315–323.

Podrid, A. (2003) HIPAA—Exceptions providing law enforcement officials and social service providers access to protected health information. National District Attorneys Association, National Center for Prosecution of Child Abuse. *Update, 16*(4). www.ndaa.org/ncpca_update_v16_no4.html

Ricci, L. R. (2011). Photodocumentation in child abuse cases. In C. Jenny (Ed.), *Child abuse and neglect* (pp. 215–221). St Louis, MO: Elsevier.

Runyon, M. K., & Urquiza, A. J. (2011). Child physical abuse: Interventions for parents who engage in coercive parenting practices and their children. In J. E. B. Myers (Ed.), *The APSAC handbook on child maltreatment* (3rd ed., pp. 195–212). Thousand Oaks, CA: Sage Publications.

Ryan, G., Leversee, T. F., & Lane, S. (2010). *Juvenile sexual offending: Causes, consequences, and correction*. Hoboken, NJ: John Wiley & Sons.

Saunders, B. E., Berliner, L., & Hanson, R. F. (Eds.). (2004). *Child physical and sexual abuse: Guidelines for treatment*. Charleston, SC: National Crime Victims Research and Treatment Center.

Schilling, E., Aseltine, R., & Gore, S. (2007). Adverse childhood experiences and mental health in young adults: A longitudinal survey. *BMC Public Health, 7*(1), 30.

Silber, S., Hermann, E., Henderson, M., & Lehman, A. (1993). Patterns of influence and response in abusing and nonabusing families. *Journal of Family Violence, 8*(1), 27–38.

Sugar, N., Taylor, J. A., Feldman, K. W., & Puget Sound Pediatric Research Network. (1999). Bruises in infants and toddlers: Those who don't cruise rarely bruise. *Archives of Pediatrics & Adolescent Medicine, 153*, 399–403.

U.S. Department of Health and Human Services. (2001). *Mental health: Culture, race, and ethnicity*. Supplement to *Mental health: A report of the Surgeon General*. Executive summary. Rockville, MD: U.S. Department of Health and Human Services, Public Health Service, Office of the Surgeon General.

U.S. Department of Health and Human Services, Administration on Children, Youth and Families. (2010). *Child maltreatment*. www.acf.hhs.gov/programs/cb/stats_research/index.htm #can

U.S. Department of Health and Human Services, Office of Civil Rights. (2003). *Summary of the HIPAA Privacy Rule*. Last revised May 2003. www.hhs.gov/ocr/privacy/hipaa/understanding /summary/privacysummary.pdf

Vickerman, K. A., & Margolin, G. (2007). Posttraumatic stress in children and adolescents exposed to family violence: II. Treatment. *Professional Psychology: Research and Practice, 38*(6), 620–628.

JEFFREY N. WHERRY, PH.D., ABPP
ERNESTINE C. BRIGGS-KING, PH.D.
ROCHELLE F. HANSON, PH.D.

2

Psychosocial Assessment in Child Maltreatment

D isclaimer #1. Beware! The following terms are confusing: Psychosocial assessment, biopsychosocial assessment, clinical intake, clinical interview, screening, mental status exam, psychological evaluation, psychiatric evaluation—these terms probably carry different meanings for nearly everyone reading this chapter. For the purposes of this chapter, we use the term *psychosocial assessment* to refer to a process for assessing the symptoms, behaviors, and treatment needs of children who have experienced maltreatment.

Disclaimer #2. Bias ahead! As licensed psychologists with an interest in psychological assessment of maltreated children, we are inclined to "sell you" on some degree of formal assessment of abused children. To be clear, it is our bias that successful treatments are informed by a good assessment. Ultimately, this requires a skilled clinician who uses data to understand a client's strengths, needs, and difficulties and for treatment planning, much as a detective uses clues in solving a mystery. In addition, in the case of child maltreatment, a good assessment should include some systematic evaluation of common symptoms associated with abuse and should utilize items that are reliable, valid, and normed.

Disclaimer #3. Limited advances in assessment. In many ways, the development of reliable, valid, and normed assessments of abuse-related symptoms has lagged behind the development of evidence-based treatments for maltreated children. This is good news and, potentially at least, bad news. The good news is that maltreated children and their families are receiving some level of assistance. The potential bad news is that, without adequate assessment, children may be receiving treatment that is not appropriate. Moreover, many of the available, psychometrically sound measures for child maltreatment focus primarily on the assessment of either sexual abuse or physical abuse and not on the co-occurring or multiple forms of abuse and neglect that are often typical (Saunders, 2003).

As you may have surmised from the disclaimers, our purpose here is to provide a comprehensive overview of psychosocial assessment for children who have experienced abuse, neglect, or some other traumatic event. Along the way we identify some of the key terms and definitions used to describe assessment, examine the components that are an essential part of good clinical practice, and discuss some of the challenges that arise in assessing the diverse needs of these children. We offer descriptions of potential measures, some final considerations, and available resources.

DEFINITION OF TERMS

Psychological Assessments

The term *psychological assessment* is usually considered more comprehensive than the term *psychological testing* (Handler & Meyer, 1998). Many psychological tests are administered, scored, and interpreted almost exclusively by psychologists (e.g., projectives such as the Rorschach Inkblot Test and cognitive tests such as the Wechsler Intelligence Scale for Children). Other assessment instruments are used by a diverse group of professionals with formal training in their ethical administration, scoring, and interpretation. Regardless of the professional affiliation of the assessor, instruments should be psychometrically sound, which includes good reliability and validity, and should be normed for the population for which they are being used (Conradi, Wherry, & Kisiel, 2011).

Reliability is the consistency of a measure, test, or tool (or its specific items). Reliability may include consistency across time (test-retest) or across independent raters (joint or inter-rater), as well as consistency within the measure itself (internal consistency).

Validity is the degree to which a measure, test, or tool (or its specific items) accurately represents a psychological construct, domain, or dimension of functioning. Various types of validity (e.g., face/construct, criterion/concurrent/predictive, content, and convergent/divergent/discriminant) contribute to determining whether an instrument is useful, meaningful, and truly measuring what it purports to measure.

Standardization of norms is the process of measuring a sufficient and representative sample along a psychological construct, domain, or dimension of functioning for the purposes of characterizing a population. For a measure to be developmentally and culturally sensitive, the standardization should represent the population for which it will be used (e.g., by age, sex, and race/ethnicity).

Screening, Assessments, Testing, Intakes, and Evaluations

Unfortunately, terms like *screening, testing, assessment, intake,* and *evaluation* may be used interchangeably or differently by clinicians. All of these terms refer to some form of assessment, incorporating one or more methods or procedures. The procedures may differ by professional discipline, by the referral questions, by the role of the clinician, and (hopefully) by the needs and unique presentation of the child and/or child population in question.

Historically, psychologists have used a comprehensive "battery" of tests administered without reflection on the specific referral questions of relevance. Moreover, referring agents often are guilty of recommending an evaluation for all abused children without a thought to the specific questions to be answered. As a result, children may be described in general terms (e.g., as having "problems with managing his anger") rather than by informed clinical opinions. Or nebulous and mysterious phrases might be used, such as "poor reality testing" (which often comes from one particular score of the Rorschach). Other slightly scientific but still vague terms might be used, such as "externalizing" and "internalizing" behavior problems (from the broad-band rating scales of the Child Behavior Checklist, CBCL; Achenbach, 1993). In the end, the helpfulness of these terms in describing and planning for children who have been abused is dubious at best.

. . .

At a time in history when we are able to refine our assessments and, by necessity, are required to control costs, an unthinking reliance on comprehensive evaluations is not the best practice. Rather, as in medicine, a stepwise approach seems warranted. For example, in a medical practice, a patient presents to the physician's office with a cluster of symptoms, a complaint, or a question. The health care staff starts with these complaints and, through a process of hypothesis testing and differential diagnosis, explores additional symptoms and underlying processes that may facilitate an accurate diagnosis and proper treatment. The need for additional tests is determined based on the presenting problem and the differential diagnoses under consideration.

The same process of hypothesis testing should occur when a child who has been abused presents as irritable, unable to concentrate, and having difficulty sleeping. Rather than a comprehensive battery of tests, the clinician should ask additional questions about symptoms, obtain a history, and consider at least the possibility of the most common abuse-related sequelae, such as posttraumatic stress disorder (PTSD), depression, anxiety, or attention-deficit / hyperactivity disorder (ADHD). Specific instruments might be used to screen efficiently for the presence of these disorders. Then, if one or more of the disorders appears likely, a unidimensional measure (assessing a single construct, such as depression) or set of measures might be used to explore one of these diagnoses more thoroughly. The use of specific tests might be indicated even though the tests are brief. This type of thoughtful approach to the assessment process is likely to yield a more accurate picture of the child's problems and functioning, which can then guide decisions regarding the need for further intervention.

COMMON SETTINGS FOR INITIAL ASSESSMENT OF ABUSED CHILDREN

Children Entering into the Care of Child Protective Services

In many states, historically, children in the child welfare system have been psychologically evaluated at the time of placement outside the home. Too often those evaluations have been "comprehensive" in scope but general in focus. They have often included cognitive assessments and projective techniques. In more recent years, there has been an increase in the use of both unidimensional measures and broadband rating scales, such as the Child Behavior Checklist (Achenbach, 1993), completed by youth as well as by caregivers, teachers, or other relevant adults. However, rarely are abuse-focused measures utilized in these child welfare assessments. For example, in a review of current clinical practices, Cashel (2002) found that 71% of psychologists used clinical interviews, and 69.8% of psychologists also used IQ or cognitive assessments; no tests of trauma symptoms were identified for use with adults, let alone children. Thus, despite increased awareness of the importance of targeted assessments in child welfare settings, global clinical or diagnostic interviews continue to be ranked as the most common forms of assessment across disciplines (Summerfeldt & Antony, 2002).

Child Welfare

Conradi, Wherry, and Kisiel (2011) suggest that it is critical that the child welfare system work with the mental health system to ensure that abused children receive trauma-focused screening and assessment and referral to the appropriate trauma-focused mental health services. The authors also note that assessment helps to identify those children who may not be candidates for trauma-focused treatment—that is, those who are not displaying trauma-related symptoms.

After years of multiple disciplines neglecting or minimizing the impact of abuse, policymakers have become increasingly attentive to "trauma" and "trauma-informed care." Unfortunately, this newfound interest and current fervor of legislators might not always be tempered or informed by the need for empirically supported assessments that lead to appropriate treatment. Thus there is the danger that uninformed clinicians will implement trauma-focused treatments with children who do not have symptoms of trauma. Arguably, the indiscriminate application of a trauma-focused, evidence-based treatment (e.g., Trauma-Focused Cognitive Behavioral Therapy, TF-CBT; Cohen, Mannarino, & Deblinger, 2006), based on an assumption that all abused children have been traumatized, is as problematic as not recognizing the impact of trauma. For example, in Texas, Senate Bill 219 (Texas Family Code § 264.015, 2011, an act relating to health and mental health services for children in foster care and kinship care) expanded the mandate for training in trauma-informed care without a clear consensus in the field on the recommended components of trauma-informed care. Thus, the legislative body has mandated training for a construct for which there is little specific agreement.

Consistent with this argument, Wilson (2012) recommends that children and their families must be properly assessed as a key step in the delivery of evidence-based practices to address trauma and abuse. To accomplish this, Wilson suggests that referral agents, brokers, or gatekeepers become more educated about referral sources.

Children's Advocacy Centers

Children's advocacy centers (CACs) have been operational since the late 1980s. CACs represent a collection of multidisciplinary team members who normally are tasked with the investigation and prosecution of child abuse cases and treatment of abused children. The centerpiece for years has been the forensic interview of the child. More recently, extended forensic interviews were developed to meet the needs of children who made incomplete or vague disclosures in the initial forensic interview. Though mental health services always have been a necessary component of services available through a CAC, only recently have the identification and treatment of abuse-related symptoms received focus. This important development runs in parallel with advancements in the science of assessment and the availability of evidence-based treatments for abused children and their nonoffending parents. This development is owed to leaders in the field and at the National Children's Alliance (NCA; this membership organization represents more than 750 CACs across the nation) and the realization that the success of CACs should be defined more by improvements in functioning for children than by rates of prosecution.

Several challenges continue to impact the delivery of mental health services, generally, and assessments, specifi-

cally, in CACs. First, only about 30% of CACs provide assessment and treatment services within the agency. The majority of centers continue to rely on mental health professionals in the community. However, in a recent survey, only about 35% of CAC executive directors agreed or strongly agreed that there were adequate numbers of providers for treatment and assessment within their communities (Wherry, Huey, & Medford, 2013). This is particularly concerning because Wherry, Baldwin, Junco, and Floyd (in press) found that 34% of an outpatient CAC treatment-seeking sample experienced suicidal thinking.

In this same survey, when executive directors were asked if there were adequate numbers of service providers/clinicians in their communities with experience in assessing, specifically, PTSD symptoms, 12.6% strongly disagreed, 33.0% disagreed, 18.7% were uncertain, 30.2% agreed, and 5.5% strongly agreed. When directors were asked to identify various assessment instruments as helpful, the three highest response rates were to the Trauma Symptom Checklist for Young Children (TSCYC; Briere, 2005), the Trauma Symptom Checklist for Children (TSCC; Briere, 1999), and broadband rating scales (e.g., the Child Behavior Checklist [Achenbach 2000; Achenbach & Rescorla, 2001] and the Behavioral Assessment System for Children, Second Edition, BASC-2 [Reynolds & Kamphaus, 2006]). While identification of the TSCC and TSCYC as commonly used helpful tests is encouraging, the names of the tests (involving the term *trauma*) provided insight into their intended use and may have inflated the response. Moreover, since only about one-third of surveyed CAC directors agreed that there were adequate numbers of trained providers in their communities, it would seem that what is perceived as best practice may not coincide with the availability of trained professionals.

Finally, in some jurisdictions where CACs operate, prosecutors are reluctant for victims to receive an assessment of symptoms. When prosecutors are candid, they will admit that these assessments complicate the prosecution of their cases. For example, various measures (e.g., the CBLC, TSCYC) include items in which caregivers are asked to rate the frequency of lying by the child. Prosecutors are fearful that a parent's report of the child's lying may taint their case. In reality, some frequency of lying at certain ages is normative. For example, on the TSCYC (Briere, 2005), the item assessing the frequency of lying loads on the validity scale, and its complete absence may indicate a parent who is underreporting symptoms. Thus, it should be the responsibility of the prosecution to produce expert witnesses who are able to explain this normative process to the court and to jurors. Never should the "case" supersede the recovery of the individual child victim.

Other Settings

Abused children are identified in a variety of other settings, including pediatric outpatient clinics, pediatric hospitals, inpatient psychiatric hospitals, community mental health centers, and schools. Perhaps abused children would be properly identified more frequently and earlier if screening for abuse and adverse experiences was routine (Felitti et al., 1998). Use of a brief instrument to screen for both exposure and abuse-related symptoms would potentially result in the identification of children in need of treatment and, where indicated, those requiring more thorough assessments (Briggs et al., 2012; Wherry, Corson, & Hunsaker, in press).

A GOOD ASSESSMENT

Despite the increased recognition of the importance of evidence-based trauma-focused treatment, there has been less emphasis on evidence-based, abuse-related assessments in both child welfare and CAC settings. This potentially becomes problematic inasmuch as children may be misdiagnosed in child welfare settings (e.g., with a diagnosis of ADHD, bipolar disorder, or psychosis not otherwise specified) or not assessed at all in CAC settings. Thus, an important focus of this chapter is to highlight the need for a thoughtful approach to assessment for these populations that includes obtaining information from multiple sources or "raters," methods of assessment (e.g., observation, self-report, clinical interviews), and the purpose and process of conducting the assessment.

Raters

At its best, a good assessment of a child is a "snapshot" in time. Even when assessment results are integrated with history and findings from previous reports, they remain just a partial understanding or description of a child at one moment in time. To enhance the quality of the data used in an assessment, the information should come from several sources.

CAREGIVER RATINGS. Parents and/or caregivers who know the child can be helpful informants. For the abused child placed in a foster home or a residential setting, caregivers can provide a useful perspective. However, these ratings of behavior from adults, like any assessment procedure, have their potential flaws. For example, physically abusive parents may exaggerate a child's externalizing or acting-out behavior, which may reflect an attributional bias at best or a blaming of the child for his or her abuse at worst. Conversely, in clinical settings, parents occasionally "project" their own distress on their child, as evidenced by their ratings.

Professional caregivers, such as foster parents or residential staff, can provide another helpful perspective. In clinical practice, however, the ratings from foster parents or residential workers can be influenced in ways that underestimate the severity or frequency of problems assessed. In these situations, it is as though the internal norms of these professional caregivers are influenced by their experience with clinical populations. Despite the instructions and even the corrective admonishments of the evaluator, these well-intentioned caregivers may compare the child referred for assessment with other children who have lived in their home, unit, or cottage. Among residential staff, this is illustrated when staff members say something like, "He has his problems, but he's no Johnny," at which point other staff members nod in agreement. Thus, caregiver ratings, even when using instruments with outstanding psychometric qualities, may have their drawbacks.

CHILD SELF-REPORTS. For the child who is able to read and comprehend what is read, self-report measures can be informative. However, reading ability alone may not be sufficient, depending on the construct being assessed. For example, in the treatment of sexual abuse and physical abuse victims, there often is a cognitive component to therapy. One of the goals of the cognitive component is to examine and sometimes modify the cognitive attributions that give the abuse meaning. Sometimes, negative attributions result in unwarranted shame, guilt, and responsibility. While these attributions certainly develop, children—depending on their developmental status—may not have the metacognitive ability (the ability to think about their thinking) to accurately answer questions about this process or their understanding and attributions about the abuse. Thus, evaluators need to be aware that in some cases, children may not be the best informant regarding their abuse-related cognitions and attributions.

TEACHER RATINGS. Another useful source of information can be teachers, and in most cases, teachers are usually not comparing the child being evaluated with their best biological child or even their best or worst student in class. However, anecdotally, it may be true that teachers see behavior through an educational lens, where such things as inattention, distractibility, or oppositional behaviors can interfere with completion of academic assignments and positive peer relationships. Symptoms often described as internalizing (e.g., symptoms of anxiety and depression) may go unrecognized and thereby receive less attention. And importantly, there are situations where educators might wish to keep the information that the child has been abused confidential, which may negate the possibility of teacher ratings altogether.

LACK OF AGREEMENT. A final issue is that evaluators must recognize the possibility that informant ratings and child self-reports may yield discrepant results. For example, Rutter et al. (1976) found that mothers and teachers agreed on the presence of behavioral disorders in only 7% of children. Other studies have found similar low correlations (Fergusson & Horwood, 1987a, 1987b, 1989), leading some to conclude that clinicians simply should expect some degree of disagreement among informants (Lee, Elliott, & Barbour, 1994).

Methods

There is considerable variation among the many methods that have been used in assessing children. Generally, when feasible, it is best to use a multi-method approach. For example, Meyer et al. (2001) found a number of studies that reported many diagnostic errors when only one assessment measure or method was used.

UNIDIMENSIONAL VERSUS BROAD-BAND RATING SCALES. We described above the importance of obtaining information from multiple sources; including caregivers, teachers, and children's self-reports. Regarding specific areas to assess, it is recommended that caregivers, teachers, and/or other relevant adults complete broad-band rating scales that assess a wide range of behaviors and symptoms (e.g., the CBCL). While there are excellent, psychometrically sound unidimensional measures (e.g., the Children's Depression Inventory-2, CDI-2 [Kovacs, 2010]; the UCLA PTSD Reaction Index [Rodriguez, Steinberg, & Pynoos, 1999]), this focus on a single construct limits the breadth of information available to understand a child's pre-morbid and current functioning, as well as abuse-related symptoms, specifically. An additional concern about unidimensional measures is that they can force the rater to attempt to fit multiple problems into the single measure being assessed. Not surprisingly, this can result in either a false positive for the specific symptom being measured or the absence of endorsement (because the measure does not fit with the child's problems), leading the evaluator to conclude, mistakenly, that the child is exhibiting no symptoms.

PROJECTIVES. Projective tests are those in which children theoretically project their own psychology or personality into a drawing, story, or description of a stimulus. The use of these measures is rooted in the practice of psychology from as early as the 1940s or 1950s. While there is a rich tradition of using these approaches with children, their administration, scoring, and interpretation remain more art than science. That is, the chief complaint related to these approaches is one of poor reliability, if any, in scoring, as well as a lack of evidence for validity in interpretations. Seldom do these measures have norms based on age, sex, or clinical versus nonclinical status. At times, though, through the use of projectives, a child may tell his story, draw his family, or make reference to his experience, and this can be informative. Occasionally, responses occur with the use of projectives (e.g., genitalia on a drawing) that may be revealing; however, there are no studies in which specificity and sensitivity have been calculated to allow such occurrences to serve as a pathognomonic indicator for abusive events in the life of a child. Furthermore, as with drawings, anatomically detailed dolls, and even parent ratings (e.g., Child Sexual Behavior Inventory, CSBI; Friedrich, 1998), the inclusion of sexual content or aggressive responses is not diagnostic for sexual abuse or physical abuse, respectively. In the end, some of these projective drawing procedures, such as the Draw-A-Person, Kinetic Family Drawing, or House-Tree-Person tests (Murstein, 1965; Weiner & Greene,

2008), may serve as useful warm-up activities in the initial work with a child client, as long as clinicians do not over-interpret the findings.

One final mention about the Rorschach Inkblots, specifically, is warranted—especially when the test is administered, scored, and interpreted using the Exner Comprehensive System, the most common scoring system for this measure (Exner, 1993, 2002). While the Exner system is an improvement over past scoring systems, it remains a fairly complex and time-consuming procedure that may not directly assess dimensions or constructs that are helpful in understanding most abused children. And further, the reliability and validity of the Exner system have not been adequately demonstrated (Wood, Nezworski, & Stejskal, 1996).

CLINICAL INTERVIEW. The clinical interview (also called clinical intake, psychosocial interview, biopsychosocial interview, or mental status exam) is the most frequent evaluation procedure used by clinicians across all disciplines, but it, too, is not without its problems. Structured clinical interviews, often used in psychiatric studies, are time-consuming and may have components or modules with limited reliability and validity. Additionally, the use of these procedures often results in high rates of comorbidity (i.e., multiple diagnoses made), without the process of differential diagnosis. This may result in over-diagnosis or misdiagnosis and, as a result, ill-informed treatment. While semi-structured interviews allow more flexibility by the clinician, they are fraught with the same shortcomings as structured clinical interviews. A key limitation of clinical interviews is that, even for the skilled clinician, it is possible that preconceived hypotheses are the only ones explored in this process. As a result, "pet" diagnoses may be over-identified and children and adolescents may receive inappropriate treatment. Despite these shortcomings, some form of clinical interviewing, when used in conjunction with reliable, valid, and normed measures, can often elucidate descriptive findings.

A variation of semi-structured interviewing is the testing of limits when using formal assessment procedures. For example, when using a self-report measure, the clinician might administer the entire measure and score and interpret it according to the stated instructions. Then the evaluator might use the child's answers as a launching point for interviewing the child and inquiring about examples of situations associated with the endorsed thoughts, feelings, or behaviors as described by the instruments. A similar approach is possible with caregiver ratings. This "testing of limits," when done without changing formal scores, can "put clinical flesh on the assessment skeleton."

BEHAVIORAL OBSERVATIONS. Behavioral observations also can be informative. Like all other forms of assessment, however, the observations are only "a slice of life" or a picture in time and/or place and may not be representative of both the good and the "bad" behavior of a child. When overt, externalizing behaviors are identified in a home, classroom, or office, one may be able to hypothesize and test the role of various stimuli or events in the possible establishment or maintenance of behaviors. For some abused children, these same observations may provide clues to stimuli or triggers that elicit otherwise inexplicable behavior by the child. For example, a certain tone of voice, a particular look from an adult, or another sensory experience (e.g., smell or taste) may serve as a reminder of past abuse and result in a response that otherwise cannot be explained by the seemingly innocuous situation.

In the final analysis, there is no single approach or instrument that will always be superior (Verhulst, 1995). Even instruments that are reliable, valid, and normed may be rejected by children and/or caregivers or fail to delineate a clear picture of symptoms and treatment needs. Moreover, lack of agreement among raters (parents, teachers, and youth; Achenbach, 1993) may inadvertently affect case conceptualization and treatment. Thus we recommend an approach that is ongoing and includes multiple methods and informants.

Purpose

Assessments of abused children are most useful in describing a child at a given point in time. When augmented by ratings from caregivers or teachers, the picture becomes more complete. When supplemented by interview data, the image becomes still clearer. However, there are many purposes or questions that are not well-served or answered by assessments.

DID ABUSE OCCUR? No evaluation or assessment can establish definitively that a child was, in fact, abused. In reality and under most circumstances, only two people know whether abuse occurred—the victim and the perpetrator. Assessment findings may be "consistent with" a history of abuse, but results from an assessment can never definitively establish that abuse occurred.

PREDICTION. Most assessments also do a poor job of predicting the future. The best predictor of the future is always past behavior. This is true with regard to hurting others, hurting oneself, or the likelihood of reoffending (e.g., in the case of abuse perpetration). For those who refer children for assessment, remember that no clinician has a crystal ball.

NEED FOR THERAPY. Another frequent purpose for assessment invoked by caseworkers pertains to the question often stated as follows: "Will this client/child benefit from therapy?" All standardized measures that we know of assess symptoms but do not assess interest or motivation for treatment in children. One of the most frequently under-

utilized methods is for the caseworker to simply ask the child if she or he wants to participate in therapy.

PROGRAM EVALUATION. In an age when funders are looking for more from agencies than the total number served, pre- and post-treatment assessments can help demonstrate that a program is beneficial to children and their families. Pre- and post-treatment assessments by children and caregivers can provide the type of data valued and required by funders. Hersen (2004) recommends assessments before, during, and after treatment.

PLACEMENT AND OTHER QUESTIONS. At times, bureaucracies mistakenly ask clinicians to speculate about matters for which there are not always sound assessment strategies and that, in the end, rely primarily on a highly subjective interview. For example, clinicians may be asked to assess the appropriateness of placing a child of color in a home with caregivers that are not of the same race. No instrument or series of questions can reliably ascertain the answer to this placement question. The intent of the question is noble, but good intentions are not always informed by science. Although many believe it is advantageous to match foster parents or clinicians with children on the basis of race, there is little empirical evidence among children to support these assertions and evidence to the contrary with regard to forensic interviews (Springman, Wherry, & Notaro, 2006).

Process

The process of a good assessment may be determined in part by its purpose. For example, if the purpose is to screen large numbers of children, measures might be administered and interpreted without background information or even meeting the child. Obviously, such an approach has its limitations (e.g., missing a certain number of children with positive symptoms), but it may be a relatively inexpensive and efficient method for identifying children in need of further evaluation.

As noted above, the best assessment of children often involves multiple informants. It is important that both children and caregivers are engaged in and perceive some benefit from the process. At the very least, the instructions should be clear and the informant must be able to read and comprehend the nature of the rating or self-report. In working with families, it is imperative to recognize that some parents are already in a one-down situation. Even in cases of sexual abuse by someone outside the family, parents may feel unnecessarily guilty about the abuse. Recognizing this possibility and sensitively supporting that parent is an important step in engagement. For children, remember that rarely, if ever, does a child awaken one morning, come to the breakfast table, and say to her parents, "Mom and Dad, I would like to begin therapy, so let's get an assessment done." It just does not happen. At worst, children believe they have done something wrong, necessitating the appointment. At best, they have been told that the process will provide them with support and help. More likely, they have been told nothing or, at the very least, are confused by the entire process.

Of great importance, clients deserve assessment feedback. This feedback should be provided in jargon-free language that is clearly understandable. If treatment recommendations are linked to these "findings," the rationale should also be explained. Documentation of findings also deserves some mention. The level of documentation may vary with the nature of the assessment process. If the purpose is screening, the report of findings will be fairly brief. In any event, the record should be readable and jargon-free and should highlight the major findings. If there are limitations in terms of the accuracy or validity of the findings, these should be noted. In situations where the whole process is invalid (e.g., due to an inability to cooperatively engage the child or caregiver), the process should be described as such, and the choice of reporting no findings should be considered, given that any conclusions would probably be inaccurate.

SELECTING AN ASSESSMENT FOR USE WITH MALTREATED CHILDREN

Advancements in Assessment of Trauma Symptoms

A good starting point for evaluation is to use measures designed to assess symptoms that are most common among abused children, including anxiety, depression, anger, trauma symptoms (including PTSD and dissociation), and sexualized behaviors (Kendall-Tackett, Williams, & Finkelhor, 1993). However, to assess only one of these dimensions is inadequate. While it is true that virtually any symptom can result from child abuse, no single symptom is pathognomonic or diagnostic for abuse. Even sexualized behaviors are not a definitive sign of sexual abuse, as there may be alternative explanations such as the child's exposure to sexually explicit behaviors on the Internet.

The National Child Traumatic Stress Network (NCTSN), funded by the Substance Abuse and Mental Health Services Administration, has made great strides in the assessment of trauma and its impact. One example is the NCTSN Core Data Set (CDS), a Web-based data collection system that includes clinical interview components and standardized measures (e.g., CBCL, TSCC, and UCLA PTSD Reaction Index) that assess a wide array of trauma-related symptoms, functional impairments, and behavioral problems, in addition to gathering extensive information on trauma history profiles. The CDS also captures information on service utilization, treatment services, and outcomes.

One measure widely promoted throughout the NCTSN, the UCLA PTSD Reaction Index, represented, at its onset, a significant advancement. The measure is unidimensional, however, assessing only the presence or absence of PTSD

symptoms. The problem with over-reliance on the UCLA PTSD Reaction Index for assessment of abused children is the assumption that all abused children have been traumatized and will exhibit PTSD-type symptoms. Certainly abuse is negative, stressful, adverse, and potentially traumatic, but not all children who have been abused qualify for a formal diagnosis of PTSD. While the debate rages on, in our experience as clinical supervisors and trainers we have encountered individuals who routinely assign "trauma" as a diagnosis or, at least, as a descriptor when referring to any abuse. The potential danger in assuming that all children are traumatized is that this can result in misdiagnosis and subsequent referral to a trauma-focused treatment that may not be appropriate. Furthermore, over time, the public and clinicians alike might conclude that trauma-focused treatments are not effective when, in fact, the problem is that a referral was inappropriate in the first place.

For the purposes of this chapter, we reserve the term *trauma symptoms* for those symptoms that arise as a result of activation of the fight-or-flight response. Anything less could be considered frightening, alarming, stressful, negative, or adverse, but not necessarily "traumatic." The Adverse Childhood Experiences (ACE) Study provides one example of a longitudinal study of events labeled as "adverse" though not necessarily traumatic, but which, nonetheless, can have long-term negative psychological, social, and physical health effects (Felitti et al., 1998). Examples of these types of events are substance or alcohol abuse by a parent, living with a parent or family member who is mentally ill or depressed, and/or experiencing a family member going to prison. Not only are some events not necessarily traumatic (e.g., a parent going to prison, a child being placed in a foster home), but for some children, these events, especially foster home placement, may signal the transition to a safe environment. Again, when the fight-or-flight response is activated, trauma symptoms may result and may require attention even though their overall presentation does not meet the criteria for "full-blown PTSD" (Griffin et al., 2011, p. 84). And finally, even events that would not be defined as "traumatic" (i.e., those not resulting in a flight-or-flight response) may cause distress, warranting further assessment and potential intervention.

Obstacles to Assessing Child Abuse

There are several obstacles to the assessment of child abuse sequelae. Child victims may deny that the abuse event occurred (Shapiro & Dominiak, 1990), may be too ashamed about the event to report its impact (Wyatt et al., 1999), and may have difficulty with direct questioning (Perrin, Smith, & Yule, 2000). Young children may lack the metacognitive skills needed to report symptoms accurately. Therefore, as discussed above, the parents' report of symptoms is critical in the assessment of PTSD. A revised set of criteria for diagnosing PTSD among young children has been included in the fifth edition of the *Diagnostic and Statistical Manual*, due to perceived shortcomings of the fourth edition (*DSM-IV;*

American Psychiatric Association, 1994; Iselin et al., 2010; Scheeringa et al., 2003). Specifically, these shortcomings include problems related to children and their parents not endorsing avoidant cluster symptoms relative to reexperiencing and arousal symptoms. This resulted in changes to the number of required avoidant symptoms, from one of five to one of seven (Scheeringa et al., 2012).

One of the great challenges in assessing abused children, then, involves both an accurate "gathering" of symptoms present and a concise conceptualization of symptomatology, so that a coherent treatment plan might follow. Again, some children may not be traumatized and may exhibit other symptoms (e.g., sexualized behavior), and some children may have symptoms below the threshold for a diagnosis of PTSD or may be misdiagnosed with another disorder mimicking the symptoms of PTSD. An important step in the assessment process prior to the delivery of treatment is the differential diagnosis of various symptoms.

DIFFERENTIAL DIAGNOSIS

Certain behaviors, symptoms, or disorders may pre-date child abuse or co-occur by chance (e.g., psychotic symptoms, bipolar disorder, ADHD), but there is no empirical basis to conclude that child abuse precipitates or causes psychosis, bipolar disorder, or ADHD. Rather, some symptoms may be as yet unrecognized developmental equivalents of PTSD symptoms in children. The American Academy of Child and Adolescent Psychiatry's (2010) "Practice Parameter for the Assessment and Treatment of Children and Adolescents with Posttraumatic Stress Disorder" recommends that "the psychiatric assessment should consider differential diagnoses of other psychiatric disorders and physical conditions that may mimic PTSD" (p. 420). A good history, including the time of onset and duration of symptoms, is necessary to make the distinctions required for a good differential diagnosis. Specifically, details about abuse often are discovered years later but coincide with the onset of other symptoms misdiagnosed during an earlier period in the child's life. The following are presentations of symptoms that may serve the same developmentally sensitive and functional purpose (i.e., alarming, promoting safety) as PTSD symptoms (reexperiencing, arousal, and avoidance) and, as a result, can lead to misdiagnosis.

Reexperiencing Symptoms

PSYCHOSIS. Rather than psychosis, it is far more likely that maltreated children may demonstrate behavior inconsistent with the demands of a given situation because unknown stimuli are triggering a conditioned, anxious response.

VISUAL HALLUCINATIONS. Rather than having visual hallucinations, a child may have reexperiencing symptoms of trauma, which, when described, mimic visual hallucinations (Carter & Wherry, 2007). Hypnopompic and hypnogogic hallucinations (dream states) may be misinterpreted, especially by inexperienced clinicians, as visual hallucinations.

Arousal Symptoms

BIPOLAR DISORDER. Children may be emotionally dysregulated due to chronic activation of the fight-or-flight response; these children probably should not be considered for a diagnosis of bipolar disorder (Wherry, Carter, et al., 2008). The same children may exhibit sexualized behaviors, which certainly should not be misconstrued as manic symptoms of sexual indiscretions like those evidenced among adults.

PANIC DISORDER. Rather than panic disorder, children may present with anxiety that rises to the level of panic; however, in some cases, the anxiety may be "triggered" by a stimulus unknown, unidentified, or symbolic in nature. For example, a relationship may have characteristics similar to a formerly abusive relationship, and those characteristics (e.g., controlling, demanding) may result in panic even though there is no physical or sexual abuse in the current relationship.

ADHD. Concentration problems alone do not warrant a diagnosis of ADHD. Concentration problems can be symptomatic of PTSD hyperarousal or symptoms of depression secondary to abuse.

Avoidance Symptoms

SEPARATION ANXIETY / SCHOOL PHOBIA. Rather than having separation anxiety or school phobia, young children who are reluctant to separate from a safe parent may be exhibiting adaptive avoidant behavior designed to protect the child from an undetected abuser (Berres et al., 2007; Wherry & Marrs, 2008).

SOMATIZATION. In some families, somatic symptoms serve a purpose similar to those found among children with separation anxiety features. That is, somatic symptoms (as mild as headaches or stomachaches and as extreme as conversion disorders of "paralysis") may bring a safe parent to the child's side or, in the extreme case, cause the child to be removed from an unsafe home and admitted to a hospital (Wherry, McMillan, & Hutchison, 1991).

SUBSTANCE ABUSE. Substance abuse has been documented as a coping strategy for adolescents with PTSD who have been sexually abused (Hawke, Jainchill, & Leon, 2000; Kilpatrick et al., 2000; Raghavan & Kingston, 2006). While this can be effective in nullifying the PTSD symptoms of arousal and reexperiencing, the additional problems in functioning can be debilitating.

EVALUATION OF MULTIPLE SYMPTOMS ASSOCIATED WITH ABUSE

Other common symptoms that abused children experience include anger, anxiety, and depression. For sexually abused children, a subset may also experience sexualized behavior or sexual concerns. Because of the diverse and often complex presentation among many abused/traumatized children, there is a need for trauma-focused measures that can capture this complexity. Examples include the TSCC (Briere, 1996) and the TSCYC (Briere, 2005).

TRAUMA SYMPTOM CHECKLIST FOR CHILDREN (TSCC). The TSCC is designed for use with children and adolescents ages 8–16. It is a 54-item, self-report measure with a validity scale that examines both under-reporting (Underresponse) and over-reporting (Hyperresponse) of symptoms. Raw scores, t-scores, and percentile scores are reported for each of the following scales: Anxiety, Depression, Anger/Aggression, Posttraumatic Stress, Dissociation (Overt and Fantasy), and Sexual Concerns (Preoccupation and Distress). The alpha coefficients for clinical scales range from 0.77 to 0.89 in the standardization sample. Adequate convergent, discriminant, and predictive validity have been demonstrated in normative and clinical samples. Normative data were derived from a nonclinical sample of 3,008 children; 53% were female, and the racial distribution was 44% Caucasian, 27% black, and 22% Hispanic/Latino.

TRAUMA SYMPTOM CHECKLIST FOR YOUNG CHILDREN (TSCYC). The TSCYC is a 90-item caregiver rating scale completed for children ages 3–12. It also utilizes two scales for assessment of under-reporting (Response Level) and atypical responses (Atypical Response). The raw scores, t-scores, and percentile scores are reported for each of the following scales: Anxiety, Depression, Anger/Aggression, Posttraumatic Stress—Intrusion, Posttraumatic Stress—Avoidance, Posttraumatic Stress—Arousal, Posttraumatic Stress—Total, Dissociation, and Sexual Concerns. In Briere's (1999) initial study, the clinical scales had good reliability, with alphas ranging from 0.81 to 0.93. Additionally, TSCYC scales were predictive of exposure to sexual abuse, physical abuse, and witnessing domestic violence. Subsequent studies have demonstrated the convergent validity of the TSCYC with other parent ratings (e.g., the Child Behavior Checklist, Child Sexual Behavior Inventory, and UCLA PTSD Reaction Index). The convergent validity of the TSCYC and the TSCC has been found to be moderate (Lanktree et al., 2008) to weak (Wherry, Graves, & Rhodes, 2008), perhaps illustrating the lack of agreement often found between children and caregivers and further highlighting the need for a multi-informant approach to screening and assessment of abused children. The TSCYC also has been used in screening children for PTSD with a model correctly classifying 100% of the PTSD-negative and 72.7% of the PTSD-positive participants. These findings suggest that the TSCYC may

be used as an economical and time-efficient screening device for PTSD (Pollio, Glover-Orr, & Wherry, 2008). The TSCYC has been normed with a sample of 750 parents stratified to match U.S. Census data by region, parent's educational level, and child's age, race, ethnicity, and gender. The one limitation of the TSCC and TSCYC is that they have not been particularly sensitive to treatment changes, making it difficult to use these measures as a way to assess treatment progress.

EVALUATION OF SINGLE CONSTRUCTS USING UNIDIMENSIONAL MEASURES

When a measure such as the TSCC or TSCYC indicates the presence of significantly elevated frequencies of symptoms for depression, PTSD, sexual concerns, anger, anxiety, or dissociation, there may be value in using a unidimensional measure to further understand the nature of that elevated symptom. For maltreated children, several unidimensional measures can be useful, including the Child Sexual Behavior Inventory (sexual concerns; Friedrich, 1998), the UCLA PTSD Reaction Index (Steinberg et al., 2004), and the Child Dissociative Checklist (CDC; dissociation; Putnam, Helmers, & Trickett, 1993).

Sexualized Behavior

CHILD SEXUAL BEHAVIOR INVENTORY (CSBI). The CSBI, a 38-item instrument completed by caregivers for children ages 2–12, assesses sexualized behavior in children. Studies indicate that it is reliable and valid, and it has been normed by age and sex. However, there is no validity scale. The measure has two subscales—Developmentally Related Sexual Behavior (DRSB) and Sexual Abuse Specific Items (SASI)—and a CSBI Total score. The DRSB includes behaviors that at age 3 might be normative but at age 12 would be highly unlikely, unusual, or atypical. The SASI subscale includes items consistent with behaviors that may be exhibited by sexually abused children. An elevation of the SASI Scale score, however, does *not* indicate or prove that a child has been sexually abused. According to the developer, William Friedrich, these sexualized behaviors might be due to other family behaviors such as watching movies with explicit sexual content, family nudity, or observing parents having sex (Friedrich, 1998). An alpha coefficient of 0.72 was obtained for the CSBI Total score, indicating good internal consistency. Test-retest reliability was 0.91 when the retest was administered an average of two weeks later. Inter-rater reliability for mother-father pairs was 0.83. The manual cites data supporting the convergent, discriminant, and construct validity of the CSBI. The measure was standardized on a nonclinical sample of 1,114 children and on a primarily Caucasian (76%) clinical sample of 512 children.

CHILD SEXUAL BEHAVIOR CHECKLIST—REVISED (CSBC-R). Johnson (2003) developed the CSBC-R for the assessment of sexualized behavior. The instrument has not been normed, however, and there are no studies related to its reliability and validity. Thus, the instrument probably should be used as a semi-structured interview with caregivers. Biological parents, foster parents, or staff may observe the same sexualized behaviors but report them with different frequencies. These discrepancies may result from caregivers' different roles and/or the varied settings in which the child is observed. Additionally, interpretations of sexual behavior may vary as a function of overall feelings about the child or because of cultural differences such as religious beliefs. According to T. C. Johnson (personal communication, February 20, 2013), "The discussion of the differences [in scores] is extremely rich clinical material and can then be developed into treatment goals."

ADOLESCENT CLINICAL SEXUAL BEHAVIOR INVENTORY—SELF-REPORT (ACSBI-S). The ACSBI-S (Friedrich et al., 2004) is a 45-item self-report scale for assessing a broad range of sexual behaviors and attitudes among adolescents. Adolescent participants respond to items on a three-point scale ranging from 0 (not true) to 2 (very true), reflecting their perceived level of sexual knowledge, sexual interest, sexual risk behavior, and sexual discomfort. Two research studies have produced (1) a five-factor solution (Sexual Knowledge/Interest, Sexual Risk/Misuse, Divergent Sexual Interest, Concerns about Appearance, and Fear/Discomfort), accounting for 37.6% of the total variance (Friedrich et al., 2004); and (2) a three-factor solution (Sexual Knowledge/Interest, Sexual Risk/Misuse, and Concerns about Appearance), accounting for 41.58% of the variance (Wherry et al, 2009). Research suggested that each scale has adequate internal consistency, with alpha coefficients ranging from 0.65 to 0.84, with the exception of the Fear/Discomfort Scale, which had an alpha of 0.45. Test-retest reliability at one week was 0.74. The ACSBI-S total score was correlated with the CBCL's Delinquency subscale ($r = 0.25$), ASCQ (Adolescent Sexual Concern Questionnaire) sexual concerns items ($r = 0.72$), and the TSCC subscales of Sexual Concerns ($r = 0.73$), Sexual Concerns—Distress ($r = 0.54$), and Sexual Concerns—Preoccupation ($r = 0.68$). The ACSBI-S has no norms, however, and the samples used to date have been homogeneous with regard to race and ethnicity.

PTSD

UCLA PTSD REACTION INDEX (UCLA PTSD-RI). Unidimensional measures for assessing PTSD in children are somewhat limited. The UCLA PTSD Reaction Index for *DSM-IV* is available for completion by children, adolescents, and caregivers. Internal consistency for the full scales is excellent ($\alpha = 0.90$). Test-retest reliability is reported at 0.84 after a median of seven days. Convergent validity is good, though, to date, there are no published norms for this instrument.

CHILDREN'S PTSD INVENTORY. This instrument (Saigh, 2003) is a semi-structured interview that consists of five subscales. Moderate (0.58) to high (0.89) alphas are reported, and the internal consistency for the overall diagnosis is a Cronbach's alpha of 0.95. Inter-rater reliability and test-retest reliability are good. The author reports moderate to high sensitivity and specificity, good convergent validity, and discriminant validity. Two small clinical samples (n = 150; n = 42) were used to establish the psychometric properties.

Dissociation

CHILD DISSOCIATIVE CHECKLIST (CDC), VERSION 3.0. The CDC (Putnam, Helmers, & Trickett, 1993) is a 20-item parent rating scale. Items are rated on a scale from 0 (not true) to 2 (very true). These ratings are summed, and a cutoff score equal to or greater than 12 is considered "clinically meaningful," particularly in older children. The CDC has a one-year test-retest reliability coefficient of rho = 0.69 (N = 73, $p = 0.0001$) in a sample that included sexually abused girls and a nonabused comparison group. Putman and colleagues (1993) reported good discriminant validity. Concurrent validity with other measures of externalizing behavior has been demonstrated (Wherry et al., 1994).

ADOLESCENT DISSOCIATIVE EXPERIENCES SCALE (A-DES). The A-DES (Armstrong et al., 1997) is a screening instrument developed to detect dissociative behavior in children and adolescents between 11 and 17 years of age. Its reliability and validity have been demonstrated in at least two different studies (Armstrong et al., 1997; Steven & Carlson 1996), but no normative data are available.

Assessing Events

ABUSE DIMENSIONS INVENTORY (ADI). The ADI (Chaffin et al., 1997) is an instrument designed to measure the severity of physical and sexual abuse. Also recorded are duration of abuse, number of most severely rated incidents, total number of incidents, abuser's reaction to disclosure, use of force or coercion to gain submission or compliance, use of force or coercion to gain secrecy, and relationship of the abuser to the victim. The ordering of items in terms of severity was obtained by surveying a national sample of mental health professionals who belonged to a national organization for professionals working in the child abuse field. Coefficients of concordance for orderings averaged 0.87. Inter-rater reliability of the scales based on a semi-structured interview with nonaccused parents ranged from 0.84 to 0.99, and factor analysis of the instrument produced a four-factor solution with separate factors for physical abuse behaviors, sexual abuse behaviors, number and duration of physical abuse events, and number and duration of sexual abuse events (Chaffin et al., 1997).

Screening for Other Traumatic Events

A number of instruments, checklists, and interviews are available to screen for exposure to traumatic events other than the referent child abuse allegation. We know from research that the various forms of child maltreatment often co-occur (Saunders, 2003) and that interpersonal family violence or domestic violence is frequently present where there is child maltreatment. Since effective treatment is more likely when children can first be protected from the many forms of abuse they experience, it is important to conduct a thorough assessment of potentially traumatic events aside from the initial referent event.

Table 2.1 lists several additional instruments (checklists, procedures, and interviews) that can be used to screen for a history of traumatic events as well as symptoms of depression and anxiety (we acknowledge that this is a representative, not exhaustive, list of all available measures). For the trauma screening measures, it is important to acknowledge that reliability and validity studies can be difficult to conduct with these instruments, and endorsement of items by children or parents cannot be used as forensic evidence to establish that these events have happened. Rather, the value of these instruments is for the clinician tasked with treating these children and families.

Regarding measurement of anxiety and depression, there are many self-report and parent ratings that can be used to assess these constructs more thoroughly (see table 2.1). These measures have particular value after children are first screened or assessed and evidence of these constructs is found.

Broad-Band Rating Scales

Broad-band rating scales are measures, often lengthy, completed by caregivers, teachers, or adolescents. They have value in screening maltreated children because of the breadth of the domains assessed. However, these measures do not assess specifically for trauma-related symptoms such as PTSD, and they may have very few items devoted to the assessment of sexualized behaviors or concerns. One of the primary benefits of these scales is identifying symptoms that otherwise might not have been reported or detected in screening for abuse-related symptoms. These newly identified symptoms may not be a focus of the treatment for abuse but may require treatment from another provider.

Two broad-band rating scales are used primarily in clinical and school settings. They have been studied extensively and possess outstanding psychometric qualities (reliability, validity, and excellent normative samples). The Child Behavior Checklist (CBCL; Achenbach & Rescorla, 2001) is often used in clinical settings, and the Behavioral Assessment Scale for Children, Second Edition (BASC-2; Reynolds & Kamphaus, 2002) is often used in school settings, though they work equally well in either setting. The reliability and validity of both are well established. An example of a free, easily accessible, brief measure is the Strengths and Diffi-

Table 2.1. Self-report and Parent Rating Measures

Area of Assessment	Instrument
Trauma screening	Traumatic Events Screening Inventory—Child Report Form—Revised (TESI-CRF-R), Parent Report—Revised (TESI-PRR; Ford, 2002a; Ghosh-Ippen et al., 2002), and Self-report Revised (TESI-SRR; Ford, 2002b)
	UCLA PTSD Reaction Index for *DSM-IV* (UCLA PTSD-RI)—Child, Adolescent, and Parent Versions (Rodriguez, Steinberg, & Pynoos, 1999)
	Adolescent Self-Report Trauma Questionnaire (Horowitz, Weine, & Jekel, 1995)
	Children's PTSD Inventory (Saigh, 2003)
	Childhood PTSD Interview—Child (CPTSDI-C) / Childhood PTSD Interview—Parent (CPTSDI-P; Fletcher, 1996)
	The Adolescent Trauma History Checklist and Interview (Habib & Labruna, 2006)
	Lifetime Incidence of Traumatic Events (LITE Student Form; LITE Parent Form; Greenwald & Rubin, 1999)
	When Bad Things Happen (Fletcher, 1996)
	My Worst Experiences Scale (Hyman, 1996)
	Childhood Trauma Questionnaire (Bernstein et al., 1994)
	Juvenile Victim Questionnaire (Finkelhor et al., 2005)
Anxiety	Beck Anxiety Inventory—Youth (BAI-Y; A. T. Beck & Steer, 1993; J. S. Beck et al., 2005)
	Social Anxiety Scale for Children—Revised (La Greca, 1999)
	Child Anxiety Sensitivity Index (CASI; Reiss et al., 1986)
	State Trait Anxiety Inventory for Children (Spielberger, 1973; Spielberger, Gorsuch, & Lushene, 2005)
	Multidimensional Anxiety Scale for Children (MASC-2; March, 2012)
Depression	Children's Depression Inventory-2 (CDI; Kovacs, 2010)
	Beck Depression Inventory—Youth (J. S. Beck et al. 2005)

culty Questionnaire, which is highly correlated with the CBCL.

Other Procedures

Two additional procedures deserve mention. These are not clinical procedures in the traditional sense. The Extended Forensic Evaluation (Carnes et al., 2001; Carnes, Wilson, & Nelson-Gardell, 1999) is a procedure with a defined protocol that requires specific, intensive training. It can be considered an extension of the forensic interview and should be done by individuals with training in forensic interviewing and with a mental health background. The procedure is used in some jurisdictions as a follow-up to a forensic interview that might have resulted in a partial or vague disclosure of abuse.

A second procedure is the Child and Adolescent Needs and Strengths—Trauma Version (CANS-Trauma; Kisiel et al., 2009), a method for summarizing existing assessment results. The CANS-Trauma is an information-integration tool, not an assessment measure. It systematically documents trauma experiences, symptoms, functional difficulties and strengths, caregiver needs and strengths, and management and planning needs. However, as this is an information-integration tool, the results are only as helpful and accurate as the original information gathered during an assessment.

SPECIAL CONCERNS

Assessing Families

Several additional instruments deserve special mention as they relate to assessment of families.

CHILD ABUSE POTENTIAL INVENTORY (CAP-I). The CAP-I (Milner, 1986) is a parent self-report form for discriminating between physically abusive and non–physically abusive parents. The CAP-I shows good levels of internal reliability and test-retest reliability, as well as correct classification rates for physically abusive and matched comparison parents ranging from approximately 85% to 90% (Milner & Wimberley, 1980). Item factors most successfully discriminating were those associated with distress, rigidity, and unhappiness (Milner & Wimberley, 1980). Additionally, in a separate study, pretreatment CAP-I scores predicted risk of further abuse among physically abusive parents in a treatment program (Chaffin & Valle, 2003).

PARENTING STRESS INDEX (PSI). The PSI (Loyd & Abidin, 1985) consists of six Child domains: Adaptability, Acceptability, Demandingness, Mood, Distractibility/Hyperactivity, and Reinforces Parent; and seven Parent domains: Competence, Social Isolation, Attachment to Child, Health, Role Restriction, Depression, and Spouse. Test-retest reliability after three weeks was 0.82 for the Child subscales and 0.71 for the Parent subscales. Validity is well established, and the normative group included 534 parents of children in a pediatric practice and 223 Spanish-speaking mothers from a large northeastern city.

Cultural Considerations

One of the basic requirements in the field of assessment is standardization of norms using a representative sample for sex, age, and race/ethnicity. Some of the instruments have not been standardized, while others (e.g., the CSBI) were standardized on a primarily Caucasian sample. Standard interpretations of t-scores are appropriate when the family/child is among the racial or ethnic groups included in the representative sample. Unfortunately, for less-represented cultures (i.e., non-Caucasian, non–African American, and non–Hispanic/Latino), the availability of appropriate, normed measures is scant.

Several principles of cultural competence deserve mention. First, the interpretation of any behavior or event should be neither ethnocentric (i.e., based on the majority cultural norm) nor completely culturally relative. There often is as much variability within a racial group as between racial groups. Thus, it is important to learn about global and idiosyncratic cultural beliefs and practices related to child rearing, family structure, sex roles, and religious beliefs, as well as levels of acculturation. Second, while much has been written about the potential advantages of matching clinicians with children by race, little research has specifically focused on children who have been abused. One exception is a study by Springman, Wherry, and Notaro (2006), which found that race matching predicted disclosure rates in forensic interviews, but in the opposite direction to that hypothesized. That is, Caucasian children were more likely to disclose to an African American interviewer, and African American children were more likely to disclose to a Caucasian interviewer. Finally, in cases of child maltreatment, other cultural considerations may be particularly salient in affecting clients' level of trust and engagement in the assessment and treatment process—including concerns about the disproportionate representation of some racial/ethnic groups in the child welfare system, differences in rates of substantiation and out-of-home placement, and greater likelihood of other system involvement for many children of color. As noted by some researchers and public policymakers (Alliance for Racial Equality in Child Welfare, 2011; Bartholet, 2009; Drake et al., 2011), these are complex issues, confounded by factors, such as socioeconomic status and higher rates of child maltreatment among some racial/ethnic groups, that may account for this apparent disproportionality. All of this speaks to the importance of cultural sensitivity and awareness in the assessment process.

Prosecution Needs versus Mental Health Needs

In some instances, there can be resistance among prosecutors regarding assessments conducted in CACs. As we noted above, one objection hinges on items included in some of the assessment measures that can adversely affect the legal proceedings. This can be addressed by including expert testimony as part of the prosecution. Most importantly, a comprehensive assessment should never be withheld because of concerns that it will negatively influence the prosecution of a child abuse case.

Concurrent Sessions

One potential objection by therapists to the use of assessments is the belief that they will interfere with establishing a therapeutic alliance. Certainly, some parents, especially in cases of child sexual abuse, need sessions with the therapist to tell their story and to secure emotional support and direction from the therapist. Also, for some children, self-report measures may seem too much like a reading task from school, which can interfere with rapport-building. One way to address these potential problems is to complete the assessment after several sessions of rapport-building, engagement, and building of the therapeutic alliance. Another approach is to use one dedicated clinician for assessment and another for provision of therapy. One of us (Wherry) used this type of approach in a child advocacy center. The initial appointment with the therapist was followed by a coordinated appointment at which, depending on the age and circumstances of the client, the child saw the intake specialist while the parent spoke with the therapist. The next scheduled session either repeated this process or alternated, so that the child saw the therapist and the parent completed assessment information with the intake specialist. In this way, the assessment and therapy processes were kept separate, enabling the parent and child to simultaneously complete the assessment and establish rapport and a strong alliance with the clinician delivering the treatment.

In addition to splitting these assessment and treatment responsibilities among clinical staff, it is often helpful to demystify the process of assessment and treatment by informing caregivers before the appointment about what to expect, addressing questions or logistical barriers, and creating a safe environment for children and their families. Mary McKay has written extensively about how to enhance engagement so that the clinical staff and the families served can partner to achieve optimal outcomes (e.g., McKay & Bannon, 2004).

Report Writing

When assessments primarily describe child symptoms and a treatment plan (in contrast to a description of the abuse), clinicians should consider sharing these reports with the parents. This requires the clinician to write the report with limited jargon and in a manner that makes it readable and understandable. One of the chief complaints often heard from caseworkers is about the clinician who will cut and paste results into the same report format—sometimes without making corrections for the current case, and even using the wrong name. A variant of this poor practice is the clinician who copies interpretive statements from a software scoring program and pastes these into a report.

If assessment instruments are used in routine screening for trauma and symptoms among many children, it may be impossible to write highly individualized reports. This is the tradeoff. However, screening large numbers of children and then making referrals for full evaluations when scale scores are elevated may be effective, efficient, and economical in the long term.

New Modalities

With each passing day there seem to be significant advances in technology that affect the way business is conducted. For many years, test publishers have made computer scoring programs available for a number of products (e.g., the TSCC, TSCYC, CBCL, BASC, and BASC-2). These can speed the process of scoring and interpretation. Another advance that followed was the ability to purchase design software that, with the test publisher's contractual agreement, allowed the test to be loaded onto a tablet, such as the Apple iPad, to facilitate

administration, scoring, and data entry. More recently, test publishers are making the same features (administration, scoring, and data entry) available online for individual administration of specific tests. For many, the preferred interface with the Internet is a tablet. Each approach has its advantages. One recommendation to consider, especially for administrators, is subscribing to a system that allows the automatic downloading of information for program evaluation in order to monitor progress and satisfy funders.

"Profiles"

It is important to emphasize that no assessment profiles, in isolation, prove that a child was abused or that an alleged perpetrator is either guilty or innocent. Such profiles simply do not exist. Thus, if someone were to suggest that a child victim or alleged perpetrator did not fit the "profile," it might be wise to cease making referrals to that individual.

THE FUTURE

We noted earlier that psychologists and clinicians are unable to predict the future in their assessments of individual children. Similarly, it is impossible to predict the future in the field of assessment of abused children. As this chapter is being written, legislators and bureaucracies are defining policies for trauma-focused and abuse-focused services and assessments. Congress now requires that child welfare agencies address the issue of child trauma when developing a plan for meeting the health and mental health needs of youth in foster care (Casey Family Programs, 2011). Griffin and colleagues (2011) analyzed fourteen thousand clinical assessments from the child welfare system in Illinois and found that child welfare agencies adopt "policies requiring that mental health screenings and assessments of all youth in child welfare include measures of traumatic events and trauma-related symptoms" (p. 69). They further recommended that all state child welfare agencies update their policies and procedures. Nonetheless, while many states are considering or have enacted policies addressing trauma among their abused populations, many child welfare systems still do not routinely screen for trauma exposure or trauma-related symptoms beyond initial assessment of the precipitating event (Greeson et al., 2011). Despite good intentions, requiring clinicians to begin a process for which they have no training will have unintended, negative consequences. Similarly, the referring agents (also called "gatekeepers" or "brokers")—typically child welfare caseworkers—need training in what services, including specific assessments, are helpful.

One promising approach to training these broker professionals is Project BEST, a statewide collaborative effort in South Carolina, funded by the Duke Endowment, "to use innovative community-based dissemination, training, and implementation methods to dramatically increase the capacity of every community in South Carolina to deliver evidence-supported mental health treatments (ESTs) to every abused and traumatized child who needs them" (http://academicdepartments.musc.edu/projectbest). Project BEST makes use of a comprehensive dissemination and implementation model (the Community-Based Learning Collaborative) to train both clinicians and broker professionals (e.g., child welfare professionals, child protective service workers, guardians ad litem) in trauma-focused evidence-based practices. Clinicians learn to deliver Trauma-Focused Cognitive Behavioral Therapy (Cohen, Mannarino, & Deblinger, 2006), and brokers learn to conduct trauma-informed assessments, to be knowledgeable about trauma-focused evidence-based treatments, to make informed mental health treatment referrals, and to monitor cases to ensure successful completion of treatment. (For further details, see chapter 22.)

There are several other initiatives to improve care for abused children, either independently or in cooperation with the National Children's Alliance and the National Child Traumatic Stress Network. The NCA is a membership organization with some oversight of its 750-plus voluntary CAC members. Accredited CACs must meet certain multidisciplinary standards, including a mental health component. In the past decade there has been a significant shift in focus to more thoroughly meet the mental health needs of the children served in these settings. The NCA continues to provide leadership and improve access to care for thousands of children every year. In the future, this challenge will be embraced systematically by the health care system, educational institutions, professional associations, and licensure boards. When one considers the inadequate training provided in most graduate and professional training programs, however, many key challenges remain to the widespread use of assessment in the child abuse field. While the NCTSN has developed a core curriculum and implemented it on a limited basis in some social work programs, there is still no systematic requirement by accrediting bodies (e.g., the American Psychological Association) or licensure boards for any discipline. Training licensed professionals after graduate school is arguably an expensive and inefficient approach to training.

On a positive note, the Academy on Violence and Abuse has developed core competencies that have been endorsed by the American Academy of Pediatrics, the American Academy of Nursing, the Nursing Network on Violence against Women International, and the Gay and Lesbian Medical Association; these core competencies also are supported by the American Medical Association and the International Association of Forensic Nurses. The competencies are organized for the health system, educational institutions, and individual learners.

RESOURCES

Several websites can connect the reader to valuable resources.

- The Measures Review website of the National Child Traumatic Stress Network (www.nctsn.org/resources/online-research/measures-review). Many of the measures mentioned in this chapter, as well as others, can be found here, with a full description of psychometric properties, citations' reading level, and so forth.
- The Assessment Tools website of the California Evidence-Based Clearinghouse for Child Welfare (www.cebc4cw.org/assessment-tools). This shares many of the characteristics of the NCTSN website.
- The Academy on Violence and Abuse website (www.avahealth.org). The core competencies for training in trauma assessment are available here.

SUMMARY

The intent of this chapter is to highlight the importance and value of conducting informed, focused assessments for children and their families who have experienced trauma and abuse. Significant advances have been made in the field, with widespread recognition that informed assessments not only help to establish the credibility of a child's abuse disclosure but also inform treatment referrals and treatment planning and, by extension, increase the likelihood of successful treatment.

References

Achenbach, T. M. (1993). *Empirically based taxonomy: How to use syndromes and profile types derived from the CBCL/4-18, TRF, and YSF.* Burlington, VT: University of Vermont, Department of Psychiatry.

Achenbach, T. M. (2000). *Manual for the ASEBA preschool forms & profiles.* Burlington, VT: University of Vermont, Research Center for Children, Youth, & Families.

Achenbach, T. M., & Rescorla, L. A. (2001). *Manual for the ASEBA school-age forms & profiles.* Burlington, VT: University of Vermont, Research Center for Children, Youth, & Families.

Alliance for Racial Equality in Child Welfare. (2011). *Disparities and disproportionality in child welfare: Analysis of the research.* Washington, DC: Center for the Study of Social Policy and the Annie E. Casey Foundation.

American Academy of Child and Adolescent Psychiatry. (2010). Practice parameter for the assessment and treatment of children and adolescents with posttraumatic stress disorder. *Journal of the American Academy of Child and Adolescent Psychiatry, 49,* 414–430.

American Psychiatric Association. (1994). *Diagnostic and statistical manual of mental disorders—fourth edition.* Washington, DC: Author.

Armstrong, J. G., Putnam, F. W., Carlson, E. B., Libero, D. Z., & Smith, S. R. (1997). Development and validation of a measure of adolescent dissociation: The Adolescent Dissociative Experiences Scale. *Journal of Nervous and Mental Disease, 185*(8), 491–497.

Bartholet, E. (2009). Racial disproportionality. *Arizona Law Review, 51,* 871–932.

Beck, A. T., & Steer, R. A. (1993). *BAI: Beck Anxiety Inventory manual.* San Antonio, TX: Psychological Corporation.

Beck, J. S., Beck, A. T., Jolly, J. B., & Steer R. A. (2005). *The Beck Youth Inventories* (2nd ed.). San Antonio, TX: Harcourt Assessment.

Bernstein, D. P., Fink, L., Handelsman, L., & Foote, J. (1994). Initial reliability and validity of a new retrospective measure of child abuse and neglect. *American Journal of Psychiatry, 151*(8), 1132–1136.

Berres, A., Smith, M., Junko, K., & Wherry, J. N. (2007, October 24). *Empirical support for alternative avoidant criteria for the diagnosis of PTSD in abused children.* Poster presented at the annual conference of the American Academy of Child and Adolescent Psychiatry, Boston, MA.

Briere, J. (1996). *The Trauma Symptom Checklist for Children.* Odessa, FL: Psychological Assessment Resources.

Briere, J. (1999). *The Trauma Symptom Checklist for Young Children.* Odessa, FL: Psychological Assessment Resources.

Briere, J. (2005). *The Trauma Symptom Checklist for Young Children.* Odessa, FL: Psychological Assessment Resources.

Briggs, E. C., Fairbank, J. A., Greeson, J. K. P., Layne, C. M., Steinberg, A. M., Amaya-Jackson, et al. (2012, March 26). Links between child and adolescent trauma exposure and service use histories in a national clinic-referred sample. *Psychological Trauma: Theory, Research, Practice, and Policy.* Advance online publication. doi:10.1037/a0027312

Carnes, C. N., Nelson-Gardell, D., Wilson, C., & Orgassa, U. C. (2001). Extended forensic evaluation when sexual abuse is suspected: A multisite field study. *Child Maltreatment, 6*(3), 230–242.

Carnes, C. N., Wilson, C., & Nelson-Gardell, D. (1999). Extended forensic evaluation when sexual abuse is suspected: A model and preliminary data. *Child Maltreatment, 4,* 242–254.

Carter, C., & Wherry, J. N. (2007, October). *Co-morbidity/misdiagnosis of psychotic symptoms in abused children with PTSD.* Presentation at the American Academy of Child and Adolescent Psychiatry, Boston, MA.

Casey Family Programs. (2011, May). *Promoting Safe and Stable Families Program: Background and context.* Seattle: WA. www.casey.org

Cashel, M. L. (2002). Child and adolescent psychological assessment: Current clinical practices and the impact of managed care. *Professional Psychology: Research and Practice, 33*(5), 446–453.

Chaffin, M., & Valle, L. A. (2003). Dynamic prediction characteristics of the Child Abuse Prevention Inventory. *Child Abuse & Neglect, 27,* 463–481.

Chaffin, M., Wherry, J. N., Newlin, C., Crutchfield, A., & Dykman, R. (1997). The Abuse Dimensions Inventory: Initial data on a research measure of abuse severity. *Journal of Interpersonal Violence, 12*(4), 569–589.

Cohen, J. A., Mannarino, A. P., & Deblinger, E. (2006). *Treating trauma and traumatic grief in children and adolescents.* New York, NY: Guilford Press.

Conradi, L., Wherry, J., & Kisiel, C. (2011). Linking child welfare and mental health using trauma-informed screening and assessment practices. *Child Welfare, 90*(6), 129–147.

Drake, B., Jolley, J. M., Lanier, P., Fluke, J., Barth, R. P., & Jonson-Reid, M. (2011). Racial bias in child protection? A comparison of competing explanations using national data. *Pediatrics, 127*(3), 471–478.

Exner, J. E, (1993). *The Rorschach: A comprehensive system: Vol. I. Basic foundations* (3rd ed.). New York, NY: John Wiley & Sons.

Exner, J. E. (2002). *The Rorschach: Basic foundations and principles of interpretation* (Vol. 1). Hoboken, NJ: John Wiley & Sons.

Felitti, V. J., Anda, R. F., Nordenberg, D., Williamson, D. F., Spitz, A. M., Edwards, V., et al. (1998). Relationship of childhood abuse and household dysfunction to many of the leading causes of death in adults: The Adverse Childhood Experiences (ACE) study. *American Journal of Preventive Medicine, 14,* 245–258.

Fergusson, D. M., & Horwood, L. J. (1987a). The trait and method components of ratings of conduct disorder—Part I. Maternal and teacher evaluations of conduct disorder in young children. *Journal of Child Psychology and Psychiatry, and Allied Disciplines, 28,* 249–260.

Fergusson, D. M., & Horwood, L. J. (1987b). The trait and method components of ratings of conduct disorder—Part II. Factors related to the trait component of conduct disorder scores. *Journal of Child Psychology and Psychiatry, and Allied Disciplines, 28,* 261–272.

Fergusson, D. M., & Horwood, L. J. (1989). Estimation of method and trait variance in ratings of conduct disorder. *Journal of Child Psychology and Psychiatry, and Allied Disciplines, 30,* 365–378.

Finkelhor, D., Hamby, S. L., Ormrod, R., & Turner, H. (2005). The Juvenile Victimization Questionnaire: Reliability, validity, and national norms. *Child Abuse & Neglect, 29*(4), 383–412.

Fletcher, K. (1996). *Preliminary psychometrics of four new measures of childhood PTSD.* Paper presented at the International Research Conference on Trauma and Memory, University of New Hampshire, Durham, NH.

Ford, J. (2002a) *Traumatic Events Screening Inventory—Parent Report Revised (TESI).*Unpublished manuscript. University of Connecticut, Storrs, CT.

Ford, J. (2002b). *Traumatic Events Screening Inventory—Self Report Revised (TESI).* Unpublished manuscript. University of Connecticut, Storrs, CT.

Friedrich, W. N. (1998). *The Child Sexual Behavior Inventory professional manual.* Odessa, FL: Psychological Assessment Resources.

Friedrich, W. N., Lysne, M., Sim, L., & Shamos, S. (2004). Assessing sexual behavior in high-risk adolescents with the Adolescent Clinical Sexual Behavior Inventory (ACSBI). *Child Maltreatment, 9,* 239–250.

Ghosh-Ippen, C., Ford, J., Racusin, R., Acker, M., Bosquet, K., Rogers, C., et al. (2002). *Trauma Events Screening Inventory—Parent Report revised.* San Francisco, CA: Child Trauma Research Project of Early Trauma Network and National Center for PTSD, Dartmouth Child Trauma Research Group.

Greenwald, R., & Rubin, A. (1999, January). Brief assessment of children's post-traumatic symptoms: Development and preliminary validation of parent and child scales. *Research on Social Work Practice, 9*(1), 61–76.

Greeson, J. K. P., Briggs, E. C., Kisiel, C. L., Layne, C. M., Ake, G. S., Ko, S. J., et al. (2011). Complex trauma and mental health in children and adolescents placed in foster care: Findings from the National Child Traumatic Stress Network. *Child Welfare, 90*(6), 91–108.

Griffin, G., McClelland, G., Holzberg, M., Stolbach, B., Maj, N., & Kisiel, C. (2011). Addressing the impact of trauma before diagnosing mental illness in child welfare. *Child Welfare, 90*(6), 69–89.

Habib, M., & Labruna, V. (2006). *The adolescent trauma history checklist and interview.* Unpublished measure.

Handler, L., & Meyer, G. J. (1998). The importance of teaching and learning personality assessment. In L. Handler & M. J. Hilsenroth (Eds.), *Teaching and learning personality assessment.* Mahwah, NJ: Lawrence Erlbaum Associates.

Hawke, J. M., Jainchill, N., & Leon, G. D. (2000). The prevalence of sexual abuse and its impact on the onset of drug use among adolescents in therapeutic community drug treatment. *Journal of Child and Adolescent Substance Abuse, 9,* 35–49.

Hersen, M. (2004). *Psychological assessment in clinical practice: A pragmatic guide.* New York, NY: Brunner-Routledge.

Horowitz, K., Weine, S., & Jekel, J. (1995, October). PTSD symptoms in urban adolescent girls: Compounded community trauma. *Journal of American Academy of Adolescent Psychiatry, 34*(10), 1353–1361.

Hyman, I. (1996). Psychometric reviews of My Worst Experience and My Worst School Experience Scale. In B. Stamm (Ed.), *Measurement of stress, trauma, and adaptation* (pp. 212–213). Lutherville, MD: Sidran Press.

Iselin, G., LeBrocque, R., Kenardy, J., Anderson, V., & McKinlay, L. (2010). Which method of posttraumatic stress disorder classification best predicts psychosocial function in children with traumatic brain injury? *Journal of Anxiety Disorders, 24,* 774–779.

Johnson, T. C. (2003). *Child Sexual Behavior Checklist—Revised.* In assessment packet for children with sexual behavior problems. www.tcavjohn.com

Kendall-Tackett, K. A., Williams, L. M., & Finkelhor, D. (1993). Impact of sexual abuse on children: A review and synthesis of recent empirical studies. *Psychological Bulletin, 113,* 164–180.

Kilpatrick, D. G., Acierno, R., Saunders, B., Resnick, H. S., Best, C. L., & Schnurr, P. P. (2000). Risk factors for adolescent substance abuse and dependence: Data from a national sample. *Journal of Consulting and Clinical Psychology, 68,* 19–30.

Kisiel, C. L., Blaustein, M., Fogler, J., Ellis, H., & Saxe, G. (2009). Treating children with traumatic experiences: Understanding and assessing needs and strengths. In J. S. Lyons & D. A. Weiner (Eds.), *Behavioral health care: Assessment, service planning, and total clinical outcomes management.* Kingston, NJ: Civic Research Institute.

Kovacs, M. (2010). *The Child Depression Inventory 2 professional manual.* San Antonio, TX: Psychological Corporation.

La Greca, A. M. (1999). *Social anxiety scales for children and adolescents: Manual and instructions for the SASC, SASC-R, SAS-A (adolescents), and parent versions of the scales.* Miami, FL: University of Miami, Department of Psychology.

Lanktree, C. B., Gilbert, A. M., Briere, J., Taylor, N., Chen, K., Maida, C. A., & Saltzman, W. R. (2008). Multi-informant assessment of maltreated children: Convergent and discriminant validity of the TSCC and TSCYC. *Child Abuse & Neglect, 32,* 621–625.

Lee, S. W., Elliott, J., & Barbour, J. D. (1994). A comparison of cross-informant behaviour ratings in school-based diagnosis. *Behavioural Disorders, 19,* 87–97.

Loyd, B. H., & Abidin, R. R. (1985). Revision of the Parent Stress Index. *Journal of Pediatric Psychiatry, 10*(2), 169–177.

March, J. S. (2012). *Multidimensional Anxiety Scale for Children* (2nd ed.) Toronto: MultiHealth Systems.

McKay, M. M., & Bannon, W. M. (2004). Engaging families in child mental health services. *Child and Adolescent Psychiatric Clinics of North America, 13*(4), 905–921.

Meyer, G. J., Finn, S. E., Eyde, L. D., Kay, G. G., Moreland, K. L., Dies, R. R., et al. (2001). Psychological testing and psychological assessment: A review of evidence and issues. *American Psychologist, 56*(2), 128–165. doi:10.1037/0003-066X.56.2.128

Milner, J. S. (1986). *The child abuse potential inventory: Manual* (2nd ed.). Webster, NC: Psytec.

Milner, J. S., & Wimberley, R. C. (1980). Prediction and explanation of child abuse. *Journal of Clinical Psychology, 36*(4), 875–884.

Murstein, B. (1965). *Handbook of projective techniques.* New York, NY: Basic Books.

Perrin, S., Smith, P., & Yule, W. (2000). Practitioner review: The assessment of posttraumatic stress disorder in children and adolescents. *Journal of Child Psychology and Psychiatry, 41,* 277–289.

Pollio, E., Glover-Orr, E., & Wherry, J. (2008). Assessing posttraumatic stress disorder using the trauma symptom checklist for young children. *Journal of Child Sexual Abuse, 17*(2), 89–100.

Putnam, F. W., Helmers, K., & Trickett, P. K. (1993). Development, reliability, and validity of a child dissociation scale. *Child Abuse & Neglect, 17,* 731–741.

Raghavan, C., & Kingston, S. (2006). Child sexual abuse and posttraumatic stress disorder: The role of age at first use of substances and lifetime traumatic events. *Journal of Traumatic Stress, 19,* 269–278.

Reiss, S., Peterson, R. A., Gursky, D. M., & McNally, R. J. (1986). Anxiety sensitivity, anxiety frequency and the prediction of fearfulness. *Behaviour Research and Therapy, 24*(1), 1–8.

Reynolds, C. R., & Kamphaus, R. W. (2002). *The clinician's guide to the Behavior Assessment System for Children (BASC).* New York, NY: Guilford Press.

Reynolds, C. R., & Kamphaus, R. W. (2006). *BASC-2: Behavior Assessment System for Children, Second Edition.* Upper Saddle River, NJ: Pearson Education.

Rodriguez, N., Steinberg, A., & Pynoos, R. S. (1999). *UCLA PTSD Index for DSM IV instrument information: Child version, parent version, adolescent version.* Los Angeles, CA: UCLA Trauma Psychiatry Services.

Rutter, M., Tizard, J., Yule, W., Graham, P., & Whitmore, K. (1976). Isle of Wight studies, 1964–1974. *Psychological Medicine, 6*(2), 313–333.

Saigh, P. A. (2003). *The Children's Posttraumatic Stress Disorder Inventory test manual.* San Antonio, TX: Psychological Corporation.

Saunders, B. E. (2003). Understanding children exposed to violence: Toward an integration of overlapping fields. *Journal of Interpersonal Violence, 18*(4), 356–376.

Scheeringa, M. S., Myers, L., Putnam, F. W., & Zeanah, C. H. (2012). Diagnosing PTSD in early childhood: An empirical assessment of four approaches. *Journal of Traumatic Stress, 25,* 359–367.

Scheeringa, M. S., Zeanah, C. H., Myers, L., & Putnam, F. W. (2003). New findings on alternative criteria for PTSD in preschool children. *Journal of the American Academy of Child and Adolescent Psychiatry, 42,* 561–570.

Shapiro, S., & Dominiak, G. (1990). Common psychological defenses seen in the treatment of sexually abused adolescents. *American Journal of Psychotherapy, 44,* 68–74.

Spielberger, C. D. (1973). *Manual for the State-Trait Anxiety Inventory for Children.* Palo Alto, CA: Consulting Psychologists Press.

Spielberger, C. D., Gorsuch, R. L., & Lushene, R. E. (2005). *State-trait anxiety inventory.* Palo Alto, CA: Mind Garden.

Springman, R., Wherry, J., & Notaro, P. (2006). The effects of interviewer race and child race on sexual abuse disclosures in forensic interviews. *Journal of Child Sexual Abuse, 15*(3), 99–116.

Steinberg, A. M., Brymer, M. J., Decker, K. B., & Pynoos, R. S. (2004). The University of California at Los Angeles Posttraumatic Stress Disorder Reaction Index. *Current Psychiatry Reports, 6,* 96–100.

Steven, R. S., & Carlson, E. B. (1996). Reliability and validity of the Adolescent Dissociative Experiences Scale. *Dissociation, 9,* 125–129.

Summerfeldt, L. J., & Antony, M. M. (2002). Structured and semistructured diagnostic interviews. In M. M. Antony & D. H. Barlow (Eds.), *Handbook of assessment and treatment planning for psychological disorders* (pp. 3–37). New York, NY: Guilford Press.

Verhulst, F. C. (1995). Recent developments in assessment and diagnosis of child psychopathology. *European Child and Adolescent Psychiatry, 11,* 203–212.

Weiner, I., & Greene, R. (2008). *Handbook of personality assessment.* Hoboken, NJ: John Wiley & Sons.

Wetzler, S., & Katz, M. M. (1989). *Contemporary approaches to psychological assessment.* New York, NY: Brunner-Mazel.

Wherry, J. N., Baldwin, S., Junco, K., & Floyd, B. (in press). Suicidal thoughts/behaviors in sexually abused children. *Journal of Child Sexual Abuse.*

Wherry, J. N., Berres, A., Sim, L., & Friedrich, W. (2009). Factor structure of the Adolescent Clinical Sexual Behavior Inventory. *Journal of Child Sexual Abuse, 18*(3), 233–246.

Wherry, J. N., Carter, C., Bartholomew, M., Schneider, A., Van Cleave, A., Namae, E., et al. (2008, April). *Comorbidity or misdiagnosis in abused children with PTSD.* Presentation at the Southwestern Psychological Association, Kansas City, KS.

Wherry, J. N., Corson, K., & Hunsaker, S. (in press). A short form of the Trauma Symptom Checklist for Young Children using a clinical sample of sexually abused outpatients. *Journal of Child Sexual Abuse.*

Wherry, J. N., Graves, L., & Rhodes, H. (2008). The convergent validity of the Trauma Symptom Checklist for Young Children for a sample of sexually abused outpatients. *Journal of Child Sexual Abuse, 17,* 38–50.

Wherry, J. N., Huey, C., & Medford, E. (2013). *A national survey of CAC directors regarding knowledge of assessment, treatment referral, and training needs in physical and sexual abuse.* Manuscript submitted for publication.

Wherry, J. N., Jolly, J. B., Feldman, J., Adam, B., & Manjanatha, S. (1994). The Child Dissociative Checklist: Preliminary findings of a screening measure. *Journal of Child Sexual Abuse, 3*(3), 51–66.

Wherry, J. N., & Marrs, A. (2008). Anxious school refusers and symptoms of PTSD in abused children. *Journal of Child and Adolescent Trauma, 1*(2), 109–117.

Wherry, J. N., McMillan, S. L., & Hutchison, H. T. (1991). Differential diagnosis and treatment of conversion disorder and Guillain-Barre syndrome. *Clinical Pediatrics, 3*(10), 578–585.

Wilson, C. A. (2012). Special issue of Child Maltreatment on implementation: Some key developments in evidence-based models for the treatment of child maltreatment. *Child Maltreatment, 17,* 102–106.

Wood, J. M., Nezworski, T., & Stejskal, W. J. (1996). The comprehensive system for the Rorschach: A critical examination. *Psychological Science, 7*(1), 3–10.

Wyatt, G. E., Loeb, T. B., Solis, B., & Carmona, J. V. (1999). The prevalence and circumstances of child sexual abuse: Changes across a decade. *Child Abuse & Neglect, 23,* 45–60.

PART II Evidence-Based Treatments

ELISABETH POLLIO, PH.D.
MELISSA MCLEAN, LPC
LEAH E. BEHL, PH.D.
ESTHER DEBLINGER, PH.D.

3

Trauma-Focused Cognitive Behavioral Therapy

GENERAL CONSIDERATIONS

This chapter focuses on Trauma-Focused Cognitive Behavioral Therapy (TF-CBT), an evidence-based treatment designed to address the difficulties experienced by children, adolescents, and their caregivers in the aftermath of traumatic experiences. TF-CBT has the strongest empirical support among trauma treatments for children, having proven its efficacy and effectiveness in over a dozen randomized controlled trials—the gold standard of research on treatment outcomes. We discuss the theoretical framework for TF-CBT, explore its advantages and limitations, and provide a description of the treatment process. In addition, we review a number of TF-CBT studies, particularly the research involving children who have experienced sexual abuse. Given the broad range of negative and potentially long-term effects of trauma, it is important that children receive effective and timely treatment.

Trauma-Focused Cognitive Behavioral Therapy, then, is a structured, short-term, components-based treatment involving children and their nonoffending caregivers to address the negative sequelae of child maltreatment and other traumas (Cohen, Mannarino, & Deblinger, 2006; Deblinger & Heflin, 1996). TF-CBT may be the most widely disseminated evidence-based treatment to address symptoms resulting from child maltreatment (Allen & Johnson, 2012). The negative impact of child maltreatment has been well documented; sequelae include posttraumatic stress and other anxiety symptoms, depression, and behavioral difficulties (e.g., Putnam, 2003; Trickett & McBride-Chang, 1995). Such symptoms may persist into adulthood (e.g., Irish, Kobayashi, & Delahanty, 2010; Trickett & McBride-Chang, 1995). TF-CBT has been found to significantly reduce these trauma symptoms and to improve parenting skills, parental support, parental distress, and children's body safety skills. With effective ther-

apy, the negative trajectory of child maltreatment can be derailed.

THEORETICAL MECHANISMS

When children are exposed to traumatic events, they may develop problematic emotional, cognitive, physical, and/or behavioral reactions that can severely disrupt their development (e.g., Hornor, 2010; Putnam, 2003; Trickett & McBride-Chang, 1995). Children's symptoms may be linked to learning that occurred at the time of the traumatic event and in the immediate aftermath. Three learning mechanisms may significantly impact children's responses to trauma: respondent conditioning, operant conditioning, and modeling, or more simply put, learning by means of associations, consequences, and observations. Children's learned responses to trauma can significantly influence whether they "recover" optimally or continue to struggle for years after the trauma.

Children learn, for example, to associate feelings with situations. This seems to be especially relevant to situations that elicit fear. When exposed to traumatic events, children often learn to associate fear or other negative emotions they experienced at the time of the trauma with the traumatic memories and/or other reminders in the environment. Sometimes children who are abused continue to be afraid any time they are reminded of the abuse. Children experiencing symptoms of posttraumatic stress often associate feelings of fear with nondangerous cues that may have been present at the time of the abuse. For example, a child who was sexually abused in the bathroom at school may become afraid to go to that bathroom. Other examples of innocuous trauma-related cues that may come to be associated with fear and can trigger distress include darkness, nudity, men who look like the offender, basements, bedrooms, and/

or other people, places, or things associated with the original experience of abuse.

Children also learn, through consequences, which behaviors are effective in achieving desired outcomes. When children avoid the reminders of their abuse, for example, they often feel a reduction in their anxiety, so abuse-related avoidant behaviors are reinforced. Unfortunately, this avoidance pattern does not allow children to learn that nothing bad happens in the presence of innocuous abuse reminders, and thus their unrealistic fears and associated avoidant behaviors continue to be strengthened and reinforced over time. Moreover, the original fears can generalize to broader fears, such that a fear of the bathroom at school becomes a fear of all public bathrooms. Ultimately, generalized fears can increasingly interfere with children's abilities to comfortably function in life and can potentially disrupt their psychosocial development. In addition, parents may inadvertently reinforce their children's distress responses. As a result of compassion for their children in the aftermath of a trauma, parents may be overindulgent and not follow through with negative consequences for misbehavior. This pattern of parent-child interaction often inadvertently leads to increases in problematic child behaviors and a reinforcement of the child's fears, resulting in the child's continued dependence on the comforting attention of others to manage distress. The development of problematic behaviors of either an externalizing or internalizing nature, unfortunately, leaves children more prone to future escalating difficulties and potential revictimization, given the greater vulnerability of children with interpersonal problems.

Another way children learn is through modeling. When children are exposed to negative behavior, they may learn to emulate this type of behavior. For example, a sexually abused child may behave in sexually inappropriate ways toward other children or adults and/or may become more aggressive because of behavior that has been modeled in the context of abuse. Children also use modeling to make sense of what happened to them. They learn ways to cope by observing their parents' reactions to trauma. When children are traumatized, their parents—who understandably do not know how to deal with the trauma or have very negative views about what happened—may inadvertently react in ways that lead children to believe they are damaged. This learned belief can lead children to feel bad about themselves and may result in subsequent depression or behavioral problems. Alternatively, parents who respond in positive and supportive ways to their children after a trauma can enhance their children's resiliency and recovery. The parents' reactions to the trauma are an important part of how children recover and learn to respond to other stressors in their lives. Thus, TF-CBT provides coping skills as well as parenting skills training to caregivers, thereby reinforcing positive, supportive parent-child relationships. This type of relationship has been strongly correlated with positive outcomes for children who have experienced sexual abuse (Deblinger, Lippmann, & Steer, 1996). Helping parents understand their

children's behaviors and teaching them ways to correct problematic behaviors can also help parents regain their confidence. Instilling hope helps parents to be more positive role models for their children.

In TF-CBT, in addition to education and skill building, children are gradually exposed to reminders of the trauma they have experienced. Gradual exposure helps children stop avoiding the memory of the trauma by gradually introducing reminders of the trauma. This exposure helps children to learn that the memory of what happened cannot hurt them and thus they need not be afraid of memories and/or other innocuous reminders. Breaking the avoidance cycle can help eliminate the over-generalized fears a child may have developed regarding the trauma. Although the trauma narrative and processing component of TF-CBT often extinguishes unhealthy avoidance patterns, many children also benefit from in vivo exposure, particularly when avoidance extends to places and things for which the avoidance greatly interferes with their day-to-day functioning (e.g., school refusal).

When the fear of the traumatic event is decreased, children are often more able to talk about and develop a written narrative about the trauma. This narrative often includes several chapters reflecting different aspects of the traumatic experience(s) and incorporates the child's thoughts, feelings, and even physical reactions associated with the trauma(s). When the narrative is almost complete, children are encouraged to review and process their thoughts and feelings. Discussion of their thoughts related to the trauma can help identify problematic cognitions that can be addressed and challenged. The final chapter of children's trauma narrative often allows them to review their experience with a focus on what they have learned about the abuse and/or other traumas, as well as what they have discovered about their own personal strengths and the support and kindnesses of others. In addition, many children demonstrate their mastery of the trauma by ending their narratives with positive expectations for the future and with informative and encouraging messages for other children.

After careful preparation, when clinically appropriate, children and families often process these experiences in conjoint sessions during which they have an opportunity to review and acknowledge their skills and strengths while also, through sharing of the narrative, openly discussing the abuse and/or other traumas experienced. The final component of TF-CBT focuses on enhancing safety and future development. Through role plays, children learn and practice body safety skills that will help to reduce their risk of revictimization.

In sum, the principles of learning described above underlie not only the development of trauma-related symptoms but also the mechanisms by which children and their caregivers overcome trauma-related difficulties. TF-CBT emphasizes the important involvement of nonoffending caregivers as critical role models whom children are likely to observe and learn from. Education and skill building in the context of TF-CBT also use observational learning through modeling, role plays, and behavior rehearsals. Finally, through gradual exposure and, more specifically, the trauma narrative component, children effectively confront and process traumatic memories in the context of a trusting therapeutic relationship, thereby overcoming maladaptive associations and avoidant behaviors. Over the course of treatment, TF-CBT helps children and adolescents, as well as their caregivers, gain feelings of support and mastery in the face of trauma. After successfully completing TF-CBT, the experience of trauma may continue to be associated with negative emotions, but for most children those emotions are less likely to be overwhelming, and the memories often come to be associated with feelings of pride and confidence in their ability to manage and overcome difficult life stressors. In general, TF-CBT incorporates many opportunities for learning that are designed to help families grow stronger and closer in the face of trauma, empowering them with knowledge and skills that prepare them for the future.

ADVANTAGES AND LIMITATIONS

Trauma-Focused Cognitive Behavioral Therapy is a time-limited, components-based model that helps children (ages 3–17) and their families heal from traumatic events. Treatment is typically delivered in 8–20 sessions. The model addresses a wide range of difficulties, including posttraumatic stress disorder (PTSD), anxiety, depression, feelings of shame, and trauma-related behavioral difficulties in children, while also addressing the emotional reactions and skill deficits exhibited by nonoffending caregivers (Cohen, Mannarino, & Deblinger, 2006; Deblinger & Heflin, 1996). TF-CBT has been used in treating children and adolescents who have endured sexual abuse, physical abuse, traumatic grief, exposure to domestic violence, disaster, terrorism, and multiple or complex traumas, with over 25 scientific investigations documenting its efficacy. Some modifications are useful with certain populations. For example, in the case of complex trauma, the initial phase of TF-CBT may be extended, with a greater focus on developing a safe and trusting therapeutic relationship and more time devoted to skill building before the narrative work begins. As a result, TF-CBT for complex trauma may require as many as 25 sessions to accomplish the treatment goals. Although primarily tested in outpatient settings, TF-CBT is currently being used with success in residential treatment, school, and home-based settings.

Of course, like any treatment model, TF-CBT has its limitations. It is not intended for use with offending parents who have been physically abusive toward their children. For these families, we encourage the use of other evidence-based models such as Combined Parent-Child Cognitive Behavioral Therapy (CPC-CBT; Runyon & Deblinger, in press) or Alternatives for Families: Cognitive Behavioral Therapy (AF-CBT; Kolko & Swenson, 2002). In addition,

although children referred for TF-CBT need not exhibit full-blown PTSD, it is important to establish that the difficulties targeted in the context of TF-CBT stem in part from the trauma(s) suffered. TF-CBT is not appropriate for children who have not experienced trauma or have no memory of trauma(s). When addressing the trauma of sexual abuse, TF-CBT should not be initiated until the allegations have been reported and investigated according to the appropriate state laws. In addition, when abuse is suspected but not remembered by the child due to his or her young age at the time of abuse, the full course of TF-CBT may not be appropriate. Finally, TF-CBT is not recommended for children, adolescents, and/or caregivers who are actively psychotic, suicidal, or dangerous to themselves or others by virtue of their emotional and/or behavioral difficulties (e.g., fire setting, suicidal behavior, extreme aggression). However, TF-CBT may be considered for these children after such symptoms have been addressed and after a period of stabilization. In sum, although there are some clear contraindications for the use of this model, TF-CBT effectively addresses a wide range of difficulties precipitated by childhood traumatic experiences.

OVERVIEW OF TF-CBT

The core values of TF-CBT can be summarized by the acronym CRAFTS and apply to all families that come in for treatment following the experience of a traumatic event. The TF-CBT model is

- *Components-based* and provides education along with a set of skills that build on previously learned skills that are integrated in and tailored to the needs of the child and family.
- *Respectful* of cultural, individual, family, community, and religious practices, in that it seeks to understand the impact of the trauma while guiding the child and family through the healing process within their community, cultural, and religious context.
- *Adaptable and flexible* in that the therapist has the ability to be creative in implementing the components throughout the treatment to keep children and their families motivated, as well as to implement the model with diverse populations. However, it remains important to maintain adherence to the model.
- *Family focused* in that it aims to include family members who are supportive of the child. The caregivers play an integral role in treatment, as one of the primary goals is to enhance the relationship between the child and caregiver. Appropriate family members who may become involved in the child's treatment can include the parent or other caregiver and siblings or other family members, when appropriate.
- *Therapeutic relationship centered* in that the development and maintenance of a trusting, accepting, and empathic therapeutic relationship is central to the treatment

process. This helps children and caregivers develop trust and feelings of safety, enabling them to share their traumatic experiences as well as promoting their openness to learning new skill sets to heal from the trauma.

- *Self-efficacy focused* in that self-regulation of affect, behavior, and cognitions is a long-term goal within the short-term, strength-based TF-CBT model. It strives to assist the child and family in developing skills they will continue to use after completion of the therapy. Self-efficacy is encouraged through active collaboration with the child and family in planning therapy, assigning homework between sessions, noting successes in therapy, and encouraging and praising use of the TF-CBT skills (Cohen, Mannarino, & Deblinger, 2006).

TF-CBT consists of 8–20 sessions that include individual work with the caregiver and child and conjoint work in which the caregiver and child are seen together for a portion of the session. Ideally, the session duration is 90 minutes, though TF-CBT may be delivered in the standard 50- to 60-minute session length used in most community mental health clinics. At the start of treatment, more time is spent on individual work with the caregiver and child. The timing of the initiation and the number of conjoint parent-child sessions depend on the child's behavioral presentation, but most parents and children participate in at least some conjoint sessions so that information can be shared and skills can be practiced together. In the later conjoint parent-child sessions, TF-CBT therapists facilitate open parent-child communication about the trauma(s) experienced and, when clinically appropriate, the sharing of the trauma narrative.

Before commencement of TF-CBT, it is important to assess the impact of the traumatic events on the various domains of functioning for the child. Possible areas of maladjustment that TF-CBT aims to treat are also summarized by the acronym CRAFTS (Cohen, Mannarino, & Deblinger, 2006) (see table 3.1).

The measures to assess these possible areas of maladjustment are administered individually to the parent and child at the start and end of treatment. Measures are also administered during the middle phase of treatment at the clinical discretion of the therapist. The assessment measures provide a tailored treatment plan that is individualized to the child and caregiver, as well as serving as an assessment of treatment progress.

TF-CBT treatment can be conceptualized as occurring in thirds. The first third of treatment includes the engagement process, psychoeducation, parenting skills, relaxation, affective expression and modulation training, and cognitive coping. The second third includes development and processing of the trauma narrative and in vivo mastery of trauma reminders. The final third of the treatment process involves trauma-focused conjoint parent-child sessions and a focus on skill building that is designed to enhance future safety and development.

Table 3.1. Possible Areas of Maladjustment That TF-CBT Aims to Treat

Possible Areas of Maladjustment	Examples
Cognitive problems	Difficulty concentrating, learning difficulties, maladaptive patterns of thinking about self, others, and situations
Relationship problems	Increase in conflicts, poor problem-solving or social skills, hypersensitivity in interpersonal relationships, lack of ability to trust others, maladaptive strategies for making and keeping friends
Affective problems	Anxiety, sadness, anger, inability to self-soothe or regulate unwanted emotions
Family problems	Lack of effective parenting skills, poor caregiver-child communication, issues with caregiver-child attachment, disruptions in familial relationships due to violence or abuse
Traumatic behavior problems	Trauma-related, sexualized, aggressive, oppositional, or unsafe behaviors or avoidance of harmless trauma reminders
Somatic problems	Headaches, stomachaches, sleep difficulties, physical tension, hyperarousal symptoms, other physiological reactions to trauma cues

When beginning TF-CBT, it is critical to engage the child and caregiver by taking into consideration their general needs. It is also important to attend to potential obstacles that can impede or hinder the therapeutic engagement. If there are other high-priority issues following the trauma, providing the family with appropriate referrals may help to engage them in therapy once their basic needs have been met (Deblinger, Cohen, & Mannarino, 2012).

The TF-CBT components are delivered to children and caregivers in separate sessions and during conjoint parent-child sessions. The acronym PRACTICE is used to capture the components of TF-CBT (Cohen, Mannarino, & Deblinger, 2006). Each component builds on skills that were mastered in the preceding component (see table 3.2).

Psychoeducation is a component that continues throughout the treatment process. Parents and children often lack information and harbor misconceptions about the traumatic events. Psychoeducation provides accurate information that highlights factors likely to enhance optimism about treatment and recovery. Throughout treatment, psychoeducation includes educating the parent and child about the TF-CBT model and providing general information about the traumatic event, including reviewing and explaining the behavioral and emotional responses exhibited by children. Another facet of psychoeducation is providing information specific to the child's trauma experience, diagnosis, and symptom presentation (Cohen, Mannarino, & Deblinger, 2006).

Parenting skills training is another component delivered throughout the course of treatment. Caregivers who have not experienced difficulties with parenting prior to the

Table 3.2. The Components of TF-CBT: PRACTICE

Component	Goal/Rationale	Examples
Psychoeducation	To provide accurate information on trauma and its impact on the child; to enhance optimism about treatment and recovery	Use of *What do you know?* cards (Deblinger, Neubauer, et al. 2006); information hand-outs
Parenting skills	To enhance caregiver's behavior management and communication skills	Use of praise, effective instructions, reflective listening, selective attention, time-out, and contingency reinforcement schedules
Relaxation	To manage physiological stress and reduce tension that may result from trauma reminders; to quiet the mind; to manage distractions and encourage focus on the present	Focused breathing, progressive muscle relaxation exercises, and guided imagery; mindfulness and meditation exercises
Affective expression and modulation	To help the caregiver and child develop the ability to identify, express, and manage their emotions in a healthy and appropriate way	Identifying basic and trauma-related feelings words; teaching coping strategies, positive imagery, problem solving, and social skills
Cognitive coping	To provide education about the interrelationship of thoughts, feelings, and behaviors; to identify inaccurate and/or unhelpful thoughts and replace them with more accurate and productive ones	Teaching cognitive triangle; children apply skills initially to non-trauma-related problems; parents apply skills to both trauma- and non-trauma-related problems
Trauma narrative and processing	To share and process the trauma experience by identifying trauma-related thoughts, feelings, and body sensations; to assist in mastery of traumatic memories	Detailed account of trauma experience in written form or through art or play activities; challenging and reframing unhelpful/inaccurate trauma-related thoughts
In vivo mastery of trauma reminders	To target trauma-related avoidant behaviors that disrupt daily functioning	Developing plan to diminish/extinguish avoidance related to innocuous trauma cues (e.g., fear of the dark)
Conjoint parent-child sessions	To enhance the parent-child relationship; to strengthen trauma-related communication	Reviewing educational information; practicing skills with child and caregiver together; shared reading of child's narrative, if clinically appropriate
Enhancing future safety and development	To help the child feel prepared; to enhance self-efficacy; to reduce risk for revictimization	Provision of education and training in safety skills; use of role-playing and behavioral rehearsals to practice personal safety skills

traumatic event may now be challenged in this area, especially if the child is responding to the trauma with angry outbursts, aggression, or other negative behaviors (Deblinger, Cohen, & Mannarino, 2012). To effectively move through the healing process after a traumatic event, it is important to promote a sense of normalcy and consistency as it relates to rules, expectations, and routines. Even if a child is not experiencing negative behaviors, the skills can still have a positive impact on the relationship of the parent and child. Some of the skills that caregivers learn in this component are praise, selective attention, time-out, and contingency reinforcement schedules, which may include behavior charts.

Relaxation training is introduced early in treatment, as it is an effective way to help the child and caregiver manage their emotions and to reduce tension that may result from reminders of traumatic events. Focused breathing is one of the relaxation skills that can be used in any context and is easily mastered by the child and caregiver. Other relaxation skills taught are progressive muscle relaxation exercises and guided imagery. Mindfulness and meditation practices may also be used to help the child and caregiver quiet the distractions in their minds and attend to the present moment, thereby inducing relaxation.

Affective expression and modulation is particularly important, given that children may experience emotional dysregulation as a result of trauma. The goal of this component, then, is to help the caregiver and child develop the abilities to

identify and express their emotions in a healthy and appropriate way. When they are able to do this, it brings awareness of their own distressing feelings, helping the child and caregiver to manage them. The child and caregiver learn words for basic feelings, along with feelings that may be associated with the trauma. Coping strategies are also discussed with the caregiver and the child. Strategies that are less productive are discouraged and more productive ones are encouraged. Other skills introduced in this component include positive imagery, problem solving, and social skills.

Cognitive coping begins with education about the interrelationship of thoughts, feelings, and behaviors. The goals of this component are to assist the caregiver and child in identifying generally inaccurate and/or unhelpful thoughts and replacing them with more accurate and productive thoughts to help them feel better emotionally. The cognitive triangle is presented, which visually depicts the relations among thoughts, feelings, and behaviors. These skills are used in the early phase of treatment to help parents overcome dysfunctional trauma-related thoughts. Children are taught to use these skills in general at first, then later they learn to target trauma-related thoughts revealed during development of the narrative.

Trauma narrative and processing begins in the middle third of treatment. When children experience trauma, they may pair overwhelming and negative emotions with traumatic reminders, discussions, or thoughts about the experience.

The trauma narrative is created in written form or through art or play activities that allow the child to share and process his or her experience related to the trauma. The trauma-related thoughts, feelings, and body sensations are first simply elicited and later processed. Through repeated exposure to trauma narrative work, children's levels of distress decrease, in turn increasing their comfort and confidence in facing increasingly disturbing traumatic memories and reminders. Another goal during the processing of the narrative is to challenge and reframe unhelpful and inaccurate thoughts related to the trauma. This ultimately helps children and their caregivers gain a mastery over traumatic memories that emphasizes their strengths and encourages optimistic expectations for the future.

In vivo mastery of trauma reminders is critical for those children whose trauma-related avoidant behaviors disrupt their day-to-day functioning. As a result of trauma, some children may develop a generalized fear that inhibits their functioning optimally due to their avoidance of safe situations they may misperceive as threatening. This component is used when the previous gradual exposure and processing work are not sufficient to extinguish the unnecessary avoidant behaviors that the child may continue to experience. When children do not directly face their fears, they may continue to struggle with those fears for years to come. A plan for in vivo gradual exposure is developed to diminish or extinguish the avoidance related to trauma cues. The goal is for the child to develop the ability to be in the situation without unnecessary anxiety.

Conjoint parent-child sessions may begin during the initial phases of treatment, particularly when children present with acting-out behavioral problems. In the final phase of treatment, however, these sessions are used to enhance the parent-child relationship and strengthen trauma-related communication by initially reviewing educational information and practicing skills together and then reading the child's narrative, when clinically appropriate. The conjoint sessions normally occur after cognitive processing of the child's traumatic experiences by the caregiver and child in individual sessions with the therapist. TF-CBT therapists conduct a careful assessment to determine the appropriateness of trauma-focused conjoint sessions. Parents and children are prepared separately for these sessions to enhance comfort levels and success for both parent and child.

Enhancing future safety and development is typically the final therapy component. It provides education and training in safety skills to help children feel prepared and have a sense of self-efficacy should they experience an unsafe situation, as the experience of trauma may increase a child's sense of vulnerability and risk of future victimization. During this component, children learn what they can potentially do if faced with dangerous or threatening situations. Role plays and behavioral rehearsals assist children in practicing the learned personal safety skills.

Graduation from therapy is important to celebrate in the context of TF-CBT. This is an opportunity for the child and caregiver to acknowledge and review the trauma(s) of the past while simultaneously focusing on their accomplishments, progress, and strengths. Graduation should be planned with the child and caregiver as a relaxed celebration, perhaps consisting of enjoyable activities and sharing of certificates, balloons, cake, and so forth. The prospect of graduation is introduced at the start of treatment and encourages optimism and confidence about the recovery process (Cohen, Mannarino, & Deblinger, 2006).

DEVELOPMENT AND RESEARCH

As we noted above, TF-CBT has the strongest empirical base of any treatment for child trauma (Saunders, Berliner, & Hanson, 2004). Initial studies of TF-CBT were pre-post or quasi-experimental in design (Deblinger, McLeer, & Henry, 1990; Stauffer & Deblinger, 1996) and were followed by several randomized controlled trials. One of the earliest randomized trials examined the distinct benefits of children's and/or parents' participation in TF-CBT, with community treatment serving as the control condition. The findings of this investigation documented that children's direct participation in TF-CBT was critical in terms of ameliorating their PTSD symptoms, whereas parental participation in TF-CBT was critical to significantly improving parenting skills and, in turn, reducing children's externalizing behavior problems (Deblinger, Lippman, & Steer, 1996).

Another study compared TF-CBT to nondirective supportive therapy (NST) through the random assignment of 67 sexually abused preschool children (ages 3–6) and their parents (Cohen & Mannarino, 1996). Results indicated significantly greater improvements in sexual behavior problems, other behavioral difficulties, and internalizing symptoms for children in the TF-CBT group compared with the NST group. In a similar study of 49 older children (ages 7–15) who had been sexually abused, children randomly assigned to the TF-CBT group exhibited significantly greater improvements in depression and social competence compared with the NST group (Cohen & Mannarino, 1997, 1998). All three of these early randomized trials documented that the TF-CBT treatment gains were sustained at one-year follow-up assessments (Cohen & Mannarino, 1997; Cohen, Mannarino, & Knudsen, 2005; Deblinger, Steer, & Lippmann, 1999), with Deblinger et al. (1999) reporting the maintenance of treatment effects at a two-year follow-up assessment as well.

Another investigation involved the random assignment of 36 children (ages 5–17) who had been sexually abused to two TF-CBT conditions (child alone and child-parent) or a waiting-list control (WLC) condition (King et al., 2000). Children in the TF-CBT groups showed significantly greater improvements in PTSD symptoms and self-reported fear and anxiety compared with the WLC group. No significant differences were found between the child alone and child-parent TF-CBT conditions until the three-month follow-up, when children assigned to the child-parent group reported less abuse-related fear. Several randomized studies have also documented the efficacy of TF-CBT implemented in a group format (Deblinger, Stauffer, & Steer, 2001; McMullen & O'Callaghan, 2012; O'Callaghan et al., 2013). In the first multisite study of TF-CBT, 229 children (ages 8–14) who had been sexually abused and their parents were randomly assigned to TF-CBT or Child-Centered Therapy (CCT) conditions (Cohen et al., 2004). Children in the TF-CBT group showed significantly greater improvements on measures of PTSD, depression, and behavior problems compared with children in the CCT group. Children who received TF-CBT had significantly greater improvements in interpersonal trust, perceived credibility, and shame than children receiving CCT. In addition, parents in the TF-CBT group reported significantly greater improvements in their own depression, abuse-related distress, parental support, and effective parenting practices than parents in the CCT group. Between-group effect sizes were generally within the medium range. Treatment gains were maintained during the 6- and 12-month follow-up periods (Deblinger, Mannarino, et al., 2006).

A recent randomized controlled trial of TF-CBT examined the impact of the trauma narrative and treatment length (Deblinger et al., 2011). In this study, 210 children (ages 4–11) who had been sexually abused were assigned to one of four treatment conditions: 8 sessions with no trauma narrative, 8 sessions with a trauma narrative, 16 sessions with no trauma narrative, or 16 sessions with a trauma narrative. Significant improvements with large effect sizes were found within each group on all measures, which assessed a broad range of emotional and behavioral difficulties, parenting skills, and body safety skills. TF-CBT in 8 sessions with the trauma narrative seemed most effective and efficient in reducing children's abuse-related fear and generalized anxiety. TF-CBT in 16 sessions without the trauma narrative (and thus more time to focus on parenting skills) appeared most effective in improving parenting skills and reducing externalizing behavior problems. The significant improvements found at post-treatment within all conditions were sustained over the 6- and 12-month follow-up periods (Mannarino et al., 2012). Internalizing behavior problems in the much-above-average range and depressive symptoms in the above-average range at pre-treatment were predictive of the small number of children who continued to meet the full criteria for PTSD at 12 months (Mannarino et al., 2012).

The beneficial effects of TF-CBT among children in foster care also have been documented. In a quasi-experimental study, Lyons, Weiner, and Scheider (2006) found significant improvements in trauma symptoms among children in foster care treated with TF-CBT compared with those in treatment as usual. In addition, these children were about one-tenth as likely as same-age children to run away from their placements and about half as likely to have a placement disruption. Dorsey et al. (2011) investigated the impact of engagement strategies with foster parents on TF-CBT treatment. This study randomized youth (ages 6–15) and their foster parents to TF-CBT plus evidence-based engagement strategies (McKay & Bannon, 2004) or the standard delivery of TF-CBT. Significant improvements in PTSD symptoms were found across both conditions among children who completed treatment or completed at least 11 sessions. However, the children and foster parents assigned to TF-CBT plus engagement were significantly less likely to drop out prematurely and more likely to complete treatment successfully.

TF-CBT has also been used with children who have experienced other traumas. Studies have documented the positive results of TF-CBT among children who experienced traumatic grief (Cohen, Mannarino, & Staron, 2006), exposure to intimate partner violence (Cohen, Mannarino, & Iyengar, 2011), the 9/11 tragedy (CATS Consortium, 2010), and Hurricane Katrina (Jaycox et al., 2010).

CONCLUSIONS

The positive impact of TF-CBT for children who have experienced sexual abuse and other traumas has been demonstrated in numerous research studies, including over a dozen randomized controlled trials. This treatment approach has received the highest ratings for its efficacy in extensive reviews of the treatment-outcome literature sponsored by the U.S. Department of Health and Human Services (www.nrepp.samhsa.gov), the California Evidence-Based Clearinghouse for Child Welfare (www.cebc4cw.org), and the Department of Justice (Saunders, Berliner, & Hanson, 2004).

TF-CBT is an evidence-based treatment to address the negative effects of child maltreatment and other traumas, including symptoms of PTSD and other emotional and behavioral difficulties. It is a structured, short-term, components-based therapy for children that emphasizes the important involvement of nonoffending caregivers. The TF-CBT model is further described in the original treatment manuals (Cohen, Mannarino, & Deblinger, 2006; Deblinger & Heflin, 1996) and, free of charge, on Web-based introductory TF-CBT training and consultation sites (www.musc.edu/tfcbt; www.musc.edu/ctg; www.musc.edu/tfcbtconsult). Over 125,000 mental health professionals have received basic training in TF-CBT through these free-of-charge Web-based training initiatives. This treatment model will probably continue to evolve as scientific research on TF-CBT and related issues continues to inform its development and its application to a wide array of diverse, highly vulnerable, and underserved populations.

References

Allen, B., & Johnson, J. C. (2012). Utilization and implementation of Trauma-Focused Cognitive Behavioral Therapy for the treatment of maltreated children. *Child Maltreatment, 17,* 80–85.

CATS Consortium. (2010). Implementation of CBT for youth affected by the World Trade Center disaster: Matching need to treatment intensity and reducing trauma symptoms. *Journal of Traumatic Stress, 23,* 699–707.

Cohen, J. A., Deblinger, E., Mannarino, A. P., & Steer, R. (2004). A multisite, randomized controlled trial for children with sexual abuse–related PTSD symptoms. *Journal of the American Academy of Child and Adolescent Psychiatry, 43,* 393–402.

Cohen, J. A., & Mannarino, A. P. (1996). A treatment outcome study for sexually abused preschool children: Initial findings. *Journal of the American Academy of Child and Adolescent Psychiatry, 35,* 42–50.

Cohen, J. A., & Mannarino, A. P. (1997). A treatment study for sexually abused preschool children: Outcome during a one-year follow-up. *Journal of the American Academy of Child and Adolescent Psychiatry, 36,* 1228–1235.

Cohen, J. A., & Mannarino, A. P. (1998). Interventions for sexually abused children: Initial treatment outcome findings. *Child Maltreatment, 3,* 17–26.

Cohen, J. A., Mannarino, A. P., & Deblinger, E. (2006). *Treating trauma and traumatic grief in children and adolescents.* New York, NY: Guilford Press.

Cohen, J. A., Mannarino, A. P., & Iyengar, S. (2011). Community treatment of posttraumatic stress disorder in children exposed to intimate partner violence: A randomized controlled trial. *Archives of Pediatrics & Adolescent Medicine, 165,* 16–21.

Cohen, J. A., Mannarino, A. P., & Knudsen, K. (2005). Treating sexually abused children: One year follow-up of a randomized controlled trial. *Child Abuse & Neglect, 29,* 135–145.

Cohen, J. A., Mannarino, A. P., & Staron, V. R. (2006). A pilot study of modified cognitive-behavioral therapy for childhood traumatic grief (CBT-CTG). *Journal of the American Academy of Child and Adolescent Psychiatry, 45,* 1465–1473.

Deblinger, E., Cohen, J. A., & Mannarino, A. P. (2012). Introduction. In J. A. Cohen, A. P. Mannarino, & E. Deblinger (Eds.), *Trauma-focused CBT for children and adolescents: Treatment applications* (pp. 1–26). New York, NY: Guilford Press.

Deblinger, E., & Heflin, A. H. (1996). *Treating sexually abused children and their nonoffending parents: A cognitive behavioral approach.* Newbury Park, CA: Sage Publications.

Deblinger, E., Lippmann, J., & Steer, R. (1996). Sexually abused children suffering posttraumatic stress symptoms: Initial treatment outcome findings. *Child Maltreatment, 1,* 310–321.

Deblinger, E., Mannarino, A. P., Cohen, J. A., Runyon, M. K., & Steer, R. A. (2011). Trauma-focused cognitive behavioral therapy for children: Impact of the trauma narrative and treatment length. *Depression and Anxiety, 28,* 67–75.

Deblinger, E., Mannarino, A. P., Cohen, J. A., & Steer, R. A. (2006). A follow-up study of a multisite, randomized, controlled trial for children with sexual abuse–related PTSD symptoms. *Journal of the American Academy of Child and Adolescent Psychiatry, 45,* 1474–1484.

Deblinger, E., McLeer, S. V., & Henry, D. (1990). Cognitive behavioral treatment for sexually abused children suffering post-traumatic stress: Preliminary findings. *Journal of the American Academy of Child and Adolescent Psychiatry, 29,* 747–752.

Deblinger, E., Neubauer, F., Runyon, M., & Baker, D. (2006). *What do you know?* Stratford, NJ: CARES Institute.

Deblinger, E., Stauffer, L., & Steer, R. (2001). Comparative efficacies of supportive and cognitive behavioral group therapies for young children who have been sexually abused and their nonoffending mothers. *Child Maltreatment, 6,* 332–343.

Deblinger, E., Steer, R. A., & Lippmann, J. (1999). Two-year follow-up study of cognitive behavioral therapy for sexually abused children suffering post-traumatic stress symptoms. *Child Abuse & Neglect, 23,* 1371–1378.

Dorsey, S., Cox, J. R., Conover, K. L., & Berliner, L. (2011). Trauma-Focused Cognitive Behavioral Therapy for children and adolescents in foster care. *Children, Youth, and Family News.* www.apa.org/pi/families/resources/newsletter/index .aspx

Hornor, G. (2010). Child sexual abuse: Consequences and implications. *Journal of Pediatric Health Care, 24,* 358–364.

Irish, L., Kobayashi, I., & Delahanty, D. L. (2010). Long-term consequences of childhood sexual abuse: A meta-analytic review. *Journal of Pediatric Psychology, 35,* 450–461.

Jaycox, L. H., Cohen, J. A., Mannarino, A. P., Walker, D. W., Langely, A. K., Gegenheimer, K. L., et al. (2010). Children's mental health care following Hurricane Katrina: A field trial of trauma-focused psychotherapies. *Journal of Traumatic Stress, 23,* 223–231.

King, N. J., Tonge, B. J., Mullen, P., Myerson, N., Heyne, D., Rollings, S., et al. (2000). Treating sexually abused children with posttraumatic stress symptoms: A randomized clinical trial. *Journal of the American Academy of Child and Adolescent Psychiatry, 39,* 1347–1355.

Kolko, D. J., & Swenson, C. C. (2002). *Assessing and treating physically abused children and their families: A cognitive behavioral approach.* Thousand Oaks, CA: Sage Publications.

Lyons, J. S., Weiner, D. A., & Scheider, A. (2006). *A field trial of three evidence-based practices for trauma with children in state custody.* Report to the Illinois Department of Children and Family Services. Evanston, IL: Mental Health Resources Services and Policy Program, Northwestern University.

Mannarino, A., Cohen, J. A., Deblinger, E., Runyon, M. K., & Steer, R. A. (2012). Trauma-Focused Cognitive Behavioral Therapy for children: Sustained impact of treatment 6 and 12 months later. *Child Maltreatment, 17,* 231–241.

McKay, M. M., & Bannon, W. M., Jr. (2004). Engaging families in child mental health services. *Child and Adolescent Psychiatric Clinics of North America, 13,* 905–921.

McMullen, J., & O'Callaghan, P. (2012). *An RCT of Trauma-Focused Cognitive Behavioral Therapy with child soldiers in the DRC.* Manuscript submitted for publication. Belfast, Ireland: Queens College. Clinical Trials ID NCT01483261.

O'Callaghan, P., McMullen, J., Shannon, C., Rafferty, H., & Black, A. (2013). A randomized controlled trial of Trauma-Focused Cognitive Behavioral Therapy for sexually exploited, war-affected Congolese girls. *Journal of the American Academy of Child and Adolescent Psychiatry, 52*(4), 359–369.

Putnam, F. W. (2003). Ten-year research update review: Child sexual abuse. *Journal of the American Academy of Child and Adolescent Psychiatry, 42,* 269–278.

Runyon, M. K., & Deblinger, E. (in press). *Combined parent-child cognitive behavioral therapy (CPC-CBT): An approach to empower families at-risk for child physical abuse.* New York, NY: Oxford University Press.

Saunders, B. E., Berliner, L., & Hanson, R. F. (Eds.). (2004, April 26). *Child physical and sexual abuse: Guidelines for treatment* (Revised report). Charleston, SC: National Crime Victims Research and Treatment Center.

Stauffer, L. B., & Deblinger, E. (1996). Cognitive behavioral groups for nonoffending mothers and their young sexually abused children: A preliminary treatment outcome study. *Child Maltreatment, 1,* 65–76.

Trickett, P. K., & McBride-Chang, C. (1995). The developmental impact of different forms of child abuse and neglect. *Developmental Review, 15,* 311–337.

CHRISTOPHER CAMPBELL, PH.D.
MARK CHAFFIN, PH.D.
BEVERLY W. FUNDERBURK, PH.D.

4

Parent-Child Interaction Therapy in Child Welfare Settings

Parent training programs are the most common type of service prescribed for parents in the child welfare system. Parent-Child Interaction Therapy (PCIT) is an evidence-based model originally developed as a parent-mediated treatment for disruptive behavior problems in preschool-age children. The model has been adapted to treat maltreating behavior in parents. PCIT uses behavioral principles to (1) increase positive parenting skills, (2) enhance the parent-child relationship, (3) establish effective and consistent behavior management strategies, and (4) decrease child behavior problems. The adapted version of PCIT, which includes a motivational enhancement component, has been found to significantly reduce parents' child welfare recidivism in two randomized trials, including one conducted in a frontline field setting. Other studies document mental health and behavior benefits among children in the child welfare system, including foster children. The PCIT model is flexible and has been extended to home-based services or combined with trauma treatment elements. The fact that PCIT robustly delivers two types of benefits (reduced recidivism and improved child behavior) in one compact and focused intervention makes it particularly appealing for child welfare service systems. This chapter describes PCIT and its adaptations for the treatment of abusive parents. The chapter also touches on cross-cultural adaptations of PCIT and summarizes implementation and scale-up issues.

TRADITIONAL AND EVIDENCE-BASED PARENTING MODELS IN CHILD WELFARE

In a large, nationally representative sample of child welfare cases, parenting programs were the single most common type of services offered to maltreating parents (NSCAW Research Group, 2005). This should come as no surprise, given that child maltreatment is inherently and primarily a parenting problem. Reliance on parenting programs by child welfare systems has a long but not necessarily successful history. Traditional parent training models often relied on didactic presentations of abstract parenting principles, developing insight into childhood underpinnings of current parenting behavior, or unstructured class discussions. Evaluations concluded that the results were disappointing (Cohn & Daro, 1987). More recently, focus has shifted to adapting evidence-based behavioral skills–oriented parent training interventions, originally designed as parent-mediated treatments for disruptive child behavior problems, for use with caregivers in child welfare. Examples of evidence-based behavioral parenting programs applied to child welfare include The Incredible Years (Webster-Stratton, 2011), Triple-P (Sanders, 2012), and Parent-Child Interaction Therapy (Eyberg & Boggs, 1998). (See also California Evidence-Based Clearinghouse for Child Welfare, 2009; Centers for Disease Control and Prevention, 2004.) In contrast to traditional parenting models that emphasize how parenting is conceptualized, understood, or talked about, these newer evidence-based models focus on parenting as it is behaviorally delivered. The newer models may target fewer parenting principles and skills, but they target them with far greater detail, specificity, repetition, and intensity. Rather than teaching an abstract parenting concept and then leaving it to parents to translate that concept into parenting behavior, these models teach the parenting behavior directly and, in the case of PCIT, until the parent meets an objective criterion for demonstrating skill competency.

Several meta-analyses of these newer behavioral parent training programs exist, including studies focused on the elements contained in specific parenting programs (e.g., Cedar & Levant, 1990; Thomas & Zimmer-Gembeck, 2007), orientations and approaches (e.g., Maughan et al., 2005; Serketich

& Dumas, 1996), delivery settings (e.g., Sweet & Appelbaum, 2004), and case mix variations (e.g., Lundahl, Nimer, & Parsons, 2006; Lundahl, Risser, & Lovejoy, 2006; Reyno & McGrath, 2006). The overall pattern in the meta-analyses is a consistent and clinically meaningful positive effect for improving parenting behaviors and for reducing early behavior problems (e.g., Kaminski et al., 2008; Lundahl, Risser, & Lovejoy, 2006; Maughan et al., 2005; Reyno & McGrath, 2006; Serketich & Dumas, 1996).

None of the interventions listed above were originally designed for child welfare populations or to reduce child maltreatment recidivism. These models were originally developed as parent-mediated treatments for children with disruptive behavior disorders, and their adoption as treatments intended to reduce parental maltreating behavior constitutes a significant departure from this original purpose. In a child welfare context, they are often used as *parent* treatments, not *child* treatments. Caregivers in child welfare are typically referred to parenting programs primarily to achieve *parent* behavior change, not *child* behavior change, and parenting programs are used regardless of whether children actually have behavior management problems (e.g., Barth et al., 2005; Pinkston & Smith, 1998). In other applications, such as within foster care, the models may remain closer to their original design and intent. Of course, parenting models may be used to deliver both types of outcomes simultaneously—reduced recidivism risk among parents and improved well-being and reduced behavior problems among children.

Commonalities between etiological models for child behavior problems and child maltreatment may suggest a framework for understanding how a single intervention can deliver outcomes in both domains. The majority of parent-to-child violence occurs within the context of exaggerated child discipline or corporal punishment. Caregivers who physically harm their children often feel as though nothing short of harsh or violent disciplinary strategies will "work" with their children, whom they perceive (accurately or inaccurately) as having unmanageable behavior problems (Crouch & Behl, 2001). Many physically abusive caregivers self-report their behavior as discipline rather than as child abuse. Child behavior problems and parent-to-child violence may share a common and reciprocal developmental process described by Patterson's coercive cycle model (Patterson, 1976; Urquiza & McNeil, 1996). In this model, harsh discipline in response to real or perceived child defiance is reinforced by short-term child compliance, which in turn increases the caregiver's reliance on harsh discipline, potentially escalating to the point of seriously violent parent-to-child behaviors, particularly among at-risk caregivers (e.g., caregivers with depression, high distress, high anger, high emotional reactivity, or low emotional regulation). In this cycle, negative interactions tend to escalate and positive exchanges tend to diminish. In the absence of positive interactions, a hostile parent-child relationship develops that can be categorized by negative caregiver attributions, unrealistic expectations, disengagement,

inconsistent and harsh discipline, and failure to respond to the child's appropriate or prosocial behaviors. In fact, unresponsiveness to appropriate child behavior or child needs, a deteriorated relationship, and withdrawn or weak parent-child attachments form the relational context for both child physical abuse and neglect (Stith et al., 2009), which are highly comorbid problems. PCIT and related evidence-based behavioral parenting models directly target and interrupt coercive cycles, relationship deterioration, and disengaged aspects of parent-child interactions by creating or enhancing two sets of incompatible replacement behaviors: positive parent-child interaction skills and a consistent step-by-step approach to nonviolent discipline.

PARENT-CHILD INTERACTION THERAPY

Origin and Influences

PCIT is one member of a family of parent-mediated models derived from Constance Hanf's (1969) two-stage model. Hanf and colleagues at the University of Oregon School of Medicine broke with traditional child psychotherapy approaches of the day and began involving parents directly in child clinical practices, incorporating elements of developmental theory, social learning theory, behavioral principles, and interactional play techniques (Reitman & McMahon, 2012). Since its inception, variants of the Hanf model have been widely used and researched, including Helping the Noncompliant Child (McMahon & Forehand, 2003) and The Incredible Years (Webster-Stratton, 2005). Two-stage models correspond to a parenting orientation similar to Baumrind's (1967) authoritative parenting style, with the first phase developing nurturance and warmth in the parent-child relationship and the second phase developing a consistent, developmentally appropriate limit-setting and discipline strategy.

Structure and Format

Following this template, PCIT is delivered in two phases, called Child-Directed Interaction (CDI) and Parent-Directed Interaction (PDI). Each phase begins with one didactic or teaching session where PCIT skills are introduced, explained, modeled, and role-played with the caregiver(s). Teaching sessions are followed by multiple live, therapist-coached dyadic sessions where skills are practiced and refined in vivo. Live, real-time, coached skill practice and feedback during parent-child interactions is perhaps the hallmark of PCIT and a distinguishing feature of the model. During coaching sessions, therapists use prompting, modeling, reinforcement, and selective attention to shape each caregiver's acquisition and refinement of PCIT skills (Brinkmeyer & Eyberg, 2003). Standard PCIT coaching sessions are conducted with the therapist behind a one-way mirror, observing parent-child interactions. Variations of this delivery format, including home-based, in-room, and remote delivery formats, have been used with some success. The planned length of treatment intervention is a compact 14 sessions—one teaching session and approximately six coaching sessions per treatment phase (Callahan, Stevens, & Eyberg, 2010).

The primary goal of the first, CDI phase is to develop and strengthen the caregiver-child relationship and to use the relationship in positive ways to shape behavior. The relationship-strengthening skills are described under the acronym PRIDE, consisting of five elements:

- *Praise*, used to recognize and encourage prosocial behaviors, particularly labeled praise (e.g., "You did a good job picking up the toys")
- *Reflection*, used to improve active listening and verbal communication
- *Imitation* or modeling of appropriate behaviors while enjoying time with children
- *Description*, used to convey interest in positive behaviors
- *Enjoyment*, setting an affective tone for the interaction (Eyberg & Funderburk, 2011)

Differential social attention is another technique that parents are coached to use. Differential attention involves attending to appropriate child behaviors (e.g., sharing, using manners, playing appropriately) and actively ignoring attention-seeking or inappropriate child behaviors (e.g., whining, playing roughly, temper tantrums) so long as they do not cause any safety concerns (Herschell & McNeil, 2005). Studies with parents involved in child welfare services demonstrate that these skills tend to be learned quickly and fairly uniformly and result in rapid improvement in observable in-session parent-child interaction (Hakman et al., 2009).

The overarching task for caregivers in the CDI phase is to follow the *child's lead*. During the CDI phase, caregivers are coached to avoid behaviors that can take away the lead from their child, such as questioning, giving commands, criticism, sarcasm, and physically negative behavior or tone of voice. These elements of negative interaction are often common among abusive parents prior to treatment. For example, before treatment, abusive parents may be as likely to respond to a positive child behavior with criticism, sarcasm, questioning, or commands as with praise (Hakman et al., 2009). During the CDI phase, parents would be expected both to eliminate the responding to positive child behavior with negatives and to increase their use of labeled praise when their child behaves well. Before progressing to the second phase of PCIT, parents must meet a CDI mastery criterion of giving at least 10 labeled praises, 10 behavioral descriptions, 10 reflective statements, no more than a total of 3 questions, commands or criticisms, and no sarcasm or physical negatives during a five-minute observation period (Bell & Eyberg, 2002).

The second phase, PDI, focuses on discipline. The goals of PDI are to teach caregivers to give effective commands, set consistent and fair limits, and follow through with reasonable, age-appropriate, consistent consequences for misbehavior while maintaining an overall positive relationship

tone (Herschell & McNeil, 2005). During the PDI phase, caregivers learn a step-by-step time-out procedure for responding to noncompliance and severe misbehavior. With older school-age children, rather than time-out, logical consequences are substituted. As the PDI phase progresses, increased emphasis is placed on practicing and generalizing PCIT skills outside the clinic environment (e.g., to home, shopping mall, grocery store) to facilitate real-world mastery (Callahan, Stevens, & Eyberg, 2010). For parents whose children are in foster care, these later-stage practice and generalization opportunities may be limited, and findings suggest that a long delay between receiving PCIT and return of children to the home is associated with reduced treatment benefits (Chaffin et al., 2009).

The PDI phase requires caregivers to reach mastery criteria during a five-minute observation period. Parents must (1) give at least 75% "effective," or properly stated, commands and (2) show at least 75% correct follow-through (i.e., labeled praise for compliance, appropriate use of the time-out warning/procedures for noncompliance). Successful completion of the entire PCIT intervention requires that (1) caregivers meet mastery criteria in both CDI and PDI skills; (2) the child's behavior, as rated on the Eyberg Child Behavior Inventory, is equal to or less than a raw score of 114; and (3) caregivers express confidence in their abilities to appropriately manage their child's behaviors on their own (Callahan, Stevens, & Eyberg, 2010).

Efficacy for Reducing Child Behavior Problems

A long series of studies have demonstrated the model's effectiveness in decreasing children's disruptive behaviors (e.g., Eisenstadt et al., 1993; McNeil et al., 1999), increasing children's compliance with parental requests (e.g., Eyberg & Robinson, 1982), improving the parent-child relationship (e.g., Eyberg, Boggs, & Algina, 1995), and reducing parental stress (e.g., Schuhmann et al., 1998). Improvements in child behavior have been found to generalize from the controlled clinic setting to the home environment (e.g., Schuhmann et al., 1998), as well as from the home to school classrooms and from treated children in the family to untreated siblings (McNeil et al., 1991). In a recent review of 17 PCIT outcome studies (a total of 368 children who participated in PCIT), statistically significant improvements of child behavior problems were found across all studies (Gallagher, 2003). In fact, Gallagher (2003) reported clinical significance in 82% (14 of 17) of the studies, with *clinical significance* defined as changing behavior problems from the clinically significant range at pre-treatment to within the normal range at post-treatment.

Long-Term Maintenance of Gain

Follow-up studies evaluating the maintenance of treatment gains from PCIT have shown lasting benefits. For example, treatment gains in the home setting have been maintained one and two years post-treatment (Eyberg et al., 2001). Funderburk and colleagues (1998) found that PCIT gains in a clinic setting generalized to the classroom (without direct classroom intervention), and these improvements were maintained up to one year post-treatment and, to a lesser extent, at the 18-month follow-up. Boggs and colleagues (2004) found that families who completed PCIT maintained gains in both child and family functioning for one to three years post-treatment. In the study by Hood and Eyberg (2003), parent-child interactions continued to improve and mothers' confidence in controlling their child's behavior was maintained at three to six years post-treatment.

Efficacy across Case Mix Variations

PCIT has been successfully adapted for services with a range of child populations. Examples include children with developmental delays (Bagner & Eyberg, 2007; McDiarmid & Bagner, 2005), separation anxiety disorder (Pincus et al., 2005), chronic illness (Bagner, Fernandez, & Eyberg, 2004), and histories of child maltreatment (Timmer et al., 2005). Benefits also have been found across a range of caregiver populations, including nontraditional caregivers such as foster caregivers, adoptive parents, and kinship caregivers (e.g., McNeil et al., 2005; Timmer et al., 2006).

Delivery Approach

Dual-phase parenting models share substantial content. What varies most among this family of models is the delivery approach. The critical delivery element that distinguishes PCIT is individual in vivo skills *coaching*. Direct coaching has been called "both the heart and art" of PCIT (McNeil & Hembree-Kigin, 2010, p. 8). Historically, parent training has relied on a variety of indirect approaches (e.g., didactics, modeling, rehearsal) in which caregivers are taught certain skills apart from their children, then instructed to implement those skills on their own and report problems in subsequent sessions. In PCIT, live, in vivo coaching is done using a wireless earphone or "bug-in-the-ear" (earbud) over which the therapist coaches the parent's behavior while the parent interacts with the child, to shape and reinforce skills acquisition. This is most often accomplished by a therapist who is observing the parent-child interaction from behind a one-way mirror in a clinic specially equipped for PCIT (see figure 4.1).

Direct coaching of parent-child interactions has several advantages over traditional training methods, including (1) the ability to correct errors quickly, before caregivers consistently practice incorrect techniques; (2) the opportunity for the therapist to adapt as idiosyncratic problems arise and to model problem-solving skills for caregivers; (3) increased parental confidence as new skills are encouraged and supported through coaching; (4) potentially faster learning resulting from immediate feedback; (5) the opportunity for parents to implement suggestions immediately and to experience success; and (6) decreased reliance on self-reports or secondhand information that may not accurately reflect how skills are employed and responded to (McNeil & Hembree-Kigin, 2010).

Delivery elements of parenting programs were examined in a meta-analysis by Kaminski and colleagues (2008),

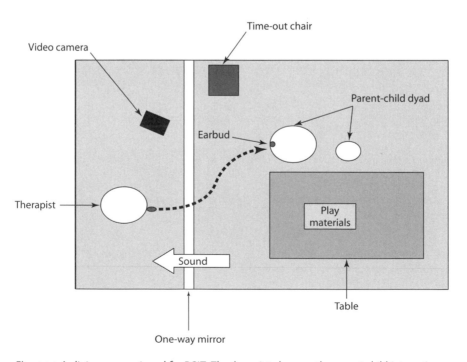

Figure 4.1. A clinic room equipped for PCIT. The therapist observes the parent-child interaction from behind a one-way mirror and can coach the parent through a wireless earphone.

who were able to identify specific program components that were associated with larger effect sizes. Programs where caregivers practiced new skills with their own child in vivo during clinic sessions yielded significantly larger effect sizes, regardless of content differences. Among a range of content and delivery elements examined, direct skills practice with the parent's own child was one of the single most powerful predictors of a larger effect size. This is a particularly salient point when it comes to serving parents in the child welfare system, where large effects are often necessary. The benefits of live coached delivery do come with a price in terms of delivery or implementation challenges—live coached delivery is labor intensive and equipment intensive, may involve scheduling challenges, is vulnerable to failed appointments, and may involve logistical challenges, given that both parent and child need to be present. Cost-effectiveness analyses have nonetheless found that the cost savings from reduced child welfare recidivism more than offset the added therapy cost (Lee, Aos, & Miller, 2008).

HOW PCIT FITS WITHIN CHILD WELFARE SERVICE SYSTEMS

As service purchasers, child welfare systems are interested in services that achieve measurable, concrete outcomes—safety, permanency, and well-being. Moreover, because child welfare systems serve the public interest and expend public monies, providing services that are demonstrably effective in yielding objective, measurable outcomes is consistent both with child welfare's mission and with public accountability requirements (Chaffin & Friedrich, 2004). PCIT is a good match for public service systems such as child welfare in a number of ways. Child maltreatment is inherently a "parenting" problem, and PCIT is inherently a parenting treatment. The peak ages for child maltreatment are in the preschool and early school-age years (U.S. Department of Health and Human Services, 2005), which corresponds well with standard PCIT inclusion criteria (although adaptations for children up to age 12 have been developed and tested). PCIT has rigorous evidence that it delivers benefits simultaneously in two of the three benchmark child welfare outcome domains: safety (i.e., reduced recidivism) and child well-being (i.e., reduced behavior problems). Because it is a compact intervention, it also may speed transitions to permanency, which is child welfare's third benchmark outcome domain. The model does not require collateral services or additional treatments in order to be effective—in fact, some evidence suggests that the model works sufficiently, or works even better, when families are not inundated with multiple concurrent therapies (Chaffin et al., 2004; Kaminski et al., 2008). PCIT has proved effective among physically abusive parents as well as in chronic child welfare cases with long histories of both abuse and neglect, which are the most common types of maltreatment in child welfare.

Child welfare also serves children in the foster care system, where child well-being is a benchmark outcome goal.

Entry into the foster care system alone increases the likelihood that children will develop mental health or behavior problems (Lawrence, Carlson, & Egeland, 2006), and as many as 50% or more of foster children may exhibit clinical problem levels (Clausen et al., 1998; Leslie et al., 2004). Behavior problems in foster care are perhaps the single largest cause of disrupted foster care placements. Children with behavior problems are more likely to have foster care placement disruptions, and foster care placement disruptions may create more behavior problems, potentially creating an escalating and pernicious cycle, not infrequently eventuating in more restrictive psychiatric or residential placements (e.g., Cook, 1994; James et al., 2006; Newton, Litrownik, & Landsverk, 2000; Timmer et al., 2006). The work of Timmer, Urquiza, and others has focused on helping children in foster and kinship care settings. Findings suggest that PCIT can enhance the quality of the foster caregiver-child relationship and improve foster caregivers' parenting skills, which in turn can improve the stability of foster placement and child mental health outcomes (e.g., McNeil et al., 2005; Timmer et al., 2006). PCIT for foster parents may offer additional advantages—skills might generalize from current to future foster children, and reliance on psychotropic medication to control foster child behavior might be reduced. Delivery and implementation adaptations of the PCIT model have been suggested specifically for serving foster care systems, including combinations of group-based and in-home PCIT delivery approaches (Mersky, personal communication, 2012).

PCIT has been found to reduce child welfare recidivism across a broad range of maltreatment types. This includes cases of physical abuse, neglect, and mixed physical abuse and neglect. It includes new entries into child welfare and repetitive child welfare cases; parents retaining all children in their home and parents with all children removed from their home; court-involved parents and parents diverted into differential response. The exception is that the model has not been tested with sexually abusive parents. Sexual abuse is quite different in etiology from neglect and physical abuse, and it is conceptually questionable whether a treatment such as PCIT, oriented toward relationship enhancement and discipline skills, would fit the needs or risks of a sexually abusive parent or the needs of a sexually abused child.

Motivational Adaptations for Parents Who Maltreat

In standard PCIT for child behavior problems, caregivers are usually voluntary consumers who are self-motivated to seek services. This is contextually different from caregivers in child welfare, who are typically coerced into services and may or may not be motivated. This difference may pose an obstacle for PCIT, because PCIT requires active practice and the demonstration of in vivo skills, along with active completion of homework and application of skills outside the sessions. Some types of parenting programs, such as didactic groups, can be passively consumed, but PCIT cannot. When

PCIT was initially adapted from a voluntary parent-mediated treatment for child behavior problems to a treatment for possibly coerced abusive parents, the main adaptation focused on motivation. The initial randomized trial with abusive parents included a pre-treatment motivational intervention based on motivational interviewing principles, before beginning PCIT. Elements of the motivational package included a testimonial from a treatment completer, examination of the parent's ability and readiness to change parenting practices, and exercises to develop the discrepancy between the current and the desired parenting relationship and family circumstances. The overall Motivation + PCIT package reduced downstream child welfare recidivism from 49% to 19% compared with a traditional group parenting class (Chaffin et al., 2004). A subsequent trial used a dismantling design to test the relative contribution of the motivational adaptation to overall recidivism reduction. Chaffin and colleagues (2009, 2011) found that combining the self-motivation component with PCIT yielded better program retention rates (85% vs. 61% cumulative program retention). The recidivism reduction effect found in the first study was replicated and was dependent on the Motivation + PCIT combination (i.e., the Motivation + PCIT cell of the 2 × 2 experimental design). PCIT without the motivational adaptation did not reduce recidivism relative to a traditional parenting group program. Conversely, the motivational intervention had effects only when combined with PCIT. Thus, combining the two appears to be necessary for achieving results among parents in child welfare.

In both of the published randomized trials, the motivational adaptation was delivered using a group format, which was selected to match the group format used by the traditional parenting group comparison. In clinical practice, the group format may not be ideal, and practitioners should consider individually delivered motivational adaptations keyed to parents' readiness, which is the more usual Motivational Interviewing practice. Individualized Motivational Interviewing approaches have been found to improve parent training outcomes outside child welfare populations (Nock & Kazdin, 2005), and we might expect individual motivational adaptations to perform well within child welfare populations. Some findings suggest that it may be unwise to deliver a fixed motivational protocol to all parents, particularly those who already are motivated. Although many PCIT practitioners are successfully using standard PCIT for treating child behavior problems in child welfare settings, reduction of maltreatment recidivism may require adding a motivational adaptation.

Other Adaptations for Parents Who Maltreat

Some maltreating parents have additional problems that may require adaptations of PCIT. These include problems with self-control, insensitivity, negative attributions, and anger control. A series of smaller adaptations were made to address these. In most respects, the adapted PCIT model developed for maltreating parents would be easily and immediately recognizable as PCIT by any standard PCIT practitioner. Remaining virtually unchanged are the fundamental elements, techniques, and structure of the model, including (1) the overarching two-phase approach (CDI and PDI), (2) PRIDE skills, (3) command training, (4) basic time-out protocol, (5) generalization guidelines, (6) expected dose, (7) setting, (8) in vivo coaching techniques and technology, (9) theory base, (10) coding schemes, (11) measures, (12) reliance on competency criteria, (13) homework assignments, and (14) treatment materials. Adaptations were made to some aspects of CDI coaching to make it more parent focused rather than child focused, such as selectively reinforcing parental self-control or sensitivity toward the child. The time-out protocol for young children is modified in three ways. First, steps are added to boost parental self-control (e.g., coaching parents to stop, take a breath, monitor their stress level, and relax or count to 10 before executing the time-out process). Second, the protocol uses only nonphysical "backups" for time-out escape. Finally, greater emphasis is placed on educating parents about developmentally normal child challenges and expectations. Adaptations may also be required for parents whose children are in foster care and parents who have limited opportunities to practice skills or complete homework. These can include using role plays, practicing CDI during scheduled visits, or practicing with other children in the home. Based on clinical experience in studies that treated noncustodial caregivers, PCIT is not recommended as a treatment modality unless the caregiver has ready access to practice with the child at least three times per week, in addition to the treatment session. We do not recommend starting PCIT if the child in foster care is unlikely ever to return home or if return may be delayed until well after PCIT is completed, because delays have been found to be associated with loss of treatment benefit (Chaffin et al., 2011).

Adaptations for Parents of School-Age Children (up to about age 12)

One of the key differences between standard PCIT for early childhood behavior problems and adapted PCIT for maltreating parents is *child age range*. Because children in the adapted protocol are in many ways secondary or collateral participants who do not necessarily have behavior problems, a broader child-age inclusion criterion seemed reasonable. Standard PCIT is geared for children under age 7, so adaptations were required for parents of older school-age children up to age 12. This extension did not seem to have a strong impact on parent outcomes—in both of the randomized trials with maltreating parents, the age of the child did not moderate or significantly alter the recidivism reduction effect. Effectiveness of the adaptation for reducing older school-age behavior problems has not been specifically tested, but many of the adaptations parallel elements found in well-tested school-age behavior problem models.

Again, the basic PCIT framework remains intact (the two-phase CDI and PDI structure, in vivo skills coaching, and the foundational behavioral theory base). In some cases, the adaptations for older children are simply matters of degree, such as continuing to emphasize labeled praise in response to positive child behavior, but for the praise to be less frequent and less effusive or demonstrative than it might be with a preschooler. In other cases, the adaptation involves substitutions, such as substituting logical consequences or loss of privileges as a backup for time-out refusal. Substitutions use parallel elements (i.e., an older-child discipline element is substituted for a standard PCIT discipline element), and the substituted elements are drawn from techniques common to behavioral parenting programs used with older children (in models such as Barkley's Defiant Child or the Boy's Town Common Sense Parenting). No hard chronological age line is established for migrating from usual PCIT to the older-child adaptations, nor is there a requirement that the older-child adaptation be adopted whole cloth. Rather, usual PCIT is treated as the default option, and older-child adaptations are selectively applied based on the clinician's assessment of developmental fit with the individual case. The following points describe the main adaptations made for parents of older school-age children:

- Older children are included more in explaining the goals of treatment ("to help parents and children get along better and reduce arguing"), in obtaining assent, and in selecting what types of logical consequences and joint "Special Time" activities should be used.
- Children are consulted about preferred ways for parents to word the verbal skills, such as praise and reflections.
- More silence during CDI is permitted, along with less frequent and effusive praise. Drills with parents are used prior to the sessions to create more practice opportunities for these skills, given the reduced number of practice repetitions during in vivo coaching.
- Reflection is coached to rephrase or validate more complex child emotions.
- More age-appropriate CDI activities are selected, often with the child's input.
- Longer time is allowed between a command and expectation of compliance.
- The parent, child, and therapist develop a menu of nonconfrontational, reasonable consequences and loss of privileges to be used as discipline options (e.g., loss of a video game, loss of TV time) as a backup in case of time-out refusal. Care is taken to distinguish between "luxuries" that can be removed contingent on compliance (e.g., TV time) and activities that may be important to retain, irrespective of compliance, because they foster growth and positive behavior (e.g., participation in a prosocial school activity).
- Because older children have longer attention spans, consequences can be applied later in time rather than

immediately. A cap is placed on the number of privileges that can be lost in a single discipline episode.
- Time-out can shift from a time-out chair to being sent to a room.
- Physical backups to time-out are eliminated.
- During the final 5–10 minutes of the session, while the therapist gives feedback and the homework assignment to the parent, the child is allowed a choice of activities (e.g., hand-held video game, choice of a preferred toy, time on the playground). If the child refused time-out during the session, the parent can withhold increments of the child's free time, allowing consequences to be applied and coached within the clinic session.
- Given the generally better self-control of older children in session and the fact that child behavior problems are not an inclusion criterion for the adapted model, many older children are rarely noncompliant in session, and therefore parents have limited in-session practice opportunities for discipline skills. In these cases, therapists use role play in which the therapist portrays a noncompliant child to permit the parent and child to learn the procedures.

Application to Children's Internalizing Problems

Trauma-related problems are common among maltreated children, so it is encouraging to note that some early pilot findings point to the benefits of PCIT in the internalizing problem domain (e.g., depression, anxiety, posttraumatic stress disorder symptoms), in addition to the well-tested and well-supported externalizing or behavior problem domain. Although it is premature to characterize PCIT as a "trauma treatment," emerging evidence suggests some benefits. Lenze, Pautsch and Luby (2011) adapted PCIT by adding an emotional-development module focused on internalizing problems, and early small-scale controlled trial results are encouraging. Thomas and Zimmer-Gembeck (2012) report significant reductions in internalizing problems in a randomized waitlist-controlled trial of standard PCIT. Findings from uncontrolled trials of other adaptations have reported specific reductions in trauma-related symptoms (Pearl et al., 2012) and anxiety symptoms (Puliafico, Comer, & Pincus, 2012). At this point, although findings do suggest benefits in the internalizing problem domain, it remains unclear (1) how robust these findings will be to replication in rigorous trials and how durable they will prove with longer follow-up; (2) whether adaptations to standard PCIT improve or are necessary for outcomes in this domain; and (3) whether PCIT would be a good choice when internalizing problems are primary rather than secondary to externalizing problems. Recent work in evidence-based treatments (EBTs) implementation suggests that it may be both feasible and desirable to "blend" modularized elements from established internalizing and externalizing EBTs based on a structured assessment-driven algorithm (Weisz et al., 2012). Under this type of approach, therapists deliver elements of multiple

EBTs simultaneously, an approach that might be particularly suitable in cases where both internalizing and externalizing features are prominent.

Implementation and Scale-up

Implementing evidence-based models in field settings involves far more than simple "train-and-hope" methods such as workshops or distribution of treatment manuals (Fixsen et al., 2005). Indeed, implementing EBTs may be more challenging than developing them. A full discussion of implementation practicalities and conceptual models is beyond the scope of our discussion here, but suffice it to say that multiple systems, complexities, and hurdles invariably are involved (Aarons, Hurlburt, & Horowitz, 2011). Of these hurdles, initial provider training may be the simplest to tackle, even if this alone is insufficient for achieving sustained and high-quality implementation.

Few studies have examined how PCIT is taken up or how it performs in scaled-up settings. In the absence of field-based effectiveness studies, there are no assurances that evidence-based models will retain the efficacy enjoyed in usually smaller and more tightly quality-controlled research settings (Shirk, 2004). Adapted PCIT for child welfare parents has been tested in an authentic but still small-scale field setting with some success, which is encouraging (Chaffin et al., 2011), but this has not been replicated, and to our knowledge, no full-scale implementations have been tested for their impact on child welfare outcomes.

PCIT does pose implementation challenges. For example, special equipment may be required, such as one-way mirrors, remote coaching transmitters and receivers, and sound equipment. Nontraditional adaptations such as home-based PCIT have been explored, but most PCIT is still a clinic-based service and this, by itself, can pose a major obstacle to widespread penetration of the client population, especially among the population segments served by child welfare systems (Kazdin & Blase, 2011). Relative to parenting classes, PCIT is costly and labor intensive to deliver. And, as for all EBTs, there are initial training requirements and ongoing provider-competency development and quality control issues that must be addressed for the model to succeed in the field on a larger scale.

PCIT began, and for many years was practiced, almost exclusively in a few university-based clinics. In 2009, PCIT International was incorporated as a governing body dedicated to maintaining the quality and fidelity of PCIT. Provider and trainer competency standards were established, along with guidelines for agency readiness. Traditionally, training in PCIT was conducted within a university-based doctoral psychology program through a mentoring model. A novice PCIT therapist first learned the model by observing an experienced expert therapist, then conducted sessions under co-therapy, and then conducted sessions under live supervision. This mentored training model, while perhaps ideal and still feasible for students in a doctoral pro-

gram, is far less feasible for large-scale implementation. It may be challenging even for an established PCIT service agency, given the required amount of trainer or coach time that might not be reimbursed under the unit-rate billing schemes on which many service agencies depend.

Current PCIT International (2009) guidelines require the same skills attainment for aspiring PCIT therapists whether training is conducted in co-therapy or in workshop format. A minimum of 40 hours of training is required, extended over approximately one year and including adherence to the uniform treatment protocol and behavioral coding system. Trainees are expected to maintain a minimum of monthly contact with a PCIT trainer until they meet skills mastery requirements and successfully graduate two PCIT cases. Training standards for PCIT Master Trainers (experienced PCIT trainers who have indicated a willingness to promote fidelity to the treatment model) have been established, as have training guidelines for other trainers, who maintain contact with Master Trainers to maintain uniform training and practice standards for the treatment. Several online training programs have been developed to augment face-to-face PCIT training. Ongoing PCIT studies are testing alternative implementation strategies in controlled multiagency trials. For example, Funderburk and colleagues are comparing ongoing therapist consultation and coaching under a live video feed with post-hoc telephone consultation. Herschell and colleagues are comparing three competing approaches—learning collaboratives, train-the-trainer, and Web-based strategies—in a multiagency controlled trial.

Cross-Cultural Extensions

Despite challenges in agency preparation and therapist training, PCIT appears to be remarkably robust across diverse populations. Applications of the model with no adaptation or very minor adaptations have been successful cross-culturally. PCIT is being disseminated worldwide, with implementations in Puerto Rico, Germany, the Netherlands, Norway, South Korea, China, and Australia. A Latino cultural adaptation, Project Gana, was tested in a controlled trial and found to be superior to usual care and equal to standard PCIT in effectiveness (McCabe & Yeh, 2009). An American Indian cultural translation of PCIT—Honoring Children: Making Relatives—incorporates the language and concepts of traditional American Indian cultures into standard PCIT treatment (Bigfoot & Funderburk, 2011) and has been replicated at multiple tribal service sites across North America. The robust nature of the treatment cross-culturally may derive from its focus on very young children and on the fact that the basic tenets of nurturance and limit setting are compatible with cross-cultural general principles of attachment and child development. Efficacy and deliverability across a range of cultures is important for state or county child welfare service systems because these systems are charged with serving diverse populations. In other contexts, such as tribal child welfare systems, it may be important to the community and the service system that evidence-based models consider local culture and are acceptable within their local community.

SUMMARY

Parent training programs continue to represent the single most common type of services offered to parents who have maltreated their children. More recently, the focus has shifted to adapting evidence-based behavioral skills–oriented parent training interventions for use with caregivers in child welfare. Originally designed as a parent-mediated treatment for disruptive child behavior problems, PCIT has demonstrated significant empirical success over the past three decades. Findings from over a hundred research articles (including eight randomized controlled trials) show that (1) PCIT is a theoretically based, efficacious treatment that is widely applicable and effective across diverse populations; (2) the treatment gains are maintained over long periods of time in a variety of environments; and (3) the PCIT protocol has been successfully adapted to match client and/or population characteristics. A recently adapted version of PCIT for use with maltreating parents has robustly delivered two types of benefits—reduced recidivism risk among abusive parents and improved well-being and behavior among children—making it particularly appealing for child welfare service systems. Additional work in foster care systems also appears promising, as does the potential for the model to improve trauma or internalizing symptoms or to be blended with specific trauma-informed treatments. Scaled-up implementation of EBTs such as PCIT systems presents several challenges, and future efforts may need to focus on aspects of implementation and on testing how well the model performs on a larger scale.

References

Aarons, G. A., Hurlburt, M., & Horwitz, S. M. (2011). Advancing a conceptual model of evidence-based practice implementation in public service sectors. *Administration and Policy in Mental Health and Mental Health Services Research, 38*, 4–23. doi:10.1007/s10488-010-0327-7

Bagner, D. M., & Eyberg, S. M. (2007). Parent-Child Interaction Therapy for disruptive behavior in children with mental retardation: A randomized control trial. *Journal of Clinical Child and Adolescent Psychology, 36*, 418–429. doi:10.1080/15374410701448448

Bagner, D. M., Fernandez, M. A., & Eyberg, S. M. (2004). Parent-Child Interaction Therapy and chronic illness: A case study. *Journal of Clinical Psychology in Medical Settings, 11*, 1–6. doi:10.1023/B:JOCS.0000016264.02407.fd

Barth, R. P., Landsverk, J., Chamberlain, P., Reid, J. B., Rolls, J. A., Hurlburt, M. S., et al. (2005). Parent-training programs in child welfare services: Planning for a more evidence-based approach to serving biological parents. *Research on Social Work Practice, 15*, 353–371. doi:10.1177/1049731505276321

Baumrind, D. (1967). Childcare practices anteceding three patterns of preschool behavior. *Genetic Psychology Monographs, 75*, 43–88.

Bell, S., & Eyberg, S. M. (2002). Parent-Child Interaction Therapy. In L. Vandecreek, S. Knapp, & T. L. Jackson (Eds.), *Innovations in clinical practice: A source book* (Vol. 20). Sarasota, FL: Professional Resource Press.

Bigfoot, D. S., & Funderburk, B. W. (2011). Honoring children, making relatives: The cultural translation of Parent-Child Interaction Therapy for American Indian and Alaska Native families. *Journal of Psychoactive Drugs, 43*, 309–318. doi:10.1080/02791072.2011.628924

Boggs, S., Eyberg, S., Edwards, D., Rayfield, A., Jacobs, J., Bagner, D., & Hood, K. (2004). Outcomes of Parent-Child Interaction Therapy: A comparison of treatment completers and study dropouts one to three years later. *Child & Family Behavior Therapy, 26*, 1–22. doi:10.1300/J019v26n04_01

Brinkmeyer, M. Y., & Eyberg, S. M. (2003). Parent-Child Interaction Therapy. In A. Kazdin & J. Weisz (Eds.), *Evidence-based psychotherapies for children and adolescents* (pp. 204–223). New York, NY: Guilford Press.

California Evidence-Based Clearinghouse for Child Welfare. (2009). *Usage guide for the CEBC.* www.cachildwelfareclearinghouse.org

Callahan, C. L., Stevens, M. L., & Eyberg, S. M. (2010). Parent-Child Interaction Therapy. In C. E. Schaefer (Ed.), *Play therapy for preschool children* (pp. 199–221). Washington, DC: American Psychological Association.

Cedar, B., & Levant, R. F. (1990). A meta-analysis of the effects of Parent Effectiveness Training. *American Journal of Family Therapy, 18*, 373–384. doi:10.1080/01926189008250986

Centers for Disease Control and Prevention, National Center for Injury Prevention and Control. (2004). *Using evidence-based parenting programs to advance CDC efforts in child maltreatment prevention: Research brief.* Atlanta, GA: Author.

Chaffin, M., & Friedrich, W. (2004). Evidence-based practice in child abuse and neglect. *Children and Youth Services Review, 26*, 1097–1113.

Chaffin, M., Funderburk B., Bard, D., Valle, L., & Gurwitch, R. (2011). A combined motivation and Parent-Child Interaction Therapy package reduces child welfare recidivism in a randomized dismantling field trial. *Journal of Consulting and Clinical Psychology, 79*, 84–95. doi:10.1037/a0021227

Chaffin, M., Silovsky, J., Funderburk, B., Valle, L. A., Brestan, E. V., Balachova, T., et al. (2004). Parent-child interaction therapy with physically abusive parents: Efficacy for reducing future abuse reports. *Journal of Consulting and Clinical Psychology, 72*, 500–510. doi:10.1037/0022-006X.72.3.500

Chaffin, M., Valle, L. A., Funderburk, B., Gurwitch, R., Silovsky, J., Bard, D., et al. (2009). A motivational intervention can improve retention in PCIT for low-motivation child welfare clients. *Child Maltreatment, 14*, 356–368. doi:10.1177/1077559509332263

Clausen, J. M., Landsverk, J., Ganger, W., Chadwick, D., & Litrownik, A. (1998). Mental health problems of children in foster care. *Journal of Child and Family Studies, 7*, 283–296.

Cohn, A. H., & Daro, D. (1987). Is treatment too late: What ten years of evaluative research tell us. *Child Abuse & Neglect, 11*, 433–442. doi:10.1016/0145-2134(87)90016-0

Cook, R. J. (1994). Are we helping foster care youth prepare for the future? *Children and Youth Services Review, 16*, 213–229. doi:10.1016/0190-7409(94)90007-8

Crouch, J. L., & Behl, L. E. (2001). Relationships among parental beliefs in corporal punishment, reported stress, and physical child abuse potential. *Child Abuse & Neglect, 25*, 413–419. doi:10.1016/S0145-2134(00)00256-8

Eisenstadt, T. H., Eyberg, S., McNeil, C. B., Newcomb, K., & Funderburk, B. (1993). Parent-Child Interaction Therapy with behavior problem children: Relative effectiveness of two stages and overall treatment outcome. *Journal of Clinical Child Psychology, 22*, 42–51. doi:10.1207/s15374424jccp2201_4

Eyberg, S. M., & Boggs, S. R. (1998). Parent-Child Interaction Therapy: A psychosocial intervention for the treatment of young conduct-disordered children. In C. E. Schaefer & J. M. Briesmeister (Eds.), *Handbook of parent training: Parents as co-therapists for children's behavior problems* (2nd ed., pp. 61–97). New York, NY: John Wiley & Sons.

Eyberg, S. M., Boggs, S., & Algina, J. (1995). Parent-Child Interaction Therapy: A psychosocial model for the treatment of young children with conduct problem behavior and their families. *Psychopharmacology Bulletin, 31*, 83–91.

Eyberg, S. M., & Funderburk, B. W. (2011). *Parent-Child Interaction Therapy International protocol*. www.pcit.org

Eyberg, S. M., Funderburk, B. W., Hembree-Kigin, T., McNeil, C. B., Querido, J., & Hood, K. K. (2001). Parent-Child Interaction Therapy with behavior problem children: One- and two-year maintenance of treatment effects in the family. *Child & Family Behavior Therapy, 23*, 1–20. doi:10.1300/J019v23n04_01

Eyberg, S. M., & Robinson, E. A. (1982). Parent-child interaction training: Effects on family functioning. *Journal of Clinical Child Psychology, 11*, 130–137. doi:10.1207/s15374424jccp1102_6

Fixsen, D. L., Naoon, S. F., Blase, K. A., Friedman, R. M., & Wallace, F. (2005). *Implementation research: A synthesis of the literature*. Tampa, FL: University of South Florida, Louis de la Parte Florida Mental Health Institute, National Implementation Research Network.

Funderburk, B., Eyberg, S. M., Newcomb, K., McNeil, C. B., Hembree-Kigin, T., & Capage, L. (1998). Parent-Child Interaction Therapy with behavior problem children: Maintenance of treatment effects in the school setting. *Child and Family Behavior Therapy, 20*, 17–38. doi:10.1300/J019v20n02_02

Gallagher, N. (2003). Effects of Parent-Child Interaction Therapy on young children with disruptive behavior disorders. *Bridges: Practice-Based Research Syntheses, 1*(4), 1–17.

Hakman, M., Chaffin, M., Funderburk, B., & Silovsky, J. F. (2009). Change trajectories for parent-child interaction sequences during Parent-Child Interaction Therapy for child physical abuse. *Child Abuse & Neglect, 33*, 461–470. doi:10.1016/j.chiabu.2008.08.003

Hanf, C. A. (1969). *A two-stage program for modifying maternal controlling during mother-child (M-C) interaction*. Paper presented at the meeting of the Western Psychological Association, Vancouver, BC.

Herschell, A. D., & McNeil, C. B. (2005). Parent-Child Interaction Therapy for children experiencing externalizing behavior problems. In L. A. Reddy, T. M. Files-Hall, & C. E. Schaefer (Eds.), *Empirically based play interventions for children*. Washington, DC: American Psychological Association.

Hood, K. K., & Eyberg, S. M. (2003). Outcomes of Parent-Child Interaction Therapy: Mothers' reports on maintenance three to six years after treatment. *Journal of Clinical Child and Adolescent Psychology, 32*, 419–429. doi:10.1207/S15374424JCCP3203_10

James, S., Leslie, L. K., Hurlburt, M. S., Slymen, D. J., Landsverk, J., Davis, I., et al. (2006). Children in out-of-home care: Entry into intensive or restrictive mental health and residential care placements. *Journal of Emotional and Behavioral Disorders, 14*, 196–208. doi:10.1177/10634266060140040301

Kaminski, J. W., Valle, L. A., Filene, J. H., & Boyle, C. L. (2008). A meta-analytic review of components associated with parent training program effectiveness. *Journal of Abnormal Child Psychology, 36*, 567–589. doi:10.1007/s10802-007-9201-9

Kazdin, A. E., & Blase, S. L. (2011). Rebooting psychotherapy research and practice to reduce the burden of mental illness. *Perspectives on Psychological Science, 6*, 21–37. doi:10.1177/1745691610393527

Lawrence, C., Carlson, E., & Egeland, B. (2006). The impact of foster care on development. *Development and Psychopathology, 18*, 57–76. doi:10.1017/S0954579406060044

Lee, S., Aos, S., & Miller, M. (2008). *Evidence-based programs to prevent children entering and remaining in the child welfare system* (Document 08-07-3901). Olympia, WA: Washington State Institute for Public Policy.

Lenze, S. N., Pautsch, J., & Luby, J. (2011). Parent-Child Interaction Therapy Emotion Development: A novel treatment for depression in preschool children. *Depression and Anxiety, 28*, 153–159. doi:10.1002/da.20770

Leslie, L. K., Hurlburt, M. S., Landsverk, J., Barth, R., & Slymen, D. J. (2004). Outpatient mental health services for children in foster care: A national perspective. *Child Abuse & Neglect, 28*, 697–712. doi:10.1016/j.chiabu.2004.01.004

Lundahl, B. W., Nimer, J., & Parsons, B. (2006). Preventing child abuse: A meta-analysis of parent training programs. *Research on Social Work Practice, 16*, 251–262. doi:10.1177/1049731505284391

Lundahl, B. W., Risser, H. J., & Lovejoy, M. C. (2006). A meta-analysis of parent training: Moderators and follow-up effects. *Clinical Psychology Review, 26*, 86–104. doi:10.1016/j.cpr.2005.07.004

Maughan, D. R., Christiansen, E., Jenson, W. R., Olympia, D., & Clark, E. (2005). Behavioral parent training as a treatment for externalizing behaviors and disruptive behavior disorders: A meta-analysis. *School Psychology Review, 34*, 267–286.

McCabe, K., & Yeh, M. (2009). Parent-Child Interaction Therapy for Mexican Americans: A randomized clinical trial. *Journal of Clinical Child and Adolescent Psychology, 38*, 753–759. doi:10.1080/15374410903103544

McDiarmid, M. D., & Bagner, D. M. (2005). Parent-Child Interaction Therapy for children with disruptive behavior and developmental disabilities. *Education and Treatment of Children, 28*, 130–141.

McMahon, R. J., & Forehand, R. L. (2003). *Helping the noncompliant child: Family-based treatment for oppositional behavior* (2nd ed.). New York, NY: Guilford Press.

McNeil, C. B., Capage, L. C., Bahl, A., & Blanc, H. (1999). Importance of early intervention for disruptive behavior problems: Comparison of treatment and waitlist-control groups. *Early Education & Development, 10*, 445–454. doi:10.1207/s15566935eed1004_2

McNeil, C. B., Eyberg, S. M., Eisendstadt, T. H., Newcomb, K., & Funderburk, B. W. (1991). Parent-Child Interaction Therapy with behavior problem children: Generalization of treatment effects to the school setting. *Journal of Clinical Child Psychology, 20*, 140–151. doi:10.1207/s15374424jccp2002_5

McNeil, C. B., & Hembree-Kigin, T. L. (2010). *Parent-Child Interaction Therapy* (2nd ed.). New York, NY: Springer.

McNeil, C. B., Herschell, A. D., Gurwitch, R. H., & Clemens-Mowrer, L. C. (2005). Training foster parents in Parent-Child Interaction Therapy. *Education and Treatment of Children, 28*, 182–196.

Newton, R. R., Litrownik, A. J., & Landsverk, J. A. (2000). Children and youth in foster care: Disentangling the relationship between problem behaviors and number of placements. *Child Abuse & Neglect, 24*, 1363–1374. doi:10.1016/S0145-2134(00)00189-7

Nock, M. K., & Kazdin, A. E. (2005). Randomized trial of a brief intervention for increasing participation in parent management training. *Journal of Consulting and Clinical Psychology, 73*, 872–879. doi:10.1037/0022-006X.73.5.872

NSCAW Research Group. (2005, April). *National Survey of Child and Adolescent Well-being (NSCAW) CPS sample component wave 1 data analysis report*. Washington, DC: U.S. Department of

Health and Human Services, Administration for Children, Youth and Families.

Patterson, G. R. (1976). The aggressive child: Victim and architect of a coercive system. In E. Mash, L. A. Hamerlynch, & L. C. Handy (Eds.), *Behavior modification and families: I. Theory and research. II. Applications and developments* (pp. 265–316). New York, NY: Brunner-Mazel.

PCIT International. (2009). *Training guidelines for Parent-Child Interaction Therapy.* www.pcit.org.

Pearl, E., Thieken, L., Olafson, E., Boat, B., Connelly, L., Barnes, J., & Putnam, F. (2012). Effectiveness of community dissemination of Parent-Child Interaction Therapy. *Psychological Trauma: Theory, Research, Practice, and Policy, 4,* 204–213. doi:10.1037/a0022948

Pincus, D. B., Choate, M. L., Eyberg, S. M., & Barlow, D. H. (2005). Treatment of young children with separation anxiety disorder using Parent-Child Interaction Therapy. *Cognitive and Behavioral Practice, 12,* 126–135.

Pinkston, E. M., & Smith, M. D. (1998). Contributions of parent training to child welfare: Early history and current thoughts. In J. R. Lutzker (Ed.), *Handbook of child abuse research and treatment* (pp. 377–399). New York, NY: Plenum Press.

Puliafico, A. C., Comer, J. S., & Pincus, D. B. (2012). Adapting Parent-Child Interaction Therapy to treat anxiety disorders in young children. *Child and Adolescent Psychiatric Clinics in North America, 21,* 607–619. doi:10.1016/j.chc.2012.05.005

Reitman, D., & McMahon, R. J. (2012). Constance "Connie" Hanf (1917–2002): The mentor and the model. *Cognitive and Behavioral Practice.* doi:10.1016/j.cbpra.2012.02.005

Reyno, S. M., & McGrath, P. J. (2006). Predictors of parent training efficacy for child externalizing behavior problems: A meta-analytic review. *Journal of Child Psychology and Psychiatry, 47,* 99–111. doi:10.1111/j.1469-7610.2005.01544.x

Sanders, M. R. (2012). Development, evaluation, and multinational dissemination of the Triple P-Positive Parenting Program. *Annual Review of Clinical Psychology, 8,* 345–379. doi:10.1146/annurev-clinpsy-032511-143104

Schuhmann, E. M., Foote, R. C., Eyberg, S. M., Boggs, S. R., & Algina, J. (1998). Efficacy of Parent-Child Interaction Therapy: Interim report of a randomized trial with short-term maintenance. *Journal of Clinical Child Psychology, 27,* 34–45. doi:10.1207/s15374424jccp2701_4

Serketich, W. J., & Dumas, J. E. (1996). The effectiveness of behavioral parent training to modify antisocial behavior in children: A meta-analysis. *Behavior Therapy, 27,* 171–186. doi:10.1016/S0005-7894(96)80013-X

Shirk, S. R. (2004). Dissemination of youth ESTs: Ready for prime time? *Clinical Psychology: Science and Practice, 11,* 308–312. doi:10.1093/clipsy.bph086

Stith, S. M., Liu, T., Davies, L. C., Boykin, E. L., Alder, M. C., Harris, J. M., et al. (2009). Risk factors in child maltreatment: A meta-analytic review of the literature. *Aggression and Violent Behavior, 14,* 13–29. doi:10.1016/j.avb.2006.03.006

Sweet, M. A., & Appelbaum, M. I. (2004). Is home visiting an effective strategy? A meta-analytic review of home visiting programs for families with young children. *Child Development, 75,* 1435–1456. doi:10.1111/j.1467-8624.2004.00750.x

Thomas, R., & Zimmer-Gembeck, M. J. (2007). Behavioral outcomes of Parent-Child Interaction Therapy and Triple P-Positive Parenting Program: A review and meta-analysis. *Journal of Abnormal Child Psychology, 35,* 475–495. doi:10.1007/s10802-007-9104-9

Thomas, R., & Zimmer-Gembeck, M. J. (2012). Parent-Child Interaction Therapy: An evidence-based treatment for child maltreatment. *Child Maltreatment, 17,* 253–266. doi:10.1177/1077559512459555

Timmer, S. G., Urquiza, A. J., Herschell, A. D., McGrath, J. M., Zebell, N. M., Porter, A. L., & Vargas, E. C. (2006). Parent-Child Interaction Therapy: Application of an empirically supported treatment to maltreated children in foster care. *Child Welfare, 85,* 919–939.

Timmer, S. G., Urquiza, A. J., Zebell, N. M., & McGrath, J. M. (2005). Parent-Child Interaction Therapy: Application to maltreating parent-child dyads. *Child Abuse & Neglect, 29,* 825–842. doi:10.1016/j.chiabu.2005.01.003

Urquiza, A. J., & McNeil, C. B. (1996). Parent-Child Interaction Therapy: An intensive dyadic intervention for physically abusive families. *Child Maltreatment, 1,* 134–144. doi:10.1177/1077559596001002005

U.S. Department of Health and Human Services, Administration on Children, Youth and Families. (2005). *Child maltreatment 2003.* Washington, DC: U.S. Government Printing Office.

Webster-Stratton, C. (2005). The Incredible Years parents, teachers, and children training series: Early intervention and prevention programs for young children. In P. S. Jensen & E. D. Hibbs (Eds.), *Psychosocial treatments for child and adolescent disorders: Empirically based approaches* (pp. 507–556). Washington, DC: American Psychological Association.

Webster-Stratton, C. (2011). *The Incredible Years parents, teachers, and children's training series: Program content, methods, research, and dissemination, 1980–2011.* Seattle, WA: Incredible Years.

Weisz, J. R., Chorpita, B. F., Palinkas, L. A., Schoenwald, S. K., Miranda, J., Bearman, S. K., et al. (2012). Testing standard and modular designs for psychotherapy treating depression, anxiety, and conduct problems in youth: A randomized effectiveness trial. *Archives of General Psychiatry, 69,* 274–282. doi:10.1001/archgenpsychiatry.2011.147

5

SHANNON SELF-BROWN, PH.D.
ERIN MCFRY, M.P.H.
ANGELA MONTESANTI, M.P.H.
ANNA EDWARDS-GAURA, PH.D.
JOHN LUTZKER, PH.D.
JENELLE SHANLEY, PH.D.
DANIEL WHITAKER, PH.D.

SafeCare

A Prevention and Intervention Program for Child Neglect and Physical Abuse

GENERAL CONSIDERATIONS

In 2010, child protective services in the United States responded to approximately 3.6 million reports of child maltreatment, and 754,000 of those reports were substantiated as official child protection cases (U.S. Department of Health and Human Services, 2010). As indicated in figure 5.1, the most common type of substantiated maltreatment is neglect, followed by physical abuse, and co-occurrence of these forms of abuse is common. Child maltreatment experts have endorsed parent training as an overarching strategy for addressing child neglect and physical abuse (Barth et al., 2005; Whitaker, Lutzker, & Shelley, 2005). This approach is warranted because in approximately four-fifths (81.3%) of substantiated cases of maltreatment, the parent, either alone or with someone else, is the perpetrator of abuse (U.S. Department of Health and Human Services, 2010).

The two most commonly discussed approaches to prevention of child maltreatment in the scientific literature are behavioral parent training programs (Chaffin, Funderburk, et al., 2011; Chaffin, Silovsky, et al., 2004; Prinz et al., 2009; Whitaker, Lutzker, & Shelley, 2005) and home visiting programs (e.g., Chaffin, 2004; Duggan et al., 2004; Hahn et al., 2005). SafeCare is a unique child maltreatment prevention program that merges these two highly recommended strategies for prevention of child neglect and physical abuse. The SafeCare model targets three risk factors strongly associated with child neglect and physical abuse, parent-child/infant interaction, child health, and home safety. For over 30 years, Dr. John Lutzker, developer of SafeCare, and his colleagues have facilitated important developmental and dissemination research on this model. This research has culminated in SafeCare being identified by the California Evidence-Based Clearinghouse for Child Welfare (2012)

as a program "supported by research evidence" for prevention of child abuse and neglect. SafeCare trainings have been conducted in 15 states across the United States and have been actively implemented throughout England. The current hub for SafeCare training and research is the National SafeCare Training and Research Center (NSTRC) at Georgia State University.

The purpose of this chapter is to describe the SafeCare intervention, the supporting research evidence for the model, the types of families for whom this intervention is most relevant, and the overall advantages and disadvantages of the SafeCare approach in treating families at risk for child neglect and physical abuse.

THE SAFECARE INTERVENTION

SafeCare is a home visiting program that consists of three modules: Parent-Child/Parent-Infant Interactions, Child Health, and Home Safety. These three modules target deficits in parenting skills and the home environment that often lead to child neglect or physical abuse referrals. Each module is approximately 6 sessions, yielding a total of 18 sessions. Sessions typically range from 1 to 1.5 hours each. Providers who deliver SafeCare have a range of educational training, from master's level therapists to paraprofessionals; however, all SafeCare providers have participated in a standardized training and certification process designated by the NSTRC (www.nstrc.org), which includes an in-person workshop and strict fidelity monitoring of providers' work with families.

The SafeCare modules are conducted sequentially, with providers beginning with the module that addresses the area of greatest need, or the presenting problem, for a given family. SafeCare delivery involves a structured approach that is consistent across the modules and includes (1) an

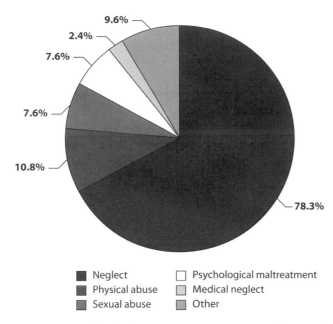

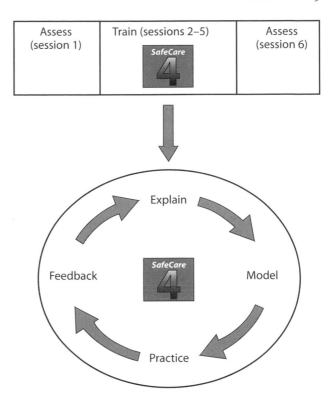

Figure 5.1. Types of child abuse. Percentages sum to more than 100% because a child may have suffered more than one type of maltreatment. *Source.* U.S. Department of Health and Human Services.

Figure 5.2. The SafeCare module structure

initial baseline assessment, (2) four to five training sessions, and (3) an end-of-module assessment (as illustrated in figure 5.2). Each module has validated observational tools that are used for the baseline assessment (completed during session 1 of each module) and end-of-module assessments (completed in the final session of each module), as well as ongoing assessments to evaluate progress during parent training sessions. The purpose of the baseline assessment is for the provider to assess the parent's current level of skill or functioning in the targeted skill areas. Once parent training begins, observational assessments continue so that the provider can determine the parent's progress and acquisition of skills. Finally, the end-of-module assessment occurs after all training sessions are complete and allows the provider to determine whether the parent has mastered the requisite skills. Importantly, SafeCare assessments are observations of behavior, not simply parental self-reports.

SafeCare parent training sessions are based on the "SafeCare 4" principles:

1. *Explain* the desired skills. The provider describes for the parent the targeted skills, why they are important, and how they might be beneficial to the parent and the child.
2. *Model* each skill. The provider physically demonstrates the skills for the parent. For example, in the parent-child interaction, the provider may show the parent how to play with a young child using positive verbalizations. In home safety, the provider might demonstrate how to secure or remove a home hazard.
3. *Practice* the skill(s). The parent is directed to practice the targeted skills in a variety of settings during the sessions.

4. *Feedback.* The provider gives positive and corrective feedback to the parent on his or her use of the targeted skills.

The provider continues this explain-model-practice-feedback process as needed until the parent demonstrates consistency and ease in using the module's target skills.

Parent-Child / Parent-Infant Interactions Module

The parent-child interaction module includes two different curricula: one for parents with infants (Parent-Infant Interaction, or PII) and another for parents with children ages 1 (walking) to 5 years (Parent-Child Interaction, or PCI), both of which are delineated below.

PARENT-INFANT INTERACTION. The goal for parents in PII is to increase positive parent-infant bonding behaviors. SafeCare providers train the parent in target skills for PII using the assess-train-assess approach described above.

Assess (PII, session 1). Two validated measures are used in the PII module. First, the Daily Activities Checklist is administered to help the parent identify which routine activities (e.g., diapering, meal time) are most challenging in daily life with the infant. The Infant-Parent Activities Training Checklist (iPAT) is an observational instrument used by the provider to score the parent on the target behaviors listed in table 5.1. During the baseline session, the provider scores the parent on the iPAT as she engages in the two daily activities that she has identified as challenging.

Table 5.1. iPAT Checklist of Parent Behaviors

LoTTS of Bonding	
Looking	Face the infant with open eyes.
Talking	Talk about what you are doing, using simple words. Use appropriate tone of voice. Use loving words and praise.
Touching	Pat, kiss, tickle, and provide affectionate/gentle contact.
Smiling	Look at the infant and turn your mouth up, laughing.
Other Bonding Behaviors	
Holding	Completely lift the infant off the surface; provide warm and direct contact.
Imitating	Imitate vocalizations or movements; be respectful.
Rocking	Gently move the infant back and forth.

Train (PII, sessions 2–5). Parent training focuses on several target skills that are related to parent-infant interaction. PII target skills (see table 5.1) include *looking, talking, touching,* and *smiling,* or the "LoTTS of Bonding" skills. Each of these core skills can be used by the parent to engage and promote bonding with the infant during daily activities. The parent is also trained in other bonding behaviors, which may vary across contexts and stages of infant development, including *imitating, holding,* and *rocking* the infant. In the training sessions, the provider uses the SafeCare 4 process to train the parent in the PII skills: explaining and modeling the targeted skills, observing the parent practice the skills during challenging daily activities (e.g., using eye contact and talking in a positive tone while dressing a squirming baby), and providing positive and corrective feedback as needed. Training sessions continue until the parent masters skill utilization in a variety of daily activities with the infant. During the training session, the provider also provides education to the parent on important topics such as the five physiological states of infants (asleep, drowsy, calm-alert, excited, and upset), developmental milestones, and a variety of engaging activities that can be used during playtime with the infant.

Assess (PII, session 6). The iPAT is used to reassess the three activities that were the focus of training to evaluate the parent's mastery, skill retention, and skill generalization.

PARENT-CHILD INTERACTION. The primary goal of the PCI module is to increase parents' positive interaction with children and to train parents in how to effectively manage child behavior. The module helps parents increase parental consistency and promote predictable and reliable expectations for the child.

Assess (PCI, session 1). The initial assessment in PCI is completed by using the Child Planned Activities Training Checklist (cPAT) to observe which of the PAT skills the parent is already employing with the child in two activities the parent identifies as challenging.

Train (PCI, sessions 2–5). After the baseline session is completed, the parent proceeds through the PCI training sessions in which the provider teaches the parent to promote positive interactions with his child and to increase structure during play and two daily activities. Session 2 begins with explaining and modeling the PAT skills described in table 5.2, including but not limited to discussing rules and consequences prior to the activity, using incidental teaching to teach simple skills and promote language development during the activity (e.g. "See the red car? This is red."), and providing positive feedback and attention after the activity is over. Next, the parent is prompted to practice the newly introduced skills while engaging in a play activity with his child, while the provider observes. During and after the activity, the provider offers positive and corrective feedback to the parent. Training sessions continue, with a focus on training the parent to use the PAT skills during additional daily activities and the child's independent play. During the training session, the provider also provides education to the parent on important topics such as developmental milestones and a variety of engaging age-appropriate activities that can be used during playtime.

Assess (PCI, session 6). The cPAT is used to reassess the three activities (play, two daily activities) that were the fo-

Table 5.2. Definition of cPAT Skills

Before
Prepare in advance
- Gets supplies/toys ready in advance (includes items already present)
- Informs the child that the activity is going to happen

Explain activity
- Gets the child's attention
- Explains the activity

Explain rules and consequences
- Gives 1+ positively stated rule
- Gives 1+ positive consequence

During
Talk about what you and your child are doing
- Talks warmly about the activity
- Uses incidental teaching

Use good physical interaction skills
- Gets on the child's level
- Uses good eye contact

Talk about what you and your child are doing
- Lets the child have 2+ choices during activity

Praise desired behaviors
- Uses 2+ labeled praises

Ignore minor misbehavior
- Ignores minor misbehavior

Provide consequences
- Follows through with stated positive and/or negative consequences as appropriate

End
Wrap up and give feedback
- Informs the child that activity is ending
- Describes what the child did well
- Lets child know what to do better next time (if applicable)

cus of training to obtain a final confirmation of mastery, skill retention, and skill generalization.

Child Health Module

The goals of the health module are to train parents to prevent childhood illnesses, identify symptoms of childhood illnesses and injuries, and provide and seek appropriate treatment for their children. The health module relies heavily on scenarios for role-playing and educates parents in a structured decision-making process (illustrated in figure 5.3) related to common childhood illnesses and injuries. In response to health role-play scenarios, parents are trained to make effective decisions based on whether to care for their child at home, call a nurse helpline or doctor's office, or go directly to the emergency room.

Assess (Child Health, session 1). The validated measure included in the health module is the Sick and Injured Child Checklist (SICC). In the baseline assessment session, three different types of role-play scenarios are administered—Care at Home, Doctor's Appointment, and Emergency Treatment—and the SICC is used to assess and score the parent's responses during role-play scenarios.

Train (Child Health, sessions 2–5). After the baseline session is completed, the parent proceeds through the health training sessions in which the provider and parent make use of various health scenarios that describe health conditions common in childhood. In each scenario, the provider describes symptoms of a common condition and then elicits responses from the parent about the condition (i.e., describe what is going on with the child) and how the parent would evaluate and address the condition. As the parent is trained, she is expected to correctly assess the symptoms and arrive at the optimal response (care at home, schedule a doctor's appointment, or go to the emergency room). During each scenario, the provider explains the symptoms, has the parent determine the condition and course of action to take, role-plays what to do in a scenario, and provides corrective feedback. The SafeCare Health Manual is a health reference document that provides information to assist parents in identifying and triaging symptoms. Included in the manual is a "Symptom and Illness Guide" that allows the parent to look up specific symptoms and provides additional information to help the parent determine the best course of action (see figure 5.3). In addition to training with the role-play scenarios, the parent also receives education on a variety of preventive health topics that are relevant in caring for children. Sample topics include helpful medical supplies to have at home, properly taking temperatures, hygiene, regular medical checkups and immunizations, sleep safety, and sudden infant death syndrome (SIDS) prevention.

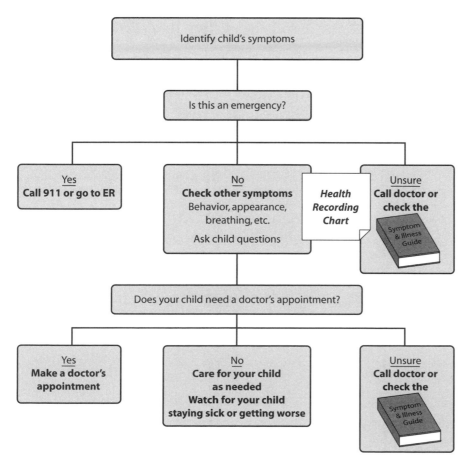

Figure 5.3. Child Health Module decision-making process

Assess (Child Health, session 6). In the final health session, the SICC is used to reassess the parent's responses to the three different types of role-play scenarios to confirm her mastery of the targeted skills.

Home Safety Module

The safety module seeks to prevent unintentional injuries by helping parents make their homes safe and encouraging parental supervision. SafeCare defines an accessible hazard as one that is both reachable by the child and unsecured, meaning in an unlocked container or space, and is without a childproof cap. The SafeCare categories of hazards are listed in table 5.3.

Assess (Home Safety, session 1). The initial safety baseline assessment focuses on three rooms and includes a thorough search for accessible hazards. The selection of rooms for assessment is based on where children spend most of their time. The validated safety measure is the Home Accident Prevention Inventory (HAPI), a checklist that helps the provider document the number of hazards accessible to children in a room. Before gathering baseline data during session 1, the provider obtains written permission from the parent to assess three rooms in the home. The consent form details how the assessment process will be conducted, including that the provider will need to look in such places as cabinets and drawers. The parent is given the opportunity to decline any portion of the assessment or to specify places where he does not want the provider to look. The parent is also invited to participate in the assessment.

Following the consent and description of the assessment process, the provider measures the eye level and reach of the tallest child to determine which items are accessible. We assume that a child can climb onto anything that is at or below eye level. The provider begins in one room and moves around the room in a clockwise fashion to find all hazardous items within reach of the child. Accessible hazards are recorded on the HAPI. At the end of the assessment of one room, the number of hazards is tallied to yield a total hazard score for the room. A new HAPI is used for every room assessed; thus, by the end of the assessment process, the provider will have completed three HAPIs.

Train (Home Safety, sessions 2–5). The training sessions focus on providing education and explanation about the 10 hazard categories, how to determine whether hazards are accessible to the child, and strategies to remove or reduce hazards. The provider gives feedback about the HAPI scores in each of the rooms assessed and works with the parent during the training sessions to identify and address each hazard by using a childproof latch or lock, placing the object out of the child's reach, or cleaning the hazard area. The responsibility for identifying and removing hazards gradually shifts from the provider to the parent. As the parent practices, the provider gives positive and corrective feedback, as well as modeling, when appropriate. For a variety of reasons (e.g., other adults living in the home, hazards beyond the parent's control to remedy), it is often difficult to reach zero hazards. However, typically, drastic reductions in hazards can take place, thus achieving a successful outcome (marked improvement from baseline). When all hazards cannot be removed, the provider emphasizes the importance of parental supervision around the remaining hazards. During the training session, the provider also discusses additional hazards with parents, such as burns and scalding water, food storage and preparation, lead poisoning, fire safety, car safety, and so on.

Assess (Home Safety, session 6). The HAPI is used to reevaluate how well the parent has maintained the safety gains in the three rooms assessed at baseline. Problem solving for the identification and removal of future hazards also occurs.

UNDERLYING RATIONALE AND THEORETICAL FRAMEWORK

The SafeCare model is based on Bandura's (1977) social learning theory and techniques described by Latham and Saari (1979), along with applied behavior analysis (Lutzker & Chaffin, 2012). Like other behavioral parent training programs, SafeCare is based on the assumption that child neglect and physical abuse are caused by parenting skill deficits that can be improved by providing parents with training in a repertoire of skills, using a specific instructional format that includes (1) provider's instruction to the parent on targeted skills, (2) provider's behavioral modeling of targeted skills, (3) parent's practice of skills through role plays and live practice with the child, and (4) provider's feedback to the parent (Shaffer et al., 2001). Importantly, these skills

Table 5.3. Hazard Categories

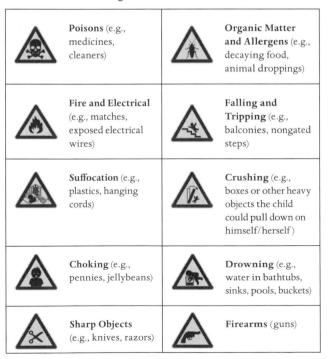

Poisons (e.g., medicines, cleaners)	**Organic Matter and Allergens** (e.g., decaying food, animal droppings)
Fire and Electrical (e.g., matches, exposed electrical wires)	**Falling and Tripping** (e.g., balconies, nongated steps)
Suffocation (e.g., plastics, hanging cords)	**Crushing** (e.g., boxes or other heavy objects the child could pull down on himself/herself)
Choking (e.g., pennies, jellybeans)	**Drowning** (e.g., water in bathtubs, sinks, pools, buckets)
Sharp Objects (e.g., knives, razors)	**Firearms** (guns)

were found to be critical to changes in parent behavior in a meta-analysis of parent training programs by Kaminski and colleagues (2008).

EVIDENCE BASE / EMPIRICAL SUPPORT

Effectiveness in Child Maltreatment Recidivism

Support for SafeCare's efficacy and effectiveness has been found in several lines of research. The three SafeCare modules have undergone rigorous single-case studies to evaluate the effectiveness of each intervention module (Metchikian et al., 1991; Tertinger, Greene, & Lutzker, 1984). Three important studies conducted to date suggest that SafeCare is an effective intervention for families currently involved in the child welfare system. The first study was a quasi-experimental study by Lutzker and colleagues (Gershater-Molko, Lutzker, & Wesch, 2002) that compared families receiving SafeCare services with families receiving standard family preservation services in California. The findings indicated that Safe-Care families were significantly less likely to have a recurrence of child maltreatment reports than services-as-usual (SAU) families. Recidivism rates three years after intervention were 15% for SafeCare families and 44% for SAU families.

More recently, two randomized trials demonstrated a significant benefit of SafeCare compared with SAU. First, a statewide comparative effectiveness trial of SafeCare in the Oklahoma child welfare system matched six service regions of Oklahoma and randomized each region to either continue with SAU (a six-month intensive family preservation program with a case management focus) or deliver SafeCare. More than 2,100 enrolled families were followed up for, on average, six years after services. The findings indicate that SafeCare reduced child maltreatment reports by about 26% (hazard ratio = 0.74), and the authors concluded that SafeCare prevented between 64 and 104 reports per 1,000 cases (assuming a recidivism rate of 45%) (Chaffin, Hecht, et al., 2012).

A recently published study examined a subsample of American Indian families from the statewide trial and also found lower child welfare recidivism rates among SafeCare families compared with SAU families (Chaffin, Bard, et al., 2012). Additionally, SafeCare was associated with greater improvement in parental depression and scores on the Child Abuse Potential Inventory among participating parents (Milner, 1986). Lastly, parents receiving SafeCare rated their services higher in cultural competency, working alliance, and satisfaction, suggesting this intervention is well received among ethnic minority groups (Chaffin, Bard, et al., 2012).

SafeCare as a Preventive Approach

Several recent trials have been conducted outside the child welfare service setting in which SafeCare was implemented as a preventive approach, with favorable results. A study focused on families residing in rural areas found greater service utilization, increased use of nonviolent discipline, and fewer child protection reports related to children's exposure to domestic violence for families in SafeCare versus SAU (Silovsky et al., 2011). Child protection reports were about one-third lower for SafeCare families (20.8%) than SAU families (31.5%) in this study; however, these differences were not statistically significant ($p = 0.19$), probably because of the small sample size used in the study (N = 105). A two-site randomized trial (Kansas and Indiana) of the parent-child interaction module of SafeCare is nearing completion. Results at six months after intervention indicate that, compared with control parents, parents receiving the SafeCare parenting module showed more positive parenting behaviors and their children were more engaged and responsive during parent-child interaction observations (Lefever et al., in press).

Cost Effectiveness

A recent report from the highly respected Washington State Institute on Public Policy (2012) showed that SafeCare's "return on investment" was $14.85 in benefits for every $1 spent on training and implementation. The authors of the report examined findings from the recent Oklahoma statewide trial and used cost estimates from both Oklahoma and Washington State. They found that SafeCare costs $102 more per family to implement than other services. However, based on the findings from the Oklahoma statewide trial, SafeCare yielded $1,501 in benefits per family. Of that total, $278 were benefits to taxpayers and $1,223 were direct benefits to participants. Though several other programs relevant to child welfare were found to have positive returns on investment (i.e., yielded more benefit than they cost), SafeCare had the highest benefit-to-cost ratio of any child welfare–relevant program.

FAMILIES SERVED BY SAFECARE

More than 500 practitioners have been trained in the Safe-Care model thus far. The bulk of these providers serve families involved in the child welfare system; however, providers who work in the justice system have also been trained, and public preventive health efforts are underway. Families involved in these systems are very diverse and can most succinctly be described as families with a variety of risk factors for child maltreatment, such as low socioeconomic status, multiple young children, single parents, and adolescent parents (Brown et al., 1998; Lee & Goerge, 1999; Murphey & Braner, 2000). In a recent qualitative research study, SafeCare providers experienced in implementing SafeCare with diverse populations reported that the model works well with families from a variety of ethnic backgrounds, and they did not recommend making systematic cultural adaptations to the model for specific populations

(Self-Brown et al., 2011). Findings from this qualitative study are further supported by the recent work of Chaffin and colleagues (Chaffin, Bard, et al., 2012), which, as discussed above, showed reduced recidivism and high consumer ratings for the intervention among American Indian families.

ADVANTAGES AND DISADVANTAGES

Advantages

The success of the SafeCare model can be attributed to several characteristics that, as supported by previous research, have proved effective in preventing child maltreatment.

1. *Services provided in the home.* To eliminate logistical barriers for families, SafeCare providers work with parents in the family's home setting to deliver parenting services. This delivery strategy offers service providers an increased opportunity to understand factors in the ecological context of the home environment that influence parents' decision making and behavior (Lutzker & Bigelow, 2002). Further, Huynen and colleagues (1996) demonstrated that teaching skills in the home, or in situ, increases the likelihood of generalization of the acquired skills.

2. *Application of behavioral parent training program.* Unlike other existing home visiting programs, the SafeCare curriculum and skills training are consistent with behavioral parent training programs typically offered in the clinic setting. By assessing parents' skills and behaviors and by providing direct intervention strategies such as instruction, behavioral modeling, and repeated parent practice, the Safe-Care program teaches parents targeted skills that promote safe, stable, and nurturing parent-child relationships (Lutzker & Bigelow, 2002).

3. *Curriculum focused on child neglect and physical abuse.* To satisfy its primary objective of preventing child maltreatment, the SafeCare model was designed to focus on three distinct areas: parent-child interaction, child health, and home safety. In contrast to other home visiting programs that focus on proxy risk factors, mostly targeting child well-being, and other behavioral parent training programs that exclusively focus on parent-child interaction, SafeCare's unique combination of modules specifically targets direct risk factors for child neglect and physical abuse, including child health risks related to deficiencies in parents' health care skills and home safety, in addition to psychosocial risks resulting from inadequate parenting skills and parent-child interactions (Edwards-Gaura et al., 2011).

4. *Targeting of families with children in the age group at greatest risk for maltreatment.* As reported by the U.S. Department of Health and Human Services (2012), children ages 0–5 are at the greatest risk for fatality as the result of maltreatment and make up more than half of all substantiated child protection cases each year. Accordingly, the SafeCare curriculum was designed to make the greatest impact on reducing child maltreatment by focusing on the parents of children 0–5 years of age.

In sum, SafeCare offers a unique, home-delivered, behavioral approach to prevention of child maltreatment and targets the two most commonly substantiated maltreatment types with parents of children in the age range at greatest risk.

Disadvantages

The success of the program, however, does not preclude the need for improvements in several areas that will continue to strengthen the model's validity and decrease the burden of child maltreatment.

1. *Home delivery is expensive.* While previous research has highlighted the many benefits of providing one-on-one services within the family's home setting, this delivery is more expensive than some clinic-based or group approaches. However, as discussed earlier, SafeCare is considered a cost-effective program, returning more than $14 for every $1 spent, according to the recent report by the Washington State Institute on Public Policy (2012).

2. *Impact of independent modules.* The success of the SafeCare curriculum has been credited to the combination of the modules' specific concentrations, but additional research is needed to tease out the effects of each module independently. If each module were found to be independently effective, there would be great potential for abbreviating the program to more specifically address a family's primary need. This could reduce service costs and potentially enhance retention rates of the program, which have been reported to be around 50% (Damashek et al., 2011).

3. *Impact on child mental health.* There is limited knowledge on the effects of the SafeCare curriculum on child mental health outcomes, and further research is necessary to understand the program's impact on specific child diagnoses. This would allow SafeCare to be implemented in additional service systems that rely on child diagnosis for treatment reimbursement.

EXPECTED OUTCOMES

The primary expected outcomes for parents who participate in the SafeCare program are increases in the targeted parenting skills. That is, parents can be expected to engage in more positive parenting behaviors, improve the safety of their homes, and make more effective child health decisions. Each of these outcomes has been demonstrated in SafeCare research (e.g., Bigelow & Lutzker, 2000; Gershater-Molko, Lutzker, & Wesch, 2002; Metchikian et al., 1999). For example, parents who complete the PCI module have higher-quality caregiving behaviors, such as being more responsive and encouraging to their children, setting appropriate behavioral expectations, and being involved in their children's activities (Lefever et al., in press).

Additional positive effects for program participants that have been demonstrated in research include reductions in parental depression (Chaffin, Bard, et al., 2012) and improved child behavior outcomes, including reductions in externalizing and internalizing behavior problems and improvements in adaptive functioning (Lefever et al., in press). These improvements tend to be apparent immediately after the intervention and at 6 months post-intervention, suggesting a generalization of skills. Finally, as noted in our discussion of research, regions that implement the SafeCare program can expect significant reductions in child protective service reports (Chaffin et al., 2011) and increases in service enrollment and completion, as compared with standard child welfare services (Damashek et al., 2011).

References

Bandura, A. (1977). *Social learning theory*. Oxford, UK: Prentice-Hall.

Barth, R. P., Landsverk, J., Chamberlain, P., Reid, J. B., Rolls, J. A., Hurlburt, M. S., & Kohl, P. L. (2005). Parent-training programs in child welfare services: Planning for a more evidence-based approach to serving biological parents. *Research on Social Work Practice, 15*(5), 353–371.

Bigelow, K. M., & Lutzker, J. R. (2000). Training parents reported for or at risk for child abuse and neglect to identify and treat their children's illnesses. *Journal of Family Violence, 15*, 311–330.

Brown, J., Cohen, P., Johnson, J. G., & Salzinger, S. (1998). A longitudinal analysis of risk factors for child maltreatment: Findings of a 17-year prospective study of officially recorded and self-reported child abuse and neglect. *Child Abuse & Neglect, 22*(11), 1065–1078.

California Evidence-Based Clearinghouse for Child Welfare. (2012, February). *SafeCare program description*. www.cebc4cw .org/program/safecare/detailed

Chaffin, M. (2004). Is it time to rethink Healthy Start / Healthy Families? *Child Abuse & Neglect, 28*(6), 589–595.

Chaffin, M., Bard, D., Bigfoot, D. S., & Maher, E. J. (2012). Is a structured, manualized, evidence-based treatment protocol culturally competent and equivalently effective among American Indian parents in child welfare? *Child Maltreatment, 17*(3), 1–11.

Chaffin, M., Funderburk, B., Bard, D., Valle, L. A., & Gurwitch, R. (2011). A combined motivation and parent-child interaction therapy package reduces child welfare recidivism in a randomized dismantling field trial. *Journal of Consulting and Clinical Psychology, 79*(1), 84–95.

Chaffin, M., Hecht, D., Bard, D., Silovsky, J. F., & Beasley, W. H. (2012). A statewide trial of the SafeCare home-based services model with parents in child protective services. *Pediatrics, 129*(3), 509–515

Chaffin, M., Silovsky, J. F., Funderburk, B., Valle, L. A., Brestan, E. V., Balachova, T., & Bonner, B. L. (2004). Parent-child interaction therapy with physically abusive parents: Efficacy for reducing future abuse reports. *Journal of Consulting and Clinical Psychology, 72*(3), 500–510.

Damashek, A., Doughty, D., Ware, L., & Silovsky, J. (2011). Predictors of client engagement and attrition in home-based child maltreatment prevention services. *Child Maltreatment, 16*(1), 9–20.

Duggan, A., McFarlane, E., Fuddy, L., Burrell, L., Higman, S. M., Windham, A., & Sia, C. (2004). Randomized trial of a statewide home visiting program: Impact in preventing child abuse and neglect. *Child Abuse & Neglect, 28*(6), 597–622.

Edwards-Gaura, A., Whitaker, D., Lutzker, J. R., Self-Brown, S., & Lewis, E. (2011). SafeCare: Application of an evidence-based program to prevent child maltreatment. In A. Rubin (Ed.), *A clinician's guide to evidence-based practice* (pp. 259–272). Hoboken, NJ: John Wiley & Sons.

Gershater-Molko, R. M., Lutzker, J. R., & Wesch, D. (2002). Using recidivism to evaluate project SafeCare: Teaching bonding, safety, and health care skills to parents. *Child Maltreatment, 7*(3), 277–285.

Hahn, R. A., Mercy, J., Bilukha, O., & Briss, P. (2005). Assessing home visiting programs to prevent child abuse: Taking silver and bronze along with gold. *Child Abuse & Neglect, 29*(3), 215–218.

Huynen, K. B., Lutzker, J. R., Bigelow, K. B., Touchette, P. E., & Campbell, R. V. (1996). Planned activities training for mothers of children with developmental disabilities. *Behavior Modification, 20*, 406–427.

Kaminski, J. W., Valle, L. A., Filene, J. H., & Boyle, C. L. (2008). A meta-analytic review of components associated with parent training program effectiveness. *Journal of Abnormal Child Psychology, 36*(4), 567–589.

Latham, G. P., & Saari, L. M. (1979). Importance of supportive relationships in goal setting. *Journal of Applied Psychology, 64*(2), 151–156.

Lee, B. J., & Goerge, R. (1999). Poverty, early childbearing, and child maltreatment: A multinomial analysis. *Children and Youth Services Review, 21*, 755–780.

Lefever, F. E. Bigelow, K. M., Carta, J. J., & Borkowski, J. G. (in press). Prediction of early engagement and completion of a home visitation parenting intervention for preventing child maltreatment. *National Head Start Association Dialog Briefs*.

Lutzker, J. R., & Bigelow, K. M. (2002). *Reducing child maltreatment: A guidebook for parent services*. New York, NY: Guilford Press.

Lutzker, J. R., & Chaffin, M. (2012). SafeCare®: An evidence-based, widely disseminated, constantly dynamic model to prevent child maltreatment. In H. Dubowitz (Ed.), *World perspectives on child abuse* (10th ed., pp. 93–96). Aurora, CO: International Society for Prevention of Child Abuse and Neglect.

Lutzker, J. R., McGill, T., Whitaker, D. J., & Self-Brown, S. (in press). SafeCare®: Preventing child neglect through scaling-up and examining implementation issues of an evidence-based practice. In R. Alexander, N. Guterman, & S. Alexander (Eds.), *Prevention of child maltreatment*. St. Louis, MO: G. W. Medical Publishing.

Metchikian, K. L., Mink, J. M., Bigelow, K. M., Lutzker, J. R., & Doctor, R. M. (1991). Reducing home safety hazards in the homes of parents reported for neglect. *Journal of Child & Family Behavior Therapy, 21*, 23–34.

Milner, J. S. (1986). *The Child Abuse Potential Inventory: Manual* (2nd ed.). Webster, NC: Psytec.

Murphey, D. A., & Braner, M. (2000). Linking child maltreatment retrospectively to birth and home visit records: An initial examination. *Journal of Policy, Practice, and Program, 79*(6), 711–728.

Prinz, R., Sanders, M., Shapiro, C., Whitaker, D., & Lutzker, J. (2009). Population-based prevention of child maltreatment: The U.S. Triple P system population trial. *Prevention Science, 10*(1), 1–12. doi:10.1007/s11121-009-0123-3

Self-Brown, S., Frederick, K., Binder, S., Whitaker, D., Lutzker, J. R., Edwards, A., & Blankenship, J. (2011). Examining the need for cultural adaptations to an evidence-based parent training program targeting the prevention of child maltreatment. *Children and Youth Services Review, 33*(7), 1166–1172. doi:10.1016/j.childyouth.2011.02.010

Shaffer, A., Kotchick, B. A., Dorsey, S., & Forehand, R. (2001). The past, present, and future of behavioral parent training: Interventions for child and adolescent problem behavior. *Behavior Analyst Today, 2*, 91–105.

Silovsky, J., Bard, D., Chaffin, M., Hecht, D. B., Burris, L., Owora, A., & Lutzker, J. (2011). Prevention of child maltreatment in high risk rural families: A randomized clinical trial with child welfare outcomes. *Children and Youth Services Review, 33*(8), 1435–1444.

Tertinger, D. A., Greene, B. F., & Lutzker, J. R. (1984). Home safety: Development and validation of one component of an ecobehavioral treatment program for abused and neglected children. *Journal of Applied Behavioral Analysis, 17,* 159–174. doi:10.1901/jaba.1984.17-159

U.S. Department of Health and Human Services, Administration for Children and Families, Administration on Children, Youth and Families, Children's Bureau. (2010). *Child maltreatment, 2008.* Washington, DC: U.S. Government Printing Office.

U.S. Department of Health and Human Services, Administration for Children and Families, Administration on Children, Youth and Families, Children's Bureau. (2012). *Child maltreatment, 2011.* Washington, DC: U.S. Government Printing Office.

Washington State Institute on Public Policy (2012, April). *Return on investment: Evidence-based options to improve statewide outcomes.* www.wsipp.wa.gov/rptfiles/12-04-1201.pdf

Whitaker, D. J., Lutzker, J. R., & Shelley, G. A. (2005). Child maltreatment prevention priorities at the Centers for Disease Control and Prevention. *Child Maltreatment, 10*(3), 245–259.

DAVID J. KOLKO, PH.D., ABPP
MONICA M. FITZGERALD, PH.D.
JESSICA L. LAUBACH, B.S.

6

Evidence-Based Practices for Working with Physically Abusive Families

Alternatives for Families: A Cognitive Behavioral Therapy

GENERAL CONSIDERATIONS

This chapter provides an overview of Alternatives for Families: A Cognitive Behavioral Therapy (AF-CBT), giving insights into the general nature of AF-CBT, its theoretical framework, target population, expected outcomes, empirical evidence, training requirements, and possible implementation obstacles. The chapter also highlights the unique disposition of AF-CBT to integrate several therapeutic methods.

WHAT IS THE FOCUS OF AF-CBT?

Alternatives for Families: A Cognitive Behavioral Therapy is an evidence-based intervention that targets individual characteristics of the child and caregiver that give rise to conflict and coercion in the home, as well as the family context in which aggression or abuse may occur (Kolko, 1996a, 1996b; Kolko et al., 2011; Kolko & Swenson, 2002). This approach emphasizes training in intra- and interpersonal skills designed to enhance self-control and reduce violent behavior. To do so, AF-CBT targets contributors to (or "risks" for) physically aggressive or abusive incidents within the child, caregiver, family, and community domains (Kolko & Kolko, 2010). Potential contributors include negative perceptions of children and developmentally inappropriate expectations, heightened anger or hostility, and harsh parenting practices, as well as coercive family interactions and heightened stressful life events. In turn, AF-CBT targets common sequelae (or "consequences") of exposure to conflict or abuse exhibited by children and caregivers. Potential targets include aggression or behavioral dysfunction, poor social competence, trauma-related emotional symptoms, developmental deficits in relationship skills, and cognitive impairments. Due to its addressing these consequences, AF-CBT has also been used as an intervention for children with behavior problems (e.g., oppositional and aggressive behavior).

WHICH CLIENTS ARE APPROPRIATE FOR AF-CBT?

AF-CBT is designed for families referred for conflict or coercion, verbal or physical aggression by caregivers (including the threat of physical force or use of excessive physical force, as well as behavior problems in children/adolescents), or child physical abuse. The treatment program has been expanded to accommodate children and adolescents with trauma symptoms related to physical abuse or discipline, such as posttraumatic stress disorder (PTSD). Thus, AF-CBT is recommended for use with (1) caregivers whose disciplinary or management strategies range from mild physical discipline to physically aggressive or abusive behaviors or who exhibit heightened levels of anger, hostility, or explosiveness, and/or (2) children who exhibit significant externalizing or aggressive behavior (e.g., oppositionality, antisocial behavior) with or without significant physical abuse / discipline–related trauma symptoms (e.g., anger, anxiety, PTSD), and/or (3) families who exhibit heightened conflict or coercion or pose threats to personal safety.

AF-CBT addresses both the risk factors and the consequences of physical, emotional, and verbal aggression in a comprehensive manner. Thus, AF-CBT seeks to address specific clinical targets among caregivers that include heightened anger or hostility, negative perceptions or attributions of their children, and difficulties in the appropriate and effective use of parenting practices, such as ineffective or punitive parenting practices. Likewise, AF-CBT targets children's difficulties with anger or anxiety, trauma-related emotional symptoms, poor social and relationship skills, behavior problems that include aggression, and dysfunctional attributions.

At the family level, AF-CBT addresses coercive family interactions by teaching skills to improve positive family relations and reduce family conflict.

FUNDAMENTALS OF AF-CBT

The content of AF-CBT is broken down into three phases: Engagement and Psychoeducation, Individual Skill Building, and Family Applications. However, there are some fundamental components of AF-CBT that are not specific to a particular phase or content area but are helpful in successfully implementing this treatment model. While some of the "fundamentals" are procedures or guidelines that are used during every session, other procedures are used whenever they are needed. The first component is *assessment*, which is an important part of any good treatment. The goal of assessment is to identify various family and clinical features of a case in order to decide whether AF-CBT is the best approach. Without appropriate assessment, clients may be subjected to unhelpful therapeutic methods, thus wasting time and resources. Assessment approaches may be structured and formal or informal, including information gathered from standardized self-report instruments or diagnostic interviews, clinical interviews, child protective services documents and caseworker reports, medical records, and direct observations. Comprehensive assessment allows the clinician to gain a full understanding of the client's current mental health and behavior problems, family strengths and deficits, and past problems, to guide clinical decision making and determine potential therapeutic needs (see chapter 2 of this volume).

After the initial assessment, practitioners continue to collect assessment information to monitor treatment response and provide ongoing feedback to the family about progress. Clinicians also conduct a discharge assessment to provide information about the impact of the treatment and to guide future planning. AF-CBT recommends four specific assessment measures: the Alabama Parenting Questionnaire (APQ; Frick, 1991); the Brief Child Abuse Potential Inventory (B-CAP; Ondersma et al., 2005), which was derived from the Child Abuse Potential Inventory (CAP; Milner & Ayoub, 1980); the Child PTSD Symptom Scale (CPSS; Foa et al., 2001); and the Strengths and Difficulties Questionnaire (SDQ; Goodman, Meltzer, & Bailey, 1998). These measures are intended to evaluate AF-CBT's primary clinical targets: (1) parenting practices and caregivers' externalizing behaviors (e.g., verbal and physical aggression, anger/arousal, child abuse potential) and the family's level of conflict/coercion and risk for physical aggression/abuse (e.g., frequent verbal and physical escalation, safety threats) (B-CAP; Ondersma et al., 2005); (2) the child's externalizing behavior and socioemotional functioning (e.g., emotional distress, conduct problems, attention problems, poor peer relations) (SDQ; Goodman et al., 1998); and (3) the child's posttraumatic stress (CPSS; Foa et al., 2001). Information about these areas is gathered from a number of sources, besides the standardized

instruments, and AF-CBT offers a recommended screen that can be used to evaluate a family's eligibility and guide professionals' clinical decision making. After an assessment determines that AF-CBT is an appropriate treatment for a particular client, a strategy called *functional analysis of behavior* is used throughout the course of treatment to determine a specific course of action for each client and address any new behavior problems. This strategy is described later in the chapter.

AF-CBT is implemented on a weekly basis, and in each session clinicians use a procedure called CA$H: Check-ins on Attendance, Safety, and Home practice. By implementing CA$H, the therapist can (1) validate the efforts of the family in remaining committed to treatment or address barriers that lead to absences from sessions, (2) assess the family's progress and use of discipline and/or coercive, harsh, threatening parenting behaviors, and (3) follow up on previously assigned home practice of skills. Home practice assignments may help the family identify the skills that are useful to them. Parenting behaviors, weekly practice, and skills are recorded and expanded throughout the treatment, using specific tracking tools and handouts (e.g., Weekly Safety Check-In, Alternatives for Families Plan). In the event that the children or caregivers convey any safety concerns or if there is any evidence of imminent risk, it is important to develop *safety plans*, another fundamental component of AF-CBT. Safety plans should incorporate three elements: (1) immediate removal from the escalated environment to keep the child safe, (2) short-term de-escalation for the caregiver to maintain self-control, and (3) a plan to resolve the conflict. Functional analysis, CA$H, the Alternatives for Families Plan, and safety plans are all important components for addressing progress and new concerns throughout the duration of AF-CBT.

CLINICAL CONTENT

As noted above and outlined in table 6.1, the content of AF-CBT is divided into three phases: Engagement and Psychoeducation, Individual Skill Building, and Family Applications. This content is based on principles and techniques from several perspectives, including learning and behavioral theory (Walker, Bonner, & Kaufmann, 1988; Wolfe, Sandler, & Kaufmann, 1981), family systems therapy (Alexander & Parsons, 1982; Anderson & Reiss, 1982; Robin & Foster, 1989), cognitive behavioral therapy (CBT; Fleischman, Horne, & Arthur, 1983; Frankel & Weiner, 1990), developmental victimology (Finklehor, 2007), and the psychology of aggression (Buss, 1961; O'Leary, 2008; O'Leary & Cohen, 2007). It also includes lessons learned from the application of interventions in collaboration with several experts and colleagues. The skills selected for training are designed to promote the use of prosocial skills (including self-control and affect regulation, assertiveness, communication, and problem solving), among other targets, that may serve as "alternatives" to the use of coercive or aggressive coping strategies. Accordingly,

Table 6.1. An Outline of the Focus and Content of Each Phase in AF-CBT

Phase	Session	Participant(s)
Phase 1: Engagement and Psychoeducation	1. Orientation	Child and caregiver
	2. Alliance Building & Engagement	Caregiver
	3. Learning about Feelings & Family Experiences	Child
	4. Family Experiences & Psychoeducation	Caregiver
Phase 2: Individual Skill Building	5. Emotion Regulation	Caregiver
	6. Emotion Regulation	Child
	7. Restructuring Thoughts	Caregiver
	8. Restructuring Thoughts	Child
	9. Promoting Positive Behavior	Caregiver
	10. Assertiveness & Social Skills	Child
	11. Techniques for Managing Behavior	Caregiver
	12. Imaginal Exposure / Meaning Making	Child
	13. Preparation for Clarification	Caregiver
Phase 3: Family Applications	14. Verbalizing Healthy Communication	Child and caregiver
	15. Enhancing Safety through Clarification	Child and caregiver
	16. Family Problem Solving	Child and caregiver
	17. Preparation for Graduation / Relapse Prevention	Child and caregiver

AF-CBT targets child, caregiver, and family characteristics. AF-CBT has a parallel parent/caregiver component, a child component, and an integrated caregiver-child skills development component. Thus, the participants for an AF-CBT session will vary depending on the topic of the session, as some sessions focus solely on the child or caregiver and are intended to be individual sessions, whereas others are joint sessions in which the child and caregiver(s) can work together on family-related issues or skills.

The content of AF-CBT is organized into 17 sessions or topics, but the sequencing of treatment components is flexible and should be modified as necessary to address pressing clinical needs. Understandably, the time needed to administer AF-CBT varies considerably with the severity and scope of family problems, the frequency of sessions, and the degree to which the family is motivated. AF-CBT has been found to be effective in a variety of settings, including outpatient mental health clinics, schools, homes, residential treatment facilities, partial programs, and other treatment centers (Kolko et al., 2012).

For a more in-depth look at how AF-CBT is conducted, we briefly describe the goals of each phase.

Phase 1: Engagement and Psychoeducation. This phase consists of four sessions and first aims to establish a supportive and trusting relationship with the family during both joint and individual child and caregiver sessions. Past experiences with therapy as well as current situations are discussed to evaluate how the therapist can tailor the therapy to the family's particular strengths and weaknesses.

Phase 2: Individual Skill Building. The second phase consists of approximately nine individual sessions that alternate between the child and caregiver(s). Skills are taught to both child and caregiver to help identify and regulate emotions and restructure problematic and unhelpful thoughts. Children are taught how to identify their triggers/cues for anger and anxiety and learn self-control techniques and stress management skills (e.g., controlled breathing, progressive muscle relaxation, positive self-statements). Caregivers are taught to notice their children's positive behaviors and learn specific behavioral techniques for managing negative, undesirable behaviors without the use of excessive or physical force. While the caregiver's skill deficits (and strengths) are being targeted, the child is taught assertiveness and effective social skills. After the child gains adequate coping skills (e.g., identifying and regulating emotions) within a safe therapeutic environment, the clinician uses imaginal exposure techniques to teach the child to overcome his or her anxiety and fears related to disturbing traumatic memories and intrusive thoughts of prior abuse or conflict within the family. Part of the skill building for caregivers involves preparing for a "clarification" session, during which caregivers discuss the abuse incident(s), take responsibility for their actions, acknowledge the impact of the abuse on the child, and comment on future plans for preventing abuse or conflict.

Phase 3: Family Applications. The final phase consists of four sessions, all of which are joint sessions with the child and caregiver(s). During this phase, the family learns about healthy communication styles and practices effective communication skills, which are essential to prepare for the final clarification session. The clarification session makes use of prior skills training and provides an opportunity for the family to discuss the abuse or conflict. The ultimate goal is for the family to be cohesive, respectful, and attentive to its commitments to maintain a safe and loving environment. To achieve this goal, the family identifies communication obstacles and alternatives and practices new communication skills, in and outside sessions. In this phase, the family is also taught formal problem-solving skills and makes specific plans for avoiding conflict/abuse in the future. These skills are integrated with other skill techniques previously learned and reinforced throughout treatment, such as positive parenting techniques, assertiveness, and social skills with family and friends.

The cumulative goal of these three phases is not only to help families communicate about and understand their past conflicts or coercive experiences but also to provide them with the tools to manage and eventually reduce the level of family conflict and physical aggression in the future (Kolko et al., 2011).

UNDERLYING RATIONALE AND THEORETICAL FRAMEWORK

One of the unique aspects of AF-CBT is that it combines elements from a variety of theories and techniques. Because of this conceptual diversity, AF-CBT can provide an integrated treatment comprising the most successful aspects of other empirically validated interventions. Of course, the main framework of AF-CBT draws heavily on cognitive behavioral therapy and behavioral or learning theory, with its focus on functional analysis, skills training methods, and the judicious use of consequences (Fleischman et al., 1983; Frankel & Weiner, 1990; Walker, Bonner, and Kaufmann., 1988; Wolfe, Sandler, & Kaufmann, 1981). In addition, AF-CBT draws from cognitive therapy methods that articulate how beliefs and attributions influence emotional reactions and behaviors and how they can be modified through experiential exercises (Beck, 1976; Bugental, Mantyla, & Lewis, 1989). It also incorporates a systems perspective as found in family therapy models that examine patterns of interactions among family members in order to identify and alleviate problems and develop strategies to help reframe how problems are viewed (Alexander & Parsons, 1982; Anderson & Reiss, 1982; Robin & Foster, 1989). Developmental victimology (Finklehor, 2007)—which describes how the specific sequelae of exposure to traumatic or abusive experiences may vary for children at different developmental stages and across the lifespan—also contributes to the structure of AF-CBT, with its inclusion of an imaginal exposure component. AF-CBT also incorporates ideas from the psychology of aggression (Buss, 1961; O'Leary, 2008; O'Leary & Cohen, 2007), which describes the processes by which aggression and coercion develop and are maintained, thus helping the individual to understand his or her history as both a contributor to and a victim of aggressive behavior (Child Welfare Information Gateway, 2007).

Though AF-CBT melds a variety of theories and techniques, its main framework is derived from CBT. The role of assessment is central to CBT in that it guides the selection and administration of key treatment tasks—selecting goals, delivering content, and preparing for termination. The underlying model of assessment in CBT is called *functional analysis*. A functional analysis or "ABC Model" (antecedents, behavior, and consequences) includes an assessment of what occurs before (A) and after (C) the problem behavior (B), as well as a detailed description of the behavior itself. Thus, the therapist will directly intervene with the behavior itself, its antecedents, and/or its consequences. Problem behavior can broadly reflect thoughts, feelings, or actions. The therapist closely assesses the frequency, duration, intensity, and pervasiveness of the problem behavior and plans the intervention(s) collaboratively with the caregiver.

Functional analysis in AF-CBT attempts to provide a careful and objective assessment of problem behaviors exhibited by children (e.g., externalizing behaviors, avoidance of trauma reminders), caregivers (e.g., aggression), and families (e.g., conflict). The following are examples of problem behaviors and their functions/consequences that would be addressed through functional analysis in AF-CBT: (1) a child who interrupts family meals and is "punished" by being removed to his room may be seeking escape from family disagreements common at the dinner table; and (2) an adult who regularly attends mandated therapy but ignores assigned tasks may be seeking a tangible reward (such as the child protective system closing the case due to a consistent attendance record). In addition, functional analysis in AF-CBT warrants an assessment of specific antecedents (e.g., history of abuse/conflict, life stressors) and consequences (e.g., caregivers' positive and negative parenting strategies; a youth's risky behaviors, such as gang activity or substance use). To assess the impact of the interventions implemented and progress toward behavioral goals, the therapist tracks behavioral changes (frequency, intensity, duration, pervasiveness). Assessment findings determine how AF-CBT treatment components are implemented for each individual child (Kolko et. al, 2011).

EXPECTED OUTCOMES

Studies of AF-CBT have shown improved outcomes for caregivers, children, and families who participate in this treatment. In families, caregivers achieved individual treatment goals related to the use of more effective discipline methods, and caregivers reported decreased overall psychological stress, decreased child abuse potential, and less drug abuse. AF-CBT has also demonstrated positive child welfare outcomes such as a decreased rate of abuse relapse or concerns about the child being harmed. Children participating in AF-CBT show increased well-being and safety from harm, as well as decreased feelings of fear, anxiety, anger, and sadness (Kolko et al., 2011). Other demonstrated outcomes in children are reductions in parent-reported severity of externalizing behavior problems, including child-to-parent aggression and the likelihood of violating other children's privacy. Children also reported greater family cohesion, and both children and parents reported reduced family conflict (Kolko et al., 2011).

EVIDENCE BASE / EMPIRICAL SUPPORT

Based on systematic reviews of available research, several groups of experts and federal agencies have highlighted the promise and benefits of AF-CBT as a treatment practice. This program has been featured in sources from the Chadwick Center for Children and Families, the National Child Traumatic Stress Network, the National Crime Victims Research and Treatment Center, the Center for Sexual Assault and Traumatic Stress of the U.S. Department of Justice, and the California Evidence-Based Clearinghouse for Child Welfare, and it has been approved as an evidence-based treatment by the Los Angeles County Office of Mental Health. Additionally, dissemination of AF-CBT has been included in the Effective Providers for Child Victims of Violence Program of the American Psychological Association. The accumulation of such widespread support is due to the empirical evidence supporting AF-CBT. Efforts at AF-CBT dissemination have been successful in diverse clinical and academic settings in the United States and, more recently, in other countries as well (e.g., Canada, England, Germany, Holland, Israel, Italy, Japan). Reports from trained practitioners generally indicate positive results in terms of clinical improvements (e.g., reductions in parental use of force/abusive behavior, improved parent-child relationships) and successful case closures in the child protective service system.

During the past three decades, outside investigators have evaluated many of the procedures incorporated into AF-CBT as effective in improving child, parent, and/or family functioning, as well as in promoting safety and/or reducing abuse risk or re-abuse among various populations of parents, children, and families. These procedures have included the use of stress management and anger-control training, cognitive restructuring, parenting skills training, psychoeducational information on the use and impact of physical force and hostility, social skills training, imaginal exposure, and family interventions focusing on reducing conflict (see Kolko & Swenson, 2002; Kolko & Kolko, 2010; Urquiza & Runyon, 2010).

In early studies, we found that use of the individual child/parent CBT and family therapy components now integrated into AF-CBT showed greater improvements than did routine community services in certain outcomes for children (child-to-parent aggression, child externalizing behavior), parents (child abuse potential, individual treatment targets reflecting abusive behavior, psychological distress, drug use), and families (conflict, cohesion; Kolko, 1996b). Official child welfare records for the entire study period revealed lower, albeit nonsignificantly, rates of recidivism among the adults who participated in individual CBT (5%) and family therapy (6%) compared with those in routine community services (30%). Parallel rates of recidivism were found for the identified abused children in the three conditions used in the study: CBT (10%), family therapy (12%), and routine services (30%). Both CBT and family therapy were conducted with high fidelity, had high rates of session attendance, and had high client satisfaction ratings. In a second study, we found that family reports of parental anger and use of force during treatment decreased for CBT and family therapy, but the decline was significantly faster for

CBT (Kolko, 1996a). This study provides empirical justification for monitoring and then addressing potential indicators of potential abusive behavior during treatment, using weekly session ratings (initially described as the Weekly Report of Abuse Indicators, WRAI).

A more recent study examined the long-term sustainability and outcome of AF-CBT as delivered by practitioners in a community-based child protection program who had received training in the model several years earlier (Kolko, Iselin, & Gully, 2011). The program's routine evaluation system was used to document the clinical and treatment outcomes of 52 families presenting with a physically abused child, between two and five years after receiving training with AF-CBT content. The amount of AF-CBT general and abuse-specific content delivered was found to predict several clinical and functional improvements in both children and caregivers, above and beyond the influence of the unique content of other evidence-based treatments that were used. The two AF-CBT content scores were differentially related to several of these outcomes. These novel naturalistic data document the sustainability and clinical benefits of AF-CBT in an existing community clinic serving physically abused children and their families, and the data are discussed in the context of key developments in the treatment model and dissemination literature.

There is also experimental evidence for the dissemination of AF-CBT (Kolko et al., 2012) with community practitioners in programs working in child welfare or mental health. Evidence suggests that practitioners trained in AF-CBT (vs. those who received training as usual) showed increased knowledge about CBT and its targeted population, the use of AF-CBT teaching processes, abuse-specific skills, and general psychological skills. Additionally, those trained in AF-CBT reported a high level of satisfaction with the program. However, both groups (AF-CBT training and training as usual) reported a decline in the level of morale within their organizations. Certainly, more work is needed to evaluate the relative benefits of alternative treatment training methods and the everyday issues that affect the stability of this workforce.

Parallel research has examined the effectiveness of the core content of AF-CBT and other clinical procedures with children referred for behavior problems. Recent clinical trials documented the benefits of receiving modular treatment in the clinic or the community for several outcomes (Kolko et al., 2009). In addition, AF-CBT content delivered in an on-site intervention has been found to improve access to mental health services and outcomes for children with behavior problems in primary care, relative to enhanced usual care (Kolko, Baumann, et al., 2012; Kolko, Campo, et al., 2010). For example, patients assigned to a nurse-administered intervention condition were significantly more likely to receive and complete mental health services, reported fewer service barriers and more patient satisfaction, and showed greater improvements on clinical outcomes, including remission of behavioral disorders at one-year follow-up. The incorporation of this diverse clinical content into a collaborative care approach applied in pediatric primary care offices has also been associated with several clinical improvements (including reductions in oppositional and aggressive behavior, hyperactivity, and functional impairment).

Besides this examination of the efficacy of implementing AF-CBT in the context of primary care clinics and community settings, its use has also been explored in schools (Herschell et al., 2012). The school setting is suitable for training individual students or groups of students in key AF-CBT general psychological skills, such as emotional regulation, cognitive processing, and social skills. However, challenges to applying AF-CBT services in this setting include logistical problems such as staff training, finding space and time for therapeutic work, and maintaining the appropriate level of confidentiality. Current applications are underway to tailor both the model and its implementation context for efficient use in school settings.

Based on this brief summary of a few empirical studies, emerging evidence suggests that for families involved in abuse or conflict, AF-CBT is an effective treatment in alternative settings and its positive outcomes extend to children, parents, and families. Additionally, studies show that clinicians trained in AF-CBT are provided with therapeutic methods that they use several years after training has ended.

TRAINING

Interested practitioners may want to explore the AF-CBT website (www.afcbt.org), which offers resource materials and information about clinician training. AF-CBT training is specifically suited for mental health practitioners who work with families involved in physical abuse, harsh discipline, or chronic hostility. Table 6.2 provides a brief overview of a representative training program in AF-CBT. In general, the training process begins with a three-day in-person seminar. During this seminar, the rationale and process of AF-CBT are explained, and clinicians are given an opportunity to role-play a variety of scenarios they may encounter with their clients. Behavioral rehearsal and role-playing are often used to train practitioners and to instruct clients in the use of AF-CBT, insofar as practicing skills in session may be the most effective way to teach families how to use them between sessions (see Beidas & Kendall, 2010; Herschell et al., 2010). Practitioners being trained in AF-CBT receive a session guide that highlights general concepts and provides an in-depth protocol for each of the 17 proposed sessions of AF-CBT. Practitioners also receive study materials, worksheets for clients, and handouts to illustrate the concepts of AF-CBT. After the initial three-day workshop seminar, professional training continues over the course of a year. During that time, there are monthly consultations with AF-CBT professionals so that clinicians can discuss their ongoing cases and receive feedback. In addition, practitioners submit digital audio files of recent sessions for review and structured feedback by the trainer.

Table 6.2. Representative AF-CBT Training: Typical Professional Training Program—One-year "Learning Community"

1. Agency readiness discussions to promote organizational/staff preparedness
2. Trainee background assessment and agency metrics (pre- and post-training evaluation)
3. Development of training materials (slides) and exercises tailored to agency/population; delivery of AF-CBT session guides (manual, handouts) and assessment materials
4. Basic training workshop / experiential seminar on use of AF-CBT (3 days)
5. Advanced training workshop 6 months later (half or full day; video conference)
6. Monthly case consultation calls with trainer (12 calls; 2 presentations per call)
7. Fidelity monitoring feedback based on trainer's reviews of digital audio files uploaded by each trainee to secure website (2 files per trainee).
8. Supervisor support calls (4 per year)
9. Online access to the trainer for Q&A and to receive new materials (via website)
10. Program data summary—baseline and follow-up evaluation / agency metrics

Observations and ratings based on all of this initial experience are then used to inform the conduct of a midpoint advanced training workshop, which is offered to ensure that clinicians are able to address common implementation obstacles and more fully understand how to incorporate and adapt relevant AF-CBT content into their therapy sessions.

IMPLEMENTATION CONSIDERATIONS

The diversity of family circumstances and individual problems associated with family conflict points to the need for a comprehensive treatment strategy that targets contributors to both caregivers' behavior and children's subsequent behavioral and emotional adjustment (Chadwick Center for Children and Families, 2004). Treatment approaches such as AF-CBT that focus on several aspects of the problem (e.g., a caregiver's parenting skills, a child's anger, family coercion) may have a greater likelihood of reducing re-abuse and more fully remediating mental health problems (Kolko & Swenson, 2002). However, clinicians must tailor the material to the individual needs of the family, which requires clinicians' decision making about the nature and order of the content to be administered and can complicate maintaining fidelity in implementing this intervention. Additionally, the standard of cognitive functioning required for clients to fully benefit from AF-CBT may limit which clients are most appropriate for the use of certain methods. For example, parents with psychiatric disorders that may significantly impair their general functioning or their ability to learn new skills (e.g., substance use disorders, major depression) may benefit from alternative or adjunctive interventions designed to address these problems (Chadwick Center for Children and Families, 2004). Children or parents with very limited intellectual functioning or developmental disabilities, or very young children, may require more simplified services or translations of some of the more complicated treatment concepts. Children with psychiatric disorders such as significant attention-deficit disorder or major depression may benefit from additional interventions. Children who have a recent history of sexual abuse that is associated with heightened posttraumatic stress symptoms have been shown to respond well to other intervention models, such as Trauma-Focused CBT (see Cohen et al., 2010).

CONCLUSIONS

Alternatives for Families: A Cognitive Behavioral Therapy is a unique therapy that targets both verbal and physical aggression in families, including family conflict, caregiver or child coercion or aggression, or child physical abuse. To work with this broad target population, AF-CBT teaches diverse psychological skills to children, caregivers, and families to help them find alternatives to the use of explosive anger and aggression. These procedures include the use of stress management and anger-control training, cognitive restructuring, parenting skills training, psychoeducational information on the use and impact of physical force and hostility, social skills training, imaginal exposure, and family interventions focused on reducing conflict (see Kolko & Swenson, 2002; Kolko & Kolko, 2010; Runyon & Urquiza, 2011). The implementation of several of these skills is explicitly coordinated to maximize the likelihood that they are used and encouraged by both children and caregivers. In addition, the integration of content domains and specific treatment components based on several conceptual models was designed to address the various clinical features of families involved in coercive behavior. There is emerging support indicating that these treatment elements are associated with improvements in the well-being of the child and the family and in child safety and welfare, as prior findings suggest that family members report reductions in family conflict, in aggression and hostility, and in a child's risk of harm. However encouraging these findings may be, developments are needed that can enhance the efficiency with which AF-CBT is applied and can expand its availability to ensure that the many practitioners who regularly serve these challenging families in diverse settings are supported during the course of routine practice.

Acknowledgments

Preparation of this chapter was supported, in part, by grants from the National Institute of Mental Health (074737) and the Substance Abuse and Mental Health Services Administration (SM54319). We acknowledge our AF-CBT team collaborators: Barbara Baumann, Elissa Brown, Daniel Kleiner, Kevin Rumsbarger, and Meghan Shaver.

References

Alexander, J., & Parsons, B. (1982). *Functional family therapy.* Monterey, CA: Brooks/Cole.

Anderson, C. M., & Reiss, D. (1982). Approaches to psychoeducational family therapy. *International Journal of Family Psychiatry, 3,* 501–517.

Beck, A. T. (1976). *Cognitive therapy and the emotional disorders.* New York, NY: International Universities Press.

Beidas, R. S., & Kendall, P. C. (2010). Training therapists in evidence-based practice: A critical review of studies from a systems-contextual perspective. *Clinical Psychology: Science and Practice, 17,* 1–30.

Bugental, D. B., Mantyla, S. M., & Lewis, J. (1989). Parental attributions as moderators of affective communication to children at risk for physical abuse. In D. Cicchetti & V. Carlson (Eds.), *Child maltreatment: Theory and research on the causes and consequences of child abuse and neglect* (pp. 254–259). New York, NY: Cambridge University Press.

Buss, A. H. (1961). *The psychology of aggression.* Hoboken, NJ: John Wiley & Sons.

Chadwick Center for Children and Families. (2004). *Closing the quality chasm in child abuse treatment: Identifying and disseminating best practices.* San Diego, CA: Author. www.chadwickcenter.org/Documents/Kaufman Report/ChildHosp-NCTA brochure.pdf

Child Welfare Information Gateway. (2007). *Alternatives for Families: Cognitive-Behavioral Therapy (AF-CBT).* Washington, DC: U.S. Department of Health and Human Services.

Cohen, J. A., Berliner, L., & Mannarino, A. (2010). Trauma-focused CBT with co-occurring trauma and behavior problems. *Child Abuse & Neglect, 34,* 215–224.

Finklehor, D. (2007). Developmental victimology: The comprehensive study of childhood victimizations. In R. C. Davis, A. J. Luirigio, & S. Herman (Eds.), *Victims of crime* (3rd ed, pp. 9–34). Thousand Oaks, CA: Sage Publications.

Fleischman, M., Horne, A., & Arthur, J. (1983). *Troubled families: A treatment program.* Champaign, IL: Research Press.

Foa, E. B., Johnson, K. M., Feeny, N. C., & Treadwell K. R. H. (2001). The Child PTSD Symptom Scale: A preliminary examination of its psychometric properties. *Journal of Clinical Child and Adolescent Psychology, 30*(3), 376–384.

Frankel, F., & Weiner, H. (1990). The Child Conflict Index: Factor analysis, reliability, and validity for clinic-referred and nonreferred children. *Journal of Clinical Child Psychology, 19,* 239–248.

Frick, P. J. (1991). *Alabama Parenting Questionnaire.* Tuscaloosa, AL: P. J. Frick, University of Alabama.

Goodman, R., Meltzer, H., & Bailey, V. (1998). The strengths and difficulties questionnaire: A pilot study on the validity of the self-report version. *European Child & Adolescent Psychiatry, 7*(3), 125–130.

Herschell, A. D., Kolko, D. J., Baumann, B. L., & Brown, E. J. (2012). Application of Alternatives for Families: A Cognitive-Behavioral Therapy to school settings. *Journal of Applied School Psychology, 28,* 270–293.

Herschell, A. D., Kolko, D. J., Baumann, B. L., & Davis, A. C. (2010). The role of therapist training in the implementation of psychosocial treatments: A review and critique with recommendations. *Clinical Psychology Review, 30*(4), 448–466.

Jellinek, M. S., Murphy, J. M., Little, M., Pagano, M. E., Comer, D. M., & Kelleher, K. J. (1999). Use of the Pediatric Symptom Checklist (PSC) to screen for psychosocial problems in pediatric primary care: A national feasibility study. *Archives of Pediatric and Adolescent Medicine, 153*(3):254–260.

Kolko, D. J. (1996a). Clinical monitoring of treatment course in child physical abuse: Psychometric characteristics and treatment comparisons. *Child Abuse & Neglect, 20*(1), 23–43.

Kolko, D. J. (1996b). Individual cognitive-behavioral treatment and family therapy for physically abused children and their offending parents: A comparison of clinical outcomes. *Child Maltreatment, 1,* 322–342.

Kolko, D. J., Baumann, B. L., Herschell, A. D., Hart, J. A., & Wisniewski, S. (2012). Implementation of AF-CBT by community practitioners serving mental health and child welfare: A randomized trial. *Child Maltreatment, 17,* 32–46.

Kolko, D. J., Brown, E. J., Shaver, M. E., Baumann, B. L., & Herschell, A. D. (2011). *Alternatives for Families: A Cognitive-Behavioral Therapy: Session guide* (3rd ed.). Pittsburgh, PA: University of Pittsburgh School of Medicine.

Kolko, D. J., Campo, J. V., Kelleher, K., & Cheng, Y. (2010). Improving access to care and clinical outcome for pediatric behavioral problems: A randomized trial of a nurse-administered intervention in primary care. *Journal of Behavioral and Developmental Pediatrics, 31,* 393–404.

Kolko, D. J., Dorn, L. D., Bukstein, O. G., Pardini, D., Holden, E. A., & Hart, J. D. (2009). Community vs. clinic-based modular treatment of children with early-onset ODD or CD: A clinical trial with three-year follow-up. *Journal of Abnormal Child Psychology, 37,* 591–609.

Kolko, D. J., Iselin, A. M., & Gully, K. (2011). Evaluation of the sustainability and clinical outcome of Alternatives for Families: A Cognitive-Behavioral Therapy (AF-CBT) in a child protection center. *Child Abuse & Neglect, 35,* 105–116.

Kolko, D. J., & Kolko, R. P. (2010). Psychological impact and treatment of child physical abuse. In C. Jenny (Ed.), *Child abuse and neglect: Diagnosis, treatment, and evidence* (pp. 476–489). New York, NY: Elsevier.

Kolko, D. J., & Swenson, C. C. (2002). *Assessing and treating physically abused children and their families: A cognitive behavioral approach.* Thousand Oaks, CA: Sage Publications.

Milner, J. S., & Ayoub, C. (1980) Evaluation of "at risk" parents using the Child Abuse Potential inventory. *Journal of Clinical Psychology, 36*(4), 945–948.

O'Leary, K. D. (2008). Couple therapy and physical aggression. In A. S. Gurman (Ed.), *Clinical handbook of couple therapy* (pp. 478–498). New York, NY: Guilford Press.

O'Leary, K. D., & Cohen, S. (2007). Treatment of psychological and physical aggression in a couple context. In J. Hammel & A. Nicholls (Eds.), *Family interventions in domestic violence: A handbook of gender inclusive theory and treatment.* New York, NY: Springer.

Ondersma, S. J., Chaffin, M., Simpson, S., & LeBreton, J. (2005). The Brief Child Abuse Potential inventory: Development and validation. *Journal of Clinical Child and Adolescent Psychology, 34,* 301–311.

Robin, A. L., & Foster, S. L. (1989). *Negotiating parent/adolescent conflict: A behavioral-family systems approach.* New York, NY: Guilford Press.

Runyon, M. K., & Urquiza, A. J. (2011) Child physical abuse: Interventions for parents who engage in coercive parenting practices and their children. In J. E. B. Myers (Ed.), *The APSAC handbook on child maltreatment* (pp. 195–212). Thousand Oaks, CA: Sage Publications.

Urquiza, A., & Runyon, M. (2010). Interventions for physically abusive parents and abused children. In J. E. B. Myers (Ed.), *The APSAC handbook on child maltreatment* (pp. 195–212). Thousand Oaks, CA: Sage Publications.

Walker, C. E., Bonner, B. L., & Kaufmann, K. L. (1988). *The physically and sexually abused child: Evaluation and treatment.* New York, NY: Pergamon Press.

Wolfe, D. A., Sandler, J., & Kaufmann, K. (1981). A competency based parent-training program for child abusers. *Journal of Consulting and Clinical Psychology, 49,* 633–640.

MELISSA K. RUNYON, PH.D.
COLETTE MCLEAN, LCSW

7

Empowering Families

Combined Parent-Child Cognitive Behavioral Therapy for Families at Risk for Child Physical Abuse

GENERAL CONSIDERATIONS

In 2011, the U.S. Department of Health and Human Services Administration for Children and Families reported that in 2010, approximately 695,000 children in the United States were victims of maltreatment. More than 17% of these children were physically abused. These statistics support the need for evidenced-based treatments (EBTs) developed specifically for this population. Combined Parent-Child Cognitive Behavioral Therapy (CPC-CBT): Empowering Families Who Are at Risk for Physical Abuse is one of only a few programs on the National Registry of Evidence-based Programs and Practices website (www.nrepp.samhsa.gov) that include both the parent and child in treatment to address the needs of families at risk for child physical abuse. CPC-CBT is a structured EBT for children ages 3–17 years and their parents (or caregivers) in families where parents engage in a continuum of coercive parenting strategies. CPC-CBT is designed not only for families where child physical abuse has been substantiated but also for families considered at risk for physical abuse. The program aims to reduce children's posttraumatic stress disorder (PTSD) symptoms, other internalizing symptoms, and behavior problems while improving parenting skills and parent-child relationships and reducing the use of corporal punishment by parents. This chapter presents an overview of CPC-CBT with an illustrative case example, the conceptual model underlying this therapy, research support for the model, appropriate clients, and expected outcomes associated with CPC-CBT.

CPC-CBT was initially developed as a group program (Runyon, Deblinger, & Schroeder, 2009; Runyon, Deblinger, & Steer, 2010), but it has been delivered in an individual format in Sweden (Kjellgren, Svedin, & Nilsson, in press) and the United States (Runyon, Deblinger, & Schroeder, 2010). Both formats can be delivered in 16–20 sessions across four phases: Engagement and Psychoeducation, Effective Coping Skills Building, Family Safety Planning, and Abuse Clarification. In the group setting, sessions are two hours with a maximum of five families (up to eight children) per group. Parents are in one group and their children are in a separate group, with two trained clinicians in each subgroup. For individual therapy, CPC-CBT is typically implemented in a 90-minute session but can be modified for 60-minute sessions, depending on the setting. Individual CPC-CBT can be administered by one trained clinician or by two co-clinicians sharing one family. In both group and individual formats, treatment begins with parents and children spending more time in their respective sessions, with a 5- to 10-minute joint session. Families spend progressively more time in joint meetings as treatment progresses.

The following case example illustrates a parent's response to some of the skills and exercises offered across the CPC-CBT phases. The names and details have been changed to protect the identity of the family.

> An 11-year-old girl, Mia, and her mother, Sharon, were referred for CPC-CBT due to substantiated allegations of child physical abuse (CPA) after Sharon reportedly "beat up" and tried to choke Mia, after Mia refused to complete her chores. The incident resulted in bruises on Mia's face and scratch marks around her neck. Mia tried to cover the marks, but they were discovered by the school, which then contacted child protective services (CPS). CPS subsequently required Sharon to complete an anger management and parenting program. At the initial therapy appointment, Sharon presented as unremorseful and blamed Mia for the CPS involvement. The initial assessment revealed that Mia was depressed, blamed herself for the abuse, and was exhibiting posttraumatic stress symptoms.

THE PHASES OF CPC-CBT

Engagement and Psychoeducation

Treatment programs for CPA should begin by engaging the parents, many of whom are guarded and hesitant and possibly unreceptive to mental health interventions, thus resulting in a high dropout rate for this population. The initial phase of CPC-CBT, the Engagement and Psychoeducation phase, is therefore critical. In fact, in a controlled trial examining CPC-CBT, the attrition rate was only 12% at posttreatment for families who completed the initial engagement sessions (the first three sessions; Runyon, Deblinger, & Steer, 2010). This phase involves working with parents to identify barriers that might hinder a commitment to treatment and problem solving around these barriers; eliciting parents' goals and matching them with the goals of the treatment model; communicating empathy, without condoning abusive behavior; and instilling hope for positive change. Common concrete barriers that are identified early in treatment include transportation, childcare needs for siblings during appointments, and being overwhelmed by the number of required services to attend concurrently. It is important to note that whenever possible, identifying some of these barriers prior to the initial therapy session—for example, at intake or over the phone—has improved the success rates of getting families in for treatment. Successful methods have been developed to use at the first phone contact and during the initial intake appointment to enhance engagement and thus reduce no-show rates (McKay, McCadam, & Pennington, 2002; McKay et al., 1998). Working with a family to both understand the barriers and advocate for the family's needs makes a difference in building a parent's confidence and trust in the treatment process.

The therapist initially establishes a collaborative working relationship with parents by discussing their goals, emphasizing common objectives, identifying and eliminating barriers to treatment, and conducting problem solving around immediate concerns (Runyon & Deblinger, in press; Runyon, Deblinger, & Schroeder, 2009; Runyon, Deblinger & Steer, 2010). Next, a disclosure of the referral incident is obtained from the parent to elicit thoughts and feelings before, during, and after the incident. During this exercise, the clinician has an opportunity to elicit from the parent what his or her parenting experience is like and what occurred with the child from the parent's perspective. Not only does this exercise allow the clinician to empathize with the parent and acknowledge the stress and challenges the parent experiences in relation to parenting, but it also provides an assessment of the level of responsibility the parent takes for the abusive behavior.

After the shared details of the referral incident, or of an anger-provoking parenting situation (when a specific physical discipline incident is not available), the clinician uses the consequence review, a motivational procedure, and other motivational interviewing principles (Donohue et al., 1998) to increase the parent's motivation for behavior change. During the consequence review, parents are encouraged to record and process the consequences of their abusive behavior for themselves and their children (e.g., CPS report, child removed from the home). The clinician can refer to this list of consequences during the course of treatment to help motivate the parent to change, learn new skills, enhance existing skills, and persevere in applying new approaches to parenting in an effort to avoid these consequences in the future. This gives the clinician an opportunity to empathize and align with parents around the negative consequences experienced as a result of their actions and to instill hope for change. After the consequence review, parents are asked to make a commitment to try not to use physical discipline throughout the course of treatment. The therapist explains to parents that if physical discipline is used, it will be difficult for the parents to know whether new strategies work. Clinicians should also emphasize that making this commitment reduces the risk of further consequences.

Children's sessions also involve engagement and introducing emotional expression skills. Children begin to learn a vocabulary of feeling words, strategies for appropriately expressing emotions, and emotional regulation skills. The initial joint session with the parent and child is for observational purposes. In the second joint session, the parent practices with the clinician and then gives the child permission to talk during sessions about what happened related to the referral incident, interactions with the parent(s), and home life.

This initial phase also involves psychoeducation about abuse and violence with both parents and children. First, the clinician offers psychoeducation about the three kinds of abuse (physical, sexual, and emotional) and violence. To diffuse defensiveness, this education begins by asking the parent, "Tell me about any abuse and violence that your child has been exposed to in your home or community." Parents inevitably begin by discussing their own abuse history, which gives the therapist an opportunity to examine its impact on their relationships with their own parents and their parenting style. This strategy also serves as an empathy-building exercise where parents examine parallels between their relationship with their parents and their relationship with their children. Parents also review experienced and potential consequences of CPA (short- and long-term behavioral and emotional effects) and are educated about the ineffectiveness of physical abuse in making positive, lasting changes in child behaviors. Psychoeducation also includes education for both parents and children about the continuum of coercive behavior and the impact of violent behavior on children. Parents also learn about child development and realistic expectations for children's behavior.

While Sharon recounted the stressful details of the incident of CPA associated with the treatment referral, the therapist elicited her thoughts and feelings related to the incident and empathized with the challenges of parenting Mia. Next, the therapist elicited consequences of Sharon's behavior. Sharon reported: "(1) The State is interfering with my right to discipline my child; (2) CPS is involved in my life; (3) Mia thinks she can get away with anything, because I can't discipline her; (4) I might not be able to work at the day care center; (5) My family criticizes me about coming to therapy." The therapist assisted Sharon in processing her thoughts and feelings related to these negative experiences and offered empathy. In response to the educational handouts about physical punishment, Sharon presented her Bible. She reported that she diligently looked for information to dispute what the "professionals" were saying regarding physical punishment. Instead she found passages that supported the "professional" viewpoint, including passages that discourage disciplining children in anger. Sharon identified that she was losing her temper when disciplining Mia and was allowing her anger to affect her reactions. She declared that she was "doing all the wrong things for the right reasons" to parent Mia.

Parenting skills training begins with the introduction of praise in the initial phase and continues across all phases. Clinicians also help families develop effective communication skills to increase family members' feelings of validation and cooperation with one another. Over the course of CPC-CBT, parents practice the implementation of active listening, communication skills, and positive parenting skills, first with the therapist and then in the joint session with their child. The therapist acts as a coach by offering positive reinforcement and corrective feedback to enhance these skills.

Effective Coping Skills Building

After the initial phase of therapy, clinicians move into the phase of effective coping skills, where psychoeducation and positive parenting skills are continued. There is also an emphasis on empowering parents to be effective by working collaboratively with them to develop adaptive coping skills (cognitive coping, anger management, relaxation, assertiveness, self-care, problem solving, etc.) to assist them in remaining calm while interacting with their child and in developing nonviolent conflict resolution skills, a variety of problem-solving skills related to child rearing, and noncoercive child behavior management skills. During training in cognitive coping skills, parents are taught age-appropriate expectations for their children, as well as how to consider alternative explanations for troublesome child behavior, to help change parents' automatic reactions. Parents learn to strengthen and identify ways to manage stressful and anger-provoking situations through basic techniques such as the art of "walking away" to cool down. As sessions progress, skills are integrated as clinicians use a functional analysis of the antecedents, behaviors, and consequences (ABCs) during parent-child interactions. Anger-monitoring forms are used with

parents in session. Clinicians also ask parents to implement at home, on a weekly basis, the techniques and strategies learned in session. In subsequent sessions, during review of the ABCs, new coping and parenting skills are introduced, behavior plans are developed, and individually tailored parenting strategies are added to the parent's toolbox. Throughout therapy, the parent and therapist work collaboratively. Concurrently, children are learning age-appropriate effective coping skills (e.g., cognitive coping, assertiveness, anger management, and social, empathy, relaxation, and problem-solving skills). Clinicians also may incorporate teaching children how to take no for an answer from a parent, how to make requests of their parents, and how to problem-solve school and peer situations.

During the skill-building phase, Sharon was receptive to new parenting strategies, because she identified that her use of yelling and threats with Mia was not getting her the results she wanted. She gradually embraced the benefits of using praise and saw how her relationship with Mia and Mia's self-esteem had suffered because the family treated Mia as an outsider, especially after CPS got involved. Sharon and Mia worked together to develop house rules for the entire family. Sharon practiced active listening skills with Mia during joint sessions. Each week she was asked to complete the anger-monitoring form and bring it in for review. While reviewing the forms in session, Sharon received guidance on how to handle these situations. As sessions continued, Sharon had fewer incidents of losing her temper with Mia, as she was managing her reactions with cognitive coping and anger management strategies.

Family Safety Planning

While elements of safety are discussed during every phase of CPC-CBT, general safety skills and the development of a family safety plan are introduced during the third phase. It is important to determine whether the family is ready to develop a safety plan by assessing whether the parent and child are reporting an increase in the use of positive parenting strategies, the parent is abstaining from using physical discipline, and the parent is exhibiting an increased capacity to manage anger-provoking situations. This assessment is based on the parent's report, clinical observations, and the child's report of changes in the parent and their relationship. After these changes have been noted, the therapist can introduce the family safety plan. As it is likely that the parent or other family member will become frustrated again in the future, the family safety plan is for the "just in case" moment when anger begins to escalate. It is developed collaboratively by the parent and child. The parent agrees that the safety plan can be initiated by all members of the family when there is concern about the anger level or uncertainty about how a family member will react in a given moment. The safety plan gives the parent an opportunity to gain control by taking a step back and thinking through how to address the child's problem behavior in order to get the desired response. Components of the safety plan include (1) selecting two or three code words from which the child can choose; (2) establishing places in the home where each family member will go when the code word is called; (3) determining a cool-down time period; and (4) establishing the place where everyone will reconvene so the parent can address the situation that occurred before the code word was used. Practice is the key to an effective safety plan. Therapists practice with parents and children, first separately and then together during joint sessions. Families are asked to practice the plan at home and to use the plan when needed.

> Sharon and Mia decided their code word was "Noodle," and after a few sessions practicing together, the clinician invited the other household members to a session to practice the safety plan together, both in session and at home.

Abuse Clarification

During the final phase of treatment, clinicians continue to work with parents to address challenging parenting situations and to improve implementation of the family safety plan. They begin to assist the family in healing from the referral incident. The clinician first works with the child to develop a "praise letter," an important component that lets the parent know that the child has seen the efforts the parent has made to parent differently or better over the past several weeks. The letter details changes the child can identify, such as the parent yelling less, use of time-outs when the child misbehaves, or spending more time together. The letter also includes specific or general praise for the parent and shares what the child likes about the parent, for example, "I like when you make my favorite meal" or "I love you."

After sharing the praise letter with the parent, the clinician initiates the development of the trauma narrative by obtaining a neutral narrative from the child, to help teach how to give a narrative account of traumatic experiences (Sternberg et al., 1997). Following the neutral narrative, the therapist helps the child develop a trauma narrative (Deblinger & Heflin, 1996) of the referral incident or other traumatic parenting interactions and assists the child in processing thoughts and feelings related to these experiences.

Concurrently, parents prepare a letter that demonstrates that they take responsibility for their abusive behavior and alleviates children's responsibility/self-blame. The therapist gives minimal instructions to the parent but frames this letter as the opportunity for the parent to speak to the child from the heart about the abusive experiences, as well as positive changes made in the family. The therapist offers the parent education, assistance in processing abuse-related thoughts/feelings, and constructive feedback as the parent

formulates and revises the letter. In the majority of cases, the final step in refining the clarification letter involves the child's trauma narrative being shared with the parent. This provides the parent with an opportunity to directly respond to the child's fears, dysfunctional thoughts, worries, and concerns. In the case example, the mother is asked what messages she would like to give to her daughter about what her daughter shared in the trauma narrative—specifically, the daughter's statement, "I thought she hated me." During joint sessions, parents and children communicate openly about the abusive experiences. The therapist provides the parent with coaching and feedback (both positive and constructive) to help the parent respond in a supportive way. This session is a powerful therapeutic experience, bringing healing and closure for a family around a topic they may not otherwise have discussed.

> In her trauma narrative, Mia described intense feelings of anxiety and associated physiological responses that she experienced while trying to hide her bruises from school personnel, "I felt nervous a lot and my heart was beating fast." She also detailed her fear that she would be in trouble after they found the bruises and asked her who caused them. She added that her mother must hate her because she encouraged Mia to hide the marks and did not seem to care that Mia was suffering (both emotionally and physically). In response to Mia's concerns, Sharon apologized for hurting her and wrote (in her clarification letter), "I needed someone to tell me I was wrong, that I went too far. I would have continued to get frustrated. I'm grateful that the state stepped in. I'm the reason why we have an open CPS case and it's not your fault." Sharon assured Mia that she loved her and that someone who loves her, even her mother, should never hit or hurt her in that way. During the joint sharing, Mia and Sharon processed their thoughts and feelings related to what they heard from one another. In a tearful moment, Mia leapt into her mother's lap as they hugged and reaffirmed their positive relationship and love for one another.

UNDERLYING RATIONALE AND THEORETICAL FRAMEWORK

CPC-CBT is grounded in cognitive behavioral theory; incorporates elements from empirically supported CBT models for families who have experienced CPA (Donohue et al., 1998; Kolko, 1996; Kolko & Swenson, 2002), sexual abuse (Cohen et al., 2004; Deblinger & Heflin, 1996), and domestic violence (Runyon et al., 1998); and incorporates elements from developmental, learning, family systems, trauma, and motivational theories. CPC-CBT uses cognitive behavioral theory to conceptualize the development, maintenance, and treatment of CPA by the parent and the emotional and behavioral difficulties exhibited by children. The therapeutic techniques used in the model with parents and children are based on the empirical literature and CBT principles. As is typical of a CBT approach, the methods directly address the cognitions, feelings, behaviors, and physiological responses of children and parents. This intervention targets change in all these areas with the expectation that a change in one area will produce change in other areas. The treatment techniques build on one another and flow from session to session. Skills are taught through modeling, behavioral rehearsal, praise, and corrective feedback.

The core principles of CPC-CBT are represented by the acronym EMPOWER:

- Empathize
- Manage emotions and behaviors
- Power through self-control and praise
- Offer choices and overcome abuse
- Work toward a noncoercive family environment
- Education about violence
- Reinforcers and respect

For the safety of children, it is critical to intervene with the at-risk and offending parent to decrease the ongoing cycle of coercive and abusive parenting and to replace these negative behaviors with positive parenting skills. CPA within the parent-child dyad can be conceptualized using Patterson's (1976, 1982) social learning model, according to Urquiza and McNeil (1996). When a child responds to the parent's use of hitting in a compliant manner, the parent's behavior is reinforced. Over time, the child may not respond to lower levels of coercion (e.g., empty threats of punishment, shouting), which may contribute to the use of increasing levels of coercion to gain the child's compliance (see Knutson & Bower, 1994). Additionally, parents frequently do not teach children the appropriate replacement behavior, which results in the child repeating the unwanted/inappropriate behavior and increases the likelihood of the parent using increased force to gain the child's compliance. This ongoing cycle of escalating violence highlights the need to teach parents positive parenting skills to produce long-term behavioral change in children, which then reinforces and strengthens the use of these skills by parents.

Research outcomes suggest that including the child in the treatment process may facilitate both the parent's acquisition and use of positive parenting skills (Runyon, Deblinger, & Steer, 2010; Webster-Stratton & Hammond, 1997) and the development and maintenance of positive parent-child interactions (Milner & Chilamkurti, 1991). To address these issues, CPC-CBT teaches parents a variety of nonviolent parenting strategies to gain a child's compliance. Through coaching of parent-child dyads in session, parental skills are shaped in much the same way that parents are shaping their children's behavior with parenting strategies. Effective parenting responses are reinforced by the child's compliant behavior across the treatment process and perhaps long after treatment has ended. This further reduces the likelihood of future coercive/punitive parent-child interactions.

During joint parent-child sessions, parents have the opportunity to practice positive parenting skills with their children, with the therapist acting as coach, to enhance the generalization of skills outside the therapeutic setting. At this time, parents also model prosocial behavior (e.g., assertive behavior, effective communication, praise, empathy) for their children by practicing skills during these interactions. Parents also practice communicating about daily events and difficult topics (e.g., children's behavioral problems at school, sexual activity, dating, child abuse), which decreases conflict and enhances the parent-child relationship immediately and in the long term. All of the practice and positive interactions assist in preparing parents and children for the Abuse Clarification phase of CPC-CBT, as described above. This process reduces the child's negative abuse-related beliefs and PTSD symptoms and changes the parent's interpretations about the child's behaviors, which may, in turn, enhance positive parenting. The greatest change may occur when parents are processing and responding to the child's trauma narrative as they begin to understand the emotional impact of their abusive behavior on the child (emotional awareness and processing), which increases their empathy for their child and contributes to long-term changes in parenting behavior. This is important because increased empathy for one's child has been associated with lower levels of child maltreatment (Kilpatrick & Hine, 2005).

In addition to intervening with and changing parents' interactions with the child, it is critical to include the child in treatment, given the importance of the child's emotional and behavioral responses; this will maximize positive child outcomes, particularly when the child presents with PTSD. There is evidence that parents alone may not be the most therapeutic agents in helping their children overcome PTSD (Deblinger, Lippmann, & Steer, 1996), particularly parents who are responsible for abusing and traumatizing their children. Initially, parents may be too emotionally involved and biased to assist their children in processing their abusive experiences. The therapist uses the CBT component known as gradual exposure, involving exposure and systematic desensitization, to target the child's PTSD symptoms (Deblinger & Heflin, 1996; Runyon & Deblinger, in press; Runyon et al., 2004; Runyon, Deblinger, & Schroeder, 2009). In this process, the therapist gradually exposes the child (through imaginal or in vivo exposure) to the anxiety-provoking abusive behaviors and abuse-related experiences in the context of a safe, therapeutic environment. The intensity of the child's conditioned emotional responses is expected to diminish over time, with repeated exposure to abuse-related cues. During this process, the child may identify and process dysfunctional abuse-related thoughts, which are associated with PTSD and other abuse-related symptoms in children who have experienced CPA (Deblinger & Runyon, 2005). CPC-CBT utilizes modeling, behavioral rehearsal, praise, and feedback to teach children skills (relaxation, emotional expression, cognitive coping) to prepare them for the exposure and processing components, where dysfunctional abuse-related thoughts can be identified and corrected by both the therapist and the parent during joint sessions. Hence, the process serves to reduce the child's PTSD symptoms, enhance parental empathy for the child, and strengthen the parent-child relationship.

If children's PTSD symptoms are not directly addressed in treatment, their problems may escalate, increasing the likelihood of a child victimizing others or being re-victimized. In response to ongoing stressors such as CPA, youths may initially experience externalizing symptoms such as anger and aggression, followed by PTSD symptoms (Pelcovitz et al., 1994), such as the dissociation and numbing seen in delinquent adolescents (Carrion & Steiner, 2000). Avoidant behaviors (e.g., numbing and dissociation) are adaptive for the child while being abused, but they may interfere with the ability to heal and place the youth at risk in the future. This raises concern that the parent will interpret the child's ongoing behaviors (e.g., PTSD, fearfulness, and/or aggression), if untreated, as noncompliance and respond with violent disciplining techniques

While children who do not directly participate in treatment may benefit greatly from positive, noncoercive interactions with their parents, ongoing feelings of anger and hostility and PTSD symptoms may leave children vulnerable to relying on unproductive coping strategies (aggression, substance use/abuse, and avoidance) to manage distress and conflict in their lives. Youths exposed to CPA are more likely to be hypersensitive to anger cues in their environment and to misinterpret social interactions and perceive others as threatening (see Price & Landsverk, 1998; Shackman, Shackman, & Pollak, 2007; Shields, Ryan, & Cicchetti, 2001). This hypervigilant behavior that is potentially protective in an abusive environment may only serve to increase anxiety, contribute to ongoing PTSD, and increase aggressive behaviors in response to "innocuous" reminders of abuse, further alienating the youth from peers and family. This may lead to the intergenerational transmission of violence. Studies have documented an increased risk for adult survivors of CPA to abuse their children (Crouch, Milner & Thomsen, 2001; Kaufman & Zigler, 1987) and their partners (Straus, 1979). Thus, the cycle of violence may be perpetuated if the child does not receive treatment, even though the abusive parent receives treatment and the ongoing CPA is stopped.

Given that parents' interactions with their children contribute to the acquisition and maintenance of child behavior problems, the parent is seen as the primary agent of change for such problems. Research has shown significantly less change in children's behavior problems in cases of sexual abuse (Deblinger & Heflin, 1996) and physical abuse (Swenson & Brown, 1999) when the parent is not included in treatment. Modeling by parents is a learning mechanism, which may explain the repeated finding that children who have experienced CPA have a greater tendency to use aggressive conflict resolution strategies and display poorer social

problem-solving skills than children who have not. It is likely that children learn aggressive behaviors by observing their parents' aggressive behavior and, during adulthood, may be prone to make use of coercive parenting strategies that were modeled for them by their parents (Crouch, Milner & Thomsen, 2001; Kaufman & Zigler, 1987).

The development and maintenance of abuse-related and general behavior problems are associated with contingencies in the child's environment. For instance, well-meaning parents may inadvertently reinforce negative behaviors, including aggression, in their children. This negative parental attention is often associated with physically abusive behavior and is well known to increase behavioral difficulties. As such, it is necessary to teach parents skills to enhance their interactions with their child, which, in turn, decreases their child's behavior problems. The therapist initially models the skill, then parents rehearse the skills and are offered praise and corrective feedback to shape their behavior and facilitate the acquisition of skills and positive parent-child interactions.

EVIDENCE BASE / EMPIRICAL SUPPORT

CPC-CBT was developed through a series of research studies that have documented positive outcomes for both children and parents after participation in this treatment program. CPC-CBT is one of just a few models developed for this population that have assessed and demonstrated improvements in children's PTSD symptoms (Kjellgren, Svedin, & Nilsson, in press; Runyon, Deblinger, & Schroeder, 2009, 2010; Runyon, Deblinger, & Steer, 2010), despite the association between PTSD and CPA (Saunders, Berliner, & Hanson, 2004). In a pilot study examining the feasibility of a CBT group approach that incorporated the child into the parent's therapy, both parents (n = 12) and children (n = 21) reported pre- to post-treatment improvements after their participation in CPC-CBT (Runyon, Deblinger, & Schroeder, 2009). Specifically, parents and children reported reductions in the use of physical punishment and improvements in children's PTSD symptoms. Parents reported improvements in parental anger toward their children, in consistency of parenting, and in child behavior problems (Runyon, Deblinger, & Schroeder, 2009). These pilot data suggested the potential value and feasibility of having the child and the parent who engages in abusive or punitive behavior participate in sessions together and directly discuss the abusive experiences while learning effective communication and coping skills, individually and together. However, there was no follow-up to assess the long-term benefits of children's participation.

To address the limitations of the initial pilot study, a controlled trial compared the relative efficacy of CPC-CBT (24 parents, 34 children) with parent-only CBT (20 parents, 26 children; Runyon, Deblinger, & Steer, 2010). This is the first controlled trial with this population to examine group CBT and the added benefit of including the child in the "at-risk or offending" parent's treatment. Children and parents were assessed prior to treatment, after 15 treatment sessions, and three months after the completion of treatment. When the children directly received treatment along with their parents, the children and parents showed greater improvements in resolving PTSD symptoms and in parenting skills, respectively, when compared with parent-only treatment.

Another pilot study examined pre- and post-treatment data for 24 children and their parents after completing 16–20 sessions of individual CPC-CBT. Preliminary analyses showed that children reported significant reductions in PTSD and depressive symptoms, while parents reported improvements in their levels of depression, in parenting skills, and in their children's internalizing and externalizing behavior problems (Runyon, Deblinger, & Schroeder, 2010).

CPC-CBT has also been evaluated in mental health centers and social service units in Sweden and the United States. Clinicians in four child protection and child and adolescent psychiatric social service units across Sweden were trained in CPC-CBT by the developer. As part of this dissemination project, researchers conducted a pilot study, with a majority of participants receiving individual CPC-CBT (Kjellgren, Svedin, & Nilsson, in press). After their participation, parents (n = 26) reported a significant decrease in depression, violent parenting tactics, inconsistent parenting, and children's trauma symptoms. Children (n = 25) reported significant improvements in trauma and depressive symptoms, as well as significant decreases in coercive parenting tactics and improvements in positive parenting. The authors concluded that CPC-CBT was applicable and effective for treating CPA in Sweden, where the definition of child physical abuse has a much lower threshold of coercion than in the United States.

In another dissemination project, clinicians in three agencies in Mississippi were trained in CPC-CBT using the National Child Traumatic Stress Network's Learning Collaborative framework. While a relatively small group of clinicians (N = 12) from these agencies were trained and provided CPC-CBT to families, pre- and post-training data revealed significant changes in organizational practices, clinicians' practices, and clinical outcomes for families. The families who received CPC-CBT over the course of the learning collaborative reported significant improvements in parenting, reductions in the use of corporal punishment, and improvements in severity of children's PTSD symptoms from pre- to post-treatment. Clinicians also reported significant increases in the use of several CPC-CBT components and skills during parent, child, and joint sessions after their participation in the collaborative.

WHICH CLIENTS ARE APPROPRIATE FOR CPC-CBT?

Children ages 3–17 years and their parents who are at risk for or have already engaged in physically abusive behavior toward their children are appropriate referrals for CPC-CBT. "At-risk" families are defined as those families who have had multiple referrals to CPS with no substantiation and those families who report using excessive physical punishment with their children. This may include parents who self-refer due to significant parenting stress, a concern about losing their temper with their child whose behavior is out of control, and/or distress about physical punishment not being effective.

In cases where children have been removed from the home, there should be a clear plan for reunification and contact should be permitted between parent and child (during therapy sessions, at a minimum). The identified parent must be willing to participate. Other caregivers in the home are strongly encouraged to participate. CPC-CBT is not an appropriate intervention for families where the child has been removed due to CPA, there is no plan for reunification, and the parental rights are being terminated.

Children who present with trauma symptoms, depression, poor social skills, self-esteem issues, and externalizing problems (e.g., aggressive, oppositional behaviors) may benefit from CPC-CBT. Parents who may benefit from this treatment include those who present with anger-control issues, depression, distorted perceptions of their child's behaviors, lack of knowledge about child development and positive parenting skills, and lack of empathy for their child's behavior.

Serious clinical issues may delay the initiation of CPC-CBT but do not preclude a family's benefitting from the model. For instance, imminent suicidal or homicidal behavior that requires crisis intervention, parents' substance abuse to the degree that it interferes with their ability to participate in CPC-CBT, and significant mental health issues that require stabilization with medication prior to participation—all may delay CPC-CBT. In these instances, the level of impairment is the key to deciding whether to initiate or delay the therapy. For example, a parent may be required to complete substance abuse counseling before starting CPC-CBT. In other cases, a parent may complete substance abuse counseling concurrently with CPC-CBT.

CPC-CBT is appropriate for children who have experienced multiple trauma types, with the exception of cases in which the child continues to reside with the perpetrator of sexual abuse. With regard to domestic violence, a thorough assessment should be conducted with the batterer, the adult who is being battered, and the child to ensure that all feel safe participating in treatment together. If there is a significant level of ongoing violence in the household, the batterer should complete a batterer's program before participating in CPC-CBT. Additional information on CPC-CBT for families in which domestic violence occurs is available elsewhere (Runyon & Deblinger, in press; Runyon, Deblinger, & Schroeder, 2009).

EXPECTED OUTCOMES

Based on the studies conducted to date or clinical anecdotes, the following positive outcomes are expected for parents, children, and the family system after their participation in CPC-CBT:

1. Improvements in children's PTSD and depressive symptoms, other internalizing symptoms, and externalizing behavior problems
2. Improvements in parents' depression, anger, coping skills, and problem-solving skills, as well as positive and consistent parenting skills
3. Increase in parents' knowledge of appropriate developmental expectations and decrease in their negative perceptions of children and their behavior
4. Increase in parents' empathy for children by enhancing insight into the behavioral and emotional impact of their parenting behavior and interactions on their children
5. Enhancement of the parent-child relationship through communication and positive interactions
6. Enhancement of the family system by developing a noncoercive family environment
7. Reduction in the recurrence of CPA and the use of corporal punishment by parents.

CONCLUSIONS

Combined Parent-Child Cognitive Behavioral Therapy is an evidence-based treatment associated with positive outcomes for children, parents, and the family system in families that are at risk for or have experienced child physical abuse (Kjellgren, Svedin, & Nilsson, in press; Runyon, Deblinger, & Schroeder, 2009, 2010; Runyon, Deblinger, & Steer, 2010). CPC-CBT is included in the NREPP (www.nrepp.samhsa.gov), where it received the highest possible score for readiness for dissemination. CPC-CBT has begun to be implemented at other sites in the United States and in Sweden, with positive results (Kjellgren, Svedin, & Nilsson, in press). For additional information on training or research in CPC-CBT, see the CARES Institute website (www.caresinstitute.org).

References

Carrion, V., & Steiner, H. (2000). Trauma and dissociation in delinquent adolescents. *Journal of the American Academy of Child and Adolescent Psychiatry, 39,* 353–359.

Cohen, J. A., Deblinger, E., Mannarino, A. P., & Steer, R. A. (2004). A multisite, randomized controlled trial for children with sexual abuse–related PTSD symptoms. *Journal of the American Academy of Child and Adolescent Psychiatry, 43,* 393–402.

Crouch, J. L., Milner, J. S., & Thomsen, C. (2001). Childhood physical abuse, early social support, and risk for maltreatment: Current social support as a mediator of risk for child physical abuse. *Child Abuse & Neglect, 25*(1), 93–107.

Deblinger, E., & Heflin, A. (1996). *Treating sexually abused children and their nonoffending parents: A cognitive-behavioral approach.* Thousand Oaks, CA: Sage Publications.

Deblinger, E., Lippmann, J., & Steer, R. (1996). Sexually abused children suffering posttraumatic stress symptoms: Initial treatment outcome findings. *Child Maltreatment, 1,* 310–321.

Deblinger, E., & Runyon, M. K. (2005). Understanding and treating feelings of shame in children who have experienced maltreatment. *Child Maltreatment, 10,* 364–376.

Donohue, B., Miller, E. R., Van Hasselt, V. B., & Hersen, M. (1998). An ecobehavioral approach to child maltreatment. In V. B. Van Hasselt, & M. Hersen (Eds.), *Handbook of psychological treatment protocols for children and adolescents* (pp. 279–356). Mahwah, NJ: Lawrence Erlbaum Associates.

Kaufman, J., & Zigler, E. (1987). Do abused children become abusive parents? *American Journal of Orthopsychiatry, 57,* 186–192.

Kilpatrick, K. L., & Hine, D. (2005). *Parental empathy, personality disorders and child maltreatment.* Final report for industry partner. Ashfield, NSW, Australia: New South Wales Department of Community Services.

Kjellgren, C., Svedin, C. G., & Nilsson, D. (in press). Child physical abuse: Experiences of combined treatment for children and their parents. A pilot study. *Child Care in Practice.*

Knutson, J. F., & Bower, M. E. (1994). Physically abusive parenting as an escalated aggressive response. In M. Potgel & J. F. Knutson (Eds.), *The dynamics of aggression: Biological and social processes in dyads and groups* (pp. 195–225). Hillsdale, NJ: Lawrence Erlbaum Associates.

Kolko, D. J. (1996). Individual cognitive-behavioral treatment and family therapy for physically abused children and their offending parents: A comparison of clinical outcomes. *Child Maltreatment, 1,* 322–342.

Kolko, D. J., & Swenson, C. (2002). *Assessing and treating physically abused children and their families: A cognitive-behavioral approach.* Thousand Oaks, CA: Sage Publications.

McKay, M., McCadam, K., & Pennington, J. (2002). Predicting child mental health service utilization by urban families: A preliminary study of child, family, environmental, and system factors. *Journal of Behavioral Health Services and Research, 19,* 1–10.

McKay, M., Stoewe, J., McCadam, K., & Gonzales, J. (1998). Increasing access to child mental health services for urban children and their caregivers. *Health and Social Work, 23,* 9–15.

Milner, J. S., & Chilamkurti, C. (1991). Physical child abuse perpetrator characteristics: A review of the literature. *Journal of Interpersonal Violence, 6,* 345–366.

Patterson, G. R. (1976). *Living with children: New methods for parents and teachers* (Revised ed.). Champaign, IL: Research Press.

Patterson, G. R. (1982). *Coercive family process.* Eugene, OR: Castalia.

Pelcovitz, D., Kaplan, S., Goldenberg, B., Mandel, F., Lehane, J., & Guarrera, J. (1994). Post-traumatic stress disorder in physically abused adolescents. *Journal of the American Academy of Child and Adolescent Psychiatry, 33,* 305–312.

Price, J. M., & Landsverk, J. (1998). Social information-processing patterns as predictors of social adaptation and behavior problems among maltreated children in foster care. *Child Abuse & Neglect, 22,* 845–858.

Runyon, M. K., Basilio, I., Van Hasselt, V. B., & Hersen, M. (1998). Child witnesses of interparental violence: Child and family treatment. In V. B. Hasselt & M. Hersen (Eds.), *Handbook of psychological treatment protocols for children and adolescents* (pp. 203–278). Mahwah, NJ: Lawrence Erlbaum Associates.

Runyon, M. K., & Deblinger, E. (in press). *Combined parent-child cognitive behavioral therapy (CPC-CBT): An approach to empower families at-risk for child physical abuse.* New York, NY: Oxford University Press.

Runyon, M. K., Deblinger, E., Ryan, E. E., & Thakkar-Kolar, R. (2004). An overview of child physical abuse: Developing an integrated parent-child cognitive-behavioral treatment approach. *Trauma, Violence, & Abuse, 5,* 65–85.

Runyon, M. K., Deblinger, E., & Schroeder, C. M. (2009). Pilot evaluation of outcomes of combined parent-child cognitive-behavioral group therapy for families at-risk for child physical abuse. *Cognitive Behavioral Practice, 16*, 101–118.

Runyon, M. K., Deblinger, E., & Schroeder, C. M. (2010). *Preliminary analyses of pre to posttreatment changes in families after their participation in Combined Parent-Child Cognitive Behavioral Therapy.* Unpublished manuscript.

Runyon, M. K., Deblinger, E., & Steer, R. (2010). Comparison of combined parent-child and parent-only cognitive-behavioral treatments for offending parents and children in cases of child physical abuse. *Child & Family Behavior Therapy, 32*, 196–218.

Saunders, B. E., Berliner, L., & Hanson, R. F. (Eds.). (2004, April 26). *Child physical and sexual abuse: Guidelines for treatment* (Revised report). Charleston, SC: National Crime Victims Research and Treatment Center.

Shackman, J. E., Shackman, A. J., & Pollak, S. D. (2007). Physical abuse amplifies attention to threat and increases anxiety in children. *Emotion, 7*, 838–852.

Shields, A., Ryan, R. M., & Cicchetti, D. (2001). Narrative representations of caregivers and emotion dysregulation as predictors of maltreated children's rejection by peers. *Developmental Psychology, 37*, 321–337.

Sternberg, K. J., Lamb, M. E., Hershkowitz, I., Yudilevitch, L., Orbach, Y., Esplin, P. W., & Hovav, M. (1997). Effects of introductory style on children's abilities to describe experiences of sexual abuse. *Child Abuse & Neglect, 21*(11), 1133–1146.

Straus, M. A. (1979). Measuring intrafamily conflict and violence: The Conflict Tactics Scale (CTS). *Journal of Marriage and Family, 41*, 75–88.

Swenson, C. C., & Brown, E. J. (1999). Cognitive-behavioral group treatment for physically abused children. *Cognitive and Behavioral Practice, 6*, 612–620.

Urquiza, A. J., & McNeil, C. B. (1996). Parent-child interaction therapy: An intensive dyadic intervention for physically abusive families. *Child Maltreatment, 1*, 134–144.

U.S. Department of Health and Human Services, Administration for Children and Families, Administration on Children, Youth and Families, Children's Bureau. (2011). *Child maltreatment, 2010.* www.acf.hhs.gov/programs/cb/stats_research /index.htm#can

Webster-Stratton, C., & Hammond, M. (1997). Treating children with early onset conduct problems: A comparison of child and parent training interventions. *Journal of Consulting and Clinical Psychology, 65*, 93–109.

LISA H. JAYCOX, PH.D.
AUDRA K. LANGLEY, PH.D.
BRADLEY D. STEIN, M.D., PH.D.
SHERYL H. KATAOKA-ENDO, M.D., M.S.H.S
MARLEEN WONG, PH.D.

8

Early Intervention for Abused Children in the School Setting

GENERAL CONSIDERATIONS

From the perspective of a clinic-based practitioner or child/family services worker, it may seem counterintuitive to intervene in the school setting for children who have been abused. Don't child welfare systems need to get involved to ensure the safety of the child? Don't families experiencing abuse of one or more of their children require intensive family intervention? Yes, we believe that both of these types of intervention are important parts of the treatment plan for children who have been abused, but school-based early mental health intervention programs can play an essential role in early detection of and treatment for many types of trauma, including abuse and neglect.

Our initial school-based trauma interventions sought to address the negative mental health and functional sequelae following children's exposure to community violence. As we screened students for exposure to community violence, however, it became apparent that many children had also experienced abuse and neglect. Refinements to our intervention program were made to ensure it was flexible enough to accommodate these children and address some of their needs related to anxious and depressive symptoms, as well as some of their behavior problems. We believe that to provide effective, early intervention in the school setting for children exposed to violence and trauma, we must be prepared to work with children who have experienced abuse and neglect and that our intervention must target some of the sequelae of abuse experiences, particularly as evidenced by changes in classroom and schoolyard behavior and disrupted classroom learning. School-based interventions are not a panacea for abused children. Rather, we see them as a way to complement and extend services provided by the child welfare, child protection, and clinic-based mental health systems and to increase access for students who may not otherwise be receiving any mental health services.

In this chapter, we describe the Cognitive Behavioral Intervention for Trauma in Schools (CBITS) program, how it addresses child abuse specifically, the theoretical rationale for the program, and the evidence supporting its effectiveness. We discuss when and why CBITS might be an appropriate intervention and the advantages and disadvantages of its use. Lastly, we address expected outcomes of CBITS program delivery. We hope that, by the end of this chapter, readers will understand the CBITS program and its potential utility for addressing the mental health needs of students who have experienced child abuse and neglect.

THE CBITS INTERVENTION

The Cognitive Behavioral Intervention for Trauma in Schools program began as an effort to intervene with recent immigrant students in the Los Angeles Unified School District who had been exposed to community violence in the United States or in their countries of origin, or both. We created a partnership in 1998 between the RAND Corporation, the University of California, Los Angeles, and the Los Angeles Unified School District to create and evaluate this program (Stein et al., 2002). In contrast to many interventions developed in academic settings and then later transported to community settings, the CBITS program was developed iteratively from the beginning in collaboration with school partners who were delivering CBITS in public schools as part of their work on school campuses, and thus the program was designed to fit school culture and be maximally flexible in addressing diverse students and diverse needs.

The primary focus of the program was on symptoms of posttraumatic stress, both because these are very common following exposure to violence (e.g., Berman et al., 1996;

Breslau et al., 1991; Horowitz, Weine, & Jekel, 1995) and because there was a good deal of evidence, developing at that time, on best practices for treating these symptoms, at least in adults (Foa & Meadows, 1997). For children, there was accruing evidence that cognitive behavioral techniques, including a focus on gradual exposure and development of a trauma narrative or detailed account of the trauma experience(s), were effective in reducing symptoms of posttraumatic stress disorder (e.g., Cohen & Mannarino, 1996; Deblinger & Heflin, 1996; March et al., 1998), and practice parameters had been developed that highlighted such techniques (Cohen & Work Group on Quality Issues, 1998). Ultimately, this process resulted in the CBITS program (Jaycox, 2003). Over the past decade, this partnership has expanded to include refinement of the program for the general multicultural student body in Los Angeles and expansion to other cities; for use with Native Americans (Goodkind, LaNoue, & Milford, 2010; Morsette, Swaney, et al., 2009; Morsette, van den Pol, et al., 2012; Ngo et al., 2008); and for broader types of trauma such as disaster (Cohen et al., 2009; Jaycox et al., 2010). It has also been adapted for special populations (Kataoka et al., 2006; Schultz et al., 2010) and for use by nonclinical staff (Jaycox et al., 2009). Originally designed for fourth- through eighth-grade students, the program has now been adapted for and disseminated for use with older teens, and an adaptation for K–5 elementary school students is underway.

CBITS consists of 10 group sessions (approximately one hour each) for children; 1–3 individual sessions for children, during which they begin talking about the details of their trauma; 2 group educational meetings for parents; and an educational session for teachers. The program incorporates evidence-based cognitive behavioral skills to combat posttraumatic stress symptoms, anxiety, and depression among children who are symptomatic following exposure to a traumatic event.

The CBITS format is group-based for six to eight participating children, delivered by a school-based mental health professional, such as a school psychologist or social worker. Each session follows the familiar cognitive behavioral format, in which a new set of techniques is introduced by a mixture of didactic presentation, use of age-appropriate activities and games to solidify concepts, and individual work on worksheets in session and between sessions. Homework is assigned in each session and reviewed at the beginning of the next session, to help generalize skills to the real world. A detailed manual is available that provides information to group leaders about overcoming obstacles to the program, such as child noncompliance with homework and challenges with using the core treatment components, as well as information on tailoring the program to the unique clinical and cultural/contextual needs of children in the group.

As an early intervention program, CBITS is designed to help youths identified with symptoms of posttraumatic stress disorder (PTSD) that may or may not be recognized by parents and teachers. The goal is that early detection and intervention will allow children to develop skills and coping strategies that reduce the psychological sequelae that commonly follow trauma exposure. CBITS has several aims: to directly reduce psychological reactions, such as symptoms of anxiety, depression, and PTSD, and thereby reduce child distress, and to mobilize resilience factors to allow the student to function more adaptively at school, at home, and socially.

As a targeted intervention, the CBITS program is intended for students who have experienced trauma and have current symptoms of PTSD. There are many possible ways to identify such students, but we generally recommend screening students on a broad scale, because symptoms of PTSD often go undetected by parents or counselors while still causing significant distress. Most of our work has screened for a range of traumas, including community violence, accidents, and disaster exposure, but not for child abuse, since schools are staffed by mandated child abuse reporters, and schools are often reluctant to screen on a broad scale for child abuse. We have found that, once a child is enrolled in CBITS, a finding of child abuse is not uncommon for those who enter the program on the basis of a different traumatic event. Another relevant method for reaching students with child abuse histories is targeted referrals from teachers or school counselors who have information about prior abuse. Although schools sometimes have concerns about embarking on a screening or referral process, wishing to avoid upsetting parents, we have found that parents are often receptive to such programming and that the parents who agree to take part rarely find these types of questions about their children "unpleasant" (Dean et al., 2004).

Regardless of the type of trauma that brings a student into the program, CBITS focuses on the most troubling traumatic event for the student at the time of the program, so long as both the interventionist and the student feel comfortable addressing that trauma in the group setting. Thus, a student might be screened into the program for exposure to community violence but later choose to work on witnessing family violence at home, or on episodes of physical or emotional abuse or neglect, or on the traumatic loss of a loved one through death or separation. Indeed, our work following hurricanes Katrina and Rita in New Orleans showed that although students were selected on the basis of hurricane-related trauma, most of them chose a different traumatic event to focus on in the groups (Langley et al., in press). Thus, even selection of a group of students who have been exposed to child abuse might, for some students, result in a focus on different traumatic events during the intervention.

UNDERLYING RATIONALE AND THEORETICAL FRAMEWORK

The overall goals of the CBITS program are to (1) reduce symptoms of PTSD and other trauma-related problems, (2) build resilience, and (3) build peer and parent support.

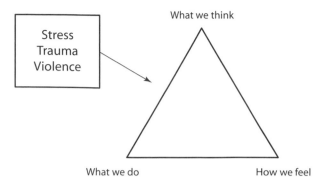

Figure 8.1. The thoughts-feelings-actions triangle

Table 8.1. How CBITS Addresses the Three Components of the Thoughts-Feelings-Action Triangle

Component	CBITS Technique
Thoughts	• Train students to notice their thoughts and evaluate their accuracy. • Train students to challenge their thinking or to challenge their unrealistic and harmful thoughts so as to have more balanced and accurate thoughts. • Train students to stop negative or problematic thoughts that are getting in their way. • Using the trauma narrative, help students make sense of their traumatic experience and reduce maladaptive thinking related to the trauma.
Feelings	• Train students in relaxation skills. • Directly reduce students' anxiety related to the trauma through imaginal exposure techniques and construction of the trauma narrative. • Directly reduce students' anxiety when they are reminded of what happened to them through in vivo exposure techniques.
Behaviors	• Train students that approaching rather than avoiding feared situations will result in more lasting anxiety reduction. • Train students that sharing painful material with supportive others can increase their sense of connection. • Train students to consider alternatives and to brainstorm solutions to problems. • Train students to develop a plan of action and to try out their desired plan. • Train students to apply these skills to real-world problems they are experiencing.

Although the treatment is delivered in a group format, the goals for each specific child are tailored to best meet his or her specific intervention needs. Here we address each goal in turn.

In terms of symptom reduction, the program builds on cognitive behavioral theory, which at a basic level posits that thoughts, feelings, and behaviors are closely related and can influence one another (see figure 8.1). Not only do they affect one another, but each is directly impacted by traumatic life events such as child abuse. For instance, thoughts or cognitions can be disrupted after an extreme trauma or experience with violence. Two general themes or schemas begin to push away normal thoughts (Foa and Jaycox, 1999): (1) "The world is dangerous. I am not safe. People cannot be trusted." (2) "I can't deal with this. I'll never be the same. I am falling apart." These are themes that would be expected to interfere with healthy growth and social development. Symptoms of PTSD include some basic alterations in feelings and behaviors as well, with heightened anxiety and startle response, hypervigilance, anxiety related to thinking or being reminded of the event, and anger and irritability, all part and parcel of the definition of the disorder (American Psychiatric Association, 1994).

We address each of the three components in different ways, as shown in table 8.1. All three components draw on a robust theoretical and empirical literature on cognitive behavioral techniques (Cahill et al., 2009). Regarding thoughts, the CBITS program builds on cognitive theory that has demonstrated how individuals can be trained to notice and change their thinking to reduce the power of habitual negative thinking. Regarding feelings, the program builds on behavioral theory that has demonstrated how the process of habituation can reduce the anxious responses to trauma reminders that result from classical and operant conditioning. In addition, CBITS provides children with tools, such as relaxation training, to calm their physiological "feelings" and reactivity. Regarding behavior, the program builds on behavioral theory that has demonstrated how approach rather than avoidance can help with the habituation process and the ability to gain mastery.

Thus, CBITS contains many of the same elements found in other empirically supported cognitive behavioral inter-

ventions for child trauma, such as Trauma-Focused CBT (TF-CBT; Cohen, Mannarino, & Deblinger, 2006). These elements include psychoeducation about trauma and common reactions, relaxation training and other anxiety reduction skills, identifying and challenging dysfunctional thinking, approaching rather than avoiding trauma reminders and triggers, assessing the safety of avoided situations, developing a trauma narrative, and social problem solving.

The importance of building resilience, another aim of CBITS, is supported by data showing that exposure to multiple forms of trauma is very common (Finkelhor et al., 2009), and in our urban schools, vulnerability to exposure to violence accrues as children age (Stein, Jaycox, Kataoka, Rhodes, & Vestal, 2003). Thus, not only do we need to address past traumatic experiences, but we also need to help build resilience for future stressful and traumatic events. Based on the empirical literature, the CBITS program focuses on building peer and parent support (Hill et al., 1996; Kliewer et al., 1998; Kuther & Fisher, 1998; Muller et al., 2000), coping strategies (Berman et al., 1996; Curle & Williams, 1996; Jeney-Gammon et al., 1993; Martini et al., 1990; Vernberg et al., 1996), and cognitive skills (Joseph et al., 1991, 1993; Kliewer et al., 1998; March, Amaya-Jackson, Murray, & Schulte, 1998; March, Amaya-Jackson, Terry, & Costanzo, 1997).

The final goal of CBITS—to build peer and parent support—warrants special mention. Child abuse tends to be relatively hidden, and students who have experienced abuse may often feel different and alone. CBITS provides an opportunity for youths to share information about their experiences with violence, trauma, or stress in a supportive environment. Participation in the group itself allows a common bond to develop among peer participants that often extends outside the group. Moreover, some of the group content aims to give students skills for appropriately sharing their experiences with violence, trauma, or stress with trusted others outside the group (including trusted friends, family members or caregivers, teachers, and/or other adults). A common theme running through the CBITS program is opening and strengthening lines of understanding and communication between parents or caregivers and their children. This is done through a variety of educational information and take-home practice assignments. To illustrate the way CBITS is operationalized for a student who has experienced child abuse, we present the (fictitious) case of Juan.

> Juan was a seventh-grader who lived with his mother, two brothers, and his maternal grandparents, who emigrated to the United States from Mexico when Juan was 2. His older brothers, both of whom were in their teens, were struggling to stay out of gang activities in their neighborhood. Juan had been physically abused by his stepfather for the past several years, beginning with harsh discipline and escalating in the past few years to severe beatings. He had been injured enough on two occasions for his mother to take him to the ER, and the abuse had been reported to authorities by the ER staff. His stepfather was living with his relatives nearby, and Juan only saw him when he was supervised by his mother.
>
> When the CBITS program was introduced at school, Juan's mother signed him up to get screened. She was aware that he'd "been through a lot" and might need some help. On the screening survey, Juan indicated that he had witnessed street violence several times, had been beaten up a few times, and had been in an earthquake. He reported moderate symptoms of PTSD and moderate symptoms of depression on the screener. When interviewed, he reported getting beaten up both at school and by his stepfather. Juan was asked to pick the traumatic event that was bothering him the most and chose to work on a shooting he had witnessed near his home, in which he saw the victim bleeding in the street before the ambulance came. He and the interviewer agreed he would start by working on this event in the CBITS groups. The interviewer spoke with Juan's mother and learned more about the abuse, then filed an additional child abuse report for the past abuse, as specified in protocols and per state law (noting that the abuse had been reported

> previously). Both Juan and his mother were eager to participate in the program.

Psychoeducation on Common Reactions to Trauma

Education about common reactions to trauma is included for all three sets of participants in CBITS (student groups, parents, and teachers). The rationale for this component is that people often do not make the connection between experiencing a past traumatic event and experiencing current symptoms. Facilitating an understanding of this connection can help people feel more in control and can motivate them to engage in the intervention to reduce symptoms. A whole range of common reactions are discussed, including symptoms of PTSD (avoidance of trauma reminders, recurrent thoughts about the trauma, sleep problems, irritability) and other common problems such as guilt or shame, depression, difficulty trusting others, and somatic symptoms.

> In Juan's first CBITS group, he stuck to the plan to work on the shooting, and when it was his turn to say why he was in the group, he said, "I saw someone get shot. I think he might have died." In Juan's second CBITS group, the students engaged in an interactive discussion in which the group leader described some common problems, and students talked about whether they had experienced those problems, and in what way. Juan also took home a handout to share with his mother and grandparents (in Spanish) describing these common reactions. He had used a highlighter in the session to mark the ones that were bothering him the most, including feeling on guard all the time when walking outside near his home, avoiding being alone, and a sense of guilt and shame. The CBITS leader noted that shame and guilt are usually more related to child abuse than to a street shooting and decided to keep an eye on Juan's other thoughts and feelings. Juan was surprised to hear that some of his peers in the group had similar reactions, and he came away from the group feeling a bit more connected to them. When Juan's mother came to one of the parent groups, she received this same handout and had an opportunity to hear about common reactions and to ask questions. Juan's teachers were also given this information, along with tips for supporting traumatized students in their classrooms that take into account some of the common reactions as a context for student behavior.

Thoughts-Feelings-Actions Triangle

At the beginning of the CBITS intervention, a triangle is presented that represents thoughts, actions, and feelings on the three vertices and explains how the three elements affect one another and guide our experience. This triangle is used throughout the course to explain what the students are learning and why and to bring together the different elements in helping each student reduce symptoms and build coping skills.

> For Juan, this triangle explained a lot. He had been feeling pretty bad about himself, especially about how nervous he felt when he was alone and how he wanted to be with his mother all the time. Seeing how trauma might make someone feel physically anxious and make them think about more bad things happening, Juan was able to put the pieces together in a new way. When the group leader asked for students to give examples, he offered, "Like, if someone is hurting you every day or every night, you might be thinking, 'What did I do now?' and feeling like you are no good at anything."

Relaxation Training

Another key component of CBITS is relaxation training, taught early in the student groups and also taught to parents in the parent meeting. The program uses a combination of imagery, guided muscle relaxation, and deep breathing so that students can find the method that works best for them, and the group leader asks them to practice every day between sessions. Students also learn a few other techniques for anxiety reduction, including thought stopping, distraction, and positive imagery.

> Juan was hesitant to try the relaxation training because his mother had been trying to get him to do something similar at home. But with the group's encouragement, he gave it a try. He didn't relax much during the group session, but he did feel pretty tired when it was over. For the homework assignment, he decided to try it at bedtime, a time when he usually wanted to go into his mother's room.

Feeling Thermometer

Students are taught how to monitor their feelings by using a "thermometer" that has a scale of 0–10, with 0 being utterly calm and relaxed, and 10 being as stressed and upset as they can ever remember being. Students use this thermometer for the remainder of the CBITS program to gauge how upset they are in different situations and to monitor changes in their feelings when they use the techniques taught in the course.

> Juan liked the feeling thermometer—simple and clear. He was surprised again to hear a couple of the other boys in the group describing high levels of stress/upset in reaction to events that didn't seem like a really big deal. He thought they looked much tougher than that.

Cognitive Therapy

Within the CBITS program, students learn to identify negative, dysfunctional thoughts related to extreme emotional responses (high ratings on the feeling thermometer) and then to challenge those thoughts to make sure they are accurate—ideally resulting in a more reasonable emotional response. Students who have experienced trauma often have extremely negative ideas about how much they can trust others or be safe in the world and about how effective or competent they are in handling stress or managing themselves in the world around them. These kinds of thoughts and beliefs can undermine their daily functioning. In CBITS groups, students learn a fun way to challenge such thoughts (the "hotseat") and to work on their own real-life examples of their thoughts in stressful situations, both within the group and as homework for the remainder of the intervention.

> Juan's CBITS group leader chose some examples that seemed to fit him pretty well when it was his turn on the "hotseat." She started with an example of someone hearing a loud noise while walking down the street, and he had to challenge the thought "Someone is shooting." A lot of kids in the group seemed to be able to relate to that one, so he got a lot of help from the others. Then, toward the end, when everyone seemed to be getting the hang of it, she gave the example of your father hitting you, and the thought, "It's my fault." At first Juan didn't know what to say, but then one student offered, "Parents should be able to control their anger and not hit." He liked that one. Then he thought of a couple of his own, like, "Even if I did something wrong, I don't deserve that" and "My father needs help."

Real-Life Exposure

CBITS also includes behavioral therapy components in which students identify things they are avoiding because they are "triggers" to anxiety, such as people, places, or things that remind them of the traumatic event. For some students, this is an easy task because many things are avoided, but for others, there may not be much avoidance. In those cases, the therapist can usually still find some social situations or other performance-related situations that make the student nervous and where he or she would like to feel more comfortable. Students learn how anxiety about a situation can increase each time the situation is avoided but diminishes with repeated and sustained exposure. Then, the group leader helps the student construct a hierarchy of situations like this and develop a plan to approach them systematically instead of avoiding them. A key aspect of this work is partnering together to ensure that the activities on the lists are safe and are not going to put the student at risk for reexposure to violence or trauma.

> For Juan, most of the things he was avoiding were related to the shooting, since his stepfather had already moved out of his home. He also avoided some things at school, related to the times he had been beaten up there. His list included the following: being outside on 37th Street alone, being behind the cafeteria after

school, going to the bathroom alone at school, and going to the neighborhood store alone on an errand. With some discussion, it seemed that these were all things that should be safe enough to do during daylight hours, or when school was in session, and that not being able to do them was making Juan feel bad and interfering with his regular activities. For his first assignment, he picked running an errand to the store. He broke it down into smaller steps, starting by going with his mother and working up to going by himself. He agreed to try going with his mother twice, then working up to going part way with his mother (she would go as far as the corner) and the rest of the way by himself. After the planning session, the CBITS leader called and spoke with his mother about the plan and the reasoning behind it, and she agreed to help him with the assignments.

Exposure to Trauma Memory and Creating a Trauma Narrative

CBITS uses a combination of individual meetings (one to three per student, depending on the student's need) and group activities to encourage the student to process or be "exposed" to the trauma memory through talking, writing, and drawing about it. In the individual meetings, time is taken to explain the reasoning behind the need to "digest" what has happened to them and how approaching the memory rather than avoiding it will ultimately decrease their anxiety. Then the student tells the story, providing feeling-thermometer ratings along the way, over and over again, with therapist assistance, until the anxiety is reduced. If the student's anxiety does not come down sufficiently within one meeting, additional meetings can be scheduled. At the end of the meeting, the therapist and student plan together how the student will continue processing a selected trauma memory in the group setting. Two sessions of the group are devoted to writing and drawing about the traumatic event and briefly sharing what is created with the group.

Juan was pretty nervous about his first individual meeting with the CBITS leader. She began by checking on which of his traumatic events he wanted to work on the most. He explained that the shooting was still popping into his mind a lot, but the memories of the physical abuse by his stepfather were also bothering him. He said he was dreaming more about the physical abuse now. Juan and the therapist agreed to start by processing the physical abuse in the individual session. In the first session, he started out feeling very anxious and nauseous, but he was able to tell the story of the "worst" incident straight through. After two sessions focused on Juan's trauma narrative of the worst time his stepfather beat him, he started to feel some relief. He found it easier to talk about and think about what happened without getting very upset, just a little bit

anxious. In planning for the group sessions, the therapist followed Juan's lead when he said he thought he'd like to write and talk about the shooting in the group sessions, not the physical abuse. In the first group session, Juan drew a picture of the shooting, using colored pencils. He deferred talking about it. In the second group session, he embellished the drawing with more color and described the picture and the event to the group without much hesitation. Juan was also able to offer other students in the group support. In particular, one other child was describing a family violence situation. Juan said to him, "Thank you for sharing that. We had stuff like that going on in our house too, so I kind of know what you mean."

Social Problem Solving

In this section of the CBITS intervention, real-life problems are addressed. The group leader encourages students to use their cognitive coping and anxiety-reduction skills in dealing with these problems, but also acknowledges that controlling the way they think and feel is only part of solving a problem. The students learn additional skills such as brainstorming and weighing pros and cons to make decisions on how to handle these events. This portion of the program brings together the various skills the students have learned and allows the therapist to work on outstanding issues that are really important to the students and would otherwise impede their recovery, such as real safety issues in the community, family problems, and peer problems.

In this section, Juan chose a couple of family situations that were giving him trouble. One had to do with his older brother, who would occasionally say things about it being Juan's fault that the stepfather had left and so they had less money now. Juan came up with a range of possible solutions, including speaking up to his brother, enlisting his mother's help, and using his own coping strategies to feel less angry. He decided to try talking to his mother, and this ultimately resulted in a good family discussion and an apology from his brother. Juan was able to report back to the group, with a smile, that things went pretty well.

EVIDENCE BASE / EMPIRICAL SUPPORT

Many youths, like Juan, have now received CBITS, which has been studied in several types of populations and found to be effective. For each population studied, the CBITS investigators have used a community-partnered approach to determine the best ways to implement the program within the cultural and community context of the population. And through a community-academic partnership, existing school staff members have delivered CBITS, which has allowed an evaluation of the intervention under "real-world" circumstances, rather than using expert developers or highly trained professionals.

In the first pilot evaluation (the Mental Health for Immigrants Program), psychiatric social workers employed by a large urban school district were trained in an eight-session version of CBITS that was delivered to immigrant students (Kataoka et al., 2003). The clinicians delivered CBITS to third- through eighth-grade students who spoke Spanish, Western Armenian, Russian, or Korean, but the evaluation focused on the largest group of students, those who spoke Spanish and who were mostly from Mexico and Central America. For this quasi-experimental evaluation of CBITS, the bilingual, bicultural, school psychiatric social workers screened a total of 879 students in nine schools for exposure to violence, posttraumatic stress, and depressive symptoms, with 31% (n = 276) reporting exposure to violence and clinically significant symptoms. Of those who were offered participation in the program, 198 students ultimately participated through the follow-up evaluation at three months. Of these, 152 were randomly assigned to receive the intervention immediately, and 46 were randomized to the waitlist group and received CBITS later in the school year.

Results showed that depressive symptoms significantly decreased (by 17%) in the CBITS group from pre- to post-test but did not change in the waitlist group. Similarly, PTSD symptoms in the CBITS group significantly decreased (by 29%) from pre- to post-test, but the reduction in the waitlist group (of 13%) was not statistically significant. Between-group comparisons showed that PTSD and depressive symptoms decreased significantly more in the CBITS group than in the waitlist control group. These differences between groups were more pronounced among students who started the program with higher levels of symptoms. Although this evaluation indicated that symptoms improved in students participating in the CBITS groups, the lack of measures of fidelity or lack of adherence to the manual, along with the quasi-experimental evaluation design, were limitations. Also, because of the low numbers of students speaking languages other than Spanish, the impact of the program on these non-Spanish-speaking students could not be assessed.

Through the academic-community partnership, several modifications were made to the intervention following that initial pilot, with key feedback from the school clinicians, such as the need to spend more time on particular sessions. The result was the current 10-session version of CBITS (Jaycox, 2003). To evaluate this 10-session version (and address some of the limitations identified in the initial pilot study), we conducted a randomized controlled study in a general sixth-grade population, with 61 students randomized to receive CBITS early in the school year and 65 students to receive CBITS later that same school year. School psychiatric social workers conducted the groups in English and audiotaped all sessions to monitor adherence to the CBITS manual. This study found that at the three-month follow-up, when the early group had completed CBITS but the delayed group had not yet started, those who had received the CBITS program reported a significantly greater reduction of PTSD symptoms than did the delayed, as yet untreated group (64% and 34% reduction of PTSD symptoms from baseline, respectively) (Stein, Jaycox, Kataoka, Wong, et al., 2003). The early CBITS group also reported significantly lower scores on symptoms of depression than did the delayed group—a 47% reduction compared with a 24% reduction from baseline. Parents of CBITS students reported significantly less psychosocial dysfunction in their children at three months compared with parents of students in the delayed group. CBITS parents reported a 35% reduction in psychosocial dysfunction from baseline in their children, compared with a 2% increase reported by control parents. No significant differences were found between the two groups in teacher-reported classroom problems of acting out or problems with shyness, anxiousness, or learning. After the delayed group also received the CBITS intervention, the six-month findings showed that students in the early group maintained their decreased symptoms and the delayed group "caught up" to the early group, such that no differences were found between groups for symptoms of PTSD and depression, parent-reported psychosocial function, or teacher-reported classroom behaviors once all students had received CBITS.

We have also examined the effects of receiving CBITS early in the school year compared with later in the school year on academic performance. In a recent preliminary study, we found that those who received CBITS early compared with those who received it later in the same school year were more likely (80% vs. 61%) to have a passing grade (C or higher) in language arts class by the end of the school year, controlling for standardized state test scores from the previous academic year, sociodemographic factors, PTSD and violence exposure, and other covariates (Kataoka et al., 2011). Thus, CBITS not only has evidence for effectively treating PTSD and depressive symptoms and improving parent-reported psychosocial functioning but may also result in better school grades.

In response to Hurricane Katrina, we conducted an evaluation comparing two effective treatments to address the trauma-related mental health symptoms resulting from the disaster, as well as other types of trauma. Youths were randomly offered either TF-CBT delivered in a local clinic or CBITS delivered in schools (Cohen et al., 2009). Students who received either treatment reported significantly decreased symptoms of PTSD following the interventions. However, a distinct difference was found in access to these two interventions. For students randomized to receive CBITS at their school, 98% of students started treatment and 91% completed it, compared with only 37% starting TF-CBT at the clinic site and 15% completing it. These results attest to the value of delivering interventions in schools rather than in the clinic (Jaycox et al., 2010) and the valuable role that a school clinician can play in bringing such interventions to students in need.

CBITS has now been disseminated to sites across the United States, with some of the sites evaluating their delivery of the treatment using nonexperimental designs. Several institutions have recognized CBITS as a best practice, including the White House Conference on Helping America's Youth, the Promising Practices Network, and the Office of Juvenile Justice and Delinquency Prevention. States, including California, have also listed CBITS as an evidence-based treatment, qualifying for reimbursement through special funding. CBITS is listed in the National Registry of Evidence-based Programs and Practices (http://nrepp.sam hsa.gov) and is a recognized evidence-based treatment as part of the National Child Traumatic Stress Network.

To assist clinicians and school districts in implementing CBITS, we have also studied some of the important factors in delivering this school-based program. We have identified key barriers to implementing these groups on campus, such as logistical barriers (i.e., space to conduct groups), lack of support from administrators and teachers, competing responsibilities, and lack of parents' engagement (Langley et al., 2010). We have found that the following can be crucial to the successful delivery of CBITS: (1) pre-implementation work (planning and consultation prior to starting CBITS groups), (2) ongoing support for clinical and logistical implementation (offered by the developers and trainers), (3) promotion of fidelity to the intervention's core components, (4) tailoring of implementation to fit the service context, and (5) placing a value on monitoring student outcomes (Nadeem et al., 2011). Some examples include using a learning collaborative approach to training and sustained consultation over time (for a further description, see Ebert et al., 2012); integrating the program into top-level school district plans and leadership, and monitoring academic outcomes; and rolling out the program through ongoing supervision and learning groups with a large school mental health system.

WHICH CLIENTS ARE APPROPRIATE FOR CBITS?

The benefit of a school-based intervention is that it can reach children who might never get specialty mental health services by providing them with access to these services directly in their daily setting. Thus, it is ideal for children exposed to traumatic events who might not otherwise be able to access mental health treatment, due to factors such as lack of health insurance, and/or barriers to intervention such as lack of transportation, time, or access to quality care in their communities, and/or low parental investment in treatment.

In our work to date, we have often been challenged to consider how to handle students with severe PTSD symptoms and whether the CBITS group would really be intense enough to address their symptoms. Given the difficulty of finding quality and timely alternative referrals for these students, however, we have always included them in the CBITS groups, while also looking for more intensive individual therapy. This has worked well, and we have come to

believe that CBITS provides a supportive environment for students to complement or augment other care, while recognizing that, alone, it may not provide the entire array of services needed.

CBITS may be particularly beneficial for students who feel isolated, different, or changed as a result of child abuse. Participation in a group of peers who have also experienced traumatic events can result in improved peer support, as well as providing a different outlook on self and future that includes an understanding of the universal nature of stress and trauma and the wealth of resilience that individuals can access to overcome them. CBITS as a supportive, skills-building approach can provide a complement to individual or family-based services offered to children who have experienced child abuse.

ADVANTAGES AND DISADVANTAGES

The opportunity to reach children through schools is a key advantage of CBITS—reaching those who are traditionally underserved. In fact, most children (75%) who receive mental health services in the United States receive them at school (Farmer et al., 2003). School-based intervention can help eliminate some of the racial/ethnic disparities in mental health services seen in other sectors (Kataoka, Stein, Nadeem, & Wong, 2007). Schools can serve as an entry point for improving access to mental health services for children (Allensworth et al., 1997; Cooper, 2008).

Another advantage of the CBITS program is its flexibility in meeting the needs of diverse students with diverse experiences. Because of the iterative development of CBITS for its initial use with recent immigrant students (Spanish-, Korean-, Russian-, and Western Armenian–speakers) and its general use with ethnically and socioeconomically diverse students, the program draws examples from the group members, thus, in effect, tailoring the groups to the participating students (Ngo et al., 2008). The same is true for the types of trauma that students address in these groups. Each group contains a mix of students who have experienced family violence, abuse, disaster, traumatic loss, accidents, and medical crises. In fact, most students have experienced several traumatic events and require help in choosing the one they want to focus on in the program. Because of this diversity of experiences, students develop a sense of the commonalities and differences in experiences, begin to understand their own reactions to trauma, and find ways to talk about themselves and support others.

The major disadvantage of CBITS is its low intensity. As a school-based group intervention, it is a less intensive intervention than many students might need. Certainly, students who are in unsafe home environments, who have complicated comorbidities, or who present a risk to themselves or others will need more intensive services. Another drawback of CBITS is that it does not engage parents to the degree that might be most desirable. For parents who want to engage, there are opportunities through homework sharing, parent groups, and communication with the therapist. Often parents are as traumatized as their children and can use more support. If this is the case, another model that more fully embraces and intervenes with the parent is preferable. But we often see that parents are not able to engage in an intervention, and the studies demonstrating the impact of CBITS have shown that it can help reduce students' symptoms even without much parent participation.

EXPECTED OUTCOMES

Expected outcomes related to CBITS are directly related to its aims. First, research has shown reductions in PTSD and depressive symptoms as a result of participation in the program, in line with its primary aim. Some measures of behavior have also been shown to improve. Second, participation in the program is expected to improve coping skills, in line with the cognitive behavioral content. Third, peer and parent support are expected to improve through the group venue and the way in which the program draws in parents to help inform them so that they can better understand and support their child. Finally, there is some evidence that academic performance may improve (Kataoka et al., 2011), a key outcome that is critically important to schools.

Acknowledgment

This work was supported by a grant from the Substance Abuse and Mental Health Services Administration's National Child Traumatic Stress Network. The Cognitive Behavioral Intervention for Trauma in Schools manual is available at www.soprislearning.com. The author of the CBITS manual, Lisa Jaycox, does not receive royalties for sales.

References

Allensworth, D., Lawson, E., Nicholson, L., & Wyche, J. (1997). *Schools and health: Our nation's investment.* Washington, DC: National Academy Press.

American Psychiatric Association. (1994). *Diagnostic and statistical manual of mental disorders—fourth edition.* Washington, DC: Author.

Berman, S. L., Kurtines, W. M., Silverman, W. K., & Serafini, L. T. (1996). The impact of exposure to crime and violence on urban youth. *American Journal of Orthopsychiatry, 66*(3), 329–336.

Breslau, N., Davis, G. C., Andreski, P., & Peterson, E. (1991). Traumatic events and posttraumatic stress disorder in an urban population of young adults. *Archives of General Psychiatry, 48*(3), 216–222.

Cahill, S. P., Rothbaum, B. O., Resick, P. A., & Follette, V. M. (2009). Cognitive-behavioral therapy for adults. In E. B. Foa, T. M. Keane, M. J. Friedman, & J. A. Cohen (Eds.), *Effective treatments for PTSD: Practice guidelines from the International Society for Traumatic Stress Studies.* New York, NY: Guilford Press.

Cohen, J. A., Jaycox, L. H., Walker, D. W., Mannarino, A. P., Langley, A. K., & DuClos, J. L. (2009). Treating traumatized children after Hurricane Katrina: Project Fleur-de-lis. *Clinical Child and Family Psychology Review, 12*(1), 55–64.

Cohen, J. A., & Mannarino, A. P. (1996). A treatment outcome study for sexually abused preschool children. *Journal of the American Academy of Child and Adolescent Psychiatry, 35,* 42–50.

Cohen, J. A., Mannarino, A. P., & Deblinger, E. (2006). *Treating trauma and traumatic grief in children and adolescents.* New York, NY: Guilford Press.

Cohen, J. A., & Work Group on Quality Issues. (1998). *Practice parameters for the assessment and treatment of children and adolescents with posttraumatic stress disorder.* Washington, DC: American Academy of Child and Adolescent Psychiatry.

Cooper, J. (2008). The federal case for school based mental health services and supports. *Journal of the American Academy of Child and Adolescent Psychiatry, 47*(1), 4–8.

Curle, C. E., & Williams, C. (1996). Post-traumatic stress reactions in children: Gender differences in the incidence of trauma reactions at two years and examination of factors influencing adjustment. *British Journal of Clinical Psychology, 35*(Pt. 2), 297–309.

Dean, K. L., Stein, B. D., Jaycox, L. H., Kataoka, S., & Wong, M. (2004). Acceptability of asking parents of traumatized children about the children's symptoms. *Psychiatric Services, 55*(8), 2985.

Deblinger, E., & Heflin, A. H. (1996). *Treating sexually abused children and their nonoffending parents: A cognitive behavioral approach.* Thousand Oaks, CA: Sage Publications.

Ebert, L., Amaya-Jackson, L., Markiewicz, J. M., Kisiel, C., & Fairbank, J. A. (2012). Use of the breakthrough series collaborative to support broad and sustained use of evidence-based trauma treatment for children in community practice settings. *Administration and Policy in Mental Health and Mental Health Services Research, 39,* 187–199.

Farmer, E. M., Burns, B. J., Phillips, S. D., Angold, A., & Costello, E. J. (2003). Pathways into and through mental health services for children and adolescents. *Psychiatric Services, 54*(1), 60–66.

Finkelhor, D., Turner, H., Ormrod, R., & Hamby, S. L. (2009). Violence, abuse, and crime exposure in a national sample of children and youth. *Pediatrics, 124*(5), 1411–1423.

Foa, E. B., & Jaycox, L. H. (1999.) Cognitive-behavioral treatment of post-traumatic stress disorder. In D. Spiegel (Ed.), *Efficacy and cost-effectiveness of psychotherapy.* Washington, DC: American Psychiatric Press.

Foa, E. B., & Meadows, E. A. (1997). Psychosocial treatments for posttraumatic stress disorder: A critical review. *Annual Review of Psychology, 48,* 449–480.

Goodkind, J. R., LaNoue, M. D., & Milford, J. (2010). Adaptation and implementation of cognitive behavioral intervention for trauma in schools with American Indian youth. *Journal of Clinical Child and Adolescent Psychology, 39*(6), 858–872.

Hill, H. M., Levermore, M., Twaite, J., & Jones, L. P. (1996). Exposure to community violence and social support as predictors of anxiety and social and emotional behavior among African American children. *Journal of Child and Family Studies, 5*(4), 399–414.

Horowitz, K., Weine, S., & Jekel, J. (1995). PTSD symptoms in urban adolescent girls: Compounded community trauma. *Journal of the American Academy of Child and Adolescent Psychiatry, 34*(10), 1353–1361.

Jaycox, L. H. (2003). *Cognitive-behavioral intervention for trauma in schools.* Longmont, CO: Sopris West Educational Services.

Jaycox, L. H., Cohen, J. A., Mannarino, A. P., Walker, D. W., Langley, A. K., Gegenheimer, K. L., et al. (2010). Children's mental health care following Hurricane Katrina: A field trial of trauma-focused psychotherapies. *Journal of Traumatic Stress, 23*(2), 223–231.

Jaycox, L. H., Langley, A. K., Stein, B. D., Wong, M., Sharma, P., Scott, M., & Schonlau, M. (2009). Support for students exposed to trauma: A pilot study. *School Mental Health, 1*(2), 49–60.

Jeney-Gammon, P., Daugherty, T. K., Finch, A. J., Belter, R. W., & Foster, K. Y. (1993). Children's coping styles and report of depressive symptoms following a natural disaster. *Journal of Genetic Psychology, 154*(2), 259–267.

Joseph, S. A., Brewin, C. R., Yule, W., & Williams, R. (1991). Causal attributions and psychiatric symptoms in survivors of the Herald of Free Enterprise disaster. *British Journal of Psychiatry, 159*, 542–546.

Joseph, S. A., Brewin, C. R., Yule, W., & Williams, R. (1993). Causal attributions and post-traumatic stress in adolescents. *Journal of Child Psychology and Psychiatry, 34*(2), 247–253.

Kataoka, S. H., Fuentes, S., O'Donoghue, V. P., Castillo-Campos, P., Bonilla, A., Halsey, K., et al. (2006). A community participatory research partnership: The development of a faith-based intervention for children exposed to violence. *Ethnicity & Disease, 16*(1, Suppl. 1), S89–97.

Kataoka, S., Jaycox, L. H., Wong, M., Nadeem, E., Langley, A., Tang, L., & Stein, B. D. (2011). Effects on school outcomes in low-income minority youth: Preliminary findings from a community-partnered study of a school-based trauma intervention. *Ethnicity & Disease, 21*, S1-71–77.

Kataoka, S. H., Stein, B. D., Jaycox, L. H., Wong, M., Escudero, P., Tu, W., et al. (2003). A school-based mental health program for traumatized Latino immigrant children. *Journal of the American Academy of Child and Adolescent Psychiatry, 42*(3), 311–318.

Kataoka, S. H., Stein, B. D., Nadeem, E., & Wong, M. (2007). Who gets care? Mental health service use following a school-based suicide prevention program. *Journal of the American Academy of Child and Adolescent Psychiatry, 46*, 1341–1348.

Kliewer, W., Lepore, S. J., Oskin, D., & Johnson, P. D. (1998). The role of social and cognitive processes in children's adjustment to community violence. *Journal of Consulting and Clinical Psychology, 66*(1), 199–209.

Kuther, T. L., & Fisher, C. B. (1998). Victimization by community violence in young adolescents from a suburban city. *Journal of Early Adolescence, 18*(1), 53–76.

Langley, A. K., Cohen, J. A., Jaycox, L. H., Mannarino, A. P., Walker, D. W., Gegenheimer, K. L., et al. (in press). Trauma exposure and mental health problems among school children 15-months post-Hurricane Katrina. *Journal of Child and Adolescent Trauma.*

Langley, A. K., Nadeem, E., Kataoka, S. H., Stein, B. D., & Jaycox, L. H. (2010). Evidence-based mental health programs in schools: Barriers and facilitators of successful implementation. *School Mental Health, 2*(3), 105–113.

March, J. S., Amaya-Jackson, L., Murray, M. C., & Schulte, A. (1998). Cognitive-behavioral psychotherapy for children and adolescents with posttraumatic stress disorder after a single-incident stressor. *Journal of the American Academy of Child and Adolescent Psychiatry, 37*(6), 585–593.

March, J. S., Amaya-Jackson, L., Terry, R., & Costanzo, P. (1997). Posttraumatic symptomatology in children and adolescents after an industrial fire. *Journal of the American Academy of Child and Adolescent Psychiatry, 36*(8), 1080–1088.

Martini, D. R., Ryan, C., Nakayama, D., & Ramenofsky, M. (1990). Psychiatric sequelae after traumatic injury: The Pittsburgh Regatta accident. *Journal of the American Academy of Child and Adolescent Psychiatry, 29*(1), 70–75.

Morsette, A., Swaney, G., Stolle, D., Schuldberg, D., van den Pol, R., & Young, M. (2009). Cognitive Behavioral Intervention for Trauma in Schools (CBITS): School-based treatment on a rural American Indian reservation. *Journal of Behavior Therapy and Experimental Psychiatry, 40*(1), 169–178.

Morsette, A., van den Pol, R., Schuldberg, D., Swaney, G., & Stolle, D. (2012) Cognitive behavioral treatment for trauma symptoms in American Indian youth: Preliminary findings and issues in evidence-based practice and reservation culture. *Advances in School Mental Health Promotion, 5*(1), 51–62.

Muller, R. T., Goebel-Fabbri, A. E., Diamond, T., & Dinklage, D. (2000). Social support and the relationship between family and community violence exposure and psychopathology among high risk adolescents. *Child Abuse & Neglect, 24*(4), 449–464.

Nadeem, E., Jaycox, L. H., Kataoka, S. H., Langley, A. K., & Stein, B. D. (2011). Going to scale: Experiences implementing a school-based trauma intervention. *School Psychology Review, 40*(4), 549–568.

Ngo, V., Langley, A., Kataoka, S. H., Nadeem, E., Escudero, P., & Stein, B. D. (2008). Providing evidence-based practice to ethnically diverse youths: Examples from the Cognitive Behavioral Intervention for Trauma in Schools (CBITS) program. *Journal of the American Academy of Child Adolescent Psychiatry, 47*(8), 858–862.

Schultz, D., Barnes-Proby, D., Chandra, A., Jaycox, L. H., Maher, E., & Pecora, P. (2010). *Toolkit for adapting Cognitive Behavioral Intervention for Trauma in Schools (CBITS) or Supporting Students Exposed to Trauma (SSET) for implementation with youth in foster care: TR722.* Santa Monica, CA: RAND Corporation.

Stein, B. D., Jaycox, L. H., Kataoka, S., Rhodes, H. J., & Vestal, K. D. (2003). Prevalence of child and adolescent exposure to community violence. *Clinical Child and Family Psychology Review, 6*(4), 247–264.

Stein, B. D., Jaycox, L. H., Kataoka, S. H., Wong, M., Tu, W., Elliott, M. N., et al. (2003). A mental health intervention for schoolchildren exposed to violence: A randomized controlled trial. *JAMA, 290*(5), 603–611.

Stein, B. D., Kataoka, S. H., Jaycox, L. H., Wong, M., Fink, A., Escudero, P., et al. (2002). Theoretical basis and program design of a school-based mental health intervention for traumatized immigrant children: A collaborative research partnership. *Journal of Behavioral Health Services and Research, 29*(3), 318–326.

Vernberg, E. M., Silverman, W. K., La Greca, A. M., & Prinstein, M. J. (1996). Prediction of posttraumatic stress symptoms in children after Hurricane Andrew. *Journal of Abnormal Psychology, 105*(2), 237–248.

SIGRID JAMES, PH.D., LCSW

9

Family Foster Care for Abused and Neglected Children

GENERAL CONSIDERATIONS

Foster care has a long tradition in the provision of care and services to maltreated and abandoned children (Kadushin & Martin, 1988). In the United States, *foster care* is often used as an umbrella term capturing all types of publicly provided child welfare placements, including family foster care, kinship care, and group home and residential care. This chapter focuses specifically on *family foster care*, which includes arrangements of children living with unrelated foster parents, with relatives, or with families who plan to adopt them. Family foster care is part of the larger child welfare system, which provides services to children and families and is governed by public policies and federal regulations. The organizational and fiscal structures of the child welfare system are complex and sometimes at odds with its overarching mission to protect children, preserve families, and enhance the well-being of the children and families it serves (e.g., D'Andrade & Berrick, 2006; Noonan et al., 2012).

Much has been written in the popular press and in academic publications about the dismal outcomes for foster youths (e.g., Allen & Vacca, 2011; Courtney et al., 2011; Leslie et al., 2010), prompting some to describe foster care as a failing system in urgent need of reform (e.g., Allen & Vacca, 2011; Eckholm, 2008; Waldock, 2011). The facts are indeed troubling, and the list of concerns and "hot-button" issues is lengthy: high rates of mental health problems and early pregnancy among foster youths; developmental, health, and educational deficits; elevated rates of homelessness, unemployment, and other poor adult psychosocial outcomes; disproportionate numbers of minority youths in foster care; frequent placement disruptions; excessive psychotropic medication use; lack of adequate developmental, academic, and mental health services, and so on.

While outcomes are not uniformly poor (e.g., Berger et al., 2009; Horowitz, Balestracci, & Simms, 2001), many background risk factors (e.g., race/ethnicity, age) along with negative experiences while in foster care (e.g., frequent placement disruptions, extended stays in care) put subgroups of foster youths at higher risk for adverse developmental outcome (Dregan & Gulliford, 2012). However, the alternatives are not ideal either. Even reunification, which remains the primary goal for achieving permanency and occurs for slightly more than half of the children in foster care, is not without problems. A 2001 study by Taussig, Clyman, and Landsverk reported that children who returned home experienced more problems across multiple domains than did children who remained in foster care, even when controlling for age and gender. Subsequent studies determined no direct effect between reunification and behavior problems, but they found that stressful life events, which were experienced with greater frequency by reunified youths, as well as mental health problems among birth parents, were prime contributors to poor behavioral outcomes (Bellamy, 2008; Lau et al., 2003). With regard to adoption, which is the second preferred permanency choice, it has been similarly reported that "many adoptees have remarkably good outcomes, but some subgroups have difficulties" (Nickman et al., 2005, p. 987; J. Coakley & Berrick, 2008). Furthermore, many children in foster care never reunify or get adopted, and thus family foster care is the only remaining option for these children outside group or residential care.

Some have suggested a return to well-run and professional institutional care—"orphanages"—in the light of the perceived failures of foster care (Allen & Vacca, 2011; McKenzie, 1998; O'Sullivan & McMahon, 2006), but these voices seem to ignore the many and well-documented problems with institutional care (Barth, 2005). As such, understanding family foster care's potential, lowering the risk for subgroups of foster youths by augmenting care through targeted services provided by other service systems (e.g., mental health, education), and finding innovative ways to train, support, and retain foster parents will remain a major focus for public child welfare systems.

This chapter cannot do justice to the ongoing critical dialogue about the benefits and shortcomings of the current foster care system or address all the complexities involved in this program. Instead, it aims to provide for an interdisciplinary audience an overview of the core features and developments in family-based foster care as a program and intervention for maltreated children.

FAMILY FOSTER CARE: SUBSTITUTE FAMILY, PLACE OF RESIDENCE, STOP-GAP OPTION, OR TREATMENT?

The Child Welfare League of America describes family foster care as "a planned, goal-directed service in which the temporary protection and nurturing of children takes place in the homes of agency-approved foster families" (www.cwla.org). This description captures a primary aspect of current U.S. child welfare policy and practice: family foster care is intended as a *time-limited* arrangement. Unlike adoption, which implies a permanent substitution of one family for another, foster families are meant to temporarily "step in" while efforts are made toward reunification with the birth family or identification of other permanency options.

Family foster care in the United States has not always been a temporary arrangement. Foster care placements of undetermined length used to be commonplace, leading to coining of the term *foster care drift* (Maas & Engler, 1959) and passage of the Adoption Assistance and Child Welfare Act of 1980 (Pub. L. No. 96-272), which put the concept of permanency at the heart of child welfare practice. Since then, permanency planning has been the central principle behind child welfare initiatives and policies. Defined as "the systematic process of carrying out within a limited period, a set of goal-directed activities designed to help children and youths live in families that offer continuity of relationships with nurturing parents or caretakers, and the opportunity to offer lifetime relationships" (Maluccio & Fein, 1983, p. 197), permanency planning redefined the purpose of foster care and the outcomes by which success should be judged (Courtney & Thoburn, 2009). The temporary nature of foster care was again ratified in the Adoption and Safe Families Act (ASFA) of 1997 (Pub. L. No. 105-89), which, by shortening the time period until the termination of parental rights could be sought, tried to balance the goal of reunification with concerns about a child's safety and well-being in the face of prolonged familial dysfunction.

While the reconceptualization of foster care as a time-limited arrangement has promoted active efforts toward establishing a plan for permanency, there is evidence that a considerable proportion of children in foster care have no permanency plan (U.S. Department of Health and Human Services, 2012), that even the termination of parental rights is no guarantee that a child will be adopted or an alternative plan for permanency will be achieved (Cushing & Greenblatt, 2009), and that about one-fifth of youths continue to spend three or more years in foster care (Cheng, 2010; U.S. Department of Health and Human Services, 2012). For these youths, the risk of placement disruptions, "aging out" of the foster care system, and experiencing adverse outcomes (e.g., homelessness, unemployment, poverty) in early adulthood is particularly high (e.g., Hook & Courtney, 2011; Leathers & Testa, 2006; Pecora et al., 2006).

The ASFA also added child well-being as an explicit focus of child welfare services (Mason, 2012), in response to voices from the practice field and a growing number of studies that documented the high rate of emotional and behavior problems among foster children and identified foster children as a high-risk population (e.g., Glisson, 1994, 1996; Pilowsky, 1995; Trupin et al., 1993). More recent studies, including findings from a nationally representative survey, the National Survey of Child and Adolescent Well-Being (Burns et al., 2004), have confirmed that between one-half and three-fourths of children entering foster care exhibit behavior or social competency problems that warrant mental health intervention (for a review of studies, see Landsverk et al., 2006). This rate is significantly higher than has been reported for community samples (U.S. Department of Health and Human Services, 1999). Although the exact causes of these higher rates are not well understood, histories of abuse and neglect and backgrounds of general family dysfunction, parental substance abuse, and poverty (DeBellis, 2001; Dube et al., 2001; Young, Boles, & Otero, 2007), coupled with the potential trauma associated with an often sudden removal from home, are all believed to contribute to foster children's high-risk status (Landsverk, Garland, & Leslie, 2002). In addition, there is evidence that instability and disruption associated with frequent placement changes while in out-of-home care adversely affect outcome (e.g., Aarons et al., 2010; Newton, Litrownik, & Landsverk, 2000).

The significant needs of foster children are not in question, but how to best address them continues to be a matter of much debate. The child welfare system has traditionally relied on the curative powers of the foster home and on the abilities of foster parents to provide a therapeutic experience for children in their care. However, traditional family foster placements are not equipped to deal with the severe emotional and behavior problems present in many foster children, and additional mental health services are needed to assess and ameliorate these problems (e.g., Burns et al., 2004; Landsverk et al., 2009). Such services have been provided, for the most part, through linkages to mental health and other agencies outside the child welfare system (Hurlburt et al., 2004; Leslie et al., 2005). The expansion of treatment or therapeutic foster homes, which are a specialized form of family-based foster care designed for foster children with significant emotional and behavior problems, has also been a direct result of the growing recognition of foster children's developmental and mental health challenges (Farmer, Dorsey, & Mustillo, 2004). Considerable efforts are currently being made to forge partnerships between service systems that would facilitate the implementation of a growing number of evidence-based interventions and promising practices now available to child welfare populations (Landsverk et al., 2009).

So what is foster care? As the discussion thus far highlights, foster care has many facets. It may provide a substitute family for some children, but in many cases it is simply just another place of residence or a stop-gap option on the way to another placement or to reunification with the primary caregiver. Lastly, for some children, foster care may in fact be treatment—in the form of a specialized treatment foster care facility, or by receiving external developmental and/or mental health services while in nonrelative foster care or in a kinship placement, or by being in the home of a particularly effective foster caregiver who is able to provide nurturing and constancy.

NUMBERS AND TRENDS

For the past two decades, child welfare initiatives and policies have in part been directed at preventing out-of-home placement altogether, by providing intensive and crisis-oriented services to biological parents and thus averting removal of a child from the home (Bagdasaryan, 2005). While the evidence for the effectiveness of such preventive family-preservation efforts has been mixed (e.g., Bagdasaryan, 2005; Ryan & Schuerman, 2004) and the reasons are probably manifold, foster care rolls have in fact declined by 29%, from a peak of 567,000 in 1999 to 400,500 by September 30, 2011 (Child Trends Data, www.childtrendsdatabank.org).

The declining trend in foster care numbers has been accompanied by a shift in the preference for available placement options. There has been a significant increase in the use of kinship placements since the mid-1990s, with concomitant decreases in nonrelative foster care placements (Ehrle & Geen, 2002; Hong et al., 2011). More recently, the explicit shift toward family-based care and the development of evidence- and community-based treatment alternatives have led to a decline in the use of group and residential placements (Budde et al., 2004; Child Trends Data, www.childtrendsdatabank.org). Finally, as noted above, placements in treatment foster care have proliferated, with the growing awareness of foster children's mental health problems and supported by a comparably strong evidence base (Burns, Hoagwood, & Mrazek, 1999).

The most recent (cross-sectional) data report published by the Children's Bureau (data for 2011) indicates that children in the general out-of-home care population had a mean age of 9.3 years (median, 8.8). Boys exceeded girls in numbers (52% vs. 48%), and African American (27%) and Hispanic/Latino (21%) children made up almost half of all children in care (U.S. Department of Health and Human Services, 2012). The disproportionality of minority youths in the foster care system continues to be a much debated topic and a focus of child welfare initiatives and policies (e.g., Mumpower, 2010). The mean number of months spent in care, according to the Children's Bureau report, was 23.9 months (median, 13.5). Across available placement options, almost half of the children (47%) were placed in nonrelative family foster care, 27% with a relative, 15% in group homes or institutions, and 4% in pre-adoptive homes. For over half of the children (52%), reunification with the biological parent or principal caretaker was the primary goal, followed by adoption (25%). Other permanency planning options included long-term foster care (6%), emancipation (5%), guardianship (4%), and living with another relative (3%).

FAMILY-BASED FOSTER CARE OPTIONS

The Placement Process

One-fifth of all children who receive child protective services in response to a child abuse report are placed into out-of-home care (U.S. Department of Health and Human Services, 2010). Once a child is considered to be in need of out-of-home placement to ensure his or her safety, several placement options (beyond emergency shelters and short-term detention centers) are available. Children can be placed in a nonrelative foster family home, with a relative, in a treatment foster home, or in a group home or larger residential facility.

Several studies have pointed out that the decision-making process involved in choosing a particular placement is often determined by resource availability, policy biases, or other factors that have little to do with the needs or best interests of the child (e.g., Crea, 2010; James, 2004) and that, too often, placements are made with only limited knowledge about the child's needs and desires. Yet there are general guidelines for placement decisions. Family-based placements are always preferred over a group home or residential care, given that a child can then participate in family life, attend community schools, and live in the community. There is general agreement among experts that group and residential care placements ought to be reserved for youths whose problems cannot be addressed in family-based care or those for whom other placement options have been exhausted (Barth, 2002, 2005). With regard to choices within family-based care, a suitable kinship placement generally takes preference over a nonrelative foster placement. In some cases, this might even imply moving a child from a stable nonrelative foster family if a kinship provider has become available (James, 2004). Treatment foster care, on the other hand, is viewed as an alternative to group and residential care and, like these settings, targets youths with serious emotional and behavior problems or other specialized needs.

The Options

There are three basic family-based foster care options: nonrelative, kinship, and treatment foster care.

Nonrelative foster care is provided in the homes of certified or licensed foster care providers according to standards established by the states. While standards vary across child welfare systems, all foster care parents are selected by means of a home study and a licensing/approval process, which aim to assess individuals' ability to provide care for someone else's child and the types of behavioral conditions they can handle or would be willing to learn how to handle. The assessment includes criminal background and child abuse and neglect registry checks for all persons in the household, references from people who can shed light on the parenting capabilities of the prospective caregiver, and an assessment of the safety and adequacy of the physical space. Nonrelative family foster care is generally sought out if a child must be placed outside the parents' home but cannot be placed with a suitable relative, and in 2011, as noted above, 47% of out-of-home care placements were with nonrelative foster caregivers. Foster caregivers may foster several children at the same time.

Relative or kinship care is the preferred form of care for children who, due to abuse or neglect, cannot live with their parents. The Child Welfare League of America defines kinship care as "the full time care, nurturing and protection of children by relatives, members of their tribes or clans, godparents, stepparents, or any adult who has a kinship bond with a child" (www.cwla.org). However, kinship care involves "substantial variations in levels of state agency involvement, financial support, types of financing mechanisms, and levels of state regulation and licensing" (Anderson, 2006, p. 717). Three kinship classifications have been identified (Geen, 2000): (1) kinship foster care, in which the child has been removed from the home through a court order; (2) voluntary kinship care, in which arrangements are made through child welfare without a court order, and (3) private kinship care, in which no contact with the child welfare system has occurred. In the context of the current discussion, the focus here is on kinship foster care placement. In 2011, 27% of child welfare placements were with relatives (U.S. Department of Health and Human Services, 2012).

The growth in kinship care has been supported by economic incentives, a shrinking foster care market, and an ideological stance that values placement with extended family and, in terms of policy, has been ratified through passage of the ASFA in 1997 and the subsequent Fostering Connections to Success and Increasing Adoptions Act of 2008 (Pub. L. No. 110-351). In contrast to nonrelative foster care, kinship care is regarded as an alternative permanency option, given that it fosters ties to the family of origin and preserves links in the child's community (Barth, 1999).

As kinship care has expanded, financial and legal complexities involved in this arrangement have become evident. Financial support for kinship families has traditionally come from Temporary Assistance for Needy Families (TANF) state funds (Ehrle, Geen, & Clark, 2001). Payments paid out through TANF tend to be smaller than Title IV-E foster care payments (caregiver subsidies) and have work requirements and time limits attached to them (Anderson, 2006). Some kinship caregivers have opted to become licensed foster parents, thus becoming eligible for regular caregiver subsidies. However, some kinship placements may not meet foster care licensing standard, while other kin caregivers may be reluctant to comply with the expectations that the foster parent role entails, such as participation in training, cooperation in implementing a case plan, and generally being subject to greater oversight by the child welfare department. The legal status of children in kinship care has also been a focus of discussion. For a number of reasons, kin caregivers are less likely to seek adoption of the child (Downs, Moore, & McFadden, 2009). To encourage long-term relationships with kin caregivers who do not wish to adopt their relatives' child, some states have experimented with subsidized guardianships as a form of permanency (www.cwla.org).

Treatment foster care is a family-based out-of-home care option for youths with emotional and behavioral disorders or other needs that require specialized care (Curtis, Alexander, & Lunghofer, 2001; Farmer, Dorsey, & Mustillo, 2004). It has emerged as a preferred alternative to more restrictive settings for youths in need of more intensive and restrictive mental health services (e.g., Meadowcroft, Thomlison, & Chamberlain, 1994). Treatment foster care combines a structured therapeutic approach with the benefits of a more normative family-based milieu, using "specially trained treatment parents as the primary implementers of therapeutic plans" (Breland-Noble et al., 2005, p. 168). While treatment foster care is generally lauded as an effective intervention (Burns, Hoagwood, & Mrazek, 1999), most of the evidence is tied to one particular model—Multidimensional Treatment Foster Care (MTFC) (Chamberlain, 2002)—which has been well tested but, as yet, has had limited penetration into the public child welfare system.

Treatment foster care has great appeal because it provides intensive and relatively short-term services (less than a year) in a least-restrictive environment, allows family-based living and community-based opportunities for learning, and provides enhanced support and training to foster caregivers, thereby increasing their satisfaction and retention rates (Chamberlain, Moreland, & Reid, 1992; Farmer et al. 2010).

OUTCOMES OF CHILDREN IN FAMILY FOSTER CARE

Any serious discussion on the outcomes of family foster care will be confounded by the fact that many foster children experience movement across placement settings over time as well as reentries into care (James, Landsverk, & Slymen, 2004; Wulczyn, Kogan, & Harden, 2003). Prevalence rates of placement disruptions vary, depending on sample and study design (Webster, Barth, & Needell, 2000; Wulczyn, Kogan, & Harden, 2003). However, we know that a significant proportion of children experience some or significant instability, moving back and forth between family-based and residential care placements. Children's movement through care makes it virtually impossible to isolate the effects of one placement type on outcomes. Nonetheless, researchers have attempted to examine outcomes by placement type.

Kinship Care versus Nonrelative Foster Care

In the light of child welfare's goals to create ongoing attachments and to provide culturally competent services, the value of kinship care is undisputed. The higher likelihood of children in kinship care to remain within their communities, to be placed with siblings, and to have more consistent contact with their birth parents contributes to the permanency of their connections (e.g., Berrick, Barth, & Needell, 1994; Chapman, Wall, & Barth, 2004; Messing, 2006), and many have described kinship placement as mutually beneficial for the child and the relative caregiver (e.g., T. Coakley et al., 2007; Dubowitz & Sawyer, 1994; Johnson-Garner & Meyers, 2003).

Research studies provide conflicting evidence about improved outcomes for children in kinship care versus foster care. Conceptual and methodological problems have contributed to often divergent results and confound current understanding of the benefits or limits of kinship care versus nonrelative foster care. Beyond differences in sample characteristics and other methodological aspects, the conceptualization and operationalization of kinship care across studies have been highly variable. Some studies use the child's first placement as a way to categorize by placement type; other studies classify children based on their "ever" spending time in kinship care or spending the majority of their out-of-home care episode in kinship care; yet another group distinguishes between placement types based on where children were placed at the time of the study. All methods of operationalizing placement type ignore a child's prior and/or subsequent placement history, and few studies control for length of time in a particular placement in relation to a child's overall length of time spent in out-of-home care.

Benefits of kinship care are relatively consistently reported in the area of placement stability. Multiple studies have shown that kinship placements are less likely than nonrelative foster care placements to be disrupted—in other words, stability is enhanced through kinship care, which in turn is believed to contribute to better developmental outcomes overall (e.g., Chamberlain et al., 2006; Cuddeback, 2004; Rubin et al., 2008). In an analysis of national survey data, Rubin and colleagues (2008) even found benefits to stability when children entered kinship care after an initial period in a nonrelative foster home. While the reasons are not entirely clear, it is likely that kinship providers have a greater commitment to their own family's offspring and perhaps greater tolerance for behaviors that might lead to disruptions in nonrelative placements. How-

ever, kinship care reduces the likelihood of reunification with the birth parent (Courtney, 1995; Koh & Testa, 2008; Scannapieco, Hegar, & McAlpine, 1997), which is a great concern because children in kinship care are more likely to leave the child welfare system without a legalized permanency arrangement (Downs, Moore, & McFadden, 2009).

Questions remain about the behavioral outcomes for children in kinship care compared with those in nonrelative placements. Some researchers have reported lower rates of behavior problems in children in kinship care at baseline (e.g., Lawrence, Carlson, & Egeland, 2006; Rubin et al., 2008; Sakai, Lin, & Flores, 2011); others found few or no differences on multiple indices of functioning (Barth et al., 2007; De Robertis & Litrownik, 2004). A recent study that examined the relationship between longer stays with kin and dimensions of adolescent well-being found greater involvement in risk behaviors—including delinquency, sexual risk behaviors, substance use, and total risk behaviors— among youths who spent more time living with kin (Taussig & Clyman, 2011). In addition, Sakai and colleagues (2011) reported seven times the rate of pregnancy and twice the risk of substance use among children in kinship care when compared with nonrelative foster care. In trying to explain these differences, Taussig and Clyman (2011) proposed that prolonged exposure to risk factors that may be associated with kinship care may have deleterious consequences over time. Kinship caregivers tend to be older and are more likely to be single, less educated, unemployed, and poor. Sakai et al. (2011) reported that the predominant form of financial support for kinship caregivers came from the TANF program.

Other studies have raised concerns about the safety of children in kinship care, given the easier and unsupervised access to sometimes abusive parents (Peters, 2005). Some experts have also raised questions about children staying within family systems that have been affected by substance abuse, poverty, and violence, all of which have intergenerational components (Ehrle & Geen, 2002; Scannapieco, Hegar, & McAlpine, 1997). Some researchers report that parenting behaviors and the quality of caregiver-child relationships are more likely to be negative in kinship foster homes than in traditional nonrelative foster homes (Chipman, Wells, & Johnson, 2002; Harden et al., 2004). Chipman and colleagues found that kinship caregivers self-reported employing corporal punishment, making a distinction between child maltreatment and physical punishment. A study that investigated parental attitudes and resources of both kinship foster caregivers (i.e., grandmothers) and traditional foster caregivers found that kinship caregivers reported greater caregiver-child conflict and displayed less warmth than traditional foster caregivers (Harden et al., 2004).

Given the socioeconomic and psychosocial needs of kinship families, the consistent findings about these families receiving less financial and emotional support from the child welfare system are disconcerting. Sakai et al. (2011) reported less parent training, less support through peer groups or respite, and less input on child welfare service plans among kinship care providers than among nonrelative foster caregivers.

Treatment Foster Care

Several studies have examined the outcomes for youths in treatment foster care. Given that treatment foster care is a program available to youths involved in child welfare, mental health, and juvenile justice systems, not all findings are relevant to this discussion. Outcomes for treatment foster care have been compared with those for youths in group or residential care, because of the similar needs and characteristics of youths in these settings (Breland-Noble et al., 2004). A few studies have reported more serious emotional and behavioral disorders among youths in residential care compared with those placed into treatment foster care (Baker et al., 2007; B. R. Lee & Thompson, 2008; McCrae et al., 2010), but both groups have more serious problems than youths in traditional nonrelative or kinship care settings (Huefner et al., 2010). There is less agreement on whether youths have better outcomes after treatment foster care or residential care. Chamberlain's (2002) MTFC model has consistently produced better results, including fewer criminal referrals and more frequent return to live with relatives. However, B. R. Lee and Thompson (2008) reported greater improvement among youths served in a teaching-family-based residential care model, such as a more favorable discharge, a greater likelihood to return home, and a reduced likelihood to experience subsequent placement in the first six months after discharge. McCrae et al. (2010) found that outcomes did not differ.

RECRUITMENT, TRAINING, AND SUPPORT OF FOSTER PARENTS

The temporary nature of foster care and the significant health, mental health, and developmental needs of the foster care population pose special challenges to foster caregivers and to the foster care system itself (Rhodes, Orme, & McSurdy, 2003). This affects how foster parents are recruited, trained, and retained, how they perceive their task, and how foster children are introduced into the family foster care setting (Hollin & Larkin, 2011).

As should be apparent by now, foster caregiving is a challenging and demanding task. Foster parents have unique roles. They are expected to function as temporary parents to children who often have histories of trauma and disrupted relationships and present with challenges in multiple domains of functioning. At the same time, they are expected to meet agency-specified responsibilities and to work within a larger system toward the implementation of a plan over which they have little or no control. Substantiated child maltreatment among foster parents is relatively rare (Drumm, 2011), but foster parents' perceptions of their roles and responsibilities often diverge from those of child welfare workers (Rhodes, Orme, & McSurdy, 2003), contributing to role confusion, unrealistic expectations, and frustration—factors that have been identified as predictors of high turnover (Hollin & Larkin, 2011; Wilson, Sinclair, & Gibbs, 2000).

The recruitment, assessment, and training of foster parents constitute a considerable investment of time and financial resources. As such, it is particularly frustrating that a majority of interested foster parents either do not complete the pre-service training or discontinue fostering after six months (Rhodes et al., 2003), leading to a well-documented shortage of suitable foster parents (Doyle & Peters, 2007). "The available evidence suggests then that a high burden of care in combination with perceived (if not actual) disempowerment, as well as dysfunctional and intrusive engagement with children's agencies, is unsustainable for many foster carers" (Murray, Tarren-Sweeney, & France, 2011, p. 151). Some research has focused on examining factors that motivate foster parents and promote their retention (e.g., Redding, Fried, & Britner, 2000; Rhodes, Orme, & Buehler, 2001; Rodger, Cummings, & Leschied, 2006). A discussion of this body of literature is beyond the scope of this chapter, but, in short, the literature indicates that unmet needs for support and training are a primary reason for high foster parent turnover (Cooley & Petren, 2011; Murray, Tarren-Sweeney, & France, 2011).

With regard to foster parent training, several reviews have noted the great variability in focus and content areas as well as in the number of training hours and the expectations involved in the training programs used by child welfare agencies (Berry, 1988; Dorsey et al., 2008; J. H. Lee & Holland, 1991; Rork & McNeil, 2011). The two most widely used programs are Model Approach to Partnership in Parenting Group Preparation and Selection of Foster and/or Adoptive Families (MAPP/GPS) and foster Parent Resources for Information, Development, and Education (PRIDE) (Dorsey et al., 2008). MAPP is primarily focused on clarifying foster/adoptive parents' new role and making sure that they know what to expect. PRIDE puts greater emphasis on the knowledge and skills required to meet the needs of foster children. Both programs have a negligible empirical base. Most of the evidence comes from MTFC, which includes both preliminary training and ongoing supervision/support for treatment foster parents. This type of training is different in that it is skills oriented, teaching foster parents specific ways to effectively respond to behavioral challenges in the child. A modified version of this training is the more recently introduced Keeping Foster Parents Trained and Supported (KEEP) foster parent training intervention (Price et al., 2009), which applies the skills-based approach of the MTFC training to regular foster care. KEEP has been tested in randomized trials and proved effective in increasing positive parenting skills and reducing child behavior problems—most importantly, in those children who typically present the greatest challenge to foster parents. KEEP also increased the rate of reunification, and the intervention was found to mitigate the disruptive effect of multiple placement changes.

CONCLUSIONS

Concerns about family foster care are justified. It is difficult to recruit and train suitable foster parents, and the complex needs of many maltreated children often exceed the capabilities of foster parents. The short-term nature of family foster care may encourage greater efforts toward making arrangements for the child that have more permanency, but it may also confound children's adjustment into these settings. The experiences of children in foster care are highly variable, and child welfare initiatives and policies should continue to be directed at stabilizing children's experiences and augmenting family foster care with targeted developmental, mental health, and educational services. Fortunately, there is a growing list of evidence-based interventions and promising practices that are now available for children in foster care and have been shown to improve outcomes for foster youths (California Evidence-Based Clearinghouse for Child Welfare, www.cebc4cw.org; Landsverk et al., 2009). The challenge at this stage is how to integrate these effective interventions into the services that are provided for children in foster care. Partnerships across service systems and supporting policies will be needed to facilitate the implementation of these interventions and to make the necessary services available to youths in foster care.

References

Aarons, G., James, S., Monn, A. R., Raghavan, R., Wells, R., & Leslie, L. K. (2010). Behavior problems and placement change in a national child welfare sample: A prospective study. *Journal of the American Academy of Child and Adolescent Psychiatry, 49*(1), 70–80.

Allen, B. S., & Vacca, J. S. (2011). Bring back orphanages—An alternative to foster care? *Children and Youth Services Review, 33*(7), 1067–1071.

Anderson, S. (2006). The impact of state TANF policy decisions on kinship care providers. *Child Welfare, 85*(4), 715–736.

Bagdasaryan, S. S. (2005). Evaluating family preservation services: Reframing the question of effectiveness. *Children and Youth Services Review, 27*(6), 615–635.

Baker, A. L., Kurland, D., Curtis, P., Alexander, G., & Papa-Lentini, C. (2007). Mental health and behavioral problems of youth in the child welfare system: Residential treatment centers compared to therapeutic foster care in the Odyssey Project population. *Child Welfare, 86*(3), 97–123.

Barth, R. (1999). After safety, what is the goal of child welfare services: Permanency, family continuity or social benefit? *International Journal of Social Welfare, 8*, 244–252.

Barth, R. (2002). *Institutions vs. foster homes: The empirical base for the second century of debate.* Chapel Hill, NC: Annie E. Casey Foundation, University of North Carolina, School of Social Work, Jordan Institute of Families.

Barth, R. (2005). Residential care: From here to eternity. *International Journal of Social Welfare, 14*, 158–162.

Barth, R., Guo, S., Green, R., & McCrae, J. (2007). Kinship care and nonkinship foster care: Informing the new debate. In R. Haskins, F. Wulczyn, & M. B. Webb (Eds.), *Child protection: Using research to improve policy and practice* (pp. 187–206). Washington, DC: Brookings Institution.

Bellamy, J. (2008). Behavioral problems following reunification of children in long-term foster care. *Children and Youth Services Review, 30*, 216–228.

Berger, L. M., Bruch, S. K., Johnson, E. I., James, S., & Rubin, D. (2009). Estimating the "impact" of out-of-home placement on child well-being: Approaching the problem of selection bias. *Child Development, 80*(6), 1856–1876.

Berrick, J. D., Barth, R. P., & Needell, B. (1994). A comparison of kinship foster homes and foster family homes: Implications for kinship foster care as family preservation. *Children and Youth Services Review, 16*(1), 33–63.

Berry, M. (1988). A review of parent training programs in child welfare. *Social Service Review, 62*, 302–323.

Breland-Noble, A. M., Elbogen, E. B., Farmer, E. M., Dubs, M. S., Wagner, H. R., & Burns, B. J. (2004). Use of psychotropic medications by youths in therapeutic foster care and group homes. *Psychiatric Services, 55*(6), 706–708.

Breland-Noble, A. M., Farmer, E. M. Z., Dubs, M. S., Potter, E., & Burns, B. J. (2005). Mental health and other service use by youth in therapeutic foster care and group homes. *Journal of Child and Family Studies, 14*(2), 167–180.

Budde, S., Mayer, S., Zinn, A., Lippold, M., Avrushin, A., Bromberg, A., et al. (2004). *Residential care in Illinois: Trends and alternatives. Final report.* Chicago, IL: Chapin Hall Center for Children at the University of Chicago.

Burns, B. J., Hoagwood, K., & Mrazek, P. J. (1999). Effective treatment for mental disorders in children and adolescents. *Clinical Child and Family Psychology Review, 2*(4), 199–254.

Burns, B. J., Phillips, S. D., Wagner, H. R., Barth, R. P., Kolko, D. J., Campbell, Y., & Landsverk, J. (2004). Mental health need and access to mental health services by youths involved with child welfare: A national survey. *Journal of the American Academy of Child and Adolescent Psychiatry, 43*, 960–970.

Chamberlain, P. (2002). Treatment foster care. In B. Burns & K. Hoagwood (Eds.), *Community treatment for youth: Evidence-based interventions for severe emotional and behavioral disorders* (pp. 117–138). New York, NY: Oxford University Press.

Chamberlain, P., Moreland, S., & Reid, K. (1992). Enhanced services and stipends for foster parents: Effects on retention rates and outcomes for children. *Child Welfare, 5*, 387–401.

Chamberlain, P., Price, J. M., Reid, J. B., Landsverk, J., Fisher, P. A., & Stoolmiller, M. (2006). Who disrupts from placement in foster and kinship care? *Child Abuse & Neglect, 30*(4), 409–424.

Chapman, M. V., Wall, A., & Barth, R. P. (2004). Children's voices: The perceptions of children in foster care. *American Journal of Orthopsychiatry, 74*(3), 293–304.

Cheng, T. C. (2010). Factors associated with reunification: A longitudinal analysis of long-term foster care. *Children and Youth Services Review, 32*(10), 1311–1316.

Chipman, R., Wells, S. J., & Johnson, M. A. (2002). The meaning of quality in kinship foster care: Caregiver, child, and worker perspectives. *Families in Society, 83*(5/6), 508–520.

Coakley, J., & Berrick, J. (2008). Research review: In a rush to permanency—Preventing adoption disruption. *Child & Family Social Work, 13*(1), 101–112.

Coakley, T. M., Cuddeback, G., Buehler, C., & Cox, M. E. (2007). Kinship foster parents' perceptions of factors that promote or inhibit successful fostering. *Children and Youth Services Review, 29*(1), 92–109.

Cooley, M. E., & Petren, R. E. (2011). Foster parent perceptions of competency: Implications for foster parent training. *Children and Youth Services Review, 33*(10), 1968–1974. doi:10.1016/j.childyouth.2011.05.023

Courtney, M. E. (1995). Reentry to foster care of children returned to their families. *Social Service Review, 69*(2), 226–241.

Courtney, M., Dworsky, A., Brown, A., Cary, C., Love, K., Vorhies, V., & Hall, C. (2011). *Midwest evaluation of the adult functioning of former foster youth: Outcomes at age 26.* Chicago, IL: Chapin Hall Center for Children at the University of Chicago.

Courtney, M., & Thoburn, J. (Eds.). (2009). *Children in state care.* Burlington, VT: Ashgate Publishing.

Crea, T. M. (2010). Balanced decision making in child welfare: Structured processes informed by multiple perspectives. *Administration in Social Work, 34*(2), 196–212.

Cuddeback, G. S. (2004). Kinship family foster care: A methodological and substantive synthesis of research. *Children and Youth Services Review, 26*(7), 623–639.

Curtis, P. A., Alexander, G., & Lunghofer, L. A. (2001). A literature review comparing the outcomes of residential group care and therapeutic foster care. *Child and Adolescent Social Work Journal, 18*(5), 377–392.

Cushing, G. G., & Greenblatt, S. B. (2009). Vulnerability to foster care drift after the termination of parental rights. *Research on Social Work Practice, 19*(6), 694–704.

D'Andrade, A., & Berrick, J. D. (2006). When policy meets practice: The untested effects of permanency reforms in child welfare. *Journal of Sociology & Social Welfare, 33*(1), 31–52.

DeBellis, M. D. (2001). Developmental traumatology: The psychobiological development of maltreated children and its implications for research, treatment, and policy. *Development and Psychopathology, 13*, 537–561.

De Robertis, M. T., & Litrownik, A. J. (2004). The experience of foster care: Relationship between foster parent disciplinary approaches and aggression in a sample of young foster children. *Child Maltreatment, 9*(1), 92–102.

Dorsey, S. S., Farmer, E. Z., Barth, R. P., Greene, K. M., Reid, J. J., & Landsverk, J. (2008). Current status and evidence base of training for foster and treatment foster parents. *Children and Youth Services Review, 30*(12), 1403–1416.

Downs S. W., Moore, E., & McFadden, E. J. (2009). *Child welfare and family services policies and practice* (8th ed.). Boston, MA: Pearson Education.

Doyle, J. J., & Peters, H. E. (2007). The market for foster care: An empirical study of the impact of foster care subsidies. *Review of Economics of the Household, 5*, 329–351.

Dregan, A. A., & Gulliford, M. C. (2012). Foster care, residential care and public care placement patterns are associated with adult life trajectories: Population-based cohort study. *Social Psychiatry and Psychiatric Epidemiology, 47*(9), 1517–1526.

Drumm, M. (2011). How widespread is abuse in foster care? *Community Care, 1872*, 32–33.

Dube, S. R., Anda, R. F., Felitti, V. J., Chapman, D. P., Williamson, D. F., & Giles, W. H. (2001). Childhood abuse, household dysfunction, and the risk of attempted suicide throughout the life span. *JAMA, 286*(24), 3089–3096.

Dubowitz, H., & Sawyer, R. J. (1994). School behavior of children in kinship care. *Child Abuse & Neglect, 18*(11), 899–911.

Eckholm, E. (2008, April 16). Bleak stories follow a lawsuit on Oklahoma foster care. *New York Times.* www.nytimes.com /2008/04/16/us/16foster.html

Ehrle, J., & Geen, R. (2002). Kin and non-kin foster care— Findings from a national survey. *Children and Youth Services Review, 24*(1), 15–35.

Ehrle, J., Geen, R., & Clark, R. L. (2001). *Children cared for by relatives: Who are they and how are they faring?* Washington, DC: Urban Institute.

Farmer, E. Z., Burns, B., Wagner, H., Murray, M., & Southerland, D. (2010). Enhancing "usual practice" treatment foster care: Findings from a randomized trial on improving youths' outcomes. *Psychiatric Services, 61*(6), 555–561.

Farmer, E. Z., Dorsey, S., & Mustillo, S. A. (2004). Intensive home and community interventions. *Child and Adolescent Psychiatric Clinics of North America, 13*(4), 857–884.

Geen, R. (2000). In the interest of children: Rethinking federal and state policies affecting kinship care. *Policy and Practice of Public Human Services, 58*(1), 19–27.

Glisson, C. (1994). The effects of services coordination teams on outcomes for children in state custody. *Administration in Social Work, 18*, 1–23.

Glisson, C. (1996). Judicial and service decision for children entering state custody: The limited role of mental health. *Social Services Review, 70*(2), 257–281.

Harden, B., Clyman, R. B., Kriebel, D. K., & Lyons, M. E. (2004). Kith and kin care: Parental attitudes and resources of foster and relative caregivers. *Children and Youth Services Review, 26*(7), 657–671.

Hollin, G., & Larkin, M. (2011). The language and policy of care and parenting: Understanding the uncertainty about key players' roles in foster care provision. *Children and Youth Services Review, 33*(11), 2198–2206.

Hong, J., Algood, C., Chiu, Y., & Lee, S. (2011). An ecological understanding of kinship foster care in the United States. *Journal of Child and Family Studies, 20*(6), 863–872.

Hook, J. L., & Courtney, M. E. (2011). Employment outcomes of former foster youth as young adults: The importance of human, personal, and social capital. *Children and Youth Services Review, 33*(10), 1855–1865.

Horowitz, S. M., Balestracci, K. M. B., & Simms, M. D. (2001). Foster care placement improves children's functioning. *Archives of Pediatrics & Adolescent Medicine, 155*, 1255–1260.

Huefner, J. C., James, S., Ringle, J., Thompson, R. W., & Daly, D. L. (2010). Patterns of movement for youth within an integrated continuum of residential services. *Children and Youth Services Review, 32*(6), 857–864.

Hurlburt, M. S., Leslie, L. K., Landsverk, J., Barth, R. P., Burns, B. J., Gibbons, R. D., et al. (2004). Contextual predictors of mental health service use among children open to child welfare services. *Archives of General Psychiatry, 61*(12), 1217–1224.

James, S. (2004). Why do foster care placements disrupt? An investigation of reasons for placement change in foster care. *Social Service Review, 78*(4), 601–627.

James, S., Landsverk, J., & Slymen, D. J. (2004). Placement movement in out-of-home care: Patterns and predictors. *Children and Youth Services Review, 26*(2), 185–206.

Johnson-Garner, M. Y., & Meyers, S. A. (2003). What factors contribute to the resilience of African-American children within kinship care? *Child and Youth Care Forum, 32*(5), 255–269.

Kadushin, A., & Martin, J. A. (1988). *Child welfare services* (4th ed.). New York, NY: Macmillan Publishing.

Koh, E., & Testa, M. F. (2008). Propensity score matching of children in kinship and nonkinship foster care: Do permanency outcomes differ? *Social Work Research, 32*(2), 105–116.

Landsverk, J., Burns, B., Stambaugh, L., & Rolls Reutz, J. (2006). *Mental health care for children and adolescents.* Seattle, WA: Casey Family Programs. www.casey.org/Resources/Publications/pdf /MentalHealthCareChildren.pdf

Landsverk, J., Burns, B., Stambaugh, L., & Rolls Reutz, J. (2009). Psychosocial interventions for children and adolescents in foster care: Review of research literature. *Child Welfare, 88*(1), 49–69.

Landsverk, J., Garland, A. F., & Leslie, L. K. (2002). Mental health services for children reported to child protective services. In J. E. B. Myers, L. Berliner, J. Briere, C. T. Hendrix, C. Jenny, & T. A. Reid (Eds.), *The APSAC handbook on child maltreatment* (2nd ed., pp. 487–507). Thousand Oaks, CA: Sage Publications.

Lau, A. S., Litrownik, A. J., Newton, R. R., & Landsverk, J. (2003). Going home: The complex effects of reunification on internalizing problems among children in foster care. *Journal of Abnormal Child Psychology, 31*(4), 345–359.

Lawrence, C. R., Carlson, E. A., & Egeland, B. (2006). The impact of foster care on development. *Development and Psychopathology, 18*(1), 57–76.

Leathers, S. J., & Testa, M. F. (2006). Foster youth emancipating from care: Caseworkers' reports on needs and services. *Child Welfare, 85*(3), 463–498.

Lee, B. R., & Thompson, R. R. (2008). Comparing outcomes for youth in treatment foster care and family-style group care. *Children and Youth Services Review, 30*(7), 746–757.

Lee, J. H., & Holland, T. P. (1991). Evaluating the effectiveness of foster parent training. *Research on Social Work Practice, 1*(2), 162–174.

Leslie, L. K., Hurlburt, M., James, S., Landsverk, J., Slymen, D. J., & Zhang, J. (2005). Entry into child welfare: A gateway to mental health services? *Psychiatric Services, 56*(8), 981–987.

Leslie, L. K., James, S., Monn, A., Kauten, M. C., Zhang, J., & Aarons, G. (2010). Health-risk behaviors in young adolescents in the child welfare system. *Journal of Adolescent Health, 47*(1), 26–34.

Maas, H., & Engler, R. (1959). *Children in need of parents.* New York, NY: Columbia University Press.

Maluccio, A., & Fein, E. (1983). Permanency planning: A redefinition. *Child Welfare, 62*(3), 195–201.

Mason, S. E. (2012). Child well-being as a federal priority in child welfare. *Families in Society, 93*(3), 155–156.

McCrae, J. S., Lee, B. R., Barth, R. P., & Rauktis, M. E. (2010). Comparing three years of well-being outcomes for youth in group care and nonkinship foster care. *Child Welfare, 89*(2), 229–249.

McKenzie, R. B. (1998). Rethinking orphanages for the 21st century: A search for reforms for the nation's child-welfare. *Spectrum: Journal of State Government, 71*(2), 8–13.

Meadowcroft, P., Thomlison, B., & Chamberlain, P. (1994). Treatment foster care services: A research agenda for child welfare. *Child Welfare, 73*(5), 565.

Messing, J. (2006). From the child's perspective: A qualitative analysis of kinship care placements. *Children and Youth Services Review, 28*(12), 1415–1434.

Mumpower, J. L. (2010). Disproportionality at the "front end" of the child welfare services system: An analysis of rates of referrals, "hits," "misses," and "false alarms." *Journal of Health and Human Services Administration, 33* (3), 364–405.

Murray, L., Tarren-Sweeney, M., & France, K. (2011). Foster carer perceptions of support and training in the context of high burden of care. *Child & Family Social Work, 16*(2), 149–158.

Newton, R. R., Litrownik, A. J., & Landsverk, J. A. (2000). Children and youth in foster care: Disentangling their relationship between problem behaviors and number of placements. *Child Abuse & Neglect, 24*(10), 1363–1374.

Nickman, S. L., Rosenfeld, A. A., Fine, P., MacIntyre, J. C., Pilowsky, D. J., Howe, R., et al. (2005). Children in adoptive families: Overview and update. *Journal of the American Academy of Child and Adolescent Psychiatry, 44*(10), 987–995.

Noonan, K., Matone, M., Zlotnik, S., Hernandez-Mekonnen, R., Watts, C., Rubin, D., & Mollen, C. (2012). Cross-system barriers to educational success for children in foster care: The front line perspective. *Children and Youth Services Review, 34*(2), 403–408.

O'Sullivan, J., & McMahon, M. F. (2006). Who will care for me? The debate of orphanages versus foster care. *Policy, Politics & Nursing Practice, 7*(2), 142–148.

Pecora, P. J., Williams, J., Kessler, R. C., Hiripi, E., O'Brien, K., Emerson, J., et al. (2006). Assessing the educational achievements of adults who were formerly placed in family foster care. *Child & Family Social Work, 11*(3), 220–231.

Peters, J. J. (2005). True ambivalence: Child welfare workers' thoughts, feelings, and beliefs about kinship foster care. *Children and Youth Services Review, 27*(6), 595–614.

Pilowsky, D. (1995). Psychopathology among children placed in family foster care. *Psychiatric Services, 46*, 906–910.

Price, J. M., Chamberlain, P. P., Landsverk, J. J., & Reid, J. J. (2009). KEEP foster-parent training intervention: Model description and effectiveness. *Child & Family Social Work, 14*(2), 233–242.

Redding, R. E., Fried, C., & Britner, P. A. (2000). Predictors of placement outcomes in treatment foster care: Implications for foster parent selection and service delivery. *Journal of Child and Family Studies, 9*(4), 425–447.

Rhodes, K. W., Orme, J. G., & Buehler, C. (2001). A comparison of family foster parents who quit, consider quitting, and plan to continue fostering. *Social Service Review, 75*(1), 84–114.

Rhodes, K., Orme, J., Cox, M., & Buehler, C. (2003). Foster family resources, psychosocial functioning, and retention. *Social Work Research, 27*(3), 135–150.

Rhodes, K., Orme, J., & McSurdy, M. M. (2003). Foster parents' role performance responsibilities: Perceptions of foster mothers, fathers, and workers. *Children and Youth Services Review, 25*(12), 935–964.

Rodger, S. S., Cummings, A. A., & Leschied, A. W. (2006). Who is caring for our most vulnerable children? The motivation to foster in child welfare. *Child Abuse & Neglect, 30*(10), 1129–1142.

Rork, K. E., & McNeil, C. B. (2011). Evaluation of foster parent training programs: A critical review. *Child & Family Behavior Therapy, 33*(2), 139–170.

Rubin, D., Downes, K., O'Reilly, A., Mekonnen, R., Luan, X., & Localio, R. (2008). Impact of kinship care on behavioral well-being for children in out-of-home care. *Archives of Pediatrics & Adolescent Medicine, 162*(6), 550–556.

Ryan, J. P., & Schuerman, J. R. (2004). Matching family problems with specific family preservation services: A study of service effectiveness. *Children and Youth Services Review, 26*(4), 347–372.

Sakai, C., Lin, H., & Flores, G. (2011). Health outcomes and family services in kinship care: Analysis of a national sample of children in the child welfare system. *Archives of Pediatrics & Adolescent Medicine, 165*(2), 159–165.

Scannapieco, M. M., Hegar, R. L., & McAlpine, C. C. (1997). Kinship care and foster care: A comparison of characteristics and outcomes. *Families in Society, 78*(5), 480–488.

Taussig, H. N., & Clyman, R. B. (2011). The relationship between time spent living with kin and adolescent functioning in youth with a history of out-of-home placement. *Child Abuse & Neglect, 35*(1), 78–86.

Taussig, H. N., Clyman, R. B., & Landsverk, J. (2001). Children who return home from foster care: A 6-year prospective study of behavioral health outcomes in adolescence. *Pediatrics, 108*(1), 1–7.

Trupin, E. W., Tarico, V. S., Low, B. P., Jemelka, R., & McClellan, J. (1993). Children on child protective service caseloads: Prevalence and nature of serious emotional disturbance. *Child Abuse & Neglect, 17*(3), 345–355.

U.S. Department of Health and Human Services. (1999). *Mental health: A report of the surgeon general.* Rockville, MD: U.S. Department of Health and Human Services, Substance Abuse and Mental Health Services Administration, Center for Mental Health Services, & National Institutes of Health, National Institute of Mental Health.

U.S. Department of Health and Human Services. (2012). *The AFCARS report.* www.acf.hhs.gov/sites/default/files/cb/afcars report19.pdf

U.S. Department of Health and Human Services, Administration for Children and Families, Administration of Children, Youth and Families. (2010). *Child maltreatment 2010*. Washington DC: U.S. Government Printing Office.

Waldock, T. (2011). Enhancing the quality of care in child welfare: Our obligation under the UN Convention on the Rights of the Child. *Relational Child & Youth Care Practice, 24*(3), 50–61.

Webster, D., Barth, R. P., & Needell, B. (2000). Placement stability for children in out-of-home care: A longitudinal analysis. *Child Welfare, 79*(5), 614.

Wilson, K. K., Sinclair, I. I., & Gibbs, I. I. (2000). The trouble with foster care: The impact of stressful "events" on foster carers. *British Journal of Social Work, 30*(2), 193–209.

Wulczyn, F., Kogan, J., & Harden, B. J. (2003). Placement stability and movement trajectories. *Social Services Review, 77*(2), 212–236.

Young, N. K., Boles, S. M., & Otero, C. (2007). Parental substance use disorders and child maltreatment: Overlap, gaps, and opportunities. *Child Maltreatment, 12*(2), 137–149.

10

SUSAN J. KELLEY, RN, PH.D., FAAN
DEBORAH M. WHITLEY, M.P.H., PH.D.

Kinship Care

GENERAL CONSIDERATIONS

In 2011, approximately 2.9 million children in the United States were living under the care of someone other than a biological parent (U.S. Census Bureau, 2011). Comprising nearly 4% of the nation's 0- to 17-year-old population, these children live in a variety of caregiving arrangements, including foster care, group homes, and kinship care. *Kinship care* refers to "any living arrangement in which children do not live with either of their parents and instead are cared for by a relative or someone with whom they have had a prior relationship" (Geen, 2004, p. 132). While the term *relative* is often used interchangeably with *kin*, it is important to note that when defining kinship care, many state child welfare agencies include as kin persons that go beyond blood relatives (e.g., godparents, family friends, or someone else with close ties to the child) (Geen, 2004). Although the practice of kinship care has long been established by cultural tradition among African Americans and other racial/ethnic groups, the formal recognition of this caregiving arrangement by the U.S. government and child protective services did not occur until the latter part of the twentieth century (Brown, Cohon, & Wheeler, 2002; Koh, 2010; U.S. Department of Health and Human Services [HHS], 2000). Since that time, available data have indicated a steady increase in the use of kinship care by families and by child welfare services in need of an alternative placement for children (Cuddeback, 2004; Ehrle & Geen, 2002; HHS, 2000; Winokur, Holtan, & Valentine, 2009). Indeed, it is estimated that more than 2.3 million children currently live in a parent-absent household that is headed by a relative, representing a more than 50% increase since 1990 (U.S. Census Bureau, 2004, 2011). Recognizing this growing trend, researchers, practitioners, and child advocates have become increasingly interested in understanding not only the characteristics of these families but also the outcomes for the children in kinship care. Such research seeks to understand whether kinship care offers a suitable and viable placement option for children whose parents can no longer care for them.

EVOLUTION OF KINSHIP CARE

Although kinship care has been documented as a cultural tradition in the African American community for centuries (Brown, Cohon, & Wheeler, 2002), the factors contributing to the surge in modern-day kinship care arose relatively recently. Prior to the latter half of the last century, child welfare workers held the belief that child abuse and neglect were indicative of dysfunction in the family of origin, meaning that placement of a child with a relative of the abusive or neglectful birth parent would inevitably result in further maltreatment (HHS, 2000). However, as the number of available foster homes and child group homes decreased and the number of children needing out-of-home placement increased over the past several decades, child welfare workers were forced to reexamine the value of kin caregivers as a placement option (HHS, 2000). In doing so, practitioners began to recognize that kinship care presented several theoretical advantages to the child welfare system. Kinship care potentially provides an opportunity to reduce the level of separation trauma, maximize the preservation of the family, maintain continuity in cultural traditions and norms, and place the child with a caregiver already knowledgeable about the child's history (Swann & Sylvester, 2006).

As the prevalence of kinship care continued to increase, state and national policy began to reflect this growing trend. Title IV-E of the Social Security Act outlines federal policy requiring states to "consider giving preference to an adult relative over a non-related caregiver when determining a placement for a child, provided that the relative caregiver meets all relative State child protection standards" (Adoption and Safe Families Act [ASFA] of 1997, Pub. L. No. 105-89, Title IV-E, § 471). The Personal Responsibility and Work Opportunity Reconciliation Act of 1996 (Pub. L. No. 104-193) replaced the Aid to Families with Dependent Children program with the current Temporary Assistance to Needy Families (TANF) program, which provides child-only grants to relatives caring for a child, regardless of the caregiver's income. Additional policy support for kinship care came from the ASFA of 1997, in which states were permitted to request federal reimbursement for kinship foster care expenses. Finally, the Fostering Connection to Success and Increasing Adoptions Act of 2008, also under the Social Security Act, required states to exercise due diligence in seeking a kinship caregiver when a child requires out-of-home care. It also specifies the necessity to keep sibling groups together and provides monetary resources to support this provision. Following these federal initiatives, many states have developed policies that give relatives placement preference or that benefit kinship caregivers through modified foster care licensing standards (Child Welfare Information Gateway, 2010; Geen, 2004).

LIMITATIONS OF RESEARCH

Research examining kinship care in the United States has proliferated, but several limitations must be considered when interpreting the results of these studies. First, the term *kinship care* lacks a precise definition. Unlike foster care, a placement option in which the child is clearly under the custody of the state and is then placed in the care of a foster parent, kinship care includes a broad continuum of caregiving arrangements ranging from public to private (Geen, 2004; HHS, 2000). Broadly defined, public kinship care involves the child welfare system in placement of the child, but private kinship care does not (HHS, 2000). Substantial variation exists within these definitions, however; private kinship care, for example, may simply be an informal arrangement between the relative and the birth parent, or it may include the assistance of social service agencies (Ehrle & Geen, 2002; Geen, 2004). Resulting from this ambiguity, a second limitation in kinship care research is the lack of consistent and precise surveillance of the families involved in kinship care (HHS, 2000). While the U.S. Census estimates provide an understanding of the number of children living in households headed by a relative, these data omit important information about the involvement of the state foster care system or child protective services. As a result, additional surveillance systems, including the Adoption and Foster Care Analysis and Reporting System (AFCARS) and the National Survey of American Families (NSAF), have attempted to fill this gap. The NSAF is the only national survey that examines voluntary kinship care, which involves children who are living with relatives as a result of child welfare involvement but are not in the custody of the state (Geen, 2004). The NSAF found there were 285,000 children in voluntary kin care, compared with 200,000 in formal foster kin care and 1,800,000 in private kin care.

Smaller-scale kinship care studies that do not use these national datasets are subject to further limitations. Such studies typically employ convenience samples, due to the challenges inherent in identifying kinship care families—particularly those that are private arrangements—thus making the research subject to selection bias (Cuddeback, 2004; Winokur, Holtan, & Valentine, 2009). Furthermore, study samples from a single state significantly hamper the generalizability of practice and policy implications, given that state policies outlining the resources and support available to kinship care families differ substantially (Child Welfare Information Gateway, 2010). Together, these methodological differences hinder the ability to reach meaningful conclusions about the long-term outcomes for children and families involved in kinship care (Cuddeback, 2004; HHS, 2000; Winokur, Holtan, & Valentine, 2009). Despite these limitations, however, relatively consistent findings in the existing literature have enabled researchers to delineate some conclusions regarding the characteristics and outcomes of kinship care families.

CHARACTERISTICS OF KINSHIP CARE FAMILIES

Although kinship caregivers cannot be considered a homogeneous population, systematic research reviews have consistently demonstrated several demographic and social factors that differentiate kinship caregivers from their nonrelative foster caregiving counterparts. In general, kinship caregivers are more likely to be older, unmarried, female, African American, less educated, unemployed, and of a lower socioeconomic status (Boetto, 2010; Cuddeback, 2004; Ehrle & Geen, 2002; Winokur, Holtan, & Valentine, 2009). They are also more likely to live in city centers rather than rural or metropolitan areas (HHS, 2000). Many of these demographic characteristics are consistent in state-by-state comparisons of the kinship care population (Koh, 2010). Grandparents as caregivers of their grandchildren are of particular interest in the kinship caregiving literature. Of the 2.3 million children living in a nonparent household headed by a relative, over two-thirds are living under the care of a grandparent (U.S. Census Bureau, 2011). Considering the older age of this population, the need for increased attention to the caregivers' health care needs is frequently cited (Fuller-Thomson & Minkler, 2000; Kelley, Whitley, & Campos, 2010).

In addition to the unique characteristics of the caregivers involved in kinship care, the children under their care share some similarities. Across national estimates, African American children are more likely than their white counterparts to be placed in kinship care (Ehrle & Geen, 2002; HHS, 2000). However, a review of AFCARS state-level data from five states indicates that this distinction may vary across states. In Arizona, for example, children in kinship care were more likely to be white than children in nonrelative foster care (Koh, 2010). The gender of children in kinship care and foster care does not appear to differ significantly (Ehrle & Geen, 2002). With regard to age, however, children in public kinship care seem to be younger than those in nonkin foster care, while children in private kinship care seem to be older (Ehrle & Geen, 2002; HHS, 2000; Koh, 2010). Existing research also points to different reasons for children entering kinship care as opposed to nonkin foster care. Children in kinship care are more likely to have been removed from the home due to parental substance abuse, while children in nonkinship care are more likely to have been removed due to mental health problems of the birth parent (Cuddeback, 2004; Ehrle & Geen, 2002). Although additional research may serve to further define the population of kinship caregivers and the children under their care, practitioners and policymakers should remain mindful of the substantial heterogeneity of this population, even from state to state (Koh, 2010).

CHALLENGES

Caring for a child who has been removed from his or her family of origin presents a myriad of challenges, including navigating the child welfare system, managing the behavior of formerly maltreated children, and, in many cases, maintaining communication with the birth parents (Chipungu & Bent-Goodley, 2004). Compounding these difficulties is the finding that, when compared with nonrelative foster caregivers, kinship caregivers are often confronted with several additional challenges to ensuring the well-being of children in their care.

Support Needs

Unlike the majority of nonrelative foster caregivers, who have made a personal and informed decision to care for children needing out-of-home placement, kinship caregivers often assume responsibility of one or more children suddenly and out of immediate need (Boetto, 2010). In doing so, many kinship caregivers are unable to procure the basic necessities (e.g., beds, infant supply needs) or the training and support services necessary to help them prepare for this challenging parental role. Moreover, caregiving grandparents, in particular, often assume the responsibility for sibling groups rather than individual children, most likely multiplying the challenges facing them (Kelley, Whitley, & Campos, 2011). This lack of training and support frequently persists into the caregiving role, as the existing literature consistently indicates that kinship caregivers receive fewer resources and less support from social service agencies than nonrelative caregivers (Goodman, Potts, & Pasztor, 2007; Sakai, Lin, & Flores, 2011).

In a small-scale study of private kinship care providers, unmet service needs were found to be one of the strongest predictors of psychological distress in caregivers (Kelley et al., 2000). Corroborating these findings, a qualitative study involving kinship foster caregivers determined that a lack of resources and parenting challenges were often reported as substantial barriers to the successful fostering of kin (Coakley et al., 2007). The importance of receiving adequate training and support is a particularly salient issue among kinship caregivers caring for children with disabilities (Whitley & Kelley, 2008). Future research should determine why social service agencies are failing to meet the needs of these kinship caregivers. Some researchers point to a lack of requirements designating the provision of services to kinship caregivers not involved with the public foster care system (Ehrle & Geen, 2002). It is also possible that professionals are often not aware of the needs of kinship caregivers. The finding that almost 80% of children in any form of kinship care (private, voluntary, or formal foster care) are in private kinship care (Geen, 2004) undoubtedly contributes to this lack of access to resources.

Financial Resources

As mentioned above, kinship caregivers are more likely to be of lower socioeconomic status than nonrelative caregivers. Data from the NSAF indicate that court-involved kin caregivers were twice as likely as their nonkin counterparts to be living at less than 200% of the federal poverty level (Ehrle & Geen, 2002). In addition, there is limited evidence suggesting that kinship caregivers are also more likely to live in homes that are more crowded, less structurally sound, and located in neighborhoods connected with high crime and violence (Cuddeback, 2004).

Current research consistently finds that kinship caregivers receive significantly less public financial assistance for providing care than nonrelative caregivers (Goodman, Potts, & Pasztor, 2007; Sakai, Lin, & Flores, 2011; Winokur, Holtan, & Valentine, 2009). Partially explaining this factor is the large percentage of kinship caregivers who are not formally integrated in the state foster care system or who do not meet the same licensing standards as nonrelative foster caregivers (Ehrle & Geen, 2002). These caregivers are not eligible for full foster care payments and, as such, they often subsist on child-only TANF payments (Anderson, 2006). TANF payments are significantly lower than foster care payments and are based on the number of children under the caregiver's care, meaning that the payment amount per child decreases with each additional child in the home (HHS, 2000). Furthermore, the time limitations and work requirements upheld in some states limit the number of kinship caregivers that are eligible for TANF payments (HHS, 2000). A study examining NSAF data found that only 52% of private kinship caregivers were receiving these payments (Ehrle & Geen, 2002). Fortunately, in the past decade, several states have modified the licensing requirements for kinship foster caregivers so that they may be eligible for full foster care payments (Anderson, 2006).

Relationship with Birth Parent

Managing communication and visitation with a child's birth parents is a challenge for many nonrelative caregivers, but the familial relationship between the birth parent and a kinship caregiver may add further complications. Indeed, qualitative findings indicate that kinship caregivers more frequently report complications with the child's family of origin as a barrier to successful fostering (Coakley et al., 2007). Child welfare workers also report kinship caregivers' difficulties in establishing and maintaining boundaries with the birth parent, an obstacle responsible for many kinship care disruptions (Terling-Watt, 2001).

Health and Aging of Caregivers

Kin caregivers tend to be older than nonkin foster parents, most likely because the majority of kinship caregivers are grandparents raising their grandchildren (Koh, 2010; U.S. Census Bureau, 2011). Not surprisingly, then, the greater health needs of this generally older population are of particular concern (Kelley, Whitley, & Campos, 2013). The effects of caregiving duties on the exacerbation of chronic diseases, including diabetes and heart disease, have been reported by grandparent caregivers (Haglund, 2000; Lee et al., 2003). In addition, findings from a nationally representative survey have shown that grandparents raising their grandchildren are more likely than their noncaregiving counterparts to be limited in their ability to perform daily tasks, even when controlling for important confounding factors (Minkler & Fuller-Thomson, 1999). The effects of deteriorating physical health on the mental health of grandparents are also evident; in a convenience sample of grandmothers raising their grandchildren, physical health was found to be a significant predictor of grandmothers' psychological distress (Kelley et al., 2000). In a study comparing kinship and nonrelative foster caregivers, kinship caregivers demonstrated higher levels of depression, parental stress, and abuse potential (Timmer, Sedlar, & Urquiza, 2004). Given the financial struggles experienced by many kinship caregivers, providing access to affordable health care and mental health services should be a priority for social service and health care professionals interacting with this caregiving population.

Special Considerations for Private Kinship Care Providers

Private kinship care, as we noted above, includes those caregiving arrangements in which the child is not in the formal custody of the state. Following the practices and policies of each individual state, however, child welfare workers may still be able to provide resources and services to these families. But other families may not have any interaction with the child welfare system at all. Because of this overall lower degree of interaction with the state child welfare system, the population of private kinship caregivers is typically difficult to monitor through state databases and thus has largely been absent from existing research (Cuddeback, 2004). Nevertheless, a few studies have used convenience samples to broaden the knowledge base on this unique population. Private kinship caregivers are more likely than nonkin foster parents to be single, to be caring for sibling sets, and to have children in care for a longer period of time (Geen, 2009; Goodman et al., 2004; Strozier & Krisman, 2007). In another study, researchers found that public kinship caregivers were more likely to use a greater array of available support services (Goodman, Potts, & Pasztor, 2007). This finding is not surprising, considering public caregivers' greater degree of interaction with social service agencies. Despite the limitations inherent in research conducted with convenience samples, the findings suggest potential vulnerabilities and areas of intervention for practitioners working with private kinship caregivers.

OUTCOMES FOR CHILDREN IN KINSHIP CARE

A primary goal of much of the existing research examining kinship care is to determine whether the outcomes for children involved in kinship care are similar to or even better than those for children living in nonrelative foster care (HHS, 2000; Winokur, Holtan, & Valentine, 2009). Reaching conclusions based on the available evidence is challenging, however, because of additional limitations in this area of research. Because ethical practice prohibits the random assignment of children to kinship or nonrelative care, researchers must depend on previously established caregiving arrangements, thus subjecting studies to bias resulting from inherent differences in group membership (Winokur, Holtan, & Valentine, 2009). In addition, the findings of many studies are based on the reports of caregivers rather than those of more objective observers (HHS, 2000; Kelley, Whitley, & Campos, 2011; Messing, 2006). Keeping these shortcomings in mind, we can find some common findings on the outcomes for children in kinship care, but caution should be used when applying these findings to practice (Cuddeback, 2004; Winokur, Holtan, & Valentine, 2009).

Behavioral, Psychological, and Academic Impact

As we described above, the trend of placing children with relatives rather than foster parents emerged out of the growing need for more placement options. However, as kinship care expanded, researchers and child welfare practitioners posited several potential advantages for children placed in these caregiving arrangements, including reduced separation trauma, a greater sense of family connectedness, and an increased sense of continuity in their lives (Boetto, 2010; Cuddeback, 2004).

Evidence suggests that children in kinship care have a greater propensity for behavior and emotional problems than children in the general population (Cuddeback, 2004).

For instance, researchers found that children in the care of grandparents had higher levels of behavior problems than those in the general population (Smith & Palmieri, 2007). This elevated occurrence of behavior problems is not surprising given the reasons (e.g., abandonment, child maltreatment, death of birth parent) that these children are no longer in the care of birth parents. In a cross-sectional study of 230 African American children in kinship care with grandmothers, almost one-third had clinically elevated child behavior problems scores (Kelley, Whitley, & Campos, 2011).

A body of research is beginning to emerge that compares outcomes for children in kinship care with those for children in nonkinship foster care. While most studies suggest improved outcomes for those in kinship care (Rubin et al., 2008; Sakai, Lin, & Flores, 2011), others show conflicting or mixed results (Hegar & Rosenthal, 2009). Several studies have employed prospective methodologies, in addition to propensity matching, to account for differences in child behavior prior to entering care (Rubin et al., 2008; Sakai, Lin, & Flores, 2011; Winokur, Holtan, & Valentine, 2009). Researchers used a nationally representative sample of 1,309 children entering kinship or nonkinship foster care to prospectively examine child behavior problems. The researchers ascertained that, even when controlling for baseline behavior, placement stability, and attempted reunification, children in kinship care were less likely to exhibit behavioral issues after three years of placement (Rubin et al., 2008). These findings were corroborated by a subsequent prospective study, also employing a national sample, in which researchers found that children in kinship care were less likely than children in nonrelative foster care to have continuing behavior problems and lower social skills (Sakai, Lin, & Flores, 2011). Surprisingly, however, the children in kinship care were also found to be twice as likely to abuse substances and seven times as likely to experience a teen pregnancy.

Also using a nationally representative sample, other researchers comparing children in kinship and nonkinship foster care found that the children in kinship care had fewer behavior problems, both internalizing and externalizing, than their counterparts in nonkinship care, as reported by caregivers (Hegar & Rosenthal, 2009). Teachers, however, reported more externalizing behavior problems in the children in kinship foster care; no differences were reported on internalizing behaviors. It is possible that informant bias may account for these conflicting results, with kinship caregivers tending to rate child behaviors more positively than nonrelative caregivers (Keller et al., 2001; Winokur, Holtan, & Valentine, 2009). Regardless, other researchers determined that in a sample of 1,377 children in kinship or nonrelative foster care, the children in nonkin care were nearly six times as likely to interact with the juvenile justice system (Winokur et al. 2008). Further indication of the positive effects of kinship care is evident in studies examining the mental health of children in out-of-home care. A systematic review by Winokur et al. (2009) concluded that kinship caregivers were nearly twice as likely as nonrelative foster caregivers to report positive emotional health of the children under their care.

Given the relatively poor educational outcomes of children in foster care (Bruskas, 2008), the academic achievement of children in kinship care is of particular interest. Unfortunately, the literature is scant and the findings are inconclusive. However, nonsignificant effect sizes point to more positive outcomes among children in kinship care (Cuddeback, 2004; Winokur, Holtan, & Valentine, 2009). Future research could benefit from examining the effect of differences in placement stability on the school performance of children in kinship and nonkinship foster care.

Placement Stability and Permanence

Both placement stability (e.g., fewer changes in foster homes) throughout the duration of a child's out-of-home care and placement permanence (e.g., reunification with birth parents or adoption) are frequently recognized as goals of the U.S. foster care system (Cuddeback, 2004; HHS, 2000). Greater placement stability and less disruptive transitions into out-of-home care have been cited as benefits of kinship care, when compared with foster care, by both researchers and the children in care themselves (Cuddeback, 2004; Messing, 2006; Winokur, Holtan, & Valentine, 2009). In fact, a systematic review of studies comparing the placement stability of children in kinship care and children in nonrelative foster care determined that children in foster care were 2.6 times more likely to experience three or more placements (Winokur, Holtan, & Valentine, 2009). The greater degree of placement stability in kinship care also appears to be consistent across U.S. states, despite differences in policies guiding the reimbursement and formalization of kinship care arrangements (Koh, 2010).

The evidence on placement permanence in kinship care is less conclusive than that on placement stability; however, existing research suggests that children in kinship care achieve placement permanence at slower rates than their counterparts in nonkin care (Cuddeback, 2004; Winokur, Holtan, & Valentine, 2009). Indeed, a large retrospective study examining the time to adoption for both kin and nonkin families found that kinship caregivers waited a longer time before initiating the adoption process (Ryan et al., 2010). State-by-state comparisons of permanence rates of children in kinship care suggest that state policies regarding the ability of kin caregivers to adopt or obtain guardianship of a child may be a factor in this outcome (Koh, 2010). Another possibility is the reluctance of kinship caregivers to establish a legally binding relationship with the child under care, for fear of inciting conflict with the birth parent and adversely affecting family functioning (Ryan et al., 2010).

In addition to achieving placement permanence with the caregiver, reunification of the child with his or her birth parent is another highly examined permanence outcome. Similar to the findings for the caregiver adoption process, a body of evidence suggests that reunification occurs more slowly among kinship care arrangements (Cuddeback, 2004; Winokur, Holtan, & Valentine, 2009). Winokur et al. (2009) found that children in nonrelative foster care were twice as likely to be reunified with their birth parents. However, as some research highlights, reunification with the birth parent may not always be the most positive outcome for the child (Lau et al., 2003; Taussig, Clyman, & Landsverk, 2001). In a six-year prospective study comparing the outcomes of children who had been reunified with their parents with those of children who had not, Taussig and colleagues (2001) determined that reunified children exhibited more self-destructive behavior, substance abuse, and overall risk profiles. The children were also more likely to have been arrested, to have dropped out of school, or to have received lower grades. Research should explore the possibility that slower rates of reunification in kinship care arrangements may serve as a protective factor against negative outcomes for children and adolescents.

Long-Term Outcomes

Given the large numbers of children who are raised in kinship care, the long-term outcomes for this population are of interest. Although some evidence from small convenience samples suggests that adults who lived under kinship care as children fare better than those who lived in nonrelative foster care, methodological weaknesses render the results of these studies inconclusive (Cuddeback, 2004). A more recent study using data from the National Survey of Family Growth indicates that adult women who were in kinship care as children may have poorer outcomes in some aspects of their emotional well-being than women in the general population (Carpenter & Clyman, 2004). It is important to note that no comparisons were made with women who had been in nonkinship foster care. As we mentioned earlier, because of the adverse events associated with placement in kinship care (e.g., abandonment or maltreatment by birth parents), it is not unexpected that these individuals would experience some long-term negative outcomes. Additional prospective research using more standardized measures of well-being and more meaningful comparison groups would provide a greater understanding of these outcome findings.

INTERVENTIONS FOR KINSHIP CARE PROVIDERS AND CHILDREN

Serving the needs of kinship care families requires a sustained, coordinated effort by both public and private agencies. Services for public kinship care providers are more defined than those for private kinship care providers. Support groups, legal services, respite care, parent education, and kinship navigator services are examples of current services targeted to kinship care providers. As noted earlier, families in the public foster care system have greater access to a variety of services and resources (e.g., counseling, material aid, medical care) than families in private kinship care (Macomber, Geen, & Clark, 2001). Families involved in public foster care generally have a case manager to assist with identifying public and community-based services, while families in private kinship care may have to rely on their own assertiveness and ingenuity to access needed services. Many private kinship care providers—older grandparent caregivers, in particular—may not have the physical or emotional capacity to navigate the bureaucratic systems to acquire services, and as a result, needs go unmet. We describe here the most widely available intervention models to assist kinship caregivers. The listing is not meant to be an all-inclusive resource but is simply an overview of the most prominent intervention strategies.

Support Groups

A concern of many kinship providers is emotional stress and the sense of not being able to cope with daily challenges while caring for children. As summarized earlier, stress related to a variety of factors (e.g., inadequate financial resources, caring for multiple children, and/or caring for those with disabilities or with problematic behaviors) is common, with kinship providers feeling inadequate and unsupported. Kinship providers, specifically grandparents, often express feelings of social isolation from friends, family, and the community (Gerald, Landry-Meyer, & Roe, 2006).

Support groups are a popular intervention strategy to help kinship providers address their emotional needs in a supportive environment. Support groups generally require relatively low levels of staffing to implement, have little monetary cost, and have significant utility. As an illustration of their popularity, since 1996, the Brookdale Foundation, through its Relatives as Partners Program (RAPP), has provided seed money to local and state agencies to develop, implement, and evaluate support groups for relative caregivers, in addition to other services (Brookdale Foundation, 2007). As a result of the RAPP initiative, such groups are now offered across the country. Support groups can be offered as a component of a broader multimodal intervention for kinship care providers or as a freestanding service (Kelley et al., 2001; Strozier, 2012).

The positive effect of support groups for kinship care providers on a variety of outcomes has been reported in the literature (Smith, 2003; Strozier, 2012). A recent study by Strozier (2012) explored the effectiveness of support groups in enhancing social support for 61 participants, comparing kinship caregivers who participated in support groups and those who did not. Her findings showed that the caregivers participating in support groups experienced enhanced perceptions of social support compared with the nonparticipants. Despite the small sample size, a value of this study is that it explores the unique effects of support groups. Research on understanding the impact of support groups on family functioning is a continuing area of interest.

Children in kinship care may also benefit from peer support groups. There are limited studies on their utility, however. In a small-scale study that explored how grandparent caregivers viewed support groups for their grandchildren, the majority of respondents believed that a support group could be beneficial for their grandchildren, especially if the group addressed topics that improved the quality of the grandparent-grandchild relationship (Smith, Savage-Stevens, & Fabian, 2002). The caregivers also viewed the support groups for children as a respite resource, allowing kinship caregivers to attend their own support group meeting or socialize with family and friends.

Legal Support Services

Many private kinship care providers take on the responsibility of caring for children without considering the possible legal implications associated with this decision. Many providers do not understand that having physical care of a minor child does not give them any legal rights; the birth parents continue to have the legal right to make any and all decisions for the child. As noted earlier, many kinship providers are reluctant to pursue a legal relationship with their minor relative because of engendering possible repercussions from the birth parents or destroying the hope that the birth parents will gain the capacity to assume responsibility for their children. Yet, having a legal relationship is important. Efforts to help kinship providers determine which legal alternative meets the needs of the child and the family should take precedence.

There are a number of legal options that private kinship providers should consider. The four primary types of legal relationship are guardianship, legal custody, relative foster care, and adoption. *Guardianship* is supported by the courts, allowing an adult relative to make medical decisions, add children to medical insurance plans, or enroll them in school. Generally, adult relatives must go through a court process to acquire guardianship, which has proved prohibitive for some kinship caregivers due to time, travel, and cost.

Legal custody is similar to guardianship but is often granted by a different court. It requires court action to determine whether, in the best interest of the child, the kinship care provider should assume responsibility for the child for a period of time. In some cases, the relative caregiver may need to seek legal consultation, especially if there is a question about the capacity of the birth parents to care for their child or children. De facto custody is available in some states and does not require proving the parent is "unfit" if the relative has been raising the child for a significant length of time (American Bar Association, 2012).

Relative foster care, or public kinship foster care, occurs when a parent's rights have been suspended or terminated by the courts and the state child welfare agency has legal custody of the child. The intent is to place a child in an environment that is safe and stable and promotes family well-being. Foster care is not viewed as a permanent solution;

either reunification with the birth parent or adoption is the ultimate goal of the foster care program.

Kinship providers may consider *adoption* as the most permanent legal option. Adoptions occur after the parents' legal rights are permanently terminated. An adult relative assumes full parental responsibility for the child. Relatives caring for children previously in the care of the state may receive federal adoption subsidies to support care for children with special needs (e.g., older children, sibling groups, children with disabilities).

For information on any of the above legal services, kinship providers are encouraged to seek legal consultation. Local legal aid societies are a primary resource for kinship providers to obtain legal assistance. In some areas, local attorneys specializing in adoption may offer legal support pro bono. Area agencies on aging services are another resource that may provide legal consultation for kinship providers, but access to their services is usually limited to caregivers 60 years of age or older.

Kinship Navigator Services

A common concern of kinship care providers is a lack of awareness about what resources or services are available in communities to meet family needs. Kinship providers may have a cursory understanding about public welfare programs (e.g., food stamps, Medicaid, the Women, Infants, and Children, or WIC, program) but lack a clear understanding about how to apply for them. This is especially true for private kinship care providers. Too often, kinship providers needing financial assistance inquire at local county welfare offices about TANF and food stamps but are not informed about any specialized programs in aging or child welfare services. As a result, providers eligible for a broad spectrum of services do not receive access to them because workers in one department are unaware of services or benefits provided by other departments. Kinship navigator services are designed to address this problem; this is a coordinated effort to ensure kinship providers have broad access to available services and benefits that address the varied needs of kinship families. Navigators provide information about the public benefits and services available to kinship providers and the eligibility criteria for federal, state, and local benefits, including legal services, as well as providing assistance in completing benefit applications, when necessary. Navigator programs may also provide assistance in identifying specialized educational programs; in finding medical, mental health, and dental services; and in locating child care, parent education trainings, support groups, and respite care. In some localities, trained kinship care liaisons work on telephone warm lines; others are stationed in public welfare, child welfare, or aging services offices, providing on-site assistance to providers. Websites sponsored by state and local agencies are another resource to inform kinship providers about local services and benefits. The Family Connections Act of 2008 identified kinship navigator services as one of its primary program components. As yet, there is little evidence on the effectiveness of navigator services, because programs were just implemented in 2009. Future studies should explore not only the service outcomes of kinship providers but also the effectiveness of the navigator network with local aging, child welfare, and other service providers.

Financial Assistance

A shortage of money is a constant source of emotional stress for many kinship providers. Some providers are living on fixed incomes, while others have delayed retirement to increase their finances or have returned to work (Wang & Marcotte, 2007). Traditional welfare benefits (e.g., TANF, child-only TANF, food stamps, WIC) provide the core financial assistance package for private kinship providers and are a common source of assistance to acquire basic necessities. The amount of the TANF benefits varies by state, and generally the benefit levels do not meet a family's full financial needs.

Relative foster care subsidies, as noted earlier, are also a potential source of financial support for kinship providers. Like TANF, the subsidy amount varies across states. Some states provide the same rate for relative as for nonrelative foster parents; other states have a variable rate. Adjustments may depend on the age of the child, with providers caring for adolescent children receiving slightly higher subsidy rates than those caring for younger children. Similarly, subsidized guardianship provides temporary financial assistance to kinship providers caring for children formerly in state custody. Generally, the amount of the subsidy is based on a proportional rate of foster care payments.

Georgia has taken a unique approach to supporting grandparent caregivers over the age of 60 with their financial needs. In 2006, Georgia established the Emergency/Crisis Intervention Services Payment. The one-time payment, which is up to three times the TANF payment for a family, can be used however the provider chooses. For example, recipients can use the money to pay a utility bill, to purchase furniture or infant products, or for anything else considered an emergency by the caregiver. Another targeted benefit for kinship providers in Georgia is the Grandparents Raising Grandchildren Monthly Subsidy. Families receive $50 per child each month to assist with child care expenses. The grandparent must be 60 years of age or older; the grandchild does not have to be in state custody to receive these benefits. These resources are designed to support the most senior kinship providers, who often are the most financially needy.

Physical and Behavioral Health

The literature provides a broad array of studies that explore the health and mental health needs of kinship providers. Interventions designed to address these needs include home-based nursing support services. In a sample of 529 African American grandmothers raising their grandchildren, researchers studied the effectiveness for physical and mental health outcomes of a home-based comprehensive intervention that included registered nurse home visits (Kelley, Whitley, and Campos, 2010). Registered nurses visited participants each month to monitor health indicators such as weight, blood pressure, and cholesterol and glucose levels, as well as to review medication regimens. They also worked with clients to encourage preventive health care practices. The findings of this study suggest that the intervention had a positive effect on participants' physical vitality, mental health, and role functioning, both physical and emotional.

According to the American Academy of Pediatrics (2012), many children receive only sporadic health care prior to entering foster care, with a high prevalence of undiagnosed or undertreated chronic health problems. Of those in foster care, approximately 50% have chronic illnesses and 10% are medically fragile or have complex health needs. The academy also recognizes that children in foster care meet the federal definition of special health care needs and warrant special interventions to ensure they receive appropriate and adequate health care services. Even after entering foster care, children may not receive all necessary health care because of a variety of barriers. Findings from a qualitative study suggest that kinship care providers may have more difficulties than nonkin foster parents in finding and using primary health care services (Schneiderman, Smith, & Palinkas, 2012). To address the challenges associated with the health care needs of children in foster care, the American Academy of Pediatrics (2012) published standards of health care for these children. The academy also promotes the medical or health care home model for children in foster care, with services that include health screenings, comprehensive assessments, periodic health monitoring, and preventive care (Sanchez, Gomez, & Davis, 2010).

Given the extent of trauma previously experienced by children in kinship care and their levels of behavior problems, trauma-focused cognitive behavioral therapy is often warranted. At a minimum, children in kinship care should be thoroughly screened for behavioral issues and fully evaluated, if indicated. Because parenting traumatized children requires specialized skills, kinship care providers may need guidance and support in managing child behavior problems. School-based interventions for kinship caregivers and the children in their care are a valuable option for supporting these families (Strozier et al., 2005). Several other promising interventions are described in the literature (Pacifici et al., 2006; Price et al., 2008).

Child Development Services

Children in private and public kinship care are at an increased risk for developmental disabilities for a variety of reasons, including prior exposure to child maltreatment and substance abuse and receipt of minimal prenatal care

(Grant, 2000; Whitley & Kelley, 2008). In one cohort of children in kinship care, 67% of grandmothers were raising children under 5 years of age and 40% reported the presence of a special-needs child in their home (Grant, 2000). In an exploratory study of 74 young African American grandchildren being raised by their grandmothers, 54% had a confirmed diagnosis of a developmental delay; almost one-third of those with a confirmed diagnosis were found to have fetal alcohol syndrome or fetal alcohol spectrum disorder (Whitley & Kelley, 2008). Children with fetal alcohol spectrum disorder might display a combination of abnormalities, including failure to thrive, growth deficiency, dysmorphic facial features, and central nervous system effects.

The key to assisting these children is to ensure that each child receives an early screening, a comprehensive developmental diagnostic evaluation, and the most appropriate treatment protocol, which is monitored and updated annually. Many children with developmental delays need continuous care, in partnership with health and educational specialists. The challenge is that many kinship providers have little knowledge about developmental delays, do not know the terminology in the field of special education (e.g., IDEA, individual education plans, individual family service plans), are unfamiliar with the special-education service delivery process, and lack the confidence to assume an advocacy role to ensure their children receive adequate services. Giving young children early access to developmental evaluation and treatment services is critical to reducing the educational and social effects from developmental delays. A challenge here is to establish training and support services for kinship caregivers so they can build the confidence and capacity to become effective advocates for the children in their care.

CONCLUSIONS

Kinship care has emerged as a preferred form of substitute care when birth parents are unable or unwilling to take responsibility for their children. Despite the rapid expansion of this form of care, our knowledge on kinship care outcomes and how best to support these families is limited. Existing research, while far from conclusive, does suggest that outcomes for children in kinship care may be somewhat better than those for their counterparts in nonrelative foster care. Either way, children in kinship care remain at higher risk for elevated behavior problems than children in the general population. Therefore, to maximize their long-term outcomes, these children need greater access to therapeutic treatment modalities such as trauma-focused cognitive behavioral therapy.

The dedication of kinship caregivers is highly commendable; however, the multiple challenges they encounter may impede their ability to provide a supportive caregiving environment. The current disparities in public support for kinship caregivers are of serious concern and necessitate immediate attention. Particular consideration needs to be given to private kinship care families, who represent by far the largest proportion of children in out-of-home care and yet remain a somewhat invisible segment of the population. Better public surveillance is needed to address the numbers, characteristics, and needs of these families. Policymakers and clinicians must ensure that comprehensive policies and best practices are in place for all kinship care families, whether public or private.

References

American Academy of Pediatrics. (2012). *Healthy foster care America: Health care standards.* www2.aap.org/fostercare /health_care_standard.html

American Bar Association. (2012). Grandfamilies.org: Care and Custody—Summary & Analysis. www2.grandfamilies.org /CareandCustody/CareandCustodySummaryAnalysis.aspx

Anderson, S. G. (2006). The impact of state TANF policy decisions on kinship care providers. *Child Welfare, 85*(4), 715–736.

Boetto, H. (2010). Kinship care: A review of issues. *Family Matters, 85*, 60–67.

Brookdale Foundation. (2007). *Brookdale Foundation: Relatives as parents guidebook.* New York, NY: Author.

Brown, S., Cohon, D., & Wheeler, R. (2002). African American extended families and kinship care: How relevant is the foster care model for kinship care? *Children and Youth Services Review, 24*(1–2), 53–77. doi:10.1016/S0190-7409(01)00168-2

Bruskas, D. (2008). Children in foster care: A vulnerable population at risk. *Journal of Child and Adolescent Psychiatric Nursing, 21*(2), 70–77. doi:10.1111/j.1744-6171.2008.00134.x

Carpenter, S. C., & Clyman, R. B. (2004). The long-term emotional and physical wellbeing of women who have lived in kinship care. *Children and Youth Services Review, 26*(7), 673–686. doi:10.1016/j.childyouth.2004.02.015

Child Welfare Information Gateway. (2010). *Placement of children with relatives.* Washington, DC: U.S. Department of Health and Human Services, Administration on Children, Youth and Families, Children's Bureau. www.childwelfare.gov /systemwide/laws_policies/statutes/placement.cfm

Chipungu, S. S., & Bent-Goodley, T. B. (2004). Meeting the challenges of contemporary foster care. *Future of Children, 14*(1), 75–93.

Coakley, T. M., Cuddeback, G., Buehler, C., & Cox, M. E. (2007). Kinship foster parents' perceptions of factors that promote or inhibit successful fostering. *Children and Youth Services Review, 29*(1), 92–109. doi:10.1016/j.childyouth.2006.06.001

Cuddeback, G. S. (2004). Kinship family foster care: A methodological and substantive synthesis of research. *Children and Youth Services Review, 26*(7), 623–639. doi:10.1016/j.childyouth.2004.01.014

Ehrle, J., & Geen, R. (2002). Kin and non-kin foster care— Findings from a national survey. *Children and Youth Services Review, 24*(1–2), 15–35. doi:10.1016/S0190-7409(01)00166-9

Fuller-Thomson, E., & Minkler, M. (2000). African American grandparents raising grandchildren: A national profile of demographic and health characteristics. *Health & Social Work, 25*(2), 109–118. doi:10.1093/hsw/25.2.109

Geen, R. (2004). The evolution of kinship care policy and practice. *Future of Children, 14*(1), 131–149.

Gerald, J., Landry-Meyer, L., & Roe, J. (2006). Grandparents raising grandchildren: The role of social support in coping with caregiving challenges. *International Journal of Aging and Human Development, 62*(4), 359–383.

Goodman, C. C., Potts, M. K., & Pasztor, E. M. (2007). Caregiving grandmothers with vs. without child welfare system involvement: Effects of expressed need, formal services, and informal social support on caregiver burden. *Children and Youth Services Review, 29*(4), 428–441. doi:10.1016/j.child youth.2006.10.002

Goodman, C. C., Potts, M., Pasztor, E. M., & Scorzo, D. (2004). Grandmothers as kinship caregivers: Private arrangements compared to public child welfare oversight. *Children and Youth Services Review, 26*(3), 287–305. doi:10.1016/j.childyouth .2004.01.002

Grant, R. (2000). The special needs of children in kinship care. *Journal of Gerontological Social Work, 33,* 5–22. doi:10.1300/ J083v33n03_02

Haglund, K. (2000). Parenting a second time around: Ethnography of African American grandmothers parenting grandchildren due to parental cocaine abuse. *Journal of Family Nursing, 6*(2), 120–135. doi:10.1177/107484070000600203

Hegar, R. L., & Rosenthal, J. A. (1999). Kinship care and sibling placement: Child behaviors, family relationships, and school outcomes. *Children and Youth Services Review, 31,* 670–679. doi:10.1016/j.childyouth.2009.01.002

Keller, T. E., Wetherbee, K., Le Prohn, N. S., Payne, V., Sim, K., & Lamont, E. R. (2001). Competencies and problem behaviors of children in family foster care: Variations by kinship placement status and race. *Children and Youth Services Review, 23*(12), 915–940. doi:10.1016/S0190-7409(01)00175-X

Kelley, S. J., Whitley, D. M., & Campos, P. E. (2010). Grandmothers raising grandchildren: Results of an intervention to improve health outcomes. *Journal of Nursing Scholarship, 42*(4), 379–386. doi:10.1111/j.1547-5069.2010.01371.x

Kelley, S. J., Whitley, D. M., & Campos, P. E. (2011). Behavior problems in children raised by grandmothers: The role of caregiver distress, family resources, and the home environment. *Children and Youth Services Review, 33,* 2138–2145. doi:10.1016/j.childyouth.2011.06.021

Kelley, S. J., Whitley, D. M., & Campos, P. E. (2013). African American caregiving grandmothers: Results of an intervention to improve health indicators and health promotion behaviors. *Journal of Family Nursing, 19,* 53–73. doi:10.1177/1074840712462135

Kelley, S. J., Whitley, D., Sipe, T. A., & Crofts Yorker, B. (2000). Psychological distress in grandmother kinship care providers: The role of resources, social support, and physical health. *Child Abuse & Neglect, 24*(3), 311–321. doi:10.1016/ S0145-2134(99)00146-5

Kelley, S. J., Yorker, B. C., Whitley, D., & Sipe, T. A. (2001). A multi-modal intervention for grandparents raising grandchildren: Results of a pilot study. *Child Welfare, 80*(1), 27–50.

Koh, E. (2010). Permanency outcomes of children in kinship and non-kinship foster care: Testing the external validity of kinship effects. *Children and Youth Services Review, 32*(3), 389–398. doi:10.1016/j.childyouth.2009.10.010

Lau, A. S., Litrownik, A. J., Newton, R. R., & Landsverk, J. (2003). Going home: The complex effects of reunification on internalizing problems among children in foster care. *Journal of Abnormal Child Psychology, 31*(4), 345–358. doi:10.1023/A:1023816000232

Lee, S., Colditz, G., Berkman, L., & Kawachi, I. (2003). Caregiving to children and grandchildren and risk of coronary heart disease in women. *American Journal of Public Health, 93*(11), 1939–1944. doi:10.2105/AJPH.93.11.1939

Macomber, J. E., Geen, R., & Clark, R. (2001). *Children cared for by relatives: Who are they and how are they doing? (New federalism: National survey of America's families,* No. B-28). Washington, DC: Urban Institute.

Messing, J. T. (2006). From the child's perspective: A qualitative analysis of kinship care placements. *Children and Youth*

Services Review, 28(12), 1415–1434. doi:10.1016/j.child youth.2006.03.001

Minkler, M., & Fuller-Thomson, E. (1999). The health of grandparents raising grandchildren: Results of a national study. *American Journal of Public Health, 89*(9), 1384–1389. doi:10.2105/AJPH.89.9.1384

Pacifici, C., Delaney, R., White, L., Nelson, C., & Cummings, C. (2006). Web-based training for foster, adoptive, and kinship parents. *Children and Youth Services Review, 28,* 226–246. doi:10.1016/j.childyouth.2006.02.003

Price, J. M., Chamberlain, P., Landsverk, J., Leve, L., & Laurent, H. (2008). Effects of a foster parent training intervention on placement changes of children in foster care. *Child Maltreatment, 13*(1), 64–75.

Rubin, D. M., Downes, K. J., O'Reilly, A. L. R., Mekonnen, R., Luan, X., & Localio, R. (2008). Impact of kinship care on behavioral well-being for children in out-of-home care. *Archives of Pediatrics & Adolescent Medicine, 162*(6), 550–556. doi:10.1001/archpedi.162.6.550

Ryan, S. D., Hinterlong, J., Hegar, R. L., & Johnson, L. B. (2010). Kin adopting kin: In the best interest of the children? *Children and Youth Services Review, 32*(12), 1631–1639. doi:10.1016/j.child youth.2010.06.013

Sakai, C., Lin, H., & Flores, G. (2011). Health outcomes and family services in kinship care: Analysis of a national sample of children in the child welfare system. *Archives of Pediatrics & Adolescent Medicine, 165*(2), 159. doi:10.1001/archpediatrics .2010.277

Sanchez, K., Gomez, R., & Davis, K. (2010). Fostering connections and medical homes: Addressing health disparities among children in substitute care. *Children and Youth Services Review, 32,* 286–291. doi:10.1016/j.childyouth.2009.09.008

Schneiderman, J. U., Smith, C., & Palinkas, L. A. (2012). The caregiver as gatekeeper for accessing health care for children in foster care: A qualitative study of kinship and unrelated caregivers. *Children and Youth Services Review, 34,* 2123–2130. doi:10.1016/j.childyouth.2012.07.009

Smith, G. C. (2003). How caregiving grandparents view support groups: An exploratory study. In J. B. Hayslip & J. H. Patrick (Eds.), *Working with custodial grandparents* (pp. 69–91). New York, NY: Springer.

Smith, G. C., & Palmieri, P. A. (2007). Risk of psychological difficulties among children raised by custodial grandparents. *Psychiatric Services, 58,* 1303–1310. doi:10.1176/appi.ps.58.10.1303

Smith, G. C., Savage-Stevens, S. E., & Fabian, E. S. (2002). How caregiving grandparents view support groups for grandchildren in their care. *Family Relations, 51*(3), 274–281. doi:10.1111/j.1741-3729.2002.00274.x

Strozier, A. L. (2012). The effectiveness of support groups in increasing social support for kinship caregivers. *Children and Youth Services Review, 34,* 876–881. doi:10.1016/j.childyouth .2012.01.007

Strozier, A. L., & Krisman, K. (2007). Capturing caregiver data: An examination of kinship care custodial arrangements. *Children and Youth Services Review, 29*(2), 226–246. doi:10.1016/j.childyouth.2006.07.006

Strozier, A. L., McGrew, L, Krisman, K., & Smith, A. (2005). Kinship care connection: A school-based intervention for kinship caregivers and the children in their care. *Children and Youth Services Review, 27,* 1011–1029. doi:10.1016/j.child youth.2004.12.026

Swann, C. A., & Sylvester, M. S. (2006). Does the child welfare system serve the neediest kinship care families? *Children and Youth Services Review, 28,* 1213–1228. doi:10.1016/j.child youth.2005.11.007

Taussig, H. N., Clyman, R. B., & Landsverk, J. (2001). Children who return home from foster care: A 6-year prospective study of behavioral health outcomes in adolescence. *Pediatrics, 108*(1), e10. doi:10.1542/peds.108.1.e10

Terling-Watt, T. (2001). Permanency in kinship care: An exploration of disruption rates and factors associated with placement disruption. *Children and Youth Services Review, 23*(2), 111–126. doi:10.1016/S0190-7409(01)00129-3

Timmer, S. G., Sedlar, G., & Urquiza, A. J. (2004). Challenging children in kin versus nonkin foster care: Perceived costs and benefits to caregivers. *Child Maltreatment, 9*(3), 251–262. doi:10.1177/1077559504266998

U.S. Census Bureau. (2004). Table CH-1. Living arrangements of children under 18 years old: 1960 to present. *Current Population Survey, 2003, Annual Social and Economic Supplement.* www.census.gov/population/socdemo/hh-fam/tabCH-1.pdf

U.S. Census Bureau. (2011). Table C2. Household relationships and living arrangements of children under 18 years, by age and sex: 2011. *Current Population Survey, 2011, Annual Social and Economic Supplement.* www.census.gov/population/www/socdemo/hh-fam/cps2011.html

U.S. Department of Health and Human Services (HHS). (2000). *Report to the Congress on kinship foster care.* Washington, DC: U.S. Department of Health and Human Services, Administration for Children and Families, Administration on Children, Youth, and Families, Children's Bureau.

Wang, Y., & Marcotte, D. (2007). Golden years? The labor market effects of caring for grandchildren. *Journal of Marriage and Family, 69*(5), 1283–1296. doi:10.1111/j.1741-3737.2007.00447.x

Whitley, D. M., & Kelley, S. J. (2008). Developmental screening and evaluation results of young African American grandchildren raised by grandparents: Thoughts for research and practice. *Arete, 32*(1), 38–57.

Winokur, M., Crawford, G., Longobardi, R., & Valentine, D. (2008). Matched comparison of children in kinship care and foster care on child welfare outcomes. *Families in Society, 89*(3), 338–346. doi:0.1606/1044-3894.3759

Winokur, M., Holtan, A., & Valentine, D. (2009). Kinship care for the safety, permanency, and well-being of children removed from the home for maltreatment. *Cochrane Database of Systematic Reviews.* doi:10.1002/14651858.CD006546.pub2

PART III Special Populations and Special Topics

11

The Sanctuary Model

Rebooting the Organizational Operating System in Group Care Settings

OUTLINING THE CHALLENGES

Trauma-Organized Children

The children who arrive for placement in a residential program or group home are there because each one has problems that are exceedingly complex, that cannot be managed in a less restrictive level of care, and that pose significant difficulties for the adults in their lives. When one hears the histories of the multiple adversities to which these children have been exposed, it may be relatively easy to explain how they could come to have such problems. More challenging, however, may be trying to explain how they have survived the terrors of their lives.

The simultaneous realities of complex and interactive developmental problems that affect children's bodies, minds, and spirits alongside the resilience of individual children and of childhood itself have implications for environments that set out to help heal those bodies, minds, and spirits. In brief, children who are admitted to group care environments (1) have difficulty with maintaining safety in interpersonal relationships, largely due to disrupted attachment experiences and the erosion of trust that accompanies such experiences; (2) have significant challenges in adequately managing distressful emotions in ways that are not self-destructive, including exercising the capacities for self-discipline, self-control, and willpower; (3) are beset by cognitive problems, particularly when stress occurs and the development of essential cortical functions has not gone as smoothly as it should; (4) frequently communicate through behavior, not directly, openly, or in words; (5) feel helpless and powerless in the face of a world that they perceive has been unjust and cruel and, as a result, may be repeatedly bullied or become bullies themselves; (6) frequently lack a clear sense of social responsibility, while moral development may have been affected by disrupted attachment experi-

ences and inadequate role models; and (7) are likely to have experienced significant loss while lacking the emotional capacity to grieve, are likely to repeat the experiences that are a part of their past, and often lack any hope that the future will be any better than the past. In this way, children's lives become "trauma-organized" as their attempts to cope with unmanageable conditions lead to maladaptive coping skills and the development of problematic habits.

If we are to address the complex needs of these children, our goals must be aimed at resolving the difficulties that exposure to toxic stress creates. To accomplish this in a group setting, much is demanded of managers, therapists, caregivers, and educators. We must teach, role-model, and support the development of (1) safety skills and significant improvements in the capacity for interpersonal trust; (2) emotional management skills, including self-control, self-discipline, and the exercise of willpower; (3) cognitive skills, including identifying triggers and problematic patterns, while still being able to think in the presence of strong emotion; (4) communication skills that include rehearsals in what to say and how to say it; (5) participatory and leadership skills; (6) judgment skills, including socially acceptable and fair behavioral schemas; and (7) skills to manage grief and plan for the future.

Trauma-Organized Staff

Promoting healing in children who suffer from these kinds of interactive and complex challenges is not so much a technical problem as an adaptive one, meaning that every child is different and the moment-to-moment opportunities presented in the constant interactions between child and adult staff members offer chances for a ceaseless array of corrective emotional, cognitive, behavioral, and spiritual experiences (Bloom & Farragher, 2013). What characteristics best describe people who are able to do this complex work? They need to be secure, reasonably healthy adults who have good emotional management skills themselves. They must be intellectually and emotionally intelligent. They must be able to actively teach new skills and routines while serving as role models for what they are teaching. There are constant demands on them for patience and for empathy, so they must be able to endure intense emotional labor. To balance the demands of home and work, managers and supervisors, children and their families, they must be self-disciplined and self-controlled and must never abuse their own personal power.

Herein lie the greatest difficulties in making use of the advantages offered by residential treatment environments: the outcomes are largely dependent on the nature and quality of the relationships between children and staff, but we are faced with a workforce crisis. As a national report states, "a growing proportion of the U.S. workforce will have been raised in disadvantaged environments that are associated with relatively high proportions of individuals with diminished cognitive and social skills" (Knudsen et al., 2006, p. 10155). An expanding body of evidence indicates that the rates of exposure to childhood adversity in the general population are so high that, inevitably, a large proportion of staff members in any social service organization are likely to have their own past histories of experiences that are not entirely dissimilar to those of the children they are supposed to help, and they may have unresolved interpersonal challenges that are also not dissimilar (Esaki & Larkin, in press; Felitti & Anda, 2010).

Extraordinary demands are placed upon social service workers in the face of low salaries and inadequate funding for the organizations within which they work. Job complexity and ambiguity are high while the payoff is low, particularly for those in any type of institutional setting where the least educated, supported, trained, and supervised staff spend the most time with profoundly injured children. There is often a lack of cultural diversity and cultural sensitivity in the staff, whose composition may be ethnically and racially very different from that of the children in care.

And then there is the violence. Staff members are not safe, and this is particularly true for residential settings where the children being cared for are—by definition—the children who cannot be safely contained in less restrictive settings. Forty-eight percent of all nonfatal injuries from occupational assaults and violent acts occur in health care and social services (Occupational Safety and Health Administration, 2004). In fact, after law enforcement, the mental health sector has the highest rate of all occupations of persons employed in the sector being victimized while at work or on duty (Bureau of Justice, 2001). Much of this lack of safety has been attributed to the insufficient adoption of best practices that reduce the need for restraint and seclusion, which increase the likelihood of injury to both children and staff (LeBel, Huckshorn, & Caldwell, 2010).

Trauma-Organized Organizations

Actual rates of violence expose the problems with physical safety. But there are other safety issues as well that can be thought of as threats to psychological, social, and moral safety. Research in other industries has recorded the top workplace stressors, and although the area is insufficiently studied, anyone working in the health, education, social services, or mental health sectors can easily identify with these: too much to do in too little time; unnecessary, meaningless paperwork; random interruptions, such as telephone calls, walk-in visits, text messages, and emails; demands from supervisors; pervasive uncertainty as a result of organizational problems; unsatisfactorily explained and unannounced change; decreased funding; mistrust, unfairness, and vicious office politics; unclear policies and lack of organizational direction; career and job ambiguity resulting in feelings of helplessness and lack of control; lack of feedback, good or bad; absence of appreciation for work done; and lack of communication up and down the chain of command (Collie, 2004).

Looking at this list, it is clear that the main causes of workplace stress cannot be laid at the feet of the children and their families. In fact, as this list demonstrates, "the main sources of stress for workers are the ways in which organizations operate and the nature of the relationships that people experience within the work setting" (Bloom & Farragher, 2010, p. 70). This is not an individual problem but a social one, partly due to controllable but severe dysfunctions within those organizations and largely related to inadequate and unscientific paradigms for intervening in the lives of traumatized people, families, and communities. These multiple interactive tensions produce parallel processes, a complex group dynamic that is evident when symptomatic behavior is replicated at every level—children, families, staff, management, and organization (Alderfer & Smith, 1982).

TRAUMA-INFORMED ENVIRONMENTS: THE SANCTUARY MODEL

There are distinct advantages in treating a child within the context of a 24-hours-a-day milieu. It becomes possible to organize an entire system around the child's healing. But to effectively create that kind of helping system, certain requirements must be met: (1) an organizational mission and value system that support a culture of healing and transformation; (2) getting—and retaining—the right people for the job; (3) a universally shared, developmentally grounded, trauma-informed knowledge base that guides intervention and becomes incorporated into the organizational culture; (4) language shared by staff, children, and families; (5) thorough assessment and case formulation; (6) ongoing processes for understanding and managing individual and group dynamics; (7) individualized, trauma-informed treatment plans and processes and, where appropriate, trauma-specific treatment interventions; (8) a method for ensuring that all of the above are created, incorporated, and integrated into organizational function; and (9) a method for ensuring that it all works—that children resolve their previous wounds and get onto sounder, healthier developmental trajectories with the help and support of adults who themselves are constantly learning, adapting, and creatively expanding their own horizons.

The Sanctuary Model is an evidence-supported, developmentally grounded, trauma-informed approach to creating and sustaining an organizational culture that embraces these requirements as fundamental for any milieu setting. The Sanctuary Model is built upon what we call the Four Pillars of Sanctuary: Trauma Theory, the Sanctuary Commitments, SELF, and the Sanctuary Toolkit. Trauma Theory provides the scientific underpinning for the Sanctuary Model. The Sanctuary Commitments provide the anchoring values and are tied directly to developmentally grounded, trauma-informed treatment goals as well as the overall health of the organizational culture. SELF is a simple and easy-to-use conceptual framework that provides a "compass" allowing everyone to navigate the challenges of complex interventions, while the Sanctuary Toolkit offers practical, grounded tasks that support implementation. "Creating Sanctuary" refers to the shared experience of creating and maintaining physical, psychological, social, and moral safety within a social environment—any social environment—and thus reducing systemic violence (Bloom, 2013). The process of Creating Sanctuary begins with getting everyone on the same page—surfacing, sharing, arguing about, and finally agreeing on the basic values, beliefs, guiding principles, and philosophical principles that are to guide attitudes, decisions, problem solving, conflict resolution, and behavior (Bloom & Farragher, 2013).

Mission and Values That Support Healing

Existing institutions will have a mission, one that may have been formulated long ago. Many residential programs were originally nineteenth- or early twentieth-century orphanages, and thus the organizational mission may derive directly from a previous era, formulated decades ago by people who were then leading the organization.

Given the knowledge we now have about the way the brain works, normal child development, and the impact of toxic stress exposure, trauma, and allostatic load, most child-serving organizations need to revisit their mission. Given what we have learned in the past three decades, we now know that helping very traumatized children to heal can require significant change in organizations whose original mission was caring for and educating orphans. The work of healing complexly traumatized children is so demanding that residential programs and group homes must be mission-driven, and that mission must be constantly foremost in the minds of every staff member. Arriving at that point requires more than a statement of purpose on a boardroom wall: it requires a shared process that involves everyone in the organization, from executive leadership, through the line staff, and on to maintenance, finance, and housekeeping—that's what it means to meaningfully and consciously develop an organizational mission.

A comprehensive, developmentally grounded, and trauma-informed mission has to be anchored in a value system that can be understood, embraced, and applied by every child and adult in the system, regardless of age, experience, educational background, ethnicity, or socioeconomic class. In complex group processes that have occurred across more than three decades, seven key values have emerged, universal principles that we believe are consistent with human rights cultures around the world. We call these the seven Sanctuary Commitments. These commitments represent the guiding principles for implementation of the Sanctuary Model, the basic structural elements of the Sanctuary "operating system," and each commitment supports trauma recovery goals for children, families, staff, and the organization as a whole. The Sanctuary Commitments structure the organizational norms that determine the organizational culture, while helping the organization as a whole to promote and sustain growth and change.

The Sanctuary Commitments are designed to create a parallel process of recovery that helps to resolve the problems common to the children who enter group care environments.

1. *Commitment to Nonviolence*—to build safety skills, trust, and resilience in the face of stress
2. *Commitment to Emotional Intelligence*—to embed emotional management skills, build respect for emotional labor, and minimize the paralyzing effects of fear
3. *Commitment to Social Learning*—to build cognitive skills, improve learning and decisions, and expand awareness of problematic cognitive behavioral patterns and how to change them; to restore memory and develop the skills necessary to create and sustain a learning organization
4. *Commitment to Open Communication*—to overcome barriers to healthy communication, discuss the "undiscussables," overcome alexithymia, increase transparency, develop conflict management skills, reinforce healthy boundaries, and enable skills for resolving collective disturbances
5. *Commitment to Democracy*—to develop civic skills of self-control, self-discipline, and the exercise of healthy dissent; to learn to exercise healthy authority and leadership; to develop participatory skills that overcome learned helplessness; to develop skills for wrestling with complexity; and to honor the "voices" of self and others
6. *Commitment to Social Responsibility*—to harness the energy of reciprocity and a yearning for justice by rebuilding restorative social connection skills, establishing healthy and fair attachment relationships, and transforming vengeance into social justice

7. *Commitment to Growth and Change*—to promote the ability to work through loss in the recognition that all change involves loss; to cease repeating irrelevant or destructive past patterns of thought, feeling, and behavior; and to envision, be guided by, skillfully plan, and prepare for a different and better future.

The Sanctuary Commitments together create an ethical system and a set of checks and balances that serve as the basic skeletal system of a trauma-informed organization.

Getting the Right People for the Job

The Sanctuary Model is an organizational method for helping all staff members "get on the same page" about how we define problems, how we work together, and how we create nonviolent, therapeutic communities. Experience has demonstrated that over time, programs that implement the Sanctuary Model alter their processes for interviewing, selecting, orienting, training, and supervising staff. Primary outcomes of the implementation of the Sanctuary Model are reductions in critical incidents, reductions in child and staff injuries, improved staff morale, and reduced staff turnover, all of which contribute to the quality of care the children receive.

Universal Training

The expanding knowledge base gained across the past three decades, usually referred to as "Trauma Theory," provides the beginning of a framework for radically changing service delivery to troubled children and their families. The study of trauma gives us a lens on the workings of people under extreme conditions, but we are learning much about the entire stress continuum and the extent to which stress, particularly repetitive and toxic stressful conditions, can impact normal development. Along with the expanding field of interpersonal neuroscience, this knowledge is leading to the recognition that most of our behavior is determined by previous experiences that may have occurred even before we were born.

In the Sanctuary Model, everyone in an organization needs to have a clear understanding about how the impact of toxic stress and trauma has affected the children we work with and often the staff as well. Also vital is that everyone recognizes that stress causes us to revert to old habits that we may have overcome in the past. Learning about the psychobiology of stress, toxic stress, and trauma is liberating for people. It gives us explanatory reasons for some of the puzzling behaviors we engage in and the feelings that can come to dominate us.

Our expanding understanding about the impact of disrupted attachment, toxic stress, adversity, and trauma represents the possibility of being able to base helping and caregiving work on outcomes, a concept only rarely expected from social service and mental health organizations.

Embedded in the notion of services that truly understand the complex biopsychosocial impact of traumatic experience is the underlying premise that all people can change, even if a little bit, and that if change is not occurring, maybe this is because the service provided is not adequately matching their needs, which means *we* need to do something different instead of attributing treatment failure or lack of compliance as resistance to change or simple oppositional behavior.

Trauma theory offers an integrative, scientifically based, and developmentally grounded framework for all human systems. The psychobiology of trauma points us toward knowledge that heals the Cartesian split between mind, body, and spirit and, in doing so, "puts Humpty Dumpty back together again." The simultaneous burgeoning of knowledge about the importance of early childhood attachment and the impact of toxic stress exposure offers a developmental continuity between childhood and adulthood. Through the concept of allostatic load, we can now connect the psychobiology of trauma and disrupted attachment to many of the negative social determinants of health, such as racism, gender-based discrimination, and poverty. Never before have we had an integrative framework that allows extensive and specialized bodies of knowledge to be connected to each other within a human rights context as a public health challenge (Bloom & Farragher, 2013). We are learning how limited our freedom really is at a neurological base. As it turns out, what we call "free will" is not nearly as free as we would like to believe (Gazzaniga, 2011). At the same time, we are learning how much our social milieu can influence the brain, now known to be more malleable and "plastic" than was once assumed, and how important belief, faith, meaning, and purpose are to changing the brain (Duhigg, 2012).

To help programs accomplish universal training without having to invent those trainings on their own, we developed one training manual and accompanying training materials for all of the staff who have direct contact with children and families and another manual for all of the indirect care staff such as board members, regulators, administrative assistants, finance officers, maintenance and food service staff, and all the other people who are necessary to keep an organization functioning.

Shared Language: SELF, a Compass for the Recovery Process

In the Sanctuary Model we use SELF as a habit-changing compass for many different tasks. When faced with the complex problems that are typical of the children and families we serve, it is easy as a helper to lose your way, to focus on what is the most frightening or the easiest to understand and manage rather than on what may be the true underlying stumbling block to progress. Similarly, children in care are most likely to pay attention to whatever problems are causing the most pain for them in the immediate present, even though, from a helper's point of view, what they are doing or not doing is likely to cause them even greater suffering in the long term.

SELF is an acronym that represents the four key interdependent aspects of recovery from bad experiences. SELF provides a nonlinear, cognitive behavioral therapeutic approach for facilitating movement through the Sanctuary Commitments—regardless of whether we are talking about children, their families, staff problems, or whole organizational dilemmas. SELF is a compass that allows us to explore all four key domains of healing: *Safety, Emotions, Loss,* and *Future.* Using SELF, children, their families, and staff are able to embrace a shared, nontechnical and nonpejorative language that allows them all to see the larger recovery process in perspective. The accessible language demystifies what sometimes is seen as confusing and even insulting clinical jargon that can confound children, families, and staff, while still focusing on the aspects of pathological adjustment that pose the greatest problems for any treatment environment.

Assessment and Case Formulation

Any child who is admitted for placement in a residential program or group home is likely to have had multiple prior assessments, some focused on intellectual development, others on psychological development, although none may have included a complete developmental history. Some of those records may accompany the child, but in other cases vital information about the child's history may have been "lost along the way," particularly in cases where the child has had many previous placements. It is important that the admission team at the residential or group home obtain as many records as possible to help establish a coherent narrative of the child's experience. At the same time, it is important to recognize the possibility of profound disagreement among the records, as various adults used different "lenses" to view the child.

Diagnostic formulations are seen as a necessary element in our human service delivery systems but frequently do not offer any insight into the child's actual lived experience; nor is there usually much emphasis on the strengths the child has used to cope with his or her less-than-ideal circumstances. The trauma history of the child frequently "gets lost" too, forgotten in the demands of day-to-day challenges presented by the child's behavior. It is essential to keep the emphasis on what happened to the child, rather than what is wrong with the child, if residential staff are to achieve the desired outcomes.

All this being the case, it is important that when a child enters a new treatment setting, the staff members take it upon themselves to reassess the child and remain open to major shifts in perspectives about the child. Without such openness, the child can easily become the victim of self-fulfilling prophecies on the part of the staff, in which a child labeled with a diagnosis such as "oppositional disorder" is expected to be, therefore, oppositional. The staff then sets those expectations in interaction with the child, and the child performs oppositionally in accord with those expectations. Although currently largely ignored, research has shown that labeling people tends to create the behavior we expect to see based on the labels (Scheff, 1975).

Managing Group Dynamics: The Sanctuary Toolkit

Information about group dynamics and parallel process should be incorporated into orientation and ongoing training. Working in 24-hours-per-day settings requires specialized knowledge about the complex processes that arise in groups. People who work in group settings should have a high level of competence in understanding and utilizing group processes. These are communities, and the benefits of community should be maximized.

The Sanctuary Toolkit comprises a range of practical, routine skills that enable individuals and organizations to develop new habits and more effectively deal with difficult situations, build community, develop a deeper understanding of the effects of adversity and trauma, and build a common language and knowledge base. Community Meetings and universal Safety Plans promote a focus on social responsibility, democracy, and nonviolence on a routine, daily basis.

Many of our tools are organized around SELF, so we teach SELF Treatment Planning, SELF Psychoeducational Groups, SELF Team Meetings, and SELF Organizational Assessment, and use SELF to structure Red Flag Reviews. It helps us stay on track, keeps our focus, and provides a shared language and meaning system for everyone, regardless of their training, experience, or education. It also helps us to see the parallels between what the clients have experienced and what is going on with the staff and the organization and to intervene when we notice that a "collective disturbance" is unfolding. In doing so, we are able to see the interactive and interdependent nature of our shared lives.

Individualized, Trauma-Informed Treatment Plan and Processes

To be effective, residential treatment requires the coordination and delivery of a comprehensive array of therapeutic services, including educational and rehabilitative services that are trauma-informed. Intervention strategies must be designed to address delays in cognitive, social, and emotional development, and education must be tailored to a child's grade level, learning style, and individual capabilities (Abt Associates, 2008). As described earlier, to achieve good outcomes the staff members must be able to address children's complex and interactive problems despite the stressors coming from within themselves and simultaneously from their external environment.

The key to making this possible is fully utilizing the treatment context. Every activity and interaction has to become treatment, and that can happen only if administrators make it possible for staff members to do the challenging job of integrating many different styles, objectives, and approaches. Under the pressure of higher productivity demands and diminished resources, the failure to do this integrative work is the most glaring loss in all milieu settings. As documented more than 20 years ago, in residential settings for children, it was common to find more than 17 therapeutic approaches cobbled together without necessarily any coherence and lacking a rational linking of diagnosis, etiology, and prognosis (Wells, 1991). That situation has not changed, and if anything, under the pressures of decreased funding and increased stress, it has become far more problematic. For the purposes of reimbursement, staffing, research, and planning, treatment should be defined not as the hour spent with a clinician but as the combined efforts of clinicians guiding and supervising treatment planning and implementation that embraces the whole team, including psychiatry, direct care staff, educational staff, and indirect care staff. At the heart of these integrative efforts should be an emphasis on pattern recognition and changing traumatic reenactment scripts that inevitably unfold in the treatment setting. Providing children with the corrective experiences they require if they are to heal necessitates a wide range of responsive programming that must include trauma-specific forms of treatment and the naturally transformative expressive arts but that often begins with basic psychoeducation.

In the Sanctuary Model, treatment is structured through the use of SELF Treatment Planning, SELF Psychoeducation, and specific formats for team meetings. Similarly, the more consistent the use of the Sanctuary Commitments, the more these commitments serve as anchors for problem solving and decision making and provide internal coherence for the program. This is especially true for the Commitment to Democracy. The greater the involvement of the clients in creating more democratic environments, the more likely they are to have experiences throughout any typical day that are directly counter to many of the habits they have developed. The constant repetition of alternative ways of living and working with each other lays the groundwork for changing habits in a normal, educational and social context rather than focusing on pathology and punishment for infractions. To participate, be esteemed by others, and get recognition in a democratic environment, we have to develop skills that are in direct opposition to the skillset a person has often had to acquire to survive the rigors of a violent upbringing (Bloom & Farragher, 2013).

Integration into Organizational Function: Sanctuary Implementation

Just as a computer has an operating system that is a master program that controls a computer's basic functions and allows other programs to run on the computer *if* they are compatible with that operating system, so an organizational culture represents the operating system for an organization. Every organization has an organizational culture that represents long-held organizational patterns, routines, and habits that,

although remembered and taught to every new employee, are largely unconscious and automatic, as most habits are. The nature of the organizational culture largely determines whether or not the organization is able to fulfill its mission and reach its stated goals. Organizational culture may or may not be aligned with the actual values and mission that the organization claims to follow (Schein, 1999). Alignment of values is usually seen as management driven, if it is referred to at all, and here mental health and social service organizations are at a distinct disadvantage.

The fundamental rationale for the Sanctuary Model is to create parallel processes of recovery by radically altering the operating system for the organization as a whole and for everyone who has contact with that organization. That means intervening at the level of organizational culture in order to change the habits and routines of everyone in the organization and the organization as a whole.

The Sanctuary Model is structured around a philosophy of belief and practice that creates a process enabling organizations to dramatically shift their approach to traumatized children, adolescents, and families. To do so they must identify the habits and routines that are no longer compatible with developmentally grounded, trauma-informed care, while learning new and more useful habits. This kind of organizational change requires radical alterations in the basic mental models on which thought and action are based, and without such change, treatment is bound to fall unnecessarily short of full recovery or fail entirely. Mental models exist at the level of very basic assumptions, far below conscious awareness and everyday function, and yet they guide and determine what we can and cannot think about and act upon (Senge et al., 2000). This change in mental models must occur on the part of the clients, their families, the staff, and the leaders of the organization. We have developed a methodology to help organizations accomplish this kind of deep systemic change.

The Sanctuary Institute is a five-day intensive training experience.* Teams of five to eight people, from various levels of the organization, come together to learn from our faculty, who are colleagues from other organizations implementing Sanctuary. Together, teams begin to create a shared vision of the kind of organization they want to create. These teams will eventually become the Sanctuary Steering Committee for their organization. The training experience usually involves several organizations, and generally these organizations are very different in terms of size, scope, region, and mission. This diversity helps provide a rich learning experience for the participants.

Participants look at the change process itself and are asked to anticipate the inevitable resistance to change that is a fact of life in every organization. They look at manage-

---

*The Sanctuary Institute is a part of Andrus in Yonkers, NY (www.andruschildren.org). For more information, contact Sarah Yanosy, Director, at 914-965-2700, ext. 1117, or syanosy@jdam.org, or visit the Sanctuary Institute website at www.thesanctuaryinstitute.org.

ment styles and the way decisions are made and conflicts resolved. In the process of these discussions, they learn about what it means to engage in more democratic processes on the part of leaders, staff, and clients, especially in terms of the simultaneous increase in rights *and* responsibilities. They evaluate the existing policies and procedures that apply to staff, clients, and families and ask whether or not they are effective in achieving their shared goals. They are asked to learn about and become thoroughly familiar with the psychobiology of trauma and disrupted attachment and the multiple ways in which posttraumatic stress disorder (PTSD), complex PTSD, and other trauma-related disorders present in the children, adults, and families they work with. They are challenged to begin thinking about the implications of that knowledge for treatment. They also learn how high levels of stress in the organization can impact relationships, emotions, and decision making at every level of the organization. They develop an understanding of SELF as a conceptual tool for organizing treatment. They learn about vicarious trauma, traumatic reenactment, and the importance of understanding themselves and providing support for each other. They are introduced to the various components of the Sanctuary Toolkit.

The Sanctuary Steering Committee is instructed to go back to its organization and create a Sanctuary Core Team—a larger, multidisciplinary team that expands its reach into the entire organization. It is the members of this Core Team who will be the activators of the entire system. The Core Team should have representatives from every level of the organization to ensure that every "voice" is heard. It is vital that all key organizational leaders become actively involved in the process of change and participate in this Core Team. To assist the Core Team in structuring its activities, the team is given a Sanctuary Direct Care Staff Training Manual, a Sanctuary Indirect Staff Training Manual, a Sanctuary Implementation Manual, and several psychoeducational curricula. This team will also be able to access ongoing consultation and technical assistance from Sanctuary faculty members to guide it through the process of Sanctuary Implementation that extends over three years and leads to Sanctuary Certification. Programs that have participated in the Sanctuary Institute are enrolled in the Sanctuary Network, a community of organizations dedicated to the development of developmentally grounded, trauma-informed services. We are all committed to the belief that we can do better for our clients and our colleagues as well as our society if we can accept that the people we serve are not sick or bad but injured and that the services we provide must furnish hope, promote growth, and inspire change.

Sanctuary Certification

Sanctuary is a registered trademark, and the right to use the Sanctuary name is contingent on engagement in our certified training program and an agreement to participate in an ongoing, peer-review certification process. The Sanc-

tuary Certification process is designed to promote, sustain, and strengthen an organization's commitment to the maintenance of a healthier culture for all stakeholders. Programs usually seek Sanctuary Certification in the two- to three-year period after participation in the Sanctuary Institute. Research is underway with the hope of moving the Sanctuary Model from an "evidence-supported" to an "evidence-based" approach. In this way we hope to establish a method for guaranteeing an acceptable level of fidelity to the original model on which the research is based.*

ENSURING THAT IT WORKS: EVALUATING OUTCOMES

The impact of creating a developmentally grounded, trauma-informed culture using the Sanctuary Model should be observable and measurable. The outcomes we expect to see are applicable to all community members and include (1) less violence, including physical, verbal, and emotional forms of violence, and including but not limited to reduction in coercive forms of so-called therapeutic interventions; (2) a system-wide understanding of the complex biopsychosocial and developmental impact of trauma and abuse and what that means for the service environment; (3) less victim-blaming; (4) fewer punitive and judgmental responses; (5) clearer, more consistent boundaries, higher expectations, and linked rights and responsibilities; (6) earlier identification of and confrontation with the abusive use of power in all of its forms; (7) a better ability to articulate goals and create strategies for change; (8) an understanding and awareness of reenactment behavior, accompanied by the skills necessary to rescript reenactment, overcome resistance to change, and achieve better outcomes; (9) a more democratic environment at all levels; (10) a more diversified leadership and the embedding of leadership skills in all staff; and (11) better outcomes for children, staff, and organization.

There has been one randomized controlled trial of implementing the Sanctuary Model in children's residential settings thus far. To summarize the results, from baseline to six months there were five significant differences in the staff attitudes and behavior:

1. *Support*—how much children help and support each other; how supportive the staff is toward the children
2. *Spontaneity*—how much the program encourages the open expression of feelings by children and staff
3. *Autonomy*—how self-sufficient and independent the staff perceives the children to be in making their own decisions
4. *Personal problem orientation*—the extent to which children seek to understand their feelings and personal problems

---

*Articles about the previous Sanctuary Model research can be downloaded from www.sanctuaryweb.com. Information is also available from the Sanctuary Institute (Community Care Behavioral Health, 2011).

5. *Safety*—the extent to which staff members feel they can challenge their peers and supervisors, can express opinions in staff meetings, will not be blamed for problems, and have clear guidelines for dealing with children who are aggressive

There was also an unexpected (unexpected because of the short timeframe) but significant difference in the child outcomes and three other positive trends: *decreased verbal aggression* (significant trend), *increased internal locus of control* (significant trend), and *decreased incendiary communication and increased tension management* (significant difference) (Rivard et al., 2004).

In another study, comparing residential programs for children that were using the Sanctuary Model and programs that were not, programs using the Sanctuary Model showed a significant, positive change in organizational culture, supporting the role of the Sanctuary Model in positively affecting the culture of the workplace (McSparren & Motley, 2010).

Organizations working with troubled children have long relied on physical restraints and/or holds to prevent a child from hurting himself or others. When we looked at the first seven child-serving facilities that participated in the Sanctuary Institute and their subsequent reductions in restraints and holds, three exhibited a more than 80% decrease in the number of restraints, two had a more than 40% decrease, one had a 13% decrease, and one had a 6% drop in restraints. A three-year study of organizations using the Sanctuary Model showed reductions in physical restraints of, on average, 52.3% after the first year of implementation (Banks & Vargas, 2009a). At Andrus, within the first six years of implementation in the residential unit and school, there was a 90% decrease in critical incidents with a 54% increase in the average number of students served (Banks & Vargas, 2009b).

As part of the Pennsylvania Department of Public Welfare's efforts to reduce and eliminate restraints in children's treatment settings, the department entered into a partnership with the Sanctuary Institute to bring the Sanctuary Model to Pennsylvania in 2007. The University of Pittsburgh worked with the Pennsylvania Department of Public Welfare, the Sanctuary Institute, and 30 participating provider residential sites to conduct an open evaluation of the implementation of the model. Annual surveys were conducted from 2008 to 2010. The evaluation found that greater implementation was associated with a number of positive outcomes among staff: lower stress and higher morale, increased feelings of job competence and proficiency, and a greater investment in the individuals they serve. Implementation of the Sanctuary Model was also significantly associated with improved organizational culture and climate and a substantial decrease in the reported use of restraints by many sites (Stein et al., 2011). Additionally, an analysis of service utilization from 2007 to 2009 by children since discharged from Sanctuary Model residential treatment facilities (RTFs) versus other RTFs was conducted by Community Care Behavioral Health, a managed care company. It demonstrated that although both groups had a similar average (mean) length of stay in 2007, by 2009 the Sanctuary Model RTF providers had a substantially shorter length of stay and a somewhat greater decrease in median length of stay; a substantial increase in the percentage of discharged youths who received outpatient services in the three months following discharge; and a lower increase in the percentage of children readmitted to RTFs in the 90 days following discharge (Community Care Behavioral Health, 2011).

CONCLUSIONS

We now have a significant body of experience in watching the Sanctuary process unfold in many different kinds of organizations—more than 250 as of 2012. What we see is that adopting a trauma-sensitive organizational paradigm changes the way organizational members think and act by effecting group norms in a way that trying to influence individual behavior alone cannot accomplish. Changes in thinking change habits, and therefore change habitual routines. The SELF framework changes how people use language; the Sanctuary Commitments delineate how to best sustain interpersonal relationships; and the Sanctuary Toolkit improves the way we all actually practice. These changes create a sense of possibility and hope in our organizations, which in turn inspires hope in those who come to us for help. Changing behavior then changes the entire organization, as demonstrated in reduced turnover, improved morale, improved communication, and decreased incidents of violence. Changing the organizational behavior then changes client outcomes, resulting in the development of safety skills, improved emotional management, a greater readiness to participate in trauma-specific treatment approaches, improved social skills and relationships, more satisfactory academic or job performance, and enhanced decision making and judgment. These children are the future, and we hope that by changing client outcomes we can contribute to creating a better future for all of us.

References

Abt Associates. (2008). *Characteristics of residential treatment for children and youth with serious emotional disturbances.* Washington, DC: National Association for Children's Behavioral Health and National Association of Psychiatric Health Systems.

Alderfer, C. P., & Smith, K. K. (1982). Studying intergroup relations embedded in organizations. *Administrative Science Quarterly, 27*(1), 35.

Banks, J., & Vargas, L. A. (2009a, February). *Contributors to restraints and holds in organizations* (Andrus Center for Learning and Innovation, research brief). www.sanctuaryweb.com/PDFs_new/Banks%20and%20Vargas%20Contributors%20to%20Restraints%20and%20Holds.pdf

Banks, J., & Vargas, L. A. (2009b, March). *Sanctuary at Andrus Children's Center* (Andrus Center for Learning and Innovation, research brief). www.sanctuaryweb.com/PDFs_new/Banks%20and%20Vargas%20Sanctuary%20at%20Andrus.pdf

Bloom, S. L. (2013). *Creating sanctuary: Toward the evolution of sane societies* (2nd ed.) New York, NY: Routledge.

Bloom, S. L., & Farragher, B. (2010). *Destroying sanctuary: The crisis in human service delivery systems.* New York, NY: Oxford University Press.

Bloom, S. L., & Farragher, B. (2013). *Restoring sanctuary: A new operating system for trauma-informed systems of care.* New York, NY: Oxford University Press.

Bureau of Justice. (2001). *Violence in the workplace, 1993–99* (Bureau of Justice Statistics special report). Washington, DC: Bureau of Statistics, U.S. Department of Justice. www.ojp.usdoj.gov/bjs/pub/pdf/vw99.pdf

Collie, D. (2004, July 7). *Workplace stress: Expensive stuff.* www.emaxhealth.com/38/473.html

Community Care Behavioral Health. (2011). *Assessing the implementation of a residential facility organizational change model: Pennsylvania's implementation of the Sanctuary Model.* www.ccbh.com/pdfs/articles/Sanctuary_Model_3Pager_20110715.pdf

Duhigg, C. (2012). *The power of habit: Why we do what we do in life and business.* New York, NY: Random House.

Esaki, N., & Larkin, H. (in press). Prevalence of adverse childhood experiences among child service providers. *Families in Society.*

Felitti, V. J., & Anda, R. F. (2010). The relationship of adverse childhood experiences to adult medical disease, psychiatric disorders, and sexual behavior: Implications for healthcare. In R. Lanius, E. Vermetten & C. Pain (Eds.), *The impact of early life trauma on health and disease: The hidden epidemic* (pp. 77–87). New York, NY: Cambridge University Press.

Gazzaniga, M. (2011). *Who's in charge? Free will and the science of the brain.* New York, NY: HarperCollins.

Knudsen, E. I., Heckman, J. J., Cameron, J. L., & Shonkoff, J. P. (2006). Economic, neurobiological, and behavioral perspectives on building America's future workforce. *Proceedings of the National Academy of Sciences of the United States of America, 103*(27), 10155–10162.

LeBel, J., Huckshorn, K. A., & Caldwell, B. (2010). Restraint use in residential programs: Why are best practices ignored? *Child Welfare, 89*(2), 169–187.

McSparren, W., & Motley, D. (2010). How to improve the process of change. *Non-profit World, 28*(6), 14–15.

Occupational Safety and Health Administration. (2004). *Guidelines for preventing workplace violence for health care & social service workers.* Washington, DC: U.S. Department of Labor. www.osha.gov/Publications/osha3148.pdf

Rivard, J. C., McCorkle, D., Duncan, M. E., Pasquale, L. E., Bloom, S. L., & Abramovitz, R. (2004). Implementing a trauma recovery framework for youths in residential treatment. *Child and Adolescent Social Work Journal, 21*(5), 529–550.

Scheff, T. J. (1975). On reason and sanity: Some political implications of psychiatry thought. In T. J. Scheff (Ed.), *Labeling madness* (pp. 12–20). Englewood Cliffs, NJ: Prentice-Hall.

Schein, E. H. (1999). *The corporate culture: A survival guide—Sense and nonsense about culture change.* San Francisco, CA: Jossey-Bass.

Senge, P., Cambron-McCabe, N., Lucas, T., Smith, B., Dutton, J., & Kleiner, A. (2000). *Schools that learn: A fifth discipline fieldbook for educators, parents, and everyone who cares about education.* New York, NY: Doubleday.

Stein, B. D., Kogan, J. N., Magee, E., & Hindes, K. (2011, September 29). *Sanctuary Survey final state report.* Unpublished data, obtained from the authors.

Wells, K. (1991). Placement of emotionally disturbed children in residential treatment: A review of placement criteria. *American Journal of Orthopsychiatry, 61*(3), 345.

TATIANA DAVIDSON, PH.D.
MICHAEL DE ARELLANO, PH.D.

12

Cultural Considerations for Assessment and Treatment in Child Maltreatment Cases

PREVALENCE OF TRAUMA

The prevalence of child maltreatment is high throughout the United States: in 2011, an estimated 3.4 million referrals involving child maltreatment were received by child protective services (U.S. Department of Health and Human Services, 2012). There is also evidence to suggest significant disparities in the experience of trauma and child maltreatment among racial/ethnic minority youths, with children of African American, American Indian, or Alaska Native descent, as well as those of multiple racial descents, having the highest rates of victimization (U.S. Department of Health and Human Services, 2012). For example, in a study of trauma exposure among juvenile detainees, African American males were more likely than white males to have witnessed violence (Abram et al., 2004), and according to the current literature, American Indian and Alaska Native (AI/AN) youths are twice as likely as non-AI/AN youths to experience more severe and multiple victimizations (Pavkov et al., 2010; Stevens et al., 2005). Hispanic/Latino youths are particularly vulnerable to trauma exposure. For example, in a recent study examining the prevalence of child sexual abuse among adolescents, Newcomb, Munoz, and Carmona (2009) found that Hispanic adolescents were twice as likely as European Americans to experience child sexual abuse. And in a nationally representative study, Hispanic youths were found to report a greater number of victimization experiences than non-Hispanic white youths (Finkelhor & Dzuiba-Leatherman, 1994). In contrast, studies have consistently found that Asian Americans have the lowest reported rates of exposure to any traumatic event; however, this population has the highest rates of war-related events, compared with whites, African Americans, and Hispanics (Roberts et al., 2011).

Immigrant youths also appear to be a particularly vulnerable population, as they may have been exposed to vio-lence before, during, or after migration (Bridges et al., 2010; Guarnaccia & Lopez, 1998). For example, one study indicated that 80% of immigrant youths reported *witnessing* a violent event and 49% *directly experienced* a violent event within the past year (Jaycox et al., 2002).

Some authors have posited that the observed racial/ethnic differences are a function of the disproportionate impact of poverty and related stress and the overall economic disadvantage experienced by many racial/ethnic minority children and their families, as well as cultural stressors (Jones, Finkelhor, & Halter, 2006; Smart & Smart, 1995).

DIFFERENCES IN INCIDENT CHARACTERISTICS

Data from the National Epidemiologic Survey on Alcohol and Related Conditions indicated that African Americans and Hispanics/Latinos had significantly higher exposure to child maltreatment than whites, primarily as a result of witnessing domestic violence. Further, African Americans have significantly higher exposure to assaultive violence than whites (Roberts et al., 2011), more sibling sexual abuse, a higher likelihood of multiple abuse incidents, and more physical attacks (Davis et al., 2006; Voisin et al., 2011).

American Indians are a population that has not been widely studied in the child maltreatment literature. However, the extant literature on incident characteristics in the AI/AN adolescent population finds threat of injury and witnessing injury to be the most common forms of reported trauma (Abram et al., 2004; Deters et al., 2006). Sexual trauma (rape, sexual attack, molestation) was least commonly reported (Deters et al., 2006). A study by Gnanadesikan, Novins, and Beals (2005) found that American Indian youths who experienced sexual trauma and had multiple traumatic experiences were at particularly high risk for developing posttraumatic stress disorder (PTSD).

A major concern cited in virtually all of the aforementioned studies is that despite these high rates of trauma exposure and subsequent mental health outcomes, a vast underutilization of mental health services is observed among these racial/ethnic minority groups. This is described in greater detail below.

TRAUMA-RELATED PROBLEMS AND SERVICE UTILIZATION

Studies have consistently demonstrated that exposure to trauma increases the risk for myriad mental health problems and disorders, including PTSD, depression, anxiety disorders, externalizing problems, and substance use disorders (Danielson et al., 2005; Hanson et al., 2006). Similar to the findings on trauma prevalence, there is evidence that racial/ethnic minorities may be particularly vulnerable to developing psychopathology secondary to experiencing trauma. However, despite the rapid growth of the racial/ethnic minority population in the United States (U.S. Census, 2010), a lack of culturally and linguistically competent mental health services and providers for this population persists, which poses a significant barrier for racial/ethnic minority groups. These groups may also face additional barriers to quality mental health care.

African Americans

TRAUMA AND FUNCTIONING. Some studies show that African American and white adults have similar rates of PTSD following trauma exposure (Frueh et al., 2004), while others have found that African Americans report higher rates of PTSD and depression compared with other racial/ethnic groups (Price et al., 2013; Roberts et al., 2011). Some authors posit that perceived discrimination, race-related verbal assaults, and racial stigmatization may significantly contribute to the development of PTSD in this population (Ellis et al., 2008). Trauma experience also has been shown to affect other areas of functioning among African Americans, including decreased academic achievement (Bowen & Bowen, 1999), increased likelihood of school dropout (Porche et al., 2011), and discrimination, which can lead to greater exposure to traumatic stress (Pole et al., 2005). Additionally, histories of childhood maltreatment have been associated with substance use and risky sexual behavior among African American adolescents (Oshri, Tubman, & Burnette, 2012). Despite the differential exposure to traumatic events and the subsequent negative effects on mental health and overall well-being, African Americans have typically been found to underutilize mental health services.

AVAILABILITY AND UTILIZATION OF MENTAL HEALTH SERVICES. Cultural perspectives, availability of resources, and knowledge about mental health services have been found to significantly influence the use of mental health services among African American youths and families. Stigma attached to mental illness is highlighted as a primary barrier that prevents African Americans from accessing mental health care (Corrigan, 2004), For example, among African Americans, the notion of being seen as "crazy" or "weak" is a deterrent to participating in mental health treatment (Meinert, 2003). Different ideas of coping with mental health also may influence service utilization, with African American youths sometimes being encouraged to use willpower to withstand stressful situations (Browman, 1996). Additionally, high levels of social support, where close relationships and spirituality are used as a means of coping with stressors, are promoted as a cultural priority among many African Americans, and this could affect the use of formal mental health services (Constantine et al., 2005; Mitchell & Ronzio, 2011).

Also adversely influencing service utilization among African American youths the availability of resources for the individual and the means to obtain health care; these include transportation to remote clinics and the inconvenience of multisession treatments. African American families report more instrumental barriers than white families, such as lack of time, unavailability of child care, and limited transportation (Woodall et al., 2010). Such barriers further reduce opportunities for these families to receive education about mental health, to improve their awareness of mental health symptoms, and ultimately, to reap the benefits of treatment (Gilliss et al., 2001).

American Indians and Alaska Natives

TRAUMA AND FUNCTIONING. The few studies of these populations indicate high rates of trauma exposure, including child maltreatment, and of PTSD among American Indians and Alaska Natives (Beals et al., 2005; Manson et al., 1996). For example, a study examining the relationship between lifetime history of traumatic events and psychological functioning in a sample of American Indians found that 94% reported experiencing traumas in their lifetime, with 38% of women and 29% of men meeting the criteria for a diagnosis of PTSD (Ehlers et al., 2013). Moreover, these authors found that trauma experience was also associated with other anxiety disorders and affective disorders. Other authors have found that trauma exposure (e.g., historical trauma, violence exposure, childhood abuse) is strongly associated with early-onset substance abuse, increased risk for substance use disorders, and risky sexual behavior in the American Indian population (Bohm, Babor, & Kranzler, 2003; Hellerstedt et al., 2006; Libby et al., 2004; Whitesell et al., 2009). A study by Deters and colleagues (2006) examining the relationship between trauma and PTSD in a sample of American Indian adolescents in a residential substance abuse treatment program found that the teens in their sample reported an average of four lifetime traumas, with 10% meeting the criteria for full PTSD and 14% for partial PTSD. It is important to note, however, that while studies have generally found high rates of trauma among adult and adolescent American Indians, some authors report that only a fraction of their samples meet the criteria for PTSD.

Explanations for these discrepancies in findings include the scarcity of studies examining the effects of trauma, including child maltreatment, on mental health among American Indians and Alaska Natives; cultural variations in the experience and expression of trauma among American Indians, which may affect assessment and diagnosis of mental health disorders; stigma associated with reporting specific types of trauma (e.g., sexual abuse); and reliance on traditional healing resources within their communities (Beals et al., 2005; Deters et al., 2006). As a result, researchers have strongly advocated increased research efforts to examine the mental health outcomes among trauma-affected AI/AN individuals and the factors that may influence diagnosis and treatment.

AVAILABILITY AND UTILIZATION OF MENTAL HEALTH SERVICES. The extant, albeit limited, research indicates that American Indians and Alaska Natives do not use mental health services at rates consistent with the need for services. Moreover, AI/AN adolescents are found to be more likely than white adolescents to terminate treatment prematurely (Campbell, Weisner, & Sterling, 2006). Several reasons for these rates of service underutilization have been posited, including differential access to and limited availability of quality health care (Manson, 2000; Smedley, Stith, & Nelson, 2003), as well as the lack of health insurance (E. R. Brown et al., 2000), culturally competent service providers (Sontag & Schacht, 1993), and culturally tailored services, which are found to be associated with overall patient dissatisfaction with services (Coulter & Fitzpatrick, 2000). Cultural factors appear to be a key obstacle to service utilization among AI/AN youths, including alternative explanations of mental illness such as supernatural or spiritual forces (Cheung & Snowden, 1990), the use of self-reliance as a coping strategy (du Pré, 2000), and the use of traditional therapies (e.g., medicine men) or of members of their familial and social networks, both of which are consistent with communal values held by AI/AN families (Duran & Duran, 1995). Stigma associated with mental health treatment is also identified as a reason for service underutilization. For example, some may view treatment for emotional problems as a weakness and become concerned about how this would be viewed by others in their community (Givens & Tjia, 2002; Oetzel et al., 2006). Finally, concerns about lack of privacy, distrust of service providers, distrust of the U.S. government, and ineffective communication about emotional problems between patients and mental health providers also adversely affect service utilization (du Pré, 2000; Manson, 2000; Oetzel et al., 2006).

Asian Americans and Pacific Islanders

TRAUMA AND FUNCTIONING. Current, though limited, research suggests that Asian Americans and Pacific Islanders (AA/PIs) have a significantly lower lifetime prevalence of trauma-related PTSD and lower rates of PTSD symptoms than other racial/ethnic groups (Roberts et al., 2011). Some studies, however, indicate that AA/PIs report more severe PTSD symptoms (Friedman et al., 2004). As a possible explanation, it is important to note that the majority of studies investigating trauma among AA/PIs have focused on adults who have experienced war-related events (e.g., Friedman et al., 2004; Roberts et al., 2011), on refugee samples (Kroll, Yusuf, & Fujiwara, 2011), and on survivors of natural disasters (e.g., Siqveland, Hafstad, & Tedeschi, 2012). Moreover, studies that have sought to examine children's responses to traumatic events have used only parental reports of child symptoms. Some studies found that child maltreatment in AA/PIs can have detrimental mental health consequences into adulthood. For example, a study examining the relationship between childhood maltreatment and mental health in a sample of Indian college students found a relationship between early exposure to trauma and suicidal risk (Singh, Manjula, & Philip, 2012). Similarly, another study found that child maltreatment was associated with depression, lifetime suicidal ideation, and suicide attempts in a sample of Asian American women (Hahm et al., 2012).

Cultural factors also have been shown to influence PTSD symptoms in AA/PIs. For example, researchers have consistently demonstrated that AA/PIs tend to exhibit more emotional control as a means of avoiding shame and stigma for self and others, in order to maintain interdependence and relationship harmony (Butler, Lee, & Gross, 2007; Liu & Iwamoto, 2006; Matsumoto et al., 2005), which may account for the underreporting of symptoms. Immigration factors (e.g., poverty, separation from family) and acculturative stress (e.g., acculturation differences between children and parents) are other cultural factors that could potentially increase vulnerability to PTSD symptoms (Carr et al., 1997; Friedman et al., 2004; Hsu, Davies, & Hansen, 2004). Some investigators have suggested that culturally specific idioms of distress could influence diagnosis and subsequent treatment (Hinton et al., 2010). For example, somatic presentations of trauma such as tinnitus (buzzing in the ear), *khyâl* attacks (panic symptoms; fear of death from dysfunction of the body), or neurasthenia (mental and physical exhaustion marked by chronic fatigue, aches, and pains) could go undetected or misdiagnosed in Western psychological practices (Hinton et al., 2006; Zheng et al., 1997).

AVAILABILITY AND UTILIZATION OF MENTAL HEALTH SERVICES. Asian Americans have the lowest rates of mental health service utilization among all racial/ethnic minority groups (U.S. Department of Health and Human Services, 2001). Several barriers to the receipt of services have been identified, including stigma and shame associated with mental health problems, negative attitudes toward mental health treatment, lack of financial resources, and lack of Asian-language-proficient providers and culturally appropriate treatments (Chu, Hsieh, & Tokars, 2011; Le Meyer et al., 2009; Niv, Wong, & Hser, 2007; Ting & Hwang, 2009). It has also been shown that Asian Americans delay seeking services until their condition becomes severe (U.S. Department of Health and Human Services, 2001) and that they are likely to terminate services prematurely.

Other studies suggest that cultural factors are major contributors in the observed underutilization of services by Asian Americans. For example, S. Sue and colleagues (2012) posit that cultural bias in the conceptualization of mental health disorders can influence the reporting of symptoms by an Asian American individual, as well as influence the clinician's interpretation of the reported symptoms. Cheng, Leong, and Geist (1993) argued that Asian Americans may have different methods for coping with mental illness, such as not dwelling on uncomfortable thoughts, which could adversely affect service utilization. Acculturation, defined as the process of adapting to mainstream culture while maintaining connections with native culture (Berry, 1980), also influences the use of services by Asian Americans. Specifically, highly acculturated individuals have more positive attitudes toward seeking psychological services (Tata & Leong, 1994). Similarly, an Asian American individual's value orientation has been shown to influence service utilization. For example, adherence to more collectivistic values (i.e., emphasizing the welfare of the group over the needs of the individual; Triandis, 1988) is in conflict with the orientation of traditional mental health treatments, which place emphasis on exploring individual conflicts, potentially speaking about family problems, and having open and intimate communication with a therapist who may not be a member of the person's racial/ethnic group (Kim & Omizo, 2003; Leong & Lau, 2001; Leong, Wagner, & Kim, 1995).

Hispanics/Latinos

TRAUMA AND FUNCTIONING. Studies have consistently found that Hispanic individuals have higher rates and more severe levels of trauma-related symptoms than non-Hispanic individuals (Pole, Gone, & Kulkarni, 2008). Specifically, higher prevalence rates of PTSD and more severe levels of other types of trauma symptoms are reported in Hispanics (e.g., Marshall, Schell, & Miles, 2009; Pole et al., 2005; Pole, Gone, & Kulkarni, 2008). The experience of trauma also contributes to academic problems, school dropout, substance use, depression, and conduct problems among Hispanic youths (Alva & de Los Reyes, 1999; Oshri, Tubman, & Burnette, 2012; Porche et al., 2011; Pumariega, Rothe, & Pumariega, 2005). Cultural factors also influence the experience and manifestation of mental health disorders among Hispanics. For example, acculturation has been shown to influence mental health outcomes following a traumatic experience. Researchers found that Hispanics who strongly re-

tain their indigenous cultural norms (Kim, 2007) report more severe PTSD symptoms (Perilla, Norris, & Lavizzo, 2002). It is also important to note that Hispanics may have different conceptualizations of trauma. For example, *susto* (fright) is a culturally acceptable somatic manifestation of trauma in which an individual may exhibit nervousness, insomnia, and gastrointestinal problems. Similarly, *ataque de nervios* (attack of nerves) is a manifestation of trauma in which a person may fear dying from bodily dysfunction or may fear engaging in behaviors resulting from loss of control (Guarnaccia, Lewis-Fernández, & Rivera, 2003). When seeking treatment, Hispanic individuals may expect mental health services to treat culture-specific, trauma-related symptoms rather than treating the trauma itself. Finally, Hispanics may face additional chronic stressors that can exacerbate trauma-related symptoms, including poverty, limited access to community resources, and immigration issues (Hiott et al., 2006). For example, some Hispanic families enter the United States illegally and live with the fear of deportation (Smart & Smart, 1995), a fear that often prevents them from accessing services.

AVAILABILITY AND UTILIZATION OF MENTAL HEALTH SERVICES. Hispanic youths who have experienced trauma may face additional stressors, as mentioned above, including poverty (Bailey et al., 1999), limited access to community resources (Aguilar-Gaxiola et al., 2002), and immigration and acculturation issues (e.g., legal status, English-language proficiency) (Hiott et al., 2006)—all of which can affect access to services, as well as engagement in and completion of treatment. Indeed, Hispanics have consistently been shown to underutilize and prematurely terminate formal mental health services (Alegría et al., 2010; Goebert & Nishimura, 2011; Organista, Muñoz, & González, 1994). Several barriers to seeking and using treatment have been identified among Hispanics. Some authors cited cultural factors such as a wide use of and reliance on religious healing systems (e.g., Koss, 1980) and family support systems (Cauce et al., 2002) as possible reasons for low rates of service utilization. As such, the integration of cultural constructs into mental health services may heighten the engagement of Hispanic families. Other authors have suggested a lack of proximity to service centers (Aguilar-Gaxiola et al., 2002), limited familiarity with U.S. culture (e.g., English-language proficiency), socioeconomic status (Bailey et al., 1999), transportation problems (Miranda et al., 1996), and a limited number of bilingual counselors (D. Sue & Sue, 1999) as possible reasons for underutilization. Among immigrant populations, fear of arrest or deportation has been found to delay the use of treatment services even when available (Pumariega, Rothe, & Pumariega, 2005). Thus, addressing the potential impact of these cultural stressors (i.e., immigration history/status) is critical to providing effective, culturally relevant treatment.

. . .

Given the significant disparities in the experience of trauma among racial/ethnic minority youths, the overwhelmingly low levels of utilization of formal mental health services, and other barriers to receipt of services, novel methods of reaching this population are clearly warranted. Potential interventions developed for these families should be more culturally relevant, as this has been a noted barrier for service utilization among all the racial/ethnic minority groups described above. Additionally, successful trauma treatment requires a clinician who is aware of specific idioms of distress as well as cultural factors (i.e., immigration, acculturation, cultural values) within a client population, and one who recognizes that addressing cultural constructs will probably result in greater success in treating the trauma (Harmon, Langley, & Ginsburg, 2006). However, very little attention has been given to tailoring existing evidence-based interventions to racial/ethnic minorities so as to adequately address cultural and utilization barriers and maximize clients' engagement in and potential benefit from treatment.

EVIDENCE-BASED TREATMENT AND ETHNIC MINORITY GROUPS

Over the past several years there has been an increased awareness of the importance of cultural issues as they relate to efficacious mental health treatments for racial/ethnic minorities. Many experts (e.g., Bernal, Bonilla, & Bellido, 1995; Bernal, Jiménez-Chafey, & Domenech Rodríguez, 2009; Smith, Domenech Rodríguez, & Bernal, 2011) have emphasized the importance of evidence-based treatments (EBTs) taking into account a client's cultural contexts and values, including the integration of cultural values, collaboration with individuals familiar with the client's culture, provision of extra services to increase retention in treatment (e.g., child care), and cultural sensitivity training for professional staff (Griner & Smith, 2006; Smith, Domenech Rodríguez, & Bernal, 2011). As such, many experts have advocated the adaptation of EBTs, defined as the "systemic modification of interventions to consider the patient's culture" (Bernal, Jiménez-Chafey, & Domenech Rodríguez, 2009), to better address the specific needs of minority racial/ethnic groups. To date, various authors have adapted EBTs for use with racial/ethnic minority adults and youths (e.g., Domenech Rodríguez, Baumann, & Schwartz, 2011; McCabe et al., 2005; McCabe & Yeh, 2009; Rosselló, Bernal, & Rivera-Medina, 2008).

There is a considerable amount of research demonstrating the efficacy of treatment interventions for children and adolescents to address a range of mental health problems (e.g., Kazdin, 2000). Although some concern has been expressed about the generalizability of clinical trials to culturally diverse populations (e.g., Bernal & Scharró-del-Río, 2001; S. Sue, 1998), preliminary evidence supports the use of EBTs with racial/ethnic minority populations. For example, Huey and Polo (2008) conducted a meta-analysis of EBTs in which support was found for their use in treating anxiety-related problems, attention-deficit / hyperactivity disorder, depression, delinquency/behavior problems, substance use, trauma-related problems, mixed behavior and emotional

problems, and other psychosocial problems, and included interventions targeting problems secondary to child maltreatment and other types of trauma exposure. However, this meta-analysis included only a few studies, and these studies were not specifically designed to detect ethnic/racial differences in treatment response—which leads to a number of limitations for this analysis (for a review, see Huey & Polo, 2008). Consequently, while these findings are promising, they should be interpreted cautiously. Further research is necessary to examine the efficacy of EBTs across and within racial/ethnic groups, including studies of traditional and culture-specific mental health outcomes (e.g., somatic symptoms, culture-specific syndromes); studies of engagement in and completion of treatment; and more refined examinations of moderating/mediating factors that go beyond gross comparisons across what are assumed to be monolithic racial/ethnic groups and that can help further inform research and practice (e.g., views of mental health treatment, spirituality, acculturation).

Preliminary evidence supports a number of trauma-specific interventions, including Cognitive Behavioral Intervention for Trauma in Schools (CBITS; Jaycox, 2004; Stein et al., 2003) and Trauma-Focused Cognitive Behavioral Therapy (TF-CBT; Cohen, Mannarino, & Deblinger, 2006). Although evaluating the efficacy of these interventions across racial/ethnic groups was not the original intention of these studies, sufficient numbers of children from racial/ethnic minority groups were included in the study samples to allow examination of potential differential responses across groups. Based on the findings, the interventions demonstrated efficacy among children from diverse backgrounds.

For example, CBITS has been effectively used in schools with culturally diverse populations, including children from Latin America, Asia, and Eastern Europe, as well as with African American and Native American children. In a study involving immigrant children, CBITS was found to reduce PTSD and depressive symptoms, when compared with a waitlist group, at the initial post-treatment assessment and at follow-up (Kataoka et al., 2003; Stein et al., 2003). CBITS has been used with a wide range of acculturation levels and has been provided in Spanish, Korean, Russian, Western Armenian, and Japanese. A significant strength of CBITS is its use in school settings, which can address many of the challenges experienced by traditionally underserved populations in using and completing mental health services.

TF-CBT also has been effective in addressing mental health problems associated with child maltreatment and other types of trauma exposure among children and families from culturally diverse backgrounds. TF-CBT is a components-based, cognitive behavioral intervention that is sufficiently flexible to incorporate cultural beliefs and values while maintaining fidelity to the treatment model (Cohen, Mannarino, & Deblinger, 2006; see also chapter 3 of this volume). This treatment has been evaluated with white, African American, and Hispanic children who participated in research samples, with very limited differences in outcomes across studies (as cited in Huey and Polo, 2008). Children and caregivers report significant improvements in children's PTSD, depression, anxiety, externalizing behaviors, sexualized behaviors, feelings of shame, and mistrust, as well as parental distress and parenting practices (Cohen, Mannarino, & Deblinger, 2006).

While there is preliminary evidence supporting the use of standard EBTs for racial/ethnic minority youths, culturally modified interventions also have received support in the literature. For example, Griner and Smith (2006) found culturally adapted interventions to be effective in a review of 76 studies, with a moderate effect size ($d = 45$) averaged across all studies. In addition, interventions with culturally homogeneous groups were found to be more effective than interventions with heterogeneous groups, suggesting that interventions that are culturally specific are more efficacious than those designed to be sensitive to a broader range of cultural backgrounds.

One example of a culturally modified evidence-based treatment intervention is Honoring Children / Mending the Circle, an enhancement of TF-CBT that was developed for American Indian and Alaska Native children (Bigfoot & Schmidt, 2010). The intervention involves a careful assessment of cultural affiliation, which then leads to tailoring of TF-CBT by incorporating cultural enhancements. This tailored intervention is included in "Evidence-Based Interventions and Promising Practices," a list posted on the National Child Traumatic Stress Network website (www.nctsn.org /resources/topics/treatments-that-work/promising-practices), and case studies have been published supporting its feasibility and efficacy (e.g., Bigfoot & Schmidt, 2010).

Similarly, Culturally Modified Trauma-Focused Cognitive Behavioral Therapy (CM-TF-CBT) is based on TF-CBT and has been modified for Hispanic/Latino populations. CM-TF-CBT incorporates an assessment and a tailored integration of common cultural values, beliefs, and practices, depending on the child's and family's levels of acculturation, while maintaining treatment fidelity to the original model. This intervention is included on the National Child Traumatic Stress Network's listing of empirically supported treatments and promising practices (www.nctsn.org/resources /topics/treatments-that-work/promising-practices) and has received preliminary support for its use with trauma-exposed Hispanic/Latino children and families (de Arellano, Danielson, & Felton, 2012). For example, a pilot study of CM-TF-CBT for trauma-exposed Hispanic youths found very high retention rates and significant reductions in PTSD symptoms (Rivera & de Arellano, 2008). We discuss CM-TF-CBT in more detail later in the chapter.

CULTURALLY INFORMED ASSESSMENT

To ensure that treatments are being tailored to the individual needs of children who have suffered child maltreatment and their families, a careful assessment of trauma exposure and trauma-related problems is critical. Standard approaches to assessment may fall short of providing a clear and thorough picture of the needs and strengths of culturally diverse maltreatment victims and their families (de Arellano & Danielson, 2008). Using a culturally informed assessment, the clinician should consider a number of areas, including those specific to (1) child maltreatment (e.g., parenting practices and beliefs about corporal punishment; beliefs about sexual abuse and sex, including appropriate sexual behaviors and masturbation; views of interpersonal violence); (2) general trauma exposure (e.g., a broader range of traumatic events, such as, for immigrant populations, trauma exposure in the country of origin or during immigration or, for refugee populations, exposure to torture or war); (3) mental health outcomes (e.g., measurement of broader symptoms associated with anxiety or depression, such as somatization; measurement of culture-specific syndromes such as *ataque de nervios*); and (4) general treatment issues (e.g., views of mental health and mental health treatment, including where the family goes for help; identification of individuals who have a direct or indirect effect on parenting practices, including parents, grandparents, and other family/community members). In addition, an assessment of other general cultural constructs should include (1) spiritual beliefs (e.g., social support from religious organizations; comfort derived from spiritual practices such as prayer or meditation); (2) views of gender roles (e.g., traditional gender roles); (3) views of family (e.g., level of support); (4) language preference; and (5) individual levels of acculturation for the child and family members (de Arellano & Danielson, 2008).

INTEGRATION OF CULTURAL CONSTRUCTS

Based on the results of a culturally informed assessment, the most appropriate evidence-based treatment can be selected and tailored to meet the needs of victims of child maltreatment and their caregivers. The specific cultural views, beliefs, and practices to be considered, assessed, and appropriately integrated vary greatly across cultural groups, and the selection should be driven by a thorough understanding of the target population.

Views of Mental Health and Mental Health Treatment

Given the mental health care disparities among racial/ethnic minority groups, a significant effort should be made to engage children and caregivers in treatment. This should include gaining a better understanding of a family's views of mental health and mental health treatment, such as the use of other or preferred sources of medical or mental health care (e.g., alternative medicine, traditional folk healing practices, and/or clergy or spiritual healers). This provides the opportunity to educate the family about the mental health treatment process, given that some families have little or no experience with mental health care providers

(Schwarzbaum, 2004), as well as to assess the extent to which the family adheres to specific cultural constructs (La-Roche, 2002). Any misunderstandings or misperceptions (e.g., therapy is only for those with severe psychopathology) should be addressed by providing detailed information about treatment. For example, psychoeducational information should include a clear rationale for the treatment, estimated length of the course of treatment, overview of the therapy approach (e.g., learning additional skills to manage trauma-related distress), and the roles and responsibilities of all those involved in the treatment (e.g., parental involvement). Providing this information in a thorough manner throughout the course of treatment can help reduce incongruities in expectations between therapists and clients, which have been found to be significant predictors of treatment dropout (Schwarzbaum, 2004).

Family Involvement and Parenting Practices

For some families, focusing on one primary caregiver during treatment may be sufficient to support the child and make necessary changes to the child's environment, but additional family members may need to be involved when multiple individuals share caregiving responsibilities. Some families may have a greater sense of shared responsibility for providing care for the child, for emotional and financial support, and for decision making (e.g., Falicov, 1998; Marin & Marin, 1991; Moore & Pachon, 1985). If caregivers consistently call on other family members (e.g., grandmother, aunt) for guidance in child-rearing challenges, it can be helpful to engage those individuals in treatment, as well. For example, a phone call from the therapist to a grandmother, soliciting her opinion on how treatment can better address her grandchild's difficulties, can help engage her in supporting the primary caregiver in making changes. In addition, a thorough understanding of the caregiver's parenting views and parenting practices can help the therapist tailor the treatment to be consistent with these views. For example, some parents prefer active parenting strategies (over those perceived as passive, such as ignoring unwanted behavior) and punishment (over rewarding desired behaviors) (McCabe et al., 2005; McCabe & Yeh, 2009). And some parents report placing a high value on children obeying their caregivers as a demonstration of respect, rather than rewarding them for compliance (e.g., "I am not going to reward my child for things she should be doing; she should listen to me because I am her mother"). In such situations, interventions can be framed to be more consistent with the family's beliefs about parenting practices. Interventions such as ignoring can be framed as an active punishment (e.g., withholding wanted attention in response to inappropriate behaviors), and time-out can also be framed as a punishment (e.g., placing the child in the "chair of punishment" or at the "wall of boredom"). Behavioral interventions can also be framed as intending to increase the child's respect for parents, rather than simply focusing on increasing compliance.

Spirituality

If spirituality is important to the child and family, attempts can be made to integrate relevant beliefs and practices into the treatment. As with all cultural constructs, care should be taken to assess the importance of spirituality or religion for the child and caregivers, without assuming that these beliefs are consistent. For example, if a parent reports that spirituality is important to the family, but the child does not share the belief to the same degree, the therapist could be perceived as another adult trying to push spirituality, which could be alienating rather than engaging. For many children and families, spiritual beliefs can be a source of significant support, including social support through affiliations with organized religious institutions. Personal beliefs or individual practices (e.g., prayer) can also serve as a strength and can be used in treatment. For example, if a child draws strength or confidence from a belief that God is watching over her and providing protection, this can be referenced during treatment as a positive self-statement (e.g., "I can sleep in the dark because I know God is watching over me"), to complement a broader set of coping strategies. Similarly, if prayer brings comfort to a child, it could be integrated into strategies for relaxation and affect modulation. For families with formal religious affiliations, literature on child maltreatment and therapy that is consistent with the treatment being provided is often available from religious institutions and can be accessed online and shared with families. This approach can help to frame treatment as being congruent with a family's religious beliefs.

Appropriate Social Behavior

Cultural norms often help guide what are judged to be appropriate communication styles and social behaviors in and outside the home. Views of gender roles influence behaviors, and these can play an important role in treatment. For example, traditional gender roles that suggest males should be "tough" and not express feelings such as sadness or fear could make it challenging for a boy to express such feelings associated with his child maltreatment experiences. A strategy that can help present talking about these feelings in a more culturally congruent manner is to frame talking about happiness or anger as "easy" and discussing feelings of sadness and fear as much more challenging and thus a greater sign of toughness. This can be supported by engaging caregivers, especially male caregivers or other involved male role models, in reinforcing this notion of talking about feelings.

Another set of cultural norms that can influence treatment is one that dictates appropriate social behaviors with professionals. The traditional Hispanic/Latino value of *respeto* implies clear boundaries in relationships and is important in parenting (e.g., a child's respect for his parents) and other social interactions (e.g., how children interact with adults; the approach a caregiver takes in interacting with a mental health provider) (Santiago-Rivera, Arredondo, & Gallardo-Cooper, 2002). In addition to framing parenting practices to be more consistent with this cultural norm, the therapist needs to understand how *respeto* can potentially enhance or challenge his or her interactions with the child or caregiver. For example, *respeto* can interfere with clear and effective communication if, for the child or caregiver, asking for clarification about something in the treatment that is not fully understood or expressing a difference in opinion with the therapist is viewed as questioning authority and being disrespectful.

CULTURAL MODIFICATION OF EVIDENCE-BASED TREATMENTS

Trauma-Focused Cognitive Behavioral Therapy is an empirically supported, widely recognized treatment intervention specifically designed to treat children experiencing trauma-related symptoms and problems, such as PTSD, depression, and anxiety. TF-CBT integrates trauma-sensitive interventions, cognitive behavioral principles, attachment theory, family therapy, and humanistic therapy. The therapy is composed of core components summarized by the acronym PRACTICE: Psychoeducation and Parenting skills training, Relaxation training, Affective expression and modulation, Cognitive coping, Trauma narrative and processing, In vivo mastery of trauma reminders, Conjoint parent-child sessions, and Enhancing future safety and development (Cohen, Mannarino, & Deblinger, 2006). (See chapter 3 for a description of these components of TF-CBT.)

Several randomized controlled trials have supported the efficacy of TF-CBT for reducing symptoms of PTSD, anxiety, and depression among trauma-exposed children (E. J. Brown, Pearlman, & Goodman, 2004; Cohen et al., 2004; Cohen, Mannarino, & Iyengar, 2011; Cohen, Mannarino, & Staron, 2006; Deblinger et al., 2011). A recent meta-analysis found that TF-CBT is "probably efficacious" for racial/ethnic minority youths (Huey & Polo, 2008); however, as mentioned earlier, a significant limitation of these studies was the insufficient inclusion of racial/ethnic minority children, thus preventing generalization of treatment outcomes. To date, there is no therapeutic approach specifically designed to address the unique mental health needs of trauma-affected racial/ethnic minority youths.

Integration of Culture and Trauma Treatment: Culturally Modified TF-CBT

Trauma-Focused Cognitive Behavioral Therapy was culturally modified for trauma-affected Hispanic/Latino youths and their families on the basis of (1) theoretical and empirical literature on treatment delivery among Latinos (e.g., Cuéllar, Arnold, & Gonzáles, 1995; Fragoso & Kashubeck, 2000; Neff & Hoppe, 1993; Sabogal et al., 1987); (2) quantitative and qualitative research with trauma-affected Latino families (Bridges et al., 2010; de Arellano &

Danielson, 2008; de Arellano et al., 2005); and (3) more than 16 years of clinical work providing TF-CBT to Latino youths and their families. Culturally Modified Trauma-Focused Cognitive Behavioral Therapy integrates cultural constructs (e.g., *familismo, personalismo,* gender roles, spirituality) into each of the TF-CBT components, thus maintaining fidelity to the treatment model, and focuses on how culture influences the way children and their families view and cope with trauma. This manualized intervention allows a tailored approach in the assessment of clients' adherence to cultural constructs and in the subsequent integration of these constructs throughout treatment.

CM-TF-CBT was further developed using focus group methodology to determine the acceptability, cultural relevance, and effectiveness of the treatment. Particular attention was focused on beliefs regarding mental health and mental health treatments, views on the effects of trauma exposure, and reactions to each of the PRACTICE components of TF-CBT. Keeping in mind the vast heterogeneity within the Latino population, focus groups were conducted with Latino caregivers and providers serving Latino families in different geographic regions of the United States (e.g., Miami, San Diego, New York, several cities in Texas) (Davidson et al., 2010). Qualitative analyses of the results revealed that, in general, Latino caregivers recognized the importance of mental health treatment, particularly as it relates to trauma exposure. However, they reported a lack of knowledge about mental health services (e.g., "Is therapy for crazy people?" "What happens in therapy?") and recommended extensive psychoeducation for both caregivers and children on mental health problems and treatment. The individual PRACTICE components of TF-CBT were found to be culturally acceptable, pending the cultural appropriateness and relevance of the rationale and clinical examples provided. The caregivers emphasized that engagement in treatment would be affected by the clinician's ability to incorporate the family's cultural and belief system (e.g., spirituality, parenting practices) and to address other clinically relevant issues, including conflicts between parents and children (i.e., the acculturation gap) and difficulties associated with immigration and adjusting to a new culture.

Structure of CM-TF-CBT for Hispanics/Latinos

In CM-TF-CBT, cultural modification can be made to each of the PRACTICE components of TF-CBT. However, we should note that in addition to the suggestions and examples described below, it is ideal to integrate cultural constructs as they are identified by the family throughout treatment (e.g., prayer as a relaxation strategy) to ensure that treatment is individually tailored to meet the needs of the child and family. Furthermore, as modifications are integrated into the treatment, careful attention must be paid to staying true to the original intervention model in order to maintain treatment fidelity.

PSYCHOEDUCATION. In addition to helping to ensure that children and caregivers have a clear understanding of the rationale for treatment and congruent expectations for treatment, it may also be necessary to ensure that treatment is framed in a way consistent with the family's cultural beliefs. For example, some families for whom spirituality is very important can believe that, through a greater dedication to their faith, God will provide for their family and attending treatment is not necessary. One way to help frame treatment to be more culturally congruent with these spiritual beliefs is to suggest that perhaps the family's being referred to these treatment services is God's way of providing for the family. Another way to frame treatment in a culturally congruent way is to draw from teachings from the family's religious background in a respectful and inquiring manner, with great sensitivity to variations in belief systems. For example, the therapist can inquire about the child's and caregivers' understanding of religious teachings that may be relevant to their belief system, such as "God helps those who help themselves," as a way of framing their involvement in treatment. Another useful strategy for psychoeducation and other treatment components is the inclusion of *dichos* (proverbs) to teach various skills in a way that facilitates rapport and helps clients better relate to the materials. *Dichos* are short phrases, sentences, or rhymes that depict Spanish sayings or proverbs and are often used in common conversation (Aviera, 1996). An example of a *dicho* that might be used to instill hope during psychoeducation is "Despues de la tormenta, sale el sol entre las nubes" (English equivalent: "After the rain comes the sun").

PARENTING SKILLS TRAINING. Helping parents address child behaviors that they view as problematic can serve as an excellent opportunity to provide validation and support and some stress relief, all of which can facilitate parents' engagement in treatment. Care must be taken to validate the importance of respect, for families who identify this as a priority. And the parenting approach should be framed in a way consistent with other parental beliefs, as much as possible (e.g., focus on active parenting strategies) (McCabe et al., 2005; McCabe & Yeh, 2009).

RELAXATION TRAINING. Several authors have noted the importance of religion and spirituality among Hispanics (e.g., Campesino & Schwartz, 2006; Levin, Markides, & Ray, 1996; Neff & Hoppe, 1993). As such, religion and spirituality can be included as relaxation strategies (e.g., prayer, using religious passages as positive self-statements). It is also important to ensure that techniques are understandable and are relevant to the child's and family's experiences and knowledge. For example, imaginal scenes constructed for visualization exercises (e.g., imagining relaxing on the beach) should be relevant and familiar and easy for the child to imagine.

AFFECTIVE EXPRESSION AND MODULATION. Teaching feelings-identification skills and strategies to manage feelings can be enhanced if presented in a cultural context, such as through the use of *dichos* or *cuentos* (stories) or of books that use cultural or historical references. Another important consideration is the use of language for bilingual children. Often, bilingual children have variations in their language development, including their vocabulary for emotional expression in one language versus the other. For example, children who spoke primarily Spanish before starting school may have learned basic emotional expression in Spanish early on and may not have learned emotional expression in English in the same way in school. It can be helpful to go through simple emotion identification and expression exercises in both English and Spanish to ensure that the child fully understands the emotions being discussed. Also, as noted earlier, traditional gender roles (e.g., *machismo*) can make it more challenging for boys to express emotions such as fear and sadness. Framing discussions about these feelings as a true sign of "toughness" can be helpful. Enlisting the support of caregivers to encourage the child to talk about these feelings and to frame this as a demonstration of courage can also facilitate the child's development of affect identification and regulation skills.

COGNITIVE COPING. The integration of *cuentos* and *dichos*, as well as the inclusion of spiritual/religious references, can help develop cognitive coping skills. Numerous *cuentos* can be used to demonstrate how changing the ways we think about something can affect the ways we feel and the ways we behave (e.g., "The Little Red Ant"). The use of positive self-statements can be supplemented with common *dichos*, such as "Donde hay gana hay mana" ("Where there's a will there's a way"), and "No hay mal que por bien no venga" ("There is no misfortune from which good does not come").

TRAUMA NARRATIVE AND PROCESSING. It is often necessary to address potential barriers to direct discussion of the traumatic event, such as not wanting to share "family business" with outsiders or conservative beliefs about sex in cases of sexual abuse. There also may be a family rule that a child discussing some topics with adults, such as sex, is inappropriate. In addition, for bilingual children, being offered the opportunity to tell their story in the language they prefer can be helpful. Data suggest that information about a memory is better recalled if it is elicited in the language in which it was encoded (Javier, Barroso, & Munoz, 1993; Javier & Marcos, 1989). If a child was victimized when young and she was a monolingual Spanish-speaker at that time, working on the trauma narrative in Spanish will probably result in easier recall of the memories and perhaps a richer description.

IN VIVO MASTERY OF TRAUMA REMINDERS. There are no specific modifications for this component, but the clinician must remain respectful of the child's and family's cultural beliefs when implementing desensitization strategies. In addition, a clear rationale for the in vivo exposure is critical, and using *dichos* and *cuentos* that demonstrate the advantage of facing your fears (e.g., The Laughing Skull) can prove very useful for both in vivo exposure and the trauma narrative.

CONJOINT PARENT-CHILD SESSIONS. When preparing caregivers for the conjoint session, the therapist needs to recognize that hearing their child's narrative can be very difficult, especially for caregivers who have experienced their own trauma histories and may never have received treatment. Given the research suggesting that Hispanics may be at greater risk for victimization and less likely to access needed mental health treatment (Bridges et al., 2010; Newcomb, Munoz, & Carmona, 2009), the therapist should be sensitive to and prepared to address these issues during the gradual sharing of the child's narrative and the cognitive processing of caregivers' unhelpful thoughts.

ENHANCING FUTURE SAFETY AND DEVELOPMENT. Ideally, caregivers play an active role in this component, given their ability to influence the child's environment and to help implement strategies to reduce the risk of harm. For this reason, if the primary caregiver is not solely responsible for the care of the child, it is important to involve multiple caregivers. To help increase safety by making strategies more ecologically valid, the family and therapist can discuss safety strategies that may have been in place in the country of origin and whether these strategies could be used in their current home. Cultural values or practices that can interfere with safety should also be addressed. For example, a family that places great emphasis on *respeto* may encourage children to always comply with adults and discourage them from questioning adults. A careful discussion, with active caregiver involvement, can help children learn to distinguish when they should question the authority of adults without fear of negative consequences. An important strategy to promote safety is encouraging the child to continue to speak to the caregiver about the child maltreatment discussed in the narrative and to feel comfortable raising questions and/or concerns in the future. For cases of sexual abuse, a parent's conservative views about sex and/or social norms about whether children should be talking about sex can make it challenging to encourage this kind of communication. It is essential to help caregivers understand the importance of this strategy to help reduce risk and to engage them in the process of facilitating such communication with their child in the future.

CONCLUSIONS

There have been few evidence-based, trauma-focused interventions for child maltreatment victims from racial/ethnic minority backgrounds. This is particularly troublesome given the significant disparities in the experience of trauma and child maltreatment among racial/ethnic minority youths and the underutilization of formal mental health services consistently observed in these populations—all of which calls for novel intervention strategies to address the needs of these children. Preliminary evidence supports the efficacy of several trauma-specific interventions for racial/ethnic minority youths (Cohen, Mannarino, & Deblinger, 2006), but some methodological challenges (e.g., the limited number of racial/ethnic minority participants) limit the conclusions that can be drawn from these data.

Over the past few years, experts in the field have advocated the cultural adaptation of evidence-based treatments to improve engagement in treatment and mental health outcomes for racial/ethnic minority groups. Indeed, recent meta-analyses support the utility of cultural modification of EBTs in increasing participants' retention and engagement in treatment and increasing positive mental health outcomes among racial/ethnic minorities (Griner & Smith, 2006; Smith, Domenech Rodríguez, & Bernal, 2011). Authors advocate a careful cultural assessment prior to and during treatment, integration of cultural values, collaboration with individuals familiar with the client's culture, provision of extra services to increase client retention, and cultural sensitivity training for professional staff. Providers are encouraged to attend carefully to cultural constructs such as acculturation, specific idioms of distress, and cultural rationales (e.g., biological, spiritual) and expressions of mental health (e.g., somatization), as these have been shown to influence engagement in and completion of treatment.

To date, there are a couple of culturally modified, trauma-focused evidence-based treatments targeting racial/ethnic minority youths—Honoring Children / Mending the Circle (Bigfoot & Schmidt, 2010), an adaptation of TF-CBT for American Indian and Alaska Native youths, and Culturally Modified Trauma-Focused Cognitive Behavioral Therapy for Hispanic/Latino youths (de Arellano, Danielson, & Felton, 2012). CM-TF-CBT is an evidence-supported, trauma-focused treatment for Hispanic youths and their families; this manualized intervention integrates cultural constructs (e.g., *familismo*, spirituality) into each of the TF-CBT components, thus maintaining treatment fidelity while focusing on the role of culture as it influences how children and their families view and cope with trauma. Preliminary evidence indicates that CM-TF-CBT improves clients' engagement in treatment and reduces PTSD symptoms among Hispanic youths (Davidson et al., 2010)—thus providing further support for the need for culturally modified treatments to better serve the unique needs of trauma-affected racial/ethnic minority groups. It is our hope that this field continues to develop and to formally evaluate culturally modified EBTs, further informing the scientific community of the importance of cultural issues and the need for the integration of culture into evidence-based interventions that will better serve the mental health needs of trauma-affected racial/ethnic minority populations.

References

Abram, K. M., Teplin, L. A., Charles, D. R., Longworth, S. L., McClelland, G. M., & Dulcan, M. K. (2004). Posttraumatic stress disorder and trauma in youth in juvenile detention. *Archives of General Psychiatry, 61,* 403–411.

Aguilar-Gaxiola, S. A., Zelezny, L., Garcia, B., Edmondson, C., Alejo-Garcia, C., & Vega, W. A. (2002). Translating research into action: Reducing disparities in mental health care for Mexican Americans. *Psychiatric Services, 53,* 1563–1568.

Alegría, M., Canino, G., Stinson, F., & Grant, B. (2006). Nativity and DSM-IV psychiatric disorders among Puerto Ricans, Cuban Americans, and non-Latino whites in the United States: Results from the National Epidemiologic Survey on Alcohol and Related Conditions. *Journal of Clinical Psychiatry, 67*(1), 56–65.

Alva, S. A., & de Los Reyes, R. (1999). Psychosocial stress, internalized symptoms, and the academic achievement of Hispanic adolescents. *Journal of Adolescent Research, 14,* 343–358.

Aviera, A. (1996). "Dichos" therapy group: A therapeutic use of Spanish language proverbs with hospitalized Spanish-speaking psychiatric patients. *Cultural Diversity and Mental Health, 2*(2), 73–87.

Bailey, D. B., Skinner, D., Rodriguez, P., Gut, D., & Correa, V. (1999). Awareness, use, and satisfaction with services for Latino parents of young children with disabilities. *Exceptional Children, 65,* 367–387.

Beals, J., Manson, S. M., Whitesell, N. R., Spicer, P., Novins, D. K., Mitchell, C. M., for the AI-SUPERPFP Team. (2005). Prevalence of DSM-IV disorders and attendant help-seeking in two American Indian reservation populations. *Archives of General Psychiatry, 62,* 99–108.

Bernal, G., Bonilla, J., & Bellido, C. (1995). Ecological validity and cultural sensitivity for outcome research: Issues for the cultural adaptation and development of interventions. *Clinical Psychology: Science and Practice, 13,* 311–316.

Bernal, G., Jiménez-Chafey, M., & Domenech Rodríguez, M. (2009). Cultural adaptation of evidence-based treatments for ethno-cultural youth. *Professional Psychology: Research and Practice, 40,* 361–368.

Bernal, G., & Scharró-del-Río, M. R. (2001). Are empirically supported treatments valid for ethnic minorities? Toward an alternative approach for treatment research. *Cultural Diversity and Ethnic Minority Psychology, 7*(4), 328–342.

Berry, J. W. (1980). Acculturation as varieties of adaptation. In A. Padilla (Ed.), *Acculturation: Theory, models, and some new findings* (pp. 9–25). Boulder, CO: Westview Press.

Bigfoot, D., & Schmidt, S. R. (2010). Honoring children, mending the circle: Cultural adaptation of Trauma-Focused Cognitive-Behavioral Therapy for American Indian and Alaska Native children. *Journal of Clinical Psychology, 66*(8), 847–856.

Bohm, M. J., Babor, T. F., & Kranzler, H. R. (2003). The Alcohol Use Disorders Identification Test (AUDIT): Validation of a screening instrument for use in medical settings. *Journal of Studies on Alcohol, 56,* 423–432.

Bowen, N. K., & Bowen, G. L. (1999). Effects of crime and violence in neighborhoods and schools on the school behavior and performance of adolescents. *Journal of Adolescent Research, 14,* 319–342.

Bridges, A. J., de Arellano, M. A., Rheingold, A. A., Danielson, C., & Silcott, L. (2010). Trauma exposure, mental health, and service utilization rates among immigrant and United States–born Hispanic youth: Results from the Hispanic family study. *Psychological Trauma: Theory, Research, Practice, and Policy, 2*(1), 40–48.

Browman, C. L. (1996). The health consequences of racial discrimination: A study of African Americans. *Ethnicity & Disease, 6,* 148–153.

Brown, E. J., Pearlman, M. Y., & Goodman, R. F. (2004). Facing fears and sadness: Cognitive-behavioral therapy for childhood traumatic grief. *Harvard Review of Psychiatry, 12*(4), 187–198.

Brown, E. R., Ojeda, V. D., Wyn, R., & Levan, R. (2000). *Racial and ethnic disparities in access to health insurance and health care.* Los Angeles. CA: UCLA Center for Health Policy Research and the Henry J. Kaiser Family Foundation.

Butler, E. A., Lee, T. L., & Gross, J. J. (2007). Emotion regulation and culture: Are the social consequences of emotion suppression culture-specific? *Emotion, 7*(1), 30–48.

Campbell, C. I., Weisner, C., & Sterling, S. (2006). Adolescents entering chemical dependency treatment in private managed care: Ethnic differences in treatment initiation and retention. *Journal of Adolescent Health, 38*(4), 343–350.

Campesino, M., & Schwartz, G. E. (2006). Spirituality among Latinas/os: Implications of culture in conceptualization and measurement. *Advances in Nursing Science, 29*(1), 69–81.

Carr, V. J., Lewin, T. J., Kenardy, J. A., & Webster, R. A. (1997). Psychosocial sequelae of the 1989 Newcastle earthquake: III. Role of vulnerability factors in post-disaster morbidity. *Psychological Medicine, 27,* 179–190.

Cauce, A. M., Domenech-Rodríguez, M., Paradise, M., Cochran, B. N., Shea, J. M., Srebnik, D., & Baydar, N. (2002). Cultural and contextual influences in mental health help seeking: A focus on ethnic minority youth. *Journal of Consulting and Clinical Psychology, 70,* 44–55.

Cheng, D., Leong, F. T. L., & Geist, R. (1993). Cultural differences in psychological distress between Asian and Caucasian American college students. *Journal of Multicultural Counseling and Development, 21,* 182–190.

Cheung, F. K., & Snowden, L. R. (1990). Community mental health and ethnic minority populations. *Community Mental Health Journal, 21,* 182–190.

Chu, J. P., Hsieh, K., & Tokars, D. (2011). Help-seeking tendencies in Asian Americans with suicidal ideation and attempts. *Asian American Journal of Psychology, 2,* 25–38.

Cohen, J. A., Deblinger, E., Mannarino, A. P., & Steer, R. A. (2004). A multisite, randomized controlled trial for children with sexual abuse-related PTSD symptoms. *Journal of the American Academy of Child and Adolescent Psychiatry, 43*(4), 393–402.

Cohen, J. A., Mannarino, A. P., & Deblinger, E. (2006). *Treating trauma and traumatic grief in children and adolescents.* New York, NY: Guilford Press.

Cohen, J. A., Mannarino, A. P., & Iyengar, S. (2011). Community treatment of posttraumatic stress disorder for children exposed to intimate partner violence: A randomized controlled trial. *Archives of Pediatrics & Adolescent Medicine, 165*(1), 16–21.

Cohen, J. A., Mannarino, A. P., & Staron, V. R. (2006). A pilot study of modified cognitive-behavioral therapy for childhood traumatic grief (CBT-CTG). *Journal of the American Academy of Child and Adolescent Psychiatry, 45*(12), 1465–1473.

Constantine, M. G., Alleyne, V. L., Caldwell, L. D., McRae, M. B., & Suzuki, L. A. (2005). Coping responses of Asian, black, and Hispanic/Latina New York City residents following the September 11, 2001 terrorist attacks against the United States. *Cultural Diversity and Ethnic Minority Psychology, 11*(4), 293–308.

Corrigan, P. (2004). How stigma interferes with mental health care. *American Psychologist, 59,* 614–625.

Coulter, A., & Fitzpatrick, R. (2000). The patient's perspective regarding appropriate health care. In G. L. Albrecht, R. Fitzpatrick, & S. C. Scrimshaw (Eds.), *The handbook of social studies in health and medicine* (pp. 454–464). Thousand Oaks, CA: Sage Publications.

Cuéllar, I., Arnold, B., & González, G. (1995). Cognitive referents of acculturation: Assessment of cultural constructs in Mexican Americans. *Journal of Community Psychology, 23,* 339–356.

Danielson, C. K., de Arellano, M. A., Kilpatrick, D. G., Saunders, B. E., & Resnick, H. S. (2005). Child maltreatment in depressed adolescents: Differences in symptomatology based on history of abuse. *Child Maltreatment, 10,* 37–48.

Davidson, T. M., de Arellano, M. A., Rheingold, A. A., Danielson, C. K., & Silcott, L. (2010, November). *Cultural adaptation of an evidence-based trauma focused treatment for Latinos/as.* Paper presented at the annual meeting of the National Latino/a Psychological Association, San Antonio, Texas.

Davis, J. L., Borntrager, C., Combs-Lane, A., Wright, D., Elhai, J. D., Falsetti, S. A., et al. (2006). Comparison of racial groups on trauma and post-trauma functioning. *Journal of Trauma Practice, 5*(2), 21–36.

de Arellano, M. A., & Danielson, C. (2008). Assessment of trauma history and trauma-related problems in ethnic minority child populations: An INFORMED approach. *Cognitive and Behavioral Practice, 15*(1), 53–66.

de Arellano, M., Danielson, C., & Felton, J. W. (2012). Children of Latino descent: Culturally modified TF-CBT. In J. A. Cohen, A. P. Mannarino, & E. Deblinger (Eds.), *Trauma-Focused CBT for children and adolescents: Treatment applications* (pp. 253–279). New York, NY: Guilford Press.

de Arellano, M. A., Waldrop, A. E., Deblinger, E., Cohen, J. A., Danielson, C., & Mannarino, A. R. (2005). Community outreach program for child victims of traumatic events: A community-based project for underserved populations. *Behavior Modification, 29*(1), 130–155.

Deblinger, E., Mannarino, A. P., Cohen, J. A., Runyon, M. K., & Steer, R. A. (2011). Trauma-Focused Cognitive-Behavioral Therapy for children: Impact of the trauma narrative and treatment length. *Depression and Anxiety, 28,* 67–75.

Deters, P. B., Novins, D. K., Fickenscher, A., & Beals, J. (2006). Trauma and posttraumatic stress disorder symptomatology: Patterns among American Indian adolescents in substance abuse treatment. *American Journal of Orthopsychiatry, 76*(3), 335–345.

Domenech Rodríguez, M., Baumann, A. A., & Schwartz, A. L. (2011). Cultural adaptation of an evidence based intervention: From theory to practice in a Latino/a community context. *American Journal of Community Psychology, 47*(1–2), 170–186.

du Pré, A. (2000). *Communicating about health: Current issues and perspectives.* Mountain View, CA: Mayfield.

Duran, E., & Duran, B. (1995). *Native American postcolonial psychology.* New York. NY: State University of New York.

Ehlers, C. L., Gizer, I. R., Gilder, D. A., & Yehuda, R. (2013). Lifetime history of traumatic events in an American Indian community sample: Heritability and relation to substance dependence, affective disorder, conduct disorder and PTSD. *Journal of Psychiatric Research, 47,* 155–161.

Ellis, B. H., MacDonald, H. A., Lincoln, A. K., & Cabral, H. J. (2008). Mental health of Somali adolescent refugees: The role of trauma, stress, and perceived discrimination. *Journal of Consulting and Clinical Psychology, 76,* 184–193.

Falicov, C. (1998). *Latino families in therapy: A guide to multicultural practice.* New York, NY: Guilford Press.

Finkelhor, D., & Dzuiba-Leatherman, J. (1994). Victimization of children. *American Psychologist, 49,* 173–183.

Fragoso, J. M., & Kashubeck, S. (2000). Machismo, gender role conflict, and mental health in Mexican American men. *Psychology of Men and Masculinity, 1,* 87–97.

Friedman, M. J., Schnurr, P. P., Sengupta, A., Holmes, T., & Ashcraft, M. (2004). The Hawaii Vietnam Veterans Project: Is minority status a risk factor for posttraumatic stress disorder? *Journal of Nervous and Mental Disease, 192,* 45–50.

Frueh, B. C., Elhai, J. D., Monnier, J., Hammer, M. B., & Knapp, R. G. (2004). Symptom patterns and service use among African American and Caucasian veterans with combat-related PTSD. *Psychological Services, 1,* 22–30.

Gilliss, C. L., Lee, K. A., Gutierrez, Y., Taylor, D., Beyene, Y., Neuhaus, J., et al. (2001). Recruitment and retention of healthy minority women into community-based longitudinal research. *Journal of Women's Health and Gender Based Medicine, 10,* 77–85.

Givens, J. L., & Tjia, J. (2002). Depressed medical students' use of mental health services and barriers to use. *Academic Medicine, 77,* 918–921.

Gnanadesikan, M., Novins, D. K., & Beals, J. (2005). The relationship of gender and trauma characteristics to posttraumatic stress disorder in a community sample of traumatized Northern Plains American Indian adolescents and young adults. *Journal of Clinical Psychiatry, 66*(9), 1176–1183.

Goebert, D., & Nishimura, S. (2011). Comparison of substance abuse treatment utilization and preferences among Native Hawaiians, Asian Americans and Euro Americans. *Journal of Substance Use, 16*(2), 161–170.

Griner, D., & Smith, T. B. (2006). Culturally adapted mental health interventions: A meta-analytic review. *Psychotherapy: Theory, Research, Practice, Training, 43,* 531–548.

Guarnaccia, P. J., Lewis-Fernández, R., & Rivera, M. M. (2003). Toward a Puerto Rican popular nosology: Nervios and ataque de nervios. *Culture, Medicine, and Psychiatry, 27,* 339–366.

Guarnaccia, P. J., & Lopez, S. (1998). The mental health and adjustment of immigrant and refugee children. *Child and Adolescent Psychiatric Clinics of North America, 7,* 537–553.

Hahm, H., Kolaczyk, E., Lee, Y., Jang, J., & Ng, L. (2012). Do Asian-American women who were maltreated as children have a higher likelihood for HIV risk behaviors and adverse mental health outcomes? *Women's Health Issues, 22,* e35–43.

Hanson, R. F., Self-Brown, S., Fricker-Elhai, A., Kilpatrick, D. G., Saunders, B. E., & Resnick, H. (2006). Relations among parental substance use, violence exposure and mental health: The national survey of adolescents. *Addictive Behaviors, 31*(11), 1988–2001.

Harmon, H., Langley, A., & Ginsburg, G. S. (2006). The role of gender and culture in treating youth with anxiety disorders. *Journal of Cognitive Psychotherapy: An International Quarterly, 20*(3), 301–310.

Hellerstedt, W. L., Peterson-Hickey, M., Rhodes, K. L., & Garwick, A. (2006). Environmental, social and personal correlates of having ever had sexual intercourse among American Indian youths. *American Journal of Public Health, 96,* 2228–2234.

Hinton, D. E., Chhean, D., Pich, V., Hofmann, S. G., & Barlow, D. H. (2006). Tinnitus among Cambodian refugees: Relationship to PTSD severity. *Journal of Traumatic Stress, 19,* 541–546.

Hinton, D. E., Pich, V., Marques, L., Nickerson, A., & Pollack, M. H. (2010). Khyâl attacks: A key idiom of distress among traumatized Cambodian refugees. *Culture, Medicine, and Psychiatry, 34,* 244–278.

Hiott, A., Grzywacz, J. G., Arcury, T. A., & Qunadt, S. A. (2006). Gender differences in anxiety and depression among immigrant Hispanics. *Families, Systems, & Health, 24*(2), 137–146.

Hsu, E., Davies, C. A., & Hansen, D. J. (2004). Understanding mental health needs of Southeast Asian refugees: Historical, cultural, and contextual challenges. *Clinical Psychology Review, 24,* 193–213.

Huey, S. J., & Polo, A. J. (2008). Evidence-based psychosocial treatments for ethnic minority youth. *Journal of Clinical Child and Adolescent Psychology, 37*, 262–301.

Javier, R. A., Barroso, F., & Munoz, M. A. (1993). Autobiographical memory in bilinguals. *Journal of Psycholinguistic Research, 22*, 319–338.

Javier, R. A., & Marcos, L. R. (1989). The role of stress on the language-independence and code-switching phenomena. *Journal of Psycholinguistic Research, 18*(5), 449–472.

Jaycox, L. H. (2004). *Cognitive behavioral intervention for trauma in schools.* Longmont, CO: Sopris West Educational Services.

Jaycox, L. H., Stein, B. D., Kataoka, S. H., Wong, M., Fink, A., Escudero, P. I. A., et al. (2002). Violence exposure, posttraumatic stress disorder, and depressive symptoms among recent immigrant schoolchildren. *Journal of the American Academy of Child and Adolescent Psychiatry, 41*, 1104–1110.

Jones, L. M., Finkelhor, D., & Halter, S. (2006). Child maltreatment trends in the 1990s: Why does neglect differ from sexual and physical abuse? *Child Maltreatment, 11*, 107–120.

Kataoka, S. H., Stein, B. D., Jaycox, L. H., Wong, M., Escudero, P., Tu, W., et al. (2003). A school-based mental health program for traumatized Latino immigrant children. *Journal of the American Academy of Child and Adolescent Psychiatry, 42*(3), 311–318.

Kazdin, A. E. (2000). Developing a research agenda for child and adolescent psychotherapy. *Archives of General Psychiatry, 57*(9), 829–835.

Kim, B. S. K. (2007). Adherences to Asian and European American cultural values and attitudes toward seeking professional help among Asian American college students. *Journal of Counseling Psychology, 54*(4), 474–480.

Kim, B. S. K., & Omizo, M. M. (2003). Asian cultural values, attitudes toward seeking professional psychological help, and willingness to see a counselor. *Counseling Psychologist, 31*, 343–361.

Koss, M. P. (1980). A multivariate analysis of long-term stay in private practice psychotherapy. *Journal of Clinical Psychology, 36*, 991–993.

Kroll, J., Yusuf, A., & Fujiwara, K. (2011). Psychoses, PTSD, and depression in Somali refugees in Minnesota. *Social Psychiatry and Psychiatric Epidemiology, 46*(6), 481–493.

La Roche, M. J. (2002). Psychotherapeutic considerations in treating Latinos. *Harvard Review of Psychiatry, 10*(2), 115–122.

Le Meyer, O., Zane, N., Cho, Y., & Takeuchi, D. T. (2009). Use of specialty mental health services by Asian Americans with psychiatric disorders. *Journal of Consulting and Clinical Psychology, 77*, 1000–1005.

Leong, F., & Lau, A. (2001). Barriers to providing effective mental health services to Asian Americans. *Mental Health Services Research, 3*, 201–214.

Leong, F. T. L., Wagner, N. S., & Kim, H. H. (1995). Group counseling expectations among Asian American students: The role of culture-specific factors. *Journal of Counseling Psychology, 42*(2), 217–222.

Levin, J. S., Markides, K. S., & Ray, L. A. (1996). Religious attendance and psychological well-being in Mexican Americans: A panel analysis of three-generations data. *Gerontologist, 36*(4), 454–463.

Libby, A. M., Orton, H. D., Novins, D. K., Spicer, P., Buchwald, D., Beals, J., & Manson, S. M. (2004). Childhood physical and sexual abuse and subsequent alcohol and drug use disorders in two American-Indian tribes. *Journal of Studies on Alcohol, 65*(1), 74–83.

Liu, W. M., & Iwamoto, D. K. (2006). Asian American men's gender role conflict: The toll of Asian values, self-esteem, and psychological distress. *Psychology of Men & Masculinity, 7*(3), 153–164.

Manson, S. M. (2000). Mental health services for American Indians and Alaska Natives: Need, use, and barriers to effective care. *Canadian Journal of Psychiatry, 45*, 617–626.

Manson, S. M., Beals, J., O'Nell, T., & Piasecki, J. (1996). Wounded spirits, ailing hearts: PTSD and related disorders among Native American Indians. In A. J. Marsella, M. J. Friedman, E. T. Gerrity, & R. M. Scurfield (Eds.), *Ethnocultural aspects of posttraumatic stress disorder: Issues, research, and clinical applications* (pp. 225–283). Washington, DC: American Psychological Association.

Marín, G., & Marín, B. (1991). *Research with Hispanic populations.* Thousand Oaks, CA: Sage Publications.

Marshall, G. N., Schell, T. L., & Miles, J. V. (2009). Ethnic differences in posttraumatic distress: Hispanics' symptoms differ in kind and degree. *Journal of Consulting and Clinical Psychology, 77*, 1169–1178.

Matsumoto, D., Yoo, S. H., Hirayama, S., & Petrova, G. (2005). Development and validation of a measure of display rule knowledge: The Display Rule Assessment Inventory. *Emotion, 5*(1), 23–40.

McCabe, K., & Yeh, M. (2009). Parent-child interaction therapy for Mexican-Americans: A randomized clinical trial. *Journal of Clinical Child and Adolescent Psychology, 38*, 753–759.

McCabe, K. M., Yeh, M., Garland, A. F., Lau, A. S., & Chavez, G. (2005). The GANA program: A tailoring approach to adapting parent child interaction therapy for Mexican Americans. *Education & Treatment of Children, 28*(2), 111–129.

Meinert, J. A. (2003). Bridging the gap: Recruitment of African-American women into mental health research studies. *Academic Psychiatry, 27*, 21–28.

Miranda, J., Azocar, F., Organista, K. C., Muñoz, R. F., & Lieberman, A. (1996). Recruiting and retaining low-income Latinos in psychotherapy research. *Journal of Consulting and Clinical Psychology, 64*, 868–874.

Mitchell, S. J., & Ronzio, C. R. (2011). Violence and other stressful life events as triggers of depression and anxiety: What psychosocial resources protect African American mothers? *Maternal and Child Health Journal, 15*(8), 1272–1281.

Moore, J., & Pachon, H. (1985). *Hispanics in the United States.* Englewood Cliffs, NJ: Prentice-Hall.

Neff, J. A., & Hoppe, S. K. (1993). Race/ethnicity, acculturation, and psychological distress: Fatalism and religiosity as cultural resources. *Journal of Community Psychology, 21*(1), 3–20.

Newcomb, M. D., Munoz, D. T., & Carmona, J. (2009). Child sexual abuse consequences in community samples of Hispanic and European American adolescents. *Child Abuse & Neglect, 33*(8), 533–544.

Niv, N., Wong, E. C., & Hser, Y. (2007). Asian Americans in community-based substance abuse treatment: Service needs, utilization, and outcomes. *Journal of Substance Abuse Treatment, 33*, 313–319.

Oetzel, J., Duran, B., Lucero, J., Jiang, Y., Novins, D. K., Manson, S., et al. (2006). Rural American Indians' perspectives of obstacles in the mental health treatment process in three treatment sections. *Psychological Services, 3*, 117–128.

Organista, K. C., Muñoz, R. F., & González, G. (1994). Cognitive-behavioral therapy for depression in low-income and minority medical outpatients: Description of a program and exploratory analyses. *Cognitive Therapy and Research, 18*(3), 241–259.

Oshri, A., Tubman, J. G., & Burnette, M. L. (2012). Child maltreatment histories, alcohol and other drug use symptoms, and sexual risk behavior in a treatment sample of adolescents. *American Journal of Public Health, 102*(Suppl. 2), S250–257.

Pavkov, T. W., Travis, L., Fox, K. A., King, C., & Cross, T. L. (2010). Tribal youth victimization and delinquency: Analysis of Youth Risk Behavior Surveillance Survey data. *Cultural Diversity and Ethnic Minority Psychology, 16*(2), 123–134.

Perilla, J. L., Norris, F. H., & Lavizzo, E. A. (2002). Ethnicity, culture, and disaster response: Identifying and explaining ethnic differences in PTSD six months after Hurricane Andrew. *Journal of Social and Clinical Psychology, 21*(1), 20–45.

Pole, N., Best, S. R., Metzler, T., & Marmar, C. R. (2005). Why are Hispanics at greater risk for PTSD? *Cultural Diversity and Ethnic Minority Psychology, 11*, 144–161.

Pole, N., Gone, J. P., & Kulkarni, M. (2008). Posttraumatic stress disorder among ethnoracial minorities in the United States. *Clinical Psychology: Science and Practice, 15*, 35–61.

Porche, M. V., Fortuna, L. R., Lin, J., & Alegria, M. (2011). Childhood trauma and psychiatric disorders as correlates of school dropout in a national sample of young adults. *Child Development, 82*(3), 982–998.

Price, M., Davidson, T., Andrews, J. O., & Ruggiero, K. J. (2013). Access, use, and completion of a brief disaster mental health intervention among Hispanics, African Americans and whites affected by Hurricane Ike. *Telemedicine and Telecare, 19*, 70–74.

Pumariega, A. J., Rothe, E., & Pumariega, J. B. (2005). Mental health of immigrants and refugees. *Community Mental Health Journal, 41*, 581–597.

Rivera, S., & de Arellano, M. A. (2008). *Culturally-Modified Trauma-Focused Cognitive Behavioral Therapy.* Paper presented at the annual meeting of the San Diego International Conference on Child and Family Maltreatment, San Diego, CA.

Roberts, A. L., Gilman, S. E., Breslau, J. J., Breslau, N. N., & Koenen, K. C. (2011). Race/ethnic differences in exposure to traumatic events, development of post-traumatic stress disorder, and treatment-seeking for post-traumatic stress disorder in the United States. *Psychological Medicine, 41*(1), 71–83.

Rosselló, J., Bernal, G., & Rivera-Medina, C. (2008). Individual and group CBT and IPT for Puerto Rican adolescents with depressive symptoms. *Cultural Diversity and Ethnic Minority Psychology, 14*, 234–245.

Sabogal, F., Marín, G., Otero-Sabogal, R., Marín, B., & Peréz-Stable, E. J. (1987). Hispanic familism and acculturation: What changes and what doesn't? *Hispanic Journal of Behavioral Sciences, 9,* 397–412.

Santiago-Rivera, A. L., Arredondo, P., & Gallardo-Cooper, M. (2002). *Counseling Latinos and la familia: A practical guide.* Thousand Oaks, CA: Sage Publications.

Schwarzbaum, S. (2004). Low-income Latinos and dropout: Strategies to prevent dropout. *Journal of Multicultural Counseling and Development, 32*(extra), 296–306.

Singh, S., Manjula, M. M., & Philip, M. (2012). Suicidal risk and childhood adversity: A study of Indian college students. *Asian Journal of Psychiatry, 5*(2), 154–159.

Siqveland, J., Hafstad, G., & Tedeschi, R. G. (2012). Posttraumatic growth in parents after a natural disaster. *Journal of Loss and Trauma, 17*(6), 536–544.

Smart, J. F., & Smart, D. W. (1995). Acculturative stress of Hispanics: Loss and challenge. *Journal of Counseling and Development, 73*, 390–396.

Smedley, B. D., Stith, A. Y., & Nelson, A. R. (2003). *Unequal treatment: Confronting racial and ethnic disparities in health care.* Washington DC: Institute of Medicine, Committee on Understanding and Eliminating Racial and Ethnic Disparities in Health Care.

Smith, T. B., Domenech Rodríguez, M., & Bernal, G. (2011). Culture. *Journal of Clinical Psychology: In Session, 67*, 166–175.

Sontag, J. C., & Schacht, R. (1993). Family diversity and patterns of service utilization in early intervention. *Journal of Early Intervention, 17*, 431–444.

Stein, B. D., Jaycox, L. H., Kataoka, S. H., Wong, M., Tu, W., Elliott, M. N., & Fink, A. (2003). A mental health intervention for schoolchildren exposed to violence: A randomized controlled trial. *JAMA, 290*(5), 603–611.

Stevens, T. N., Ruggiero, K. J., Kilpatrick, D. G., Resnick, H. S., & Saunders, B. E. (2005). Variables differentiating singly and multiply victimized youth: Results from the national survey of adolescents and implications for secondary prevention. *Child Maltreatment, 10*, 211–223.

Sue, D. W., & Sue, D. (1999). *Counseling the culturally different* (3rd ed.). New York, NY: John Wiley & Sons.

Sue, S. (1998). In search of cultural competence in psychotherapy. *American Psychologist, 42*, 37–45.

Sue, S., Cheng, J., Saad, C. S., & Chu, J. P. (2012). Asian American mental health: A call to action. *American Psychologist, 67*(7), 532–544.

Tata, S. P., & Leong, F. T. L. (1994). Individualism-collectivism, social-network orientation, and acculturation as predictors of attitudes toward seeking professional psychological help among Chinese-Americans. *Journal of Counseling Psychology, 41*(3), 280–287.

Ting, J. Y., & Hwang, W. C. (2009). Cultural influences on help-seeking attitudes in Asian American students. *American Journal of Orthopsychiatry, 79*, 125–132.

Triandis, H. C. (1988). Collectivism and development. In D. Sinha & H. S. R. Kao (Eds.), *Social values and development: Asian perspectives* (pp. 285–303). New Delhi, India: Sage Publications.

U.S. Census Bureau. (2010). *Quick facts.* http://quickfacts.census.gov /qfd/states/00000.html

U.S. Department of Health and Human Services. (2001). *Mental health: Culture, race, and ethnicity* (Supplement to *Mental health: A report of the surgeon general*). Rockville MD: Office of the Surgeon General (US), Center for Mental Health Services, National Institute of Mental Health.

U.S. Department of Health and Human Services, Administration for Children and Families, Administration on Children, Youth and Families, Children's Bureau. (2012). *Child maltreatment, 2011.* www.acf.hhs.gov/sites/default/files/cb/cm11.pdf #page=18

Voisin, D. R., Bird, J. P., Hardestry, M., & Cheng Shi, S. (2011). African American adolescents living and coping with community violence on Chicago's Southside. *Journal of Interpersonal Violence, 26*(12), 2483–2498.

Whitesell, N., Beals, J., Mitchell, C. M., Manson, S. M., & Turner, R. (2009). Childhood exposure to adversity and risk of substance-use disorder in two American Indian populations: The meditational role of early substance-use initiation. *Journal of Studies on Alcohol and Drugs, 70*, 971–981.

Woodall, A., Morgan, C., Sloan, C., & Howard, L. (2010). Barriers to participation in mental health research: Are there specific gender, ethnicity and age related barriers? *BMC Psychiatry, 10*, 103.

Zheng, Y., Lin, K. M., Takeuchi, D., Kurasaki, K. S., Wang, Y. X., & Cheung, F. (1997). An epidemiological study of neurasthenia in Chinese-Americans in Los Angeles. *Comprehensive Psychiatry, 38*, 249–259.

ADAM BROWN, PSY.D.
CARRYL P. NAVALTA, PH.D.
ERIKA TULLBERG, M.P.A., M.P.H.
GLENN SAXE, M.D.

13

Trauma Systems Therapy

An Approach to Creating Trauma-Informed Child Welfare Systems

GENERAL CONSIDERATIONS

This chapter focuses on the most common context in which youths exposed to abuse and neglect come into contact with child-serving professionals: the child welfare system. Children and families involved with the child welfare system have, by definition, experienced trauma, both because of the maltreatment that brings them into contact with the system and because of the invasive nature of system involvement itself. There are important issues to consider in meeting the complex needs of youths and families within this system, and in this chapter we focus on the model of Trauma Systems Therapy.

TRAUMA SYSTEMS THERAPY

In the "real world" of service delivery—particularly within a system as complex as child welfare—many barriers are present to the implementation and sustainability of effective practices, and consequently, only a small number of child welfare–involved children and families receive needed services. We describe here an approach to assessment and intervention that has been used in a variety of settings, including child welfare settings, since 2006.

Developed by Saxe and colleagues (Ellis et al., 2012; Saxe, Ellis, & Kaplow, 2007), Trauma Systems Therapy (TST) is a comprehensive method for assessing and treating children with traumatic stress. TST adds to individually based approaches by specifically addressing social and environmental factors that are believed to be driving a child's emotional and behavior problems and has been used with children as young as 3 years old. TST conceptualizes child and adolescent traumatic stress as the interface of two conceptual axes: (1) the degree of emotional and behavioral dysregulation

Note: Drs. Brown and Navalta contributed equally to this chapter.

when a child is triggered by overt and subtle reminders or stressors; and (2) the capacity of the child's social environment to protect the child from these reminders/stressors or help the child to regulate emotions and related behavior in the face of such triggers. TST is a central organizing structure that brings together the different service systems involved in a child's care. To provide TST, a service system must be able to provide four types of services/skills: (1) individual skills-based, trauma-informed psychotherapy (emotional regulation, then cognitive/trauma processing skills); (2) home- or community-based care; (3) legal advocacy; and (4) psychopharmacology. The configuration of a team providing these services differs by community and is typically *built out of existing resources* through a survey of services already provided by a given agency that can be integrated or services that are already provided by other agencies in a region and can be integrated through interagency agreement. TST also places a strong emphasis on engaging families in treatment, using specific strategies to develop the treatment alliance and troubleshooting practical barriers to engagement in treatment. A critical element of treatment engagement is the *family's culture-based understanding* of emotion, mental health, and mental health intervention. We have a great deal of experience using TST in child welfare settings—the model is uniquely suited to address the complicated needs of youths, families, and service systems involved with child welfare because the approach explicitly addresses common implementation challenges.

KEY CLINICAL FEATURES

Identifying a Trauma System

The focus on a "trauma system" is what sets TST apart from other trauma therapy models. Most approaches for

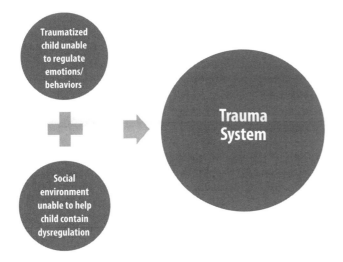

Figure 13.1. Components of a trauma system

addressing the impact of traumatic exposure on child development examine the ways in which such exposure affects adaptive functioning. TST does this by concentrating on emotional and behavioral regulation and on the role the social environment plays in triggering and maintaining this dysregulation. This dual emphasis is what is meant by a "trauma system." The TST definition of a trauma system is a traumatized youth who has difficulty regulating his or her emotions and behavior, and a social environment or system of care that is unable to help that youth to regulate or to protect him or her from threat or reminders of threat (figure 13.1).

Assessment

A child is evaluated and assessed as being in one of three categories of regulation: regulated, emotionally dysregulated, or behaviorally dysregulated. Similarly, the social environment is evaluated across a three-category designation: stable, distressed, or threatening. By determining the relationship between these two ratings (i.e., the trauma system), the clinician assesses the youth as being in one of five phases of treatment: surviving, stabilizing, enduring, understanding, or transcending. The TST Assessment Grid (table 13.1) is used to determine the phase of treatment, and each phase is

Table 13.1. Trauma Systems Therapy Assessment Grid

		Social Environmental Stability		
		Stable	Distressed	Threatening
Emotional Regulation	Regulated	Transcending	Understanding	Enduring
	Emotionally dysregulated	Understanding	Enduring	Stabilizing
	Behaviorally dysregulated	Enduring	Stabilizing	Surviving

associated with a defined set of recommended treatment interventions.

Four key factors are considered when assessing whether a child is experiencing emotional dysregulation, behavioral dysregulation, or neither. First, an episode of dysregulation is defined as changes in awareness (or consciousness), affect (or emotion), and action (or behavior)—the "3 A's"—when the child is exposed to a stressor or triggering stimulus. If these three changes do not occur, the child is not considered to be dysregulated. Second, the rate or frequency of dysregulation episodes is taken into consideration, typically by documenting the number of weekly or monthly episodes. Third, some evidence must exist that the dysregulation episode causes a problem with the child's school, family, peer relationships, or self. This problem can be related either to the dysregulation episode itself or to feelings or behaviors related to the anticipation of a dysregulation episode (i.e., an impairment or distress criterion). Fourth, when a child engages in risky or potentially dangerous behaviors during an episode (e.g., aggressive, suicidal, self-mutilatory, or otherwise impulsive behaviors), he or she is considered to be *behaviorally dysregulated*. This distinction is the most severe emotional regulation tier in the TST Assessment Grid (table 13.1). In contrast, a child is categorized as *emotionally dysregulated* when changes in the 3 A's occur but with no risky or potentially dangerous behaviors (the middle tier).

Within the framework of TST, a traumatized child who experiences a dysregulation episode transitions across four emotional states over time: regulating, revving, reexperiencing, and reconstituting—the "4 R's." Development of the TST treatment plan is dependent on designation of the child as regulated, emotionally dysregulated, or behaviorally dysregulated.

As stated above, TST conceptualizes the social environment or system of care along a three-tier continuum of stability (stable, distressed, and threatening). The constructs of *help* and *protect* are critical in distinguishing among these three levels of stability. *Help* refers to the capacity of the social environment or system of care to help the child manage emotion and emotionally motivated behavior. In contrast, *protect* pertains to the capacity of the social environment or system of care to protect the child from stressors that may lead to dysregulated emotional states, as described above. Collectively, the degree to which these capacities are present helps to precisely ascertain the stability of the social environment or system of care.

A child's social environment or system of care is considered *stable* when the following three conditions are met: (1) the child's immediate caregivers are able to help the child regulate emotion and protect him or her from stressors; (2) the child's extended family, peer group, or neighbors are able to support the child such that any limitations in the ability of the immediate caregivers to help or protect are mitigated; and (3) the child's system of care has been accessed successfully to provide needed functions that the immediate caregivers and extended family are not able to provide. In contrast, a child's social environment or system of care is considered *distressed* when neither the child's primary caregivers, extended family, nor system of care are able to help the child regulate emotional states and/or protect him from environmental stressors.

Lastly, a child's social environment or system of care is considered *threatening* when one or both of the following scenarios exist: (1) the child's caregivers pose a true threat of harm to the child; the child's extended family, peer group, or neighbors cannot adequately protect the child from this threat; and the child's system of care either has not been accessed or has not adequately protected the child from this threat, and/or (2) there is a threat of harm to the child from outside the immediate caregivers, and the child is not adequately protected from this outside threat. In sum, the use of these three constructs (stable, distressed, and threatening) will determine the extent of stability/instability of a child's social environment or system of care and will help in completion of the TST Assessment Grid (table 13.1)

Treatment Planning

Rather than including nine disparate treatment phases that correspond to each of the nine areas in the Assessment Grid, TST has only five phases of treatment that align with unique foci and themes. These phases are *Surviving, Stabilizing, Enduring, Understanding,* and *Transcending* and are rank-ordered from most intensive to least intensive in terms of the acuity of service needs. Depending on the treatment phase, one or more of the TST service modules is clinically indicated (i.e., home- and community-based care, skills-based outpatient treatment, psychopharmacology, and/or services advocacy).

1. *Surviving*—protecting the child from threatening environments and dangerous impulses and setting the stage for interventions in other phases of TST. A child in this phase is behaviorally dysregulated, and the social environment or system of care is threatening. Therefore, home- and community-based interventions are intensively used to acquire a comprehensive picture of the child's home environment and to assess the degree of threat and danger. This phase often requires working closely with social service agencies, inpatient psychiatric units, and medication-prescribing clinicians. Emotional regulation skills training and services advocacy can also be implemented, when appropriate.

2. *Stabilizing*—creating a safe social environment. Families who start in this phase usually have significant problems that will not be helped without home-based interventions. Typically, problems relate to family disorganization and/or to the child's school, peer group, and neighborhood, where stressors occur that routinely trigger the child. Interventions are delivered on-site, usually in the home or school, and are designed to help stabilize the factors in the environment that are contributing to the youth's dysregulation. Interventions in this phase often

include advocating for needed services. Many children require pharmacotherapy and advocacy for additional help and support.

3. *Enduring*—developing the skills necessary to manage emotion and respond to the establishment of a safe social environment. The child and family must be taught skills that help them endure the impact of trauma so that extreme behavior can be minimized. For skills-based psychotherapy to be effective, the youth's environment must be safe and not triggering him or her to dysregulate. The primary mode of psychotherapy in this phase of treatment is emotional regulation skills training. If treatment has started prior to this phase, home- and community-based interventions should be mostly complete. For children who start treatment in this phase, home- and community-based interventions may be required at some point.

4. *Understanding*—establishing therapeutic communication about the traumatic experience(s) so that the child and family are no longer consumed by the events. Techniques of cognitive behavioral therapy are primarily used during this phase. Emotional regulation skills training should be completed before this treatment phase so that the child has sufficient skills to manage the processing of trauma cognitions. Occasionally, medications are necessary.

5. *Transcending*—creating lasting meaning and perspective out of traumatic experiences once the trauma is over. The focus is to learn how to live in a way that is defined less by the past and more by the future. This learning includes helping the child and family say goodbye to the therapist and move beyond treatment. The child, family, and clinician work toward identifying and constructing culturally sanctioned activities that may create lasting meaning out of the child's traumatic experiences.

Intervention Modules

Interventions within TST are delivered according to a series of seven modules, used in various combinations depending on the phase of treatment in which a child and family are assessed (table 13.2). The seven treatment modules are briefly summarized here. For more detailed information on each module, please refer to our treatment manual (Saxe, Ellis, & Kaplow, 2007).

1. *Ready-Set-Go* is used with all families at the beginning of TST as a way of introducing the treatment approach, assessing the family's capacity to engage, building a treatment alliance, and working to surmount barriers to engagement.

2. *Stabilization-On-Site (SOS)* involves intensive home- and school-based services that focus on directly diminishing the sources of acute stress and traumatic reminders within the child's day-to-day environment.

3. *Services Advocacy* involves explicit work with service systems that can offer needed resources to help with emotional regulation and, particularly, with social environmental stability; such services may include housing, financial assistance, domestic violence advocacy, and so on.

Table 13.2. Trauma Systems Therapy Treatment Intervention Grid

Module	Phase				
	Surviving	Stabilizing	Enduring	Understanding	Transcending
Stabilization-On-Site (SOS)	Crisis management Connection to services Diminish triggers	Parenting skills Connections to services Diminish triggers	—	—	—
Services Advocacy	Services advocacy	Services advocacy	Services advocacy	—	—
Emotional Regulation; Cognitive Processing; Meaning Making	Emotional regulation*	Emotional regulation	Emotional regulation	Cognitive processing	Meaning making
Psychopharmacology	Psychopharmacology*	Psychopharmacology*	Psychopharmacology*	Psychopharmacology*	Psychopharmacology*

*Services that are often helpful but not essential. All other services are essential.
—=Modules not used or contraindicated.

4. *Psychopharmacology* describes the principles and practice of psychopharmacology as related to TST and the psychiatric consultant's role on a TST treatment team.

5. *Emotional Regulation* is a semi-structured, office-based therapeutic approach that helps both parents and child gain greater awareness of emotions and specific skills and strategies for regulation.

6. *Cognitive Processing* is about learning cognitive behavioral techniques of trauma processing so that the child will not become dysregulated when faced with stressors or reminders.

7. *Meaning Making* is about finding activities for the child, family, and therapist that will create lasting meaning about the traumatic event(s). These activities might include art projects, a ritual to "mark" that the child is beyond the trauma, or activities that involve helping others and are often syntonic with the cultural and religious background of the family.

Tools

THE MOMENT BY MOMENT ASSESSMENT. Within TST, gathering a clear, specific understanding of the environmental factors that trigger dysregulation is vitally important. The Moment by Moment Assessment (MMA) is the tool used to identify these triggers in the environment that lead to changes in the 3 A's and the 4 R's. To identify and accurately define areas for intervention, the TST clinical team uses the MMA to document episodes of emotional or behavioral dysregulation and the stimuli that provoke them. The following steps are used to conduct this assessment:

1. Inquire about episodes of dysregulation.
2. Understand how the 3 A's shift during these episodes.
3. Ascertain the precipitants of these episodes.
4. Understand how family members (or other members of the social environment) helped or made things worse.
5. Determine the cost of these episodes to the child and the family.

Through this process, the team gathers exquisitely detailed information about what the youth was thinking, feeling, and doing immediately before, during, and after a specified instance of dysregulation. In addition, the team gathers specific information about precise environmental conditions immediately prior to the episode. This information is obtained by interviewing the youth (once she or he is back to a regulated state), interviewing other youths who may have witnessed the event, and interviewing adults who were present as well.

PRIORITY PROBLEMS. In usual care/treatment, the clinical targets for intervention parallel the diagnostic formulation. For a child diagnosed with major depressive disorder, for example, depressive symptoms such as sad/unhappy mood, social withdrawal/isolation, and neurovegetative symptoms are the foci, and significant symptom reduction is the primary goal of treatment. In TST, however, the trauma system is the focal point of all interventions—in particular, the TST Priority Problems that precisely define the trauma system for a given child. The Priority Problems are based on the interface between the child's emotional regulation problems and stressful stimuli in the environment.

Once the information from the MMA is gathered, the TST team establishes (1) links or patterns of links between emotional/behavioral dysregulation and the stimuli that elicit it; (2) the role of members of the child's social environment in helping or hindering regulation during these patterns of links; and (3) the functional implications of these patterns of links. Then, these patterns are assigned priorities based on clinical judgment of the amount of dysfunction they cause. Such dysfunction includes, but is not limited to, problems that jeopardize physical safety, engagement in treatment, home placement, school placement, or healthy development; problems that cause significant distress to the child or family members; and problems that can be solved relatively easily and are highly meaningful to the child or family members. The TST Priority Problems are thus those patterns that are assigned the highest priorities (typically, one to four problems in all). Finally, the team formulates the TST Priority Solutions to address the corresponding Priority Problems through use of the clinically indicated treatment modules and identifies the individuals who are responsible for carrying out these solutions (e.g., child, parent, outpatient clinician, home-based therapist, advocate).

Each TST Priority Problem is constructed using the following sentence: "Signals of _____, such as _____, lead to feelings of _____, which lead to emotional and/or behavioral dysregulation, as evidenced by _____." In this sentence, designed to assist the team in creating the Priority Problem, the first blank refers to the traumatic event(s), the second refers to the specific reminders of the traumatic event(s) within the social environment, and the remaining blanks refer to the impact of these traumatic reminders on the youth's emotional and behavioral functioning.

DISSEMINATION: REAL-WORLD SETTINGS

As of early 2013, TST has been disseminated and implemented in 26 programs within 17 agencies across 10 states. Such programs include community-based outpatient programs, child welfare–mental health collaborations, foster care–mental health collaborations, shelters for unaccompanied alien minors, school-based mental health programs, residential programs, pediatric hospital-based programs, and substance abuse–mental health collaborations. Adaptations of TST have been developed for use in specialized settings, such as substance abuse programs, residential treatment, and foster care. Each adaptation adheres to key features of TST while making crucial changes necessary to meet the individualized needs of the setting—demonstrating the concept of "flexibility within fidelity" (Kendall & Beidas, 2007). The two largest-scale adaptations of TST are for child welfare and refugee trauma.

FIT FOR THE CHILD WELFARE SYSTEM

Trauma Systems Therapy addresses the *clinical and practical needs of children and families* in that treatment targets not just an individual child but a trauma system, which, again, is defined as a traumatized child who is unable to regulate his or her emotions and behavior *and* a social environment and system of care that is unable to protect that child and/ or help him or her to manage this dysregulation. TST effectively engages traumatized youth and families by using specific strategies and tools to uncover the youth's and family's "major source of pain"; identifying specific goals and solutions designed to achieve these goals; and specifying the role of all involved, including the youth, family, clinician, caseworkers, and all relevant members of the team.

TST also addresses the *organizational needs of agencies that serve traumatized youths and families* by addressing barriers that have repeatedly interfered with the dissemination of trauma-focused, evidence-based practice in frontline service settings. The development of TST has included the principle of *disseminate-ability*, or the ability of an intervention to be successfully diffused to different service sites. TST is *both* a clinical model *and* an organizational framework. The dissemination of TST requires a defined Organizational Plan, crafted in collaboration between agency leaders/stakeholders and TST trainers/developers. This Organizational Plan describes how an organization's resources will support and sustain the TST program and includes a financial plan.

TST acknowledges the *human needs of those serving youths and families* by engaging staff members at all levels as equally important members of the TST treatment team. Frontline workers often feel they have an elevated role, given that the TST assessment and treatment planning process requires their participation and, in fact, cannot be effective without the involvement of all team members at every level. TST also takes into account the impact of vicarious trauma on those providing service and incorporates an emphasis on self-care and mutual support. These concepts are embedded within the 10 TST Treatment Principles (table 13.3).

Trauma Systems Therapy has been fully developed, manualized, and successfully implemented with fidelity to the model—which is seen as critical—while allowing for flexibility so that the therapy can be adapted for use in various settings. Fidelity is based on adherence to the 10 TST Treatment Principles as a heuristic guide. These principles are based on the foundations succinctly highlighted above and fully described in the TST manual (Saxe, Ellis, & Kaplow, 2007). Sufficient fidelity to TST is anchored by these principles, and agencies that implement TST do so with training and technical support from the TST Development Team.

Since 2002, TST has had several successful large-scale implementations in child welfare agencies, with evidence to demonstrate its efficacy in these settings. Saxe et al. (2005) published the results of an open trial with 110 families comprising a cohort of children from inner city Boston and another from rural New York State. While almost 60% of families needed more intensive home- and community-based care at the beginning of treatment, only 39% of families needed this level of treatment after three months. A

Table 13.3. The 10 Trauma Systems Therapy Treatment Principles

1. Fix a broken system.
2. Put safety first.
3. Create clear, focused plans that are based on facts.
4. Don't "go" before you are "ready."
5. Put scarce resources where they'll work.
6. Insist on accountability, particularly your own.
7. Align with reality.
8. Take care of yourself and your team.
9. Build from strength.
10. Leave a better system.

more recent study showed that at 15 months post-treatment, these gains persisted and even improved (Ellis et al., 2012). Another recent article outlines a randomized controlled study of TST versus treatment as usual with an inner city sample of traumatized children (Saxe et al., 2012). The most dramatic finding after three months was that 90% of families receiving TST were still in treatment, whereas only 10% of the treatment-as-usual families were still in treatment. This suggests that TST is very effective at engagement and it highlights the importance of family engagement and integration of care within the existing services system.

TST is currently being implemented in a large child welfare agency in Kansas, which includes foster care, residential treatment, and community-based prevention services. This large-scale implementation is being evaluated by Child Trends, with support from the Annie E. Casey Foundation (results pending).

CONCLUSIONS

Trauma Systems Therapy was created as a comprehensive treatment model for traumatized children and adolescents and their families. TST also exemplifies what Kazdin designated "broad-based treatments" that "can be conceived in a modular fashion where there are separate components (modules) woven into an overall treatment plan" (Kazdin, 1997, p. 123). Although the primary treatment modules within TST are not new, a key innovation of this therapy is that the clinical model is embedded in an organizational model. That is, TST describes not only what is done clinically but also how to integrate and orchestrate different clinical interventions so that children receive the right level of care, at the right moment in time, in a tightly coordinated manner. In other words, TST provides both an organizing framework for identifying and coordinating the different service elements and a clinical model that describes exactly what providers do once they are brought together. These key features are necessary for creating effective change within the child welfare system.

The major clinical innovations of TST are a focus on engagement, a phase-based treatment strategy, and an uncompromising focus on the intersection of emotional regulation and the social environment (i.e., the trauma system). Without children and their families participating in treatment and working toward their identified treatment goals, improvement becomes unreachable. Thus, successful engagement is critical. Because TST is a phase-based model, identified services in the treatment plan for any given child are more intensive for children with higher levels of need, but they diminish in intensity as a child progresses through the course of treatment. In contrast to other intervention models that specify a set number of sessions, a child moves from one TST treatment phase to the next based on her or his progress. Such an approach allows treatment to be tailored to the unique needs of an individual child and helps agencies strategically place their resources so that the children who need the most services actually receive them. Lastly, TST is all about the trauma system—addressing both the social environment and a child's emotional regulation capacity in a genuinely collaborative manner.

References

Ellis, B. H., Fogler, J., Hansen, S., Beckman, M., Forbes, P., Navalta, C. P., et al. (2012). Trauma Systems Therapy: 15-month outcomes and the importance of effecting environmental change. *Psychological Trauma: Theory, Research, Practice, and Policy, 4*(6), 624–630. doi:10.1037/a0025192

Kazdin, A. E. (1997). A model for developing effective treatments: Progression and interplay of theory, research, and practice. *Journal of Clinical Child Psychology, 26*(2), 114–129.

Kendall, P. C., & Beidas, R. S. (2007). Smoothing the trail for dissemination of evidence-based practices for youth: Flexibility within fidelity. *Professional Psychology: Research and Practice, 38*(1), 13–20.

Saxe, G. N., Ellis, B. H., Fogler, J., Hansen, S., & Sorkin, B. (2005). Comprehensive care for traumatized children. *Psychiatric Annals, 35*(5), 443–448.

Saxe, G. N., Ellis, B. H., Fogler, J., & Navalta, C. P. (2012). Preliminary evidence for effective family engagement in treatment for child traumatic stress: Trauma Systems Therapy approach to preventing dropout. *Child and Adolescent Mental Health, 17*(1), 58–61. doi:10.1111/j.1475-3588.2011.00626.x

Saxe, G. N., Ellis, B. H., & Kaplow, J. B. (2007). *Collaborative treatment of traumatized children and teens: The Trauma Systems Therapy approach.* New York, NY: Guilford Press.

Additional Reading

Bai, Y., Wells, R., & Hillemeier, M. M. (2009). Coordination between child welfare agencies and mental health service providers, children's service use, and outcomes. *Child Abuse & Neglect, 33*(6), 372–381.

Berrick, J. D., Barth, R. P., & Needell, B. (1994). A comparison of kinship foster homes and foster family homes: Implications for kinship foster care as family preservation. *Children and Youth Services Review, 16*(1–2), 35–63.

Brown, A. D., McCauley, K., Navalta, C. P., & Saxe, G. N. (in press). Trauma Systems Therapy in residential settings: A focus on emotion regulation and the social environment of traumatized children and youth in acute care. *Journal of Family Violence.*

Burns, B. J., Phillips, S. D., Wagner, H. R., Barth, R. P., Kolko, D. J., Campbell, Y., & Landsverk, J. (2004). Mental health need and access to mental health services by youths involved with child welfare: A national survey. *Journal of the American Academy of Child and Adolescent Psychiatry, 43*(8), 960–970.

Child Welfare Information Gateway. (2012). *Child maltreatment 2010: Summary of key findings.* Washington, DC: U.S. Department of Health and Human Services, Administration for Children and Families, Administration on Children, Youth and Families, Children's Bureau.

Child Welfare Information Gateway. (2012). *Foster care statistics 2010.* Washington, DC: U.S. Department of Health and Human Services, Administration for Children and Families, Administration on Children, Youth and Families, Children's Bureau.

De Bellis, M. D., Keshavan, M. S., Clark, D. B., Casey, B. J., Giedd, J. N., Boring, A. M., et al. (1999). Developmental traumatology: Part II. Brain development. *Biological Psychology, 45,* 1271–1284.

Education Coordinating Council. (2006). *Data match results: Los Angeles Unified School District, Los Angeles Department of Children and Family Services, and Los Angeles County Probation Department.* Los Angeles, CA: Author.

Grant, B. F. (2000). Estimates of U.S. children exposed to alcohol abuse and dependence in the family. *American Journal of Public Health, 90*(1): 112–115.

Horwitz, S. M., Hurlburt, M. S., Heneghan, A., Zhang, J., Rolls-Reutz, J., Fisher, E., et al. (2012). Mental health problems in young children investigated by U.S. child welfare agencies. *Journal of the American Academy of Child and Adolescent Psychiatry, 51*(6), 572–581.

National Institute of Drug Abuse. (1994). *Substance abuse among women and parents.* http://aspe.hhs.gov/hsp/cyp/xsfamdrg.htm

Navalta, C. P. (2011). Neuropsychological aspects of child abuse and neglect. In A. S. Davis (Ed.), *Handbook of pediatric neuropsychology* (pp. 1039–1050). New York, NY: Springer Publishing.

Parrish, T., Dubois, J., Delano, C., Dixon, D., Webster, D., Berrick, J. D., & Bolus, S. (2001). *Education in foster group home children: Whose responsibility is it? Study of the educational placement of children residing in group homes.* Palo Alto, CA: American Institutes for Research.

Sedlak, A. J., Mettenburg, J., Basena, M., Petta, I., McPherson, K., Greene, A., & Li, S. (2010). *Fourth National Incidence Study of Child Abuse and Neglect (NIS-4): Report to Congress.* Executive summary. Washington, DC: U.S. Department of Health and Human Services, Administration for Children and Families.

Wulczyn, F., & Lery, B. (2007). *Racial disparity in foster care admissions* [Adobe Digital Editions version]. www.chapinhall.org/sites/default/files/old_reports/399.pdf

MONA PATEL POTTER, M.D.
SOONJO HWANG, M.D.
JEFF Q. BOSTIC, M.D., ED.D.

14

The Abused Student Cornered

School Bullying amidst Trauma

GENERAL CONSIDERATIONS

Childhood victimization, including school bullying, has been shown to alter development in the psychological, emotional, cognitive, social, and behavioral realms (Ando, Asakura, & Simons-Morton, 2005; Herman, 1997). Just as there are many ways in which children may be traumatized, there are diverse ways in which children are affected by and respond to trauma. Also important to consider is the potential risk for and impact of multiple childhood victimizations. In this chapter we review the school bullying of abused and mal-treated children to clarify shared vulnerability factors and develop an understanding of how to identify the bullying of victims of abuse in school and how to employ interventions to help this vulnerable population.

BULLYING

At any point in time, about 15%–20% of the students in elementary and secondary / junior high schools in the United States are involved in bullying as victims or bullies (Analitis et al., 2009; Olweus, 1994b). In a nationally representative study of U.S. students, ages 12–18, 32% reported bullying victimization at school. Of these victims, 21% reported being consistently made fun of, 18% said they were the subject of rumors, 11% had been pushed, shoved, tripped, or spat upon, 6% were threatened with harm, 5% were excluded from activities on purpose, and 4% were made to do things they did not want to do or had their property purposefully destroyed (U.S. Department of Education, 2010).

In many cases, children at risk for school bullying also experience other forms of trauma. Students involved in bullying, whether as bullies or victims, report more victimization in other domains, such as physical and sexual abuse, compared with students without a history of victimization

(Sharp, 1995; www.bullypolice.org). Similarly, students who report witnessing family violence are three to seven times more likely to be involved in school bullying as victims, bullies, or bully-victims (McKenna et al., 2011; Shields & Cicchetti, 2001).

Bullying is defined as aggressive behavior perpetrated by students who hold and/or try to maintain a dominant position over others, with the premeditated intention of causing mental and/or physical harm or suffering to another (Morita, 1985). Bullying is distinguished from *conflicts*, in which students of similar status (similar physical size, social status, etc.) may have disputes and arguments, but one party does not have a decided unfair advantage over the other. Moreover, unlike typical "conflicts," bullying tends to focus on repeated actions by a student or students against the victim(s) (Karna et al., 2011).

Bullying can resemble more classic *abuse* of children in which an adult has a decidedly unfair advantage over the child. While the behavior of the adult may not be intended to inflict harm on the child, sometimes the adult's behaviors toward the child reveal harm in a more insidious fashion (e.g., by exploitation of the child). Certainly, the line between disciplining a child and bullying a child can be difficult to discern; a fundamental difference is that "disciplining" typically is done with the intention of "teaching" the child better behaviors to replace more primitive ones, rather than to amplify the power the adult has over the child. The child's interpretation of the experience can also help distinguish where on the spectrum discipline falls.

Since bullying has been a familiar phenomenon throughout history, it is often considered to be "just a part of growing up." However, bullying is not normal, does not enhance skill development in those bullied (or in bullies or bystanders), and is clearly detrimental. Not only is bullying strongly associated with immediate psychological damage to students,

Table 14.1. Characteristics of Bullies and Victims

Domain	Bully	Victim
Cognitions	Negative beliefs about self and others	Negative self-related cognitions
Academic performance	May be uneven or compromised	Unusual or conspicuous strengths
Social interaction	Seeks to dominate; has trouble resolving problems with others; negatively influenced by peers	Lacks adequate social skills; may be isolated or rejected or have a small circle of friends; has difficulties solving social problems
Associated environmental variables	Family environment often characterized by conflict and poor parental monitoring; likely to perceive school as having a negative atmosphere	Often experiences a negative community, family, and/or school environment

but it also leads to long-term sequelae lasting into adulthood (Kim et al., 2006; Spivak, 2003). Individuals chronically bullied in their youth experience lower self-esteem and greater depression, which persists into adulthood (Holt, Finkelhor, & Kantor et al., 2007; Olweus, 1992). Typical characteristics of bullies and victims are listed in table 14.1 (Cook et al., 2010).

It is not uncommon for a student involved in bullying to play different roles in different circumstances. Bully-victims are students who are involved in bullying both as bullies and as victims of bullying (Schwartz, 2000); these students appear to have the most serious psychological problems (Kim, Koh, & Leventhal, 2005; Menesini, Modena, & Tani, 2009), have fewer friends, and tend to be more stigmatized by peers (Holt, 2007). Compared with students who were neither bullies nor bullying victims, both middle and high school bully-victims were found to be three to four times more likely to report seriously considering suicide, intentionally injuring themselves, being physically hurt by a family member, and witnessing violence in their family (McKenna et al., 2011).

Bystanders, or those who are not the actual bullies or targets of the aggression, also can be adversely affected by witnessing bullying experiences in school and other settings. These students may develop a sense of hopelessness in the face of inaction by school officials, perhaps leading to a deficit in empathy for those who are defenseless against bullying (Kowlaski, Limber, & Agatson, 2008). Bystanders can affect the dynamics of bullying by ignoring incidents (a passive form of accepting a bully's behavior), encouraging perpetrators (e.g., laughing at the victim, joining in), or intervening for victims (Twemlow, 2010).

While almost all states in the United States have passed anti-bullying legislation (www.bullypolice.org), wide variations exist across states in the definition of bullying, recog-

nition of bullying as a major safety/health issue, and actions required by the legislation (ranging from action encouraged, to funded, to mandated) (Srabstein, Berkman, & Pyntikova, 2008). When effective and comprehensive programs have been implemented, reports indicate significant decreases in bullying experiences among students (Olweus & Limber, 2010).

UNDERSTANDING FULL VICTIMIZATION STATUS

Experiencing multiple victimizations can contribute to differences in symptom expression and overall functioning among students; clinical focus on a single form of victimization might underestimate the impact of other victimizations (Holt, 2007; Turner, Finkelor, & Ormrod, 2010). The usually public nature of bullying may make it more apparent than other forms of victimization. Accordingly, trauma-related symptoms might be attributed to bullying if other forms of victimization are not disclosed by the victim. Table 14.2 lists factors to consider when distinguishing bullying from other forms of victimization. Assessing a student's comprehensive victimization history (see table 14.3 for sample screening questions) allows a more thorough understanding of what the student is going through and, as a result, increases the likelihood of effective interventions.

Table 14.2. Distinguishing between Bullying and Other Trauma

How Bullying Differs from Trauma	Bullying	Trauma
Other reporters	Peers or staff may have witnessed event(s)	Rarely as visible (usually occurs behind closed doors)
Assailant(s)	Other peers, often with a history of bullying others	Adults or others; "family secrets" often more common
Response to harm	Minimizing	Denial, evasion, and/or protection of adults/assailants
Description of harm	Embarrassment; redefining of bullying as "joking around"	Justification ("for my own good"; "I deserved it"; special relationship); mixed emotions ("brought it on myself, but not OK"; "will people believe me?")
How hypervigilance manifests	Avoidance of school (or parts of it, such as recess, lunchroom, bus); symptoms (e.g., somatic complaints) emerge during exposure to these places	Avoidance of being alone, even in safe places/conditions; triggered when around seemingly safe others; difficulty trusting people

Table 14.3. Sample Screening for Thorough Victimization History

Prompt: "I'm going to ask you about a number of bad things that can happen to kids. Please tell me if any of these has happened to you either recently or in the distant past."

Event	Present/ Absent	Age
Victim or witness of serious accident (car/motor-cycle, injury, fall, fire; involving serious or grotesque injury, death, or dying; known or unknown victim)		
Victim or witness of severe chronic medical illness (frequent hospitalizations or procedures, significant pain experienced by self or close other, parental substance abuse and/or mental illness)		
Witness of disaster or terrorism (flood, tornado, earthquake, hurricane, hijacking, biological weaponry)		
Victim or witness of violence (shooting, robbery, assault, discrimination, death, kidnapping, community violence)		
Victim or witness of domestic violence (physical or emotional abuse toward self, parent, or other family member; injury caused, weapon used; child protective services involved; known or unknown perpetrator)		
Victim or witness of school violence (shooting, suicide, assault, verbal and/or physical bullying, maltreatment by others, discrimination)		
Victim or witness of sexual violence (rape, attempted rape, molestation; known or unknown perpetrator; prostitution, sexual slavery, engagement in risky behavior while intoxicated)		
Displacement (homelessness, foster care, incarceration, refugee status, incarcerated or hospitalized parent)		
Victim of neglect (inadequate or grossly inappropriate care or supervision by parent or guardian, child protective services involved)		
Poverty (lack of essential resources, community violence)		
Traumatic experience while intoxicated on alcohol or drugs (sexual assault, physical and/or emotional attack)		
Other		

Source. Developed in collaboration with Katherine Boger, Ph.D.

DETECTION: IDENTIFYING STUDENTS AT RISK

Students who are victimized often report vague somatic symptoms, refuse to go to school, and experience difficulty in academic achievement before they directly report bullying experiences. When they do describe their experiences, younger victims are more inclined than older victims to turn to others for help. Girls generally are more willing to seek help than are boys (Borg, 1998; Glover et al., 2000; Hunter, Boyle, & Warden, 2004; Sharp, 1995). Victims of verbal bullying (such as name-calling) are least likely to disclose bullying, followed by those subjected to indirect bullying (e.g., being excluded, having rumors spread about them), while victims of direct bullying (e.g., physical violence, having property stolen or damaged) are most likely to tell (Seeds, Harkness, & Quilty, 2010; Twyman et al., 2010). Victims seek help from different people, including their friends, teachers, and parents, depending on their age, gender, and social situation (Klomek et al., 2009; Seeds, Harkness, & Quilty, 2010; Twyman et al., 2010). Therefore, individualization of detection and interventions targeting different sets of groups are important.

The clustering of victimizations in individuals is probably due to any combination of vulnerability factors. These include factors pertaining to socio-environmental circumstances (Cicchetti & Lynch, 1993) and characteristics of the children themselves, including biological makeup as well as emotional and behavioral concerns that can precede or follow previous victimizations (Finkelhor et al., 2009).

Specific signs to look for in victims include difficulties with emotional regulation and behavior problems, internalizing symptoms, challenges with social navigation, and trauma-related symptoms.

Difficulties with Emotional and Behavioral Regulation

The experience of school bullying and victimization can result in emotional and behavioral dysregulation in victims and bullies, which in turn can put students at increased risk of being involved in further school bullying (Bond et al., 2001; Boulton, Bucci, & Hawker, 1999). An inability to effectively titrate emotional responses to what the situation calls for can leave a student vulnerable to saying or doing something that draws negative attention his or her way and to potentially misreading and/or escalating a situation.

Internalizing Symptoms

Victims of school bullying often present with increased levels of anxiety and depression, fear of going to school, feelings of being unsafe, unhappiness at school, and low self-esteem (Salmon, James, & Smith, 1998). These students also report increased risks for developing suicidality, an eating disorder, and somatic symptoms, including headaches, stomachaches, colds, and sleep difficulties (Ryan & Smith, 2009).

Suicide and other safety issues are closely related to school bullying experiences. The risk for suicidal ideation in victims of school bullying is reported to be 1.4–5.6 times that of non-victims. Many studies have also reported an increased risk for suicidal ideation in bullies (1.4–9.0 times), and bully-victims showed the highest increased risk of suicidal ideation (1.9–10.0 times) (Kim & Leventhal, 2008). In another study, frequent bullying and victimization were associated with later suicide attempts and completed suicides, even after adjusting for baseline depression (Klomek et al., 2009). News reports covering the deaths of youths over the past five decades revealed that at least 250 reported cases of suicide death were linked to bullying or hazing (Srabstein, 2008).

Challenges with Social Navigation

Victims of bullying often suffer difficulties in many areas of socialization. They often feel isolated and socially avoided and experience lower social status than other students (Seeds, Harkness, & Quilty, 2010). Although bullies may enjoy higher social status, they can be equally avoided by other students. Again, bully-victims have the most troublesome social status, with the highest level of avoidance by others (Juvonen, Graham, & Schuster, 2003).

Victims and bully-victims generally have been characterized as being more submissive in their interactions with peers. Their lack of assertion can be detected by peers, who expect the victim to display suffering and to not retaliate (such ill treatment might not violate victims' expectations for relationships, given their past experiences [Shields & Cicchetti, 2001], or they may have an experience of learned helplessness); this then reinforces the bully's behavior. It has been theorized that these same interpersonal characteristics noted by peers are also detected by sexual assailants or abusive adults, thus increasing a victim's vulnerability to other forms of victimization. It is important to note, however, that rather than these characteristics making the child more vulnerable, the victimization experiences may contribute to the development of interaction styles that aggressors seem to target.

In addition, child victims of abuse often have difficulty in accurately recognizing emotions displayed by others (i.e., they are less socially adept), as well as experiencing challenges in regulating their own verbal and nonverbal expression, which can increase their risk of being bullied. Abused children may not "read" others accurately, so that others may be able to intimidate these children. Similarly, this lack of accurate recognition and processing of others' emotions can position these children to determine too late that they are vulnerable to bullying circumstances (Garner & Hinton, 2010).

PTSD Symptoms

Like victims of other forms of trauma, victims of school bullying may have symptoms of posttraumatic stress disorder (PTSD), appearing hypervigilant, avoiding social situations that are unstructured, deferring to others in and outside the classroom, reacting out of proportion to the circumstances, reacting dramatically to seemingly small or minor events, and perhaps even calling people by different names (flashbacks) or dissociating (Idsoe, Dyregrov, & Cosmovici-Idsoe, 2012). Repeatedly, victimized children may expect to be maltreated and therefore react to new social contexts with hyperarousal and fear; this anxious vulnerability can contribute to their risk for additional victimization (Shields & Cicchetti, 2001). Whereas arousal and vigilance may be adaptive in dangerous homes or communities, they are more likely to inhibit social functioning with peers (Shields & Cicchetti, 2001). These children may interpret neutral types of interactions as hostile and threatening and respond to them with aggression or fear, which in turn can lead to more difficulties in socialization (Dodge & Coie, 1987).

Additional Considerations

Other, less direct mechanisms may also contribute to and result from multiple trauma experiences. In these cases, multiple victimizations may be more markers than agents of a student's difficulties (Finkelhor, Ormrod, & Turner, 2007). These factors include psychiatric diagnoses, such as attention-deficit / hyperactivity disorder, autism spectrum disorder, or anxiety and depressive disorder (Twyman et al., 2010); socio-environmental factors, such as larger school size, problems with neighbors/community, or negative family factors (Bowes et al., 2009; Fonzi et al., 1999); personal characteristics, such as victims being physically weaker (Olweus, 1994a), having a different physical appearance (Farrington, 1993; Frisén, Jonsson, & Persson, 2007), or being worse at sports than others, or having chronic somatic disease (Luukkonen et al., 2010).

When victimization occurs both in the home or community and at school, these experiences can lead a child to believe this is a normal way to be treated. This not only can adversely affect the child's interactions in new social relationships but also can result in negative self-cognitions and poor self-esteem (making the child vulnerable to further victimization). In addition, given that victimization occurs in places where the child spends the majority of his or her time, the child will probably struggle with finding a "safe place" or respite.

INTERVENTIONS

Victimization, whether through school bullying, family violence, or other traumas and assaults, should be considered through the lens of the individual and also in environmental/system contexts. While individual vulnerabilities may contribute to the risk of being victimized, environmental factors also contribute to the trauma and thus require intervention.

Individual-Level Interventions

Because victims face difficulties in many aspects of their lives, they probably require a comprehensive intervention that involves multiple adults (e.g., school staff, parents, clinicians) and includes a focus on coping skills (including problem solving, emotional regulation, anger management), social skills training, attention to psychiatric disorders and trauma-related symptoms, and/or academic support. The child's evaluation of the problem and the availability of resources and support must be elicited as well (Dussich & Maekoya, 2007).

COPING SKILLS TO EFFECTIVELY MANAGE EMOTIONS. Rather than allowing emotions to drive the student, the goal is to help teach the student to experience emotions while simultaneously remaining in charge of how she or he is affected by them. Dialectical Behavioral Therapy (DBT) and cognitive behavioral therapy (CBT) techniques often can be helpful in providing these children with language and scaffolding for how to understand emotion. Students can be taught to be aware of their emotions (by naming them—sad, scared, worried, mad, etc.) in the current moment and to connect various emotions with their external experiences, internal thoughts, and resulting behaviors. They should pay attention to how that emotion affects their ability to manage situations effectively. Students should recognize how they are acting on these emotions through verbal communication, nonverbal communication / body language, and actions. They should also consider how their response to these emotions affected the situation and how different responses might have altered the course of the situation, as well as future interactions and overall functioning.

Psychiatric symptoms such as depression and anxiety can be addressed through individual and group therapy. CBT techniques can be useful to identify automatic thoughts that arise as a consequence of the traumatic experiences, and helping students challenge such thoughts can expand their thinking and provide alternative interpretations. Exposure exercises (after careful evaluation for readiness and with clear planning) can help habituate the child to uncomfortable physical and emotional experiences that arise from certain cues and triggers.

Providing a "home base" at school can help provide the student with a safe place to go when feeling distressed or in need of additional support. This can be particularly important for children who are victimized in multiple domains (e.g., school and home), as they might not get a reprieve from the victimization even when at home.

SOCIAL NAVIGATION. School staff, clinicians, and parents can help victims of abuse and bullying to cultivate social skills to engage and interact more effectively. Observing how others stand, speak, respond, and recognize when to be quiet can all be addressed so that students develop a more concrete understanding of preferred social tactics. Staff can help students identify supportive people to serve as part of their "home base" and to build connections.

Bullying is often recurrent, so a "cope ahead" plan can allay fear and impart steps to take in difficult situations. The student may identify vulnerable times and preferred interactional styles, sometimes by role-playing and rehearsing in advance. Hypothesis testing about judgments arising from victimization experiences can help students recognize that most people who engage with them will not act as an aggressor toward them.

Rehearsing with trusted adults can provide feedback to students on how to interact with peers and adults more effectively. Rehearsing with helpful/supportive peers can be even more effective, as peer influences are usually preferred by bullied youths.

Children with a past history of trauma may benefit from training to minimize their risks for bullying. They can learn how to recognize situations or subjects that disempower them or frighten them and attempt to have allies present when facing such situations.

Especially for poly-victimized students, there is a risk of developing a "victim role" or "victim identity." Helping children shift their thinking to that of a victor or survivor can give them the confidence and will to stand up for themselves. Helping them develop a sense of mastery over adversity may enable vulnerable youths to approach social encounters more confidently. Emphasizing defenses such as humor, altruism, and sublimation provides alternative, more effective ways to cope, other than denial, avoidance, or other more primitive responses.

. . .

Even when the individual develops and uses skills to manage victimization, this does not usually alter the systemic factors that allowed bullying to occur. Systems interventions are required to address the circumstances that both allowed and may perpetuate bullying incidents.

Systems Interventions

At the school level, staff discussions about bullying, inclusion of parents in discussions, and introduction of anti-bullying rules all appear to be important. Useful at the classroom level are posting, modeling, and enforcing prosocial (anti-bullying) rules and having periodic meetings with students and families. And at the individual level, supervision of student activities, meetings with students, parents, and staff, and development of plans for students affected by bullying are all helpful. Community interventions to cultivate partnerships and spread anti-bullying efforts throughout the community (from school to ball field, parks, etc.) can also be effective.

SCHOOL. Part of supporting the traumatized victim in school is to improve the school environment, moving it toward becoming a safe, respectful place to learn and interact. This decreases bullying events and also models positive ways of interacting (which might be different from what students "learn" in environments where they have been traumatized). Schools can define, practice, and reinforce the "rules of social encounters" and explain why these rules are preferred in other situations. A few anti-bullying rules that enhance social encounters among diverse individuals should be developed collaboratively by the school staff, students, and parents to increase investment in these rules. Rules should be stated in the positive—such as "Students will show respect for every other student," rather than "No student shall intimidate or threaten another student." Successful implementation requires the school system to identify desirable behaviors through specific policies and, more importantly, to model desirable behavior.

Programs conducive to prosocial interactions and to anti-bullying, such as Positive Behavioral Intervention Support (PBIS) and the Olweus anti-bullying program, have had success in decreasing school bullying (Olweus & Limber, 2010). Effective programs focus on interactions among everyone—from teaching staff to students, custodians, and other support staff—within the school.

Several school variables are associated with decreases in bullying. These include effective school leadership, professional development involving all parents and school personnel (including cafeteria staff, bus drivers, secretaries, etc.), access to mental health services for aggressors and vulnerable students, and classroom curricula that educate students to recognize bullying, provide tactics for bystanders to support victims, and develop skills in anger management, assertiveness, conflict resolution, and perspective taking. Similarly, effective school policies increase adult supervision and foster school norms against bullying by promoting "consistent, fair, and non-punitive consequences for violations." Developmental-system views toward bullying that focus on the social architecture that sustains the bullying and on the scaffolding of interventions with the individuals involved in particular incidents have a greater likelihood of successfully decreasing bullying (Pepler, 2006).

Teachers intervene when they feel sympathy for the victim and feel self-efficacy in dealing with bullying (Yoon, 2004; Yoon & Kerber, 2003). When confronted with bullying, teachers try to decide whether to punish the bullies, contact parents, foster coping skills in the victims, and/or perform conflict resolution (Limber, 2004). Adult interventions are an important part of the solution because, even when the targets of bullying enact commonly effective coping strategies, they often continue to be victimized (Kochenderfer-Ladd & Skinner, 2002).

LARGER SYSTEM. The "system" defines the limits of behaviors in social interactions and must be considered in all potential bullying situations. For example, professional athletes, from boxers to football players, often attempt to intimidate one another. In that social situation, the "rules" of bullying are drastically different from what would be tolerated in a kindergarten classroom or even the playground. As long as the system supports or tacitly encourages or just tolerates intimidation, at least in some social contexts, students will replicate such bullying roles. So any model or approach to address bullying must recognize the system as another invested "participant," defining acceptable limits to exerting power over others and sometimes intervening when those boundaries are transgressed. Much more importantly, students must be taught to recognize the various "system rules" they encounter and how to get themselves out of potentially distressing roles within these diverse systems.

What is acceptable in the "rules" that children are encouraged to practice at school compared with "outside school events" such as a sporting event or activities in a neighborhood varies widely. What is modeled and tolerated in one's neighborhood, at a sporting event, or even at home may be in clear conflict with how the student is expected to behave at school. That is, not only may the "rules" for school not apply outside the school, but the school rules may not "work" and, indeed, may leave students vulnerable if they attempt to employ what they have been asked to do at school (particularly if the school requires students to enact positive comments toward each other and they are not taught how to evade, resist, or change rules practiced in other social settings). School children may well be confused about the limits of a "rule" in diverse social situations they have not been prepared for, and they may be unable to enact what they are taught to do at school when confronted with very different behaviors modeled by others, particularly adults, who normally have the final say on the social rules in most settings.

Tactics to "Get Out of the Corner"

Perhaps more importantly, individuals rarely play only one role. In one situation a student may feel "targeted," while in another setting the same child may feel powerful or feel only like a bystander. The vitally important mission is to provide children (and adults) with tactics to use when "cornered" into any role, so that they can get out of cornered positions and navigate diverse social situations where they may be victimized, paralyzed as a bystander, inclined to intimidate another, or empowered to enact a system response to that particular situation. These techniques depend on the developmental status of the students and the developmental status of the system itself. The techniques are listed in table 14.4.

CONCLUSIONS

Victimization may occur across multiple settings and at the hands of multiple others, whether peers or adults, necessitating an investigation of trauma and bullying at school, in the neighborhood, and at home. When a student appears to have been involved in bullying outside school, it is important to consider involvement in trauma and abuse, and vice versa. Maltreatment may place some vulnerable children at risk for bullying, victimization by bullies, or both. Screening that is attentive to problems with emotional and behavioral regulation, internalizing disorders, problems with navigating social relationships or social withdrawal, and trauma-related symptoms may detect bullying and/or trauma. When developing interventions, the clinician should consider multiple domains, including systemic factors (e.g., school, family, community), interpersonal factors (e.g., peers, staff), and

Table 14.4. Developmentally Sensitive Techniques for Moving Out of the Corners

Intervention Target	Technique	Elementary School	Middle School	High School
System	Clarify rules for the system	Determine the guiding principles for social interaction; determine the importance of democratic participation vs. structured control	Specify how "diverse" or unusual students, or students who do unusual acts, will be treated; clarify the inclusion vs. exclusion "rules" of the school and how they actually operate	Clarify how the rules apply to specific situations; provide hypothetical scenarios and encourage students to comment on options and consequences
	Create policy	Create and circulate policy to invest staff, students, and parents in the "rules"	Ask staff and students to identify priorities to optimize the school culture and to minimize ostracism	Rely on staff and students to identify helpful policy and procedures, and ensure policy/procedures are well-known in the building
	Respond to allegations	Determine the process for responding to bullying incidents, and remain consistent in following up and/or fine-tuning the policy	Determine the process for responding to bullying incidents and monitor outcomes for all parties	Clarify the process for responding to bullying events, and apply it judiciously and being mindful of what principles you are seeking to teach
	Create feedback loop	Identify mechanisms for staff, students, and parents to continuously comment on potential bullying events, as well as school "rules"	Identify mechanisms for staff, students, and parents to continuously comment on potential bullying events, as well as school "rules"	Ensure that students and staff are regularly involved in evaluating bullying events and policies designed to improve school interactions
Aggressor (bully)	Ally rather than intimidate	Consider what makes good friends and how to find what others are good at that may enrich your life	Recognize that group configurations change each week; recognize the benefits/risks of including various individuals	Recognize that others can be helpful contributors to your missions and interests
	Use power for good	Consider how to make others feel good and enjoy their moments	Include others who may feel disenfranchised; model how to lead	Examine larger circles of influence and impacts on the world
	Treat others as you want to be treated	Consider how others feel	Examine impacts on those excluded; identify what you want by being in control and empowered by others	Examine how everyone should be treated so that most people can feel positive
	Identify what's triggering bullying	Examine antecedents to aggressive behaviors and alternatives that allow you to feel comfortable	Clarify what provokes aggressive behaviors and the impacts on others, at that time and later	Examine the deeper desires of the aggressor and what long-term impacts on self and others are most probable
Target (victim)	Confront aggressor	Learn how to tell aggressors to stop their current comments	Tell aggressors how to speak differently to you; learn to access peers	Label inappropriate comments by the aggressor
	Change topic	Shift the conversation if it's uncomfortable	Redirect the conversation toward appropriate topics or away from condescension	Offer conversations you will participate in or relevant appropriate topics
	Ignore aggressor	Look away, talk to others, walk away	Avoid gossip or actions that escalate conflict; instead, minimize support for aggressors	Engage in or comment about useful topics; clarify that you will leave the situation if the aggressor persists
	Access peers	Look at friends to see their reactions; ask friends to play with you	Identify different groupings of peers, which ones are of like mind to you, and other groups/members who may have helpful input	Ask peers for their perceptions and suggestions; look to peer allies for support to visit or engage the aggressor
	Access adults	Identify helpful adults and how to tell vs. "tattle"	Identify adults aware of the group "rules" in the school; seek input and appropriate actions vs. just "telling on" or "snitching"	Seek input from adults, using hypothetical situations and courses of action, if feasible, or identifying the range of students impacted by bullying

(continued)

Table 14.4. (continued)

Intervention Target	Technique	Elementary School	Middle School	High School
Observer (bystander)	Check reactions of others	Look to see others' reactions	Examine the reactions of different students and student groups	Examine and seek the perceptions of others to navigate bullying situations
	Intervene by taking positive steps	Step in, alone or with others, to confront the aggressor or to include the target	Step in, alone or with others, to address the aggressor, mindful of various group rules or dynamics	Invoke humor, redirection to good intentions gone awry, and win-win opportunities for all parties
	Change interaction	Just change the topic or "game" to something more comfortable	Shift the conversation, disallow singling out of a student, and refocus on the larger school rules or objectives	Shift the conversation or activity, label what you're observing, suggest alternatives to have an appropriate, more productive talk
	Access adults	Identify helpful adults; describe facts accurately to adults and seek input and action	Identify helpful, aware adults; seek input on options to alter the situation, including adult intervention	Identify useful adults, seek their perceptions and suggestions; discuss your options with them

intrapersonal factors (e.g., emotional regulation, self-esteem, internalizing symptoms, loneliness, social competence). Helpful interventions strengthen problem-solving and coping strategies, not only for the traumatized individual but also for the entire system.

References

Analitis, F., Velderman, M. K., Ravens-Sieberer, U., Detmar, S., Erhart, M., Herdman, M., et al., the European Kidscreen Group. (2009). Being bullied: Associated factors in children and adolescents 8 to 18 years old in 11 European countries. *Pediatrics, 123*, 569–577.

Ando, M., Asakura, T., & Simons-Morton, B. (2005). Psychosocial influences on physical, verbal, and indirect bullying among Japanese early adolescents. *Journal of Early Adolescence, 25*(3), 268–297.

Bond, L., Carlin, J. B., Thomas, L., Rubin, K., & Pattin, G. (2001). Does bullying cause emotional problems? *BMJ, 323*(7311), 480–484.

Borg, M. G. (1998). The emotional reactions of school bullies and their victims. *Educational Psychology, 18*(4), 433–444.

Boulton, M. J., Bucci, E., & Hawker, D. D. S. (1999). Swedish and English secondary school pupils' attitudes towards, and conceptions of, bullying: Concurrent links with bully/victim involvement. *Scandinavian Journal of Psychology, 40*, 277–284.

Bowes, L., Arseneault, L., Maughan, B., Taylor, A., Caspi, A., & Moffitt, T. E. (2009). School, neighborhood, and family factors are associated with children's bullying involvement: A nationally representative longitudinal study. *Journal of the American Academy of Child and Adolescent Psychiatry, 48*(5), 545–553.

Cicchetti, D., & Lynch, M. (1993). Toward an ecological/transactional model of community violence and child maltreatment: Consequences for children's development. *Psychiatry, 56*(1), 96–118.

Cook, R., Williams, K., Kim, T., Sadek, S., & Guerra, N. (2010). Predictors of bullying and victimization in childhood and adolescence: A meta-analytic investigation. *School Psychology Quarterly, 25*(2), 65–83.

Dodge, K. A., & Coie, J. D. (1987). Social-information-processing factors in reactive and proactive aggression in children's peer groups. *Journal of Personality and Social Psychology, 53*(6), 1146–1158.

Dussich, J. P., & Maekoya, C. (2007). Physical child harm and bullying-related behaviors: A comparative study in Japan, South Africa, and the United States. *International Journal of Offender Therapy and Comparative Criminology, 51*(5), 495–509.

Farrington, D. P. (1993). Understanding and preventing bullying. *Crime and Justice: A Review of Research, 17*, 381–458.

Finkelhor, D., Ormrod, R. K., & Turner, H. A. (2007). Poly-victimization: A neglected component in child victimization. *Child Abuse & Neglect, 31*(1), 7–26.

Finkelhor, D., Ormrod, R., Turner, H., & Holt, M. (2009). Pathways to poly-victimization. *Child Maltreatment, 14*(4), 316–329.

Fonzi, A., Genta, M. L., Menesini, E., Bacchini, D., Bonino, S., & Costabile, A. (1999). *The nature of school bullying: A cross-national perspective.* London, UK: Routledge.

Frisén, A., Jonsson, A., & Persson, C. (2007). Adolescents' perception of bullying: Who is the victim? Who is the bully? What can be done to stop bullying? *Adolescence, 42*(168), 749–761.

Garner P. W., & Hinton, T. S. (2010). Emotional display rules and emotional self-regulation: Associations with bullying and victimization in community-based after school programs. *Journal of Community & Applied Social Psychology, 20*, 480–496.

Glover, D., Gough, G., Johnson, M., & Cartwright, N. (2000). Bullying in 25 secondary schools: Incidence, impact and intervention. *Educational Research, 42*(2), 141–156.

Herman, J. (1997). *Trauma and recovery.* New York, NY: Basic Books.

Holt, M. (2007). Hidden forms of victimization in elementary students involved in bullying. *School Psychology Review, 36*(3), 345–360.

Holt, M. K., Finkelhor, D., & Kantor, G. K. (2007). Multiple victimization experiences of urban elementary school students: Associations with psychosocial functioning and academic performance. *Child Abuse & Neglect, 31*(5), 503–515.

Hunter, S. C., Boyle, J. M. E., & Warden, D. (2004). Help seeking amongst child and adolescent victims of peer-aggression and bullying: The influence of school-stage, gender, victimization, appraisal, and emotion. *British Journal of Educational Psychology, 74,* 375–390.

Idsoe, T., Dyregrov, A., & Cosmovici Idsoe, E. (2012). Bullying and PTSD symptoms. *Journal of Abnormal Child Psychology, 40,* 901–911.

Juvonen, J., Graham, S., & Schuster, M. A. (2003). Bullying among young adolescents: The strong, the weak, and the troubled. *Pediatrics, 112*(6), 1231–1237.

Karna, A., Voeten, M., Little, T., Poskiparta, E., Alanen, E., & Salmivalli, C. (2011). Going to scale: A nonrandomized nationwide trial of the KiVa Antibullying Program for grades 1–9. *Journal of Consulting and Clinical Psychology, 79*(6), 796–805.

Kim, Y. S., Koh, Y., & Leventhal, B. (2005). School bullying and suicidal risk in Korean middle school students. *Pediatrics, 115*(2), 357–363.

Kim, Y. S., & Leventhal, B. (2008). Bullying and suicide: A review. *International Journal of Adolescent Medicine and Health, 20*(2), 133–154.

Kim, Y. S., Leventhal, B. L., Koh, Y., Hubbard, A., & Boyce, W. T. (2006). School bullying and youth violence: Causes or consequences of psychopathologic behavior? *Archives of General Psychiatry, 63*(9), 1035–1041.

Klomek, A. B., Sourander, A., Niemelä, S., Kumpulainen, K., Piha, J., Tamminen, T., et al. (2009). Childhood bullying behavior as a risk for suicide attempts and completed suicides: A population-based birth cohort study. *Journal of the American Academy of Child and Adolescent Psychiatry, 48*(3), 254–261.

Kochenderfer-Ladd, B., & Skinner, K. (2002). Children's coping strategies: Moderators of the effects of peer victimization? *Developmental Psychology, 38*(2), 267–278.

Kowlaski, R. M., Limber, S. P., & Agatson, P. W. (2008). *Cyberbullying: Bullying in the digital age.* Malden, MA: Blackwell Publishing.

Limber, S. (Ed.). (2004). *Bullying in American schools: A social-ecological perspective on prevention and intervention.* Mahwah, NJ: Lawrence Erlbaum Associates.

Luukkonen, A., Rasanen, P., Hakko, H., Riala, K., & STUDY-70 Workgroup. (2010). Bullying behavior in relation to psychiatric disorders and physical health among adolescents: A clinical cohort of 508 underage inpatient adolescents in Northern Finland. *Psychiatry Research, 178,* 166–170.

McKenna, M., Hawk, E., Mullen, J., & Hertz, M. (2011). Bullying among middle school and high school students— Massachusetts, 2009. *MMWR Morbidity and Mortality Weekly Report, 60*(15), 465.

Menesini, E., Modena, M., & Tani, F. (2009). Bullying and victimization in adolescence: Concurrent and stable roles and psychological health symptoms. *Journal of Genetic Psychology, 170*(2), 115–133.

Morita, Y. (1985). *Sociological study on the structure of bullying group.* Osaka, Japan: Department of Sociology, Osaka City University.

Olweus, D. (1992). *Aggression and violence throughout the life span.* London, UK: Sage Publications.

Olweus, D. (1994a). *Aggressive behavior: Current perspectives.* New York, NY: Plenum Press.

Olweus, D. (1994b). Annotation: Bullying at school—Basic facts and effects of a school based intervention program. *Journal of Child Psychology and Psychiatry, 35*(7), 1171–1190.

Olweus, D., & Limber, S. P. (2010). Bullying in school: Evaluation and dissemination of the Olweus Bullying Prevention Program. *American Journal of Orthopsychiatry, 80*(1), 124–134.

Pepler, D. J. (2006). Bullying interventions: A binocular perspective. *Journal of the Canadian Academy of Child and Adolescent Psychiatry, 15*(1), 16–20.

Ryan, W., & Smith, J. D. (2009). Antibullying programs in schools: How effective are evaluation practices? *Prevention Science, 10*(3), 248–259.

Salmon, G., James, A., & Smith, D. M. (1998). Bullying in schools: Self reported anxiety, depression, and self-esteem in secondary school children. *BMJ, 317*(3), 924–925.

Schwartz, D. (2000). Subtypes of victims and aggressors in children's peer groups. *Journal of Abnormal Child Psychology, 28*(2), 181–192.

Seeds, P. M., Harkness, K. L., & Quilty, L. C. (2010). Parental maltreatment, bullying, and adolescent depression: Evidence for the mediating role of perceived social support. *Journal of Clinical Child and Adolescent Psychology, 39*(5), 681–692.

Sharp, S. (1995). How much does bullying hurt? The effects of bullying on the personal wellbeing and educational progress of secondary aged students. *Educational and Child Psychology, 12*(2), 81–88.

Shields, A., & Cicchetti D. (2001). Parental maltreatment and emotion dysregulation as risk factors for bullying and victimization in middle childhood. *Journal of Clinical Child Psychology, 30*(3), 349–363.

Spivak, H. (2003). Bullying: Why all the fuss? *Pediatrics, 112,* 1421–1422.

Srabstein, J. (2008). Deaths linked to bullying and hazing. *International Journal of Adolescent Medicine and Health, 20*(2), 235–239.

Srabstein, J. C., Berkman, B. E., & Pyntikova, E. (2008). Antibullying legislation: A public health perspective. *Journal of Adolescent Health, 42,* 11–20.

Turner, H. A., Finkelor, D., & Ormrod, R. (2010). Polyvictimization in a national sample of children and youth. *American Journal of Preventative Medicine, 38*(3), 323–330.

Twemlow, S. W. (2010). *Handbook of bullying in schools: An international perspective.* New York, NY: Routledge / Taylor & Francis Group.

Twyman, K. A., Saylor, C. F., Saia, D., Macias, M. M., Taylor, L. A., & Spratt, E. (2010). Bullying and ostracism experiences in children with special health care needs. *Journal of Developmental and Behavioral Pediatrics, 31,* 1–8.

U.S. Department of Education. (2010). *Indicators of school crime and safety: 2010.* Washington, DC: Institute of Education Sciences.

Yoon, J. (2004). Predicting teacher interventions in bullying situations. *Education and Treatment of Children, 27*(1), 37–45.

Yoon, J., & Kerber, K. (2003). Bullying: Elementary teachers' attitudes and intervention strategies. *Research in Education, 69,* 27–35.

KATHLEEN M. CHARD, PH.D.
RICH GILMAN, PH.D.

15

Cognitive Processing Therapy with Adolescents

GENERAL CONSIDERATIONS

Data from a multitude of sources indicate that a significant number of children will be exposed to a traumatic event, including abuse, car accidents, or natural disasters, to name just a few. For example, Finkelhor and colleagues (2009) found that more than 60% of American children experienced some type of violence exposure in the year prior to the survey; in an earlier survey, 22% of children had experienced four or more different types of violence (Finkelhor, Ormrod, & Turner, 2007). Although most children will recover, a sizable percentage will experience heightened levels of psychological distress, subsequently leading to a formal diagnosis of posttraumatic stress disorder (PTSD; American Academy of Child and Adolescent Psychiatry, 1998; American Psychiatric Association, 1994). As a disorder, PTSD shares a high comorbidity with depression and/or anxiety. Among school-age youths, there are also frequent observations of anger or oppositional behaviors. Thus, PTSD treatments specific to this population typically include interventions that can address these related symptoms as well.

Cognitive behavioral therapy (CBT) interventions are the most commonly researched and supported treatment models for childhood trauma. As a classification, CBT incorporates several specific models (e.g., Rationale Emotive Behavior Therapy, Prolonged Exposure), and although these models were first designed for and applied to adults, many of their techniques have been refined and modified for use with traumatized adolescents (see Kazdin & Weisz, 2003; Kendall, 2001, Silverman et al., 2008). There is substantial support for CBT interventions that target children as young as 2 years old (Stallard, 2006), although the methods used are contingent on the child's condition and cognitive level. In terms of youths diagnosed with PTSD, CBT methods typically include one or more of the following:

(1) revisiting of the traumatic material, (2) cognitive reprocessing and reframing, (3) stress management, and (4) parent treatment. Specific techniques within these methods can range from talking about the traumatic event to drawing pictures about the trauma, writing about the trauma events, or recounting the events into a tape recorder. The purpose of this chapter is to discuss the use and efficacy of a particular form of CBT, Cognitive Processing Therapy (CPT), with adolescents who have experienced trauma, as well as the advantages and disadvantages of this approach.

DESCRIPTION OF THE INTERVENTION

Cognitive Processing Therapy was created as a manualized cognitive behavioral protocol to treat PTSD and related symptoms in adult rape survivors (Resick & Schnicke, 1992). The therapy has since been adopted for all types of trauma, including child abuse, military trauma, and natural disasters (see Resick, Monson, & Chard, 2007). CPT is typically offered in 12 sessions, although shorter or longer protocols can be followed, depending on the type of trauma and the amount of distress the individual is experiencing. The treatment is multifaceted and sequentially ordered, with subsequent sessions building on skills learned in previous sessions.

In sessions 1–4, clients are given information on the theory behind CPT and are asked to write an impact statement discussing why they believe the traumatic event occurred and how the event has shaped their beliefs about self, others, and the world, particularly in the areas related to safety, trust, power/control, esteem, and intimacy. Next, individuals learn about the connection between events, thoughts, and feelings through the use of the A-B-C Sheet and begin to identify places where they have become "stuck" in their thinking. Disruptive or dysfunctional beliefs are often referred to as "stuck points," making them more concrete and thus more challengeable. Examples of stuck points include "It is my fault the event happened," "I cannot trust anyone," and "The world is not safe." Stuck points often lead to strong emotions such as shame, blame, fear, and anger that do not dissipate quickly and can adversely affect the individual's ability to function effectively and happily in society. Patterns of thinking and behaving that were established before, during, and after the abuse are discussed in detail. Then clients are taught the ways in which people can become derailed in their thinking about traumatic events, and the therapist introduces, in lay language, the underlying concepts of assimilation (taking in the new information without changing preexisting beliefs), over-accommodation (changing beliefs about the self and the world to an extreme degree), and accommodation (modifying preexisting beliefs to incorporate new information). Finally, clients write detailed accounts of the most traumatic incident, including sensory details, thoughts and feelings. (Note that in the CPT–Cognitive Only version [CPT-C], no traumatic accounts are written. The treatment remains trauma-focused but without a retelling of the traumatic event in systematic detail.) The therapist employs Socratic dialogue to help clients begin to analyze their "stuck points" and to view past events with a more balanced interpretation. In this form of questioning, the therapist feigns ignorance to elicit a client's complete knowledge on a particular topic. Incomplete or inaccurate ideas can then be corrected during follow-up questioning, which can help correct the client's misinterpretations and can lead to more realistic thought processes.

In sessions 5–7, the core cognitive therapy skills are taught, including use of the Challenging Questions Worksheet (CQW) to examine a single belief. The CQW consists of 10 questions, adapted from those created by A. T. Beck and colleagues (1979), that help clients look at the evidence for and against their belief, contextual factors that might support or refute the belief, and finally, the role of emotion in maintaining that belief. For example, a client may hold a stuck point that the traumatic event (e.g., rape, combat-related death) was "all my fault." Using the CQW, clients can begin to see that the trauma was caused by someone else or was not under their control and that although they wish the outcome had been different, there was little they could have done to prevent the end result, given the situational variables, resources, and knowledge they had at the time. The Patterns of Problematic Thinking Sheet is then introduced to allow clients to become familiar with common faulty thinking patterns that can interfere with recovery from PTSD. Each stuck point is attached to a pattern, showing clients the problematic patterns that they tend to use the most and thus allowing them to be mindful of falling into these in the future. Finally, clients learn to use the Challenging Beliefs Worksheet (CBW), which brings all of the prior worksheets together. PTSD often causes individuals to think with a narrowed view about the trauma (e.g., "I

could have prevented the event from happening"), which can then create further overgeneralized thoughts about the self, others, and the world (e.g., "I am a bad person" or "No one in authority can be trusted"). The CBW allows clients to look at their original beliefs, challenge them, and come up with alternative beliefs while also noting their change in emotions. Clients are then able to see how much relief they are likely to feel if they look at the situation more realistically instead of through the lens of PTSD. This will typically result in new thoughts such as, "I could not have prevented the trauma," "I did the best I could given the situation," "I am a good person," and "Many people in authority can be trusted."

Sessions 8–12 allow individuals to focus their thought examination in each of five key areas—safety, trust, power/control, esteem, and intimacy—using the CBW. For session 12, clients rewrite their impact statement and compare it with the version written for session 2. This allows clients to clearly recognize the changes in their thoughts, feelings, and behaviors. This is often a very powerful part of the session, with clients reporting that they were completely unaware of how much blame they were inappropriately taking for the traumatic event and how negatively they were thinking about themselves, others, and the world at the start of therapy. Finally, the therapist and client look to the future, identify any areas that may continue to be problematic, and discuss ways that the client can manage these issues.

It is important to note that when an adolescent shows some cognitive limitations, whether due to age, traumatic brain injury, substance use, or some other medical condition, the therapist should attempt to use the full protocol initially and not assume that the youth cannot do the practice assignments as written. For cases in which it becomes apparent that the client will have difficulty completing the worksheets, the authors of the CPT protocol created shortened worksheets that still help the individual examine and challenge stuck points, but with simpler forms (McIlvain, Walter, & Chard, 2013; Resick, Monson, & Chard, 2007). For example, the CQW can be shortened from 10 to 5 questions, if some of the questions are conceptually difficult for the youth to understand.

One version of Cognitive Processing Therapy, CPT for Sexual Abuse (CPT-SA), expands the therapy to 17 sessions and adds information on developmental issues and how childhood sexual abuse plays a role in shaping self-identity, attachment, self-concept, and self-esteem. In addition, the client discusses with the therapist his or her developmental interruptions and experiences, to understand the ways in which the three schematic levels most affected by sexual abuse—intra-individual, interpersonal, and worldview—are formed and reinforced through interactions with others. As the cognitions and emotions are addressed and adequately labeled by the client, subsequent CPT-SA sessions focus on seven (expanded from the five in CPT) belief areas: safety, trust, power/control, esteem, assertiveness/communication, intimacy, and social support. Although the individual's disruptive cognitions may have served as adaptive coping mechanisms during the abuse, CPT-SA helps identify disruptive schemas and incorporate more adaptive schemas that are more appropriate to current life situations.

UNDERLYING RATIONALE AND THEORETICAL FRAMEWORK

A key tenet underlying all CBT models, including CPT, is that individuals' thoughts, attitudes, and perceptions about themselves and others influence their interpretation of an external event, and this interpretation can, in turn, influence subsequent emotions and behaviors. Although integrative models have been proposed to explain the intricate relationship among thoughts (cognitions), emotions (affect), and behaviors (David & Szentagotai, 2006), factors such as personality, learned history, and access to internal (e.g., coping strategies) and external (e.g., social support systems) resources have been shown to moderate the valence of an experience. Cognitive therapists maintain that it is not an event itself but rather the cognitive interpretation of the event that establishes the probability for a given affect or behavior. Further, cognitions, affect, and behaviors are reciprocal (rather than linear) influences: as the trauma survivor avoids triggers of the event, the absence of positive experiences minimizes the probability of addressing the triggers and also reinforces avoidance. Given this interaction, CBT simultaneously targets both cognitions and behaviors.

CBT seeks to enhance an individual's awareness of cognitive misperceptions (i.e., distortions) and of the behavioral patterns that reinforce and are reinforced by these distortions. Not every distortion is targeted for therapy—only those that are creating the most distress to the individual. Thus, the task of the CBT therapist is to help the client (1) become aware of distorted cognitions, (2) identify the way these distorted cognitions are related to negative feelings and behaviors, and (3) modify distorted thinking and maladaptive behavior patterns, both of which have heretofore reinforced and maintained a negative view of self and others. It is assumed that by successfully completing these tasks, the individual will perceive and react differently to events, leading to less psychological distress and a more positive life outlook (A. T. Beck et al. 1979; J. S. Beck, 1995).

The CPT protocol was adapted from Aaron Beck's cognitive theory of depression (A. T. Beck et al., 1979). The focus on adapting a depression therapy was a departure from the work of most researchers, who were focusing on applying treatments to PTSD that had been developed for anxiety disorders, such as exposure therapy (e.g., Foa et al., 1991; Keane & Kaloupek, 1982). Specifically, in a study examining women's traumatic responses following rape, Resick and colleagues (Atkeson et al., 1982) found that such responses were frequently accompanied by depressive symptoms. Thus, PTSD was conceptualized as more than just a fear and anxiety disorder. Rather, the disorder adversely affects the individual's sense of self, view of oth-

ers, and worldviews. Resick and colleagues also found that the *perception* of danger was a more important predictor of later symptoms than was the objective danger of the situation (Girelli et al., 1986). These results suggested that the interpretation of the traumatic event was an important contributor to the traumatic response.

As a separate line of research, McCann, Sakheim, and Abrahamson (1988; see also McCann & Pearlman, 1990) recognized that people may start with a significant number of negative beliefs that may be reinforced by further traumatic events. This model focuses on the process by which trauma survivors integrate traumatic events into their overall conceptual systems (e.g., core beliefs, schemas), either by assimilating the information into existing schemas or by altering existing schemas to accommodate the new information. More specifically, *assimilation* occurs when new information, including information related to traumatic events, is congruent with prior beliefs about one's self or the world, whether positive or negative. For example, a woman with a history of child sexual abuse may quickly assimilate a later sexual trauma without effort because the information matches her previous schemas (e.g., "I am bad or dirty, therefore bad things happen to me") (Chard, Weaver, & Resick, 1997). Assimilation can also occur when individuals' memories or causal appraisals of the traumatic event are altered to be more congruent with their prior beliefs. For example, if a woman previously believed that no one she knew would rape her and then experienced acquaintance rape, she might conclude that the assault was a misunderstanding or resulted from poor communication on her part. Conversely, when events happen that are schema-discrepant and individuals adjust their schemas to incorporate this new information, this process is termed *accommodation*. An example of accommodation would be someone who says, "This happened to me but I didn't cause it" or "It happened in spite of my best effort to stop it."

Resick added assimilation and accommodation as central concepts in CPT, as well as the concept of *over-accommodation* (Resick & Schnicke, 1992, 1993)—that is, the idea that trauma survivors may alter their thinking about themselves and their world in extreme ways and develop rigid beliefs in order to feel safer or more in control (e.g., "I will never trust my judgment again" or "Everybody will try to control me"), in an attempt to prevent future victimization (Resick & Schnicke, 1992). Such over-accommodated beliefs can interfere with the processing of natural emotions that originated from the event (e.g., fear, sadness) and increase experiences of manufactured emotions, which are emotions created by the individual's inaccurate cognitions about the event (e.g., shame, anger).

McCann and Pearlman (1992) delineated trauma-related cognitive distortions in five areas: safety, trust, power/control, esteem, and intimacy. They posited that any of these five could be self-referent or other-referent disruptions in thinking. Resick included these themes as content areas of CPT and suggested that individuals could have assimilated or over-accommodated thought disruptions in any of these areas (in addition to other stuck points more clearly linked to the traumatic event).

Thus, the final CPT protocol integrates cognitive therapy and cognitive interventions with specific information on how trauma survivors process information in their schemas and the knowledge that as an individual accesses a traumatic memory, she or he experiences and extinguishes emotions attached to the event. In the past there has been some confusion that CPT is an exposure therapy, given its inclusion of a written narrative component, but the abbreviated nature of the written narrative and evidence from a dismantling study by Resick and colleagues (2008) suggest that CPT relies on cognitive restructuring, not exposure, as an agent of change.

EMPIRICAL SUPPORT

The effectiveness of Cognitive Processing Therapy has been shown in several randomized controlled trials involving individuals who had experienced a variety of traumatic events, including rape, child abuse, assault, and combat (Chard, 2005; Monson et al., 2006; Resick, Galovski, et al., 2008; Resick, Nishith, et al., 2002). Several of these studies included individuals in their late teens, with no outcome differences related to age. More recently, as noted above, Resick and colleagues (2008) conducted a dismantling study of CPT in which they found that individuals in the standard CPT protocol and in the CPT-C protocol, with no written trauma accounts, performed equally well at the completion of treatment and at follow-up; however, participants in the written-narrative-only condition did not improve as quickly, nor were the gains as significant at the completion of treatment. This study demonstrated that it is equally effective to use the full CPT protocol or the modified CPT-C (Cognitive Only) version, depending on clients' choice and their ability to cope with the revisiting of the traumatic event in great detail. Note that in CPT-C, the treatment is still trauma-focused and the event can still be discussed, albeit in less detail.

Finally, there has been one randomized controlled trial of group CPT compared with a waitlist control, conducted specifically for adolescents. Ahrens and Rexford (2002) conducted CPT with 38 adolescent males incarcerated in a youth facility. CPT was shortened to eight 60-minute sessions, primarily by condensing the final six sessions of the protocol into two sessions. The authors found that youths in the treatment condition showed a 50% improvement in their PTSD symptoms, and all individuals who received treatment had depression scores in the normal range after completion of treatment. Conversely, those in the control condition did not improve on either PTSD or depression measures until they received active treatment. It is important to note that one-third of the sample had a history of multiple traumas, over one-half had a documented history of a head injury leading to a loss of consciousness, over one-third were diagnosed with some form of attention deficit disorder, and all were incarcerated for committing a crime (e.g., assault, burglary, or drug charges). Thus, the results are even more impressive, given the complexity of the participants' histories in this study.

WHEN TO CHOOSE CPT

Research has shown that CPT can be effective for individuals suffering from a variety of traumatic events, including those with multiple traumas and complex developmental histories. That said, CPT can be offered to traumatized adolescents with a diagnosis of PTSD who have at least some memory for the traumatic event and who express some willingness to complete the practice assignments. Individuals who also have untreated mania, untreated psychosis, active suicidal intent, or a substance dependence requiring detoxification should be treated for those symptoms prior to starting CPT. Studies have revealed that individuals with chronic child abuse, personality disorders, suicidal ideation, traumatic brain injury, and substance use all do well with CPT, and these conditions should not necessarily be reasons for exclusion from the treatment (Resick, Monson, & Chard, 2007).

Many individuals who have experienced traumatic events have high levels of avoidance of people, places, and things that can remind them of the trauma, and this can overgeneralize to the therapy environment as well. As avoidance is a natural part of PTSD symptoms, it is important that the therapist and the client's parent(s) do not collude in the avoidance with the adolescent by delaying the start of trauma treatment. Instead, the avoidance should be labeled as such and the individual should be supported and encouraged to continue with the treatment plan. In addition, in clinical settings, therapists have found it effective to employ motivational interviewing techniques before therapy starts and, when avoidance is high during treatment, to continue to motivate the client to do the work required in CPT.

Finally, the therapist should be aware of the various ways in which youths can arrive at therapy and how these reasons may differ as a function of the client's age. Although adults primarily self-refer for treatment, youths are most often referred by adults (e.g., parents, guardians, and teachers). There may be instances when the child's behaviors are symptomatic of larger problems in the family that would not necessarily be ameliorated through individual CPT alone. The level and type of involvement of family members in a child's treatment can have a dramatic impact on the success of the therapy (Braswell, 1991; Kazdin, Holland, & Crowley, 1997), and for this reason there has been increased emphasis on including parents' or guardians' buy-in, support, and even participation in treatments for youths. Typically, in CPT this involves parents attending a portion of pre-treatment assessment sessions and part of session 1 so that they can hear the rationale for therapy and learn how they can support the adolescent through the process.

ADVANTAGES AND DISADVANTAGES

One of the advantages of CPT is the time-limited session length, which is often appealing, especially in our consumer-driven society. A second advantage is the possibility of shortening or lengthening the protocol as needed for a specific individual. This decision can be made midway through the therapy, allowing therapist and client to alter the course of treatment as necessary, based on the client's progress in therapy or new information that the client brings up in later sessions. A third advantage is the demonstrated efficacy of CPT for individuals with complex trauma histories and multiple psychological complaints. Thus, it is not necessary to exclude someone because of a personality disorder or substance use problem, as has often been done in standard trauma treatments in the past. It is also possible to treat someone with multiple types of trauma (e.g., child abuse and adolescent rape) without altering the treatment protocol. A fourth advantage is the possibility of omitting in-depth discussion of the traumatic event by using the CPT-C version. For individuals with limited memory of the event or those for whom focusing on the traumatic event in detail would be too overwhelming, CPT-C offers an option shown to be as effective as CPT in a comparison trial (Resick et al., 2008).

A fifth advantage of CPT is that it can be offered in group, individual, or combined group and individual formats (Chard et al., 2009). There are many advantages to using CPT in a group setting, including (1) clients can learn that they are not alone in their symptom distress; (2) group members can challenge each other regarding their cognitive distortions; (3) clients can practice their newly learned behaviors in session, under the guidance of a therapist, before trying them in the nontherapy world; and (4) clients can test hypotheses surrounding their beliefs, using feedback from other group members' experiences. The disadvantages of CPT in a group setting are similar to those for any group treatment modality. For example, clients in group therapy may feel that they do not receive enough one-on-one individualized care and that they cannot probe deeply enough into their own belief structure for fear of monopolizing the group. In addition, group dynamics can sometimes get in the way of clients' abilities or willingness to share their true thoughts, which they may do more of in individual therapy. This may be especially the case for youths, where impression management and social desirability may be more pronounced than for adults (considering that many youths are referred by teachers and parents rather than self-referred).

Although CBT, in general, has been criticized for its failure to recognize important developmental differences that may mediate its success with children (Grave & Blissett, 2004; Stallard, 2002), research indicates that modified approaches for young children can lead to improvements in both cognitive reframing and problematic behaviors (Grave & Blissett, 2004; Kendall, 2001). Further research suggests that older children (over the age of 8) have established complex higher-order reasoning skills (see Grave & Blissett, 2004),

allowing them to be aware of their cognitive distortions and the relationship among cognitions, affect, and behaviors. Thus a final advantage of CPT is that the concepts are typically easy for older children and adolescents to comprehend.

Nevertheless, developmental characteristics that are unique among this age group need to be considered by the therapist using CPT and could pose a disadvantage if not attended to during treatment. For example, the late adolescent period signifies the final stages of preparation for life beyond graduation from school (Bong, 2001) and, for many adolescents, the last ties to dependence on their parents. This awareness can lead adolescents to begin examining their identity and place in the world, and questions about their future become more salient and less ambiguous. Related to these self-appraisals is the adolescent's view of self in relation to others. Appraisals of perceived competence in handling life challenges are based on a complex system of interactions with parents, peers, romantic partners, teachers, and others at a level not usually observed among young children. This reciprocal interaction between internal thoughts and external comparisons can create a litany of potential cognitive distortions, many of which can interfere with daily functioning. Clinicians should be aware of these multiple sources when applying CPT to adolescents.

Another potential disadvantage of CPT is the reliance on practice assignments. Adolescents may be hesitant to do work outside the session, due to competing demands on their time from schoolwork or afterschool activities or for fear that someone might find their writings and read them. A final disadvantage is that the individual must know how to read and write. While some alterations to the protocol can be made using tape recorders, the treatment does require some reading, which might be aversive to some youths who are either struggling in school or have become homework-avoidant due to prior bad school experiences.

EXPECTED OUTCOMES

The research on CPT with adolescents is limited, especially for those younger than 18 years, but the existing data suggest that most individuals receiving CPT experience significant reductions in their PTSD symptoms. In addition, participants commonly report improvement in their related symptoms of depression, anxiety, low self-esteem, guilt, anger, and dissociation. No negative outcomes have been associated with CPT in research studies, and dropout rates are equal to or better than those seen in other evidence-based treatments (Resick, Monson, & Chard, 2007). Thus, CPT can be seen as a solid choice for therapists seeking evidence-based, time-limited, effective treatments for adolescents.

References

Ahrens, J., & Rexford, L. (2002). Cognitive Processing Therapy for incarcerated adolescents with PTSD. *Journal of Aggression, Maltreatment and Trauma, 6,* 201–216.

American Academy of Child and Adolescent Psychiatry. (1998). Practice parameters for the assessment and treatment of children and adolescents with posttraumatic stress disorder. *Journal of the American Academy of Child and Adolescent Psychiatry, 37*(10), 4–26S.

American Psychiatric Association. (1994). *Diagnostic and statistical manual of mental disorders* (4th ed.). Washington, DC: Author.

Atkeson, B. M., Calhoun, K. S., Resick, P. A., & Ellis, E. M. (1982). Victims of rape: Repeated assessment of depressive symptoms. *Journal of Consulting and Clinical Psychology, 50*, 96–102.

Beck, A. T., Rush, A. J., Shaw, F., & Emery, G. (1979). *Cognitive therapy of depression.* New York, NY: Guilford Press.

Beck, J. S. (1995). *Cognitive therapy: Basics and beyond.* New York, NY: Guilford Press.

Bong, M. (2001). Role of self-efficacy and task-value in predicting college students' course performance and future enrollment intentions. *Contemporary Educational Psychology, 26*, 553–570.

Braswell, L. (1991). Involving parents in cognitive-behavioral therapy with children and adolescents. In P. C. Kendall (Ed.), *Child and adolescent therapy: Cognitive-behavioral procedures* (pp. 316–351). New York, NY: Guilford Press.

Chard, K. M. (2005). An evaluation of Cognitive Processing Therapy for the treatment of posttraumatic stress disorder related to childhood sexual abuse. *Journal of Consulting and Clinical Psychology, 73*, 965–971.

Chard, K. M., Resick, P. A., Monson, C. M., & Kattar, K. (2009). *Cognitive Processing Therapy: Group manual.* Washington, DC: U.S. Department of Veterans Affairs.

Chard, K. M., Weaver, T. L., & Resick, P. A. (1997). Adapting Cognitive Processing Therapy for child sexual abuse survivors. *Cognitive and Behavioral Practice, 4*, 31–52.

David, D., & Szentagotai, A. (2006). Cognitions in cognitive-behavioral psychotherapies: Toward an integrative model. *Clinical Psychology Review, 26*, 284–298.

Finkelhor, D., Ormrod, R. K., & Turner, H. A. (2007). Poly-victimization: A neglected component in child victimization. *Child Abuse & Neglect, 31*, 7–26.

Finkelhor, D., Turner, H. A., Ormrod, R. K., & Hamby, S. L. (2009, November). Violence, crime, and exposure in a national sample of children and youth. *Pediatrics, 124*(5).

Foa, E. B., Rothbaum, B., Riggs, D., & Murdock, T. (1991). Treatment of posttraumatic stress disorder in rape victims: A comparison between cognitive-behavioral procedures and counseling. *Journal of Consulting and Clinical Psychology, 59*, 715–723.

Girelli, S. A., Resick, P. A., Marhoefer-Dvorak, S., & Hutter, C. K. (1986). Subjective distress and violence during rape: Their effects on long-term fear. *Violence and Victims, 1*, 35–46.

Grave, J., & Blissett, J. (2004). Is cognitive behavior therapy developmentally appropriate for young children? A critical review of the evidence. *Clinical Psychology Review, 24*, 399–420.

Kazdin, A. E., Holland, L., & Crowley, M. (1997). Family experience of barriers to treatment and premature termination from child therapy. *Journal of Consulting and Clinical Psychology, 65*, 453–463.

Kazdin, A. E., & Weisz, J. R. (Eds.). (2003). *Evidence-based psychotherapies for children and adolescents.* New York, NY: Guilford Press.

Keane, T. M., & Kaloupek, D. G. (1982). Imaginal flooding in the treatment of a posttraumatic stress disorder. *Journal of Consulting and Clinical Psychology, 50*, 138–140.

Kendall, P. C. (Ed.). (2001). *Child and adolescent therapy: Cognitive-behavioral procedures* (2nd ed.). New York, NY: Guilford Press.

McCann, I. L., & Pearlman, L. A. (1990). *Psychological trauma and the adult survivor: Theory, therapy, and transformation.* New York, NY: Brunner/Mazel.

McCann, I. L., & Pearlman, L. A. (1992). Constructivist self-development theory: A theoretical framework for assessing and treating traumatized college students. *Journal of American College Health, 40*, 189–196.

McCann, I. L., Sakheim, D. K., & Abrahamson, D. J. (1988). Trauma and victimization: A model of psychological adaptation. *Counseling Psychologist, 16*, 531–594.

McIlvain, S. M., Walter, K. H., & Chard, K. M. (2013). Using Cognitive Processing Therapy–Cognitive in a residential treatment setting with an OIF veteran with PTSD and a history of severe traumatic brain injury: A case study. *Cognitive and Behavioral Practice, 20*, 375–382.

Monson, C. M. Schnurr, P. P., Resick, P. A., Friedman, M. J., Young-Xu, Y., & Stevens, S. P. (2006). Cognitive Processing Therapy for veterans with military-related posttraumatic stress disorder. *Journal of Consulting and Clinical Psychology, 74*, 898–907.

Resick, P. A., Galovski, T. E., Uhlmansiek, M. O., Scher, C. D., Clum, G. A., & Young-Xu, Y. (2008). A randomized clinical trial to dismantle components of Cognitive Processing Therapy for posttraumatic stress disorder in female victims of interpersonal violence. *Journal of Consulting and Clinical Psychology, 76*, 243–258.

Resick, P. A., Monson, C. M., & Chard, K. M. (2007). *Cognitive Processing Therapy: Veteran/military manual.* Washington, DC: U.S. Department of Veterans Affairs.

Resick, P. A., Nishith, P., Weaver, T. L., Astin, M. C., & Feuer, C. A. (2002). A comparison of Cognitive Processing Therapy with prolonged exposure therapy and a waiting list condition for the treatment of chronic posttraumatic stress disorder in female rape victims. *Journal of Consulting and Clinical Psychology, 70*, 867–879.

Resick, P. A., & Schnicke, M. K. (1992). Cognitive Processing Therapy for sexual assault victims. *Journal of Consulting and Clinical Psychology, 60*, 748–756.

Resick, P. A., & Schnicke, M. K. (1993). *Cognitive Processing Therapy for rape victims: A treatment manual.* Newberry Park, CA: Sage Publications.

Silverman, W. K., Ortiz, C. D., Viswesvaran, C., Burns, B. J., Kolko, D. J., Putnam, F. W., & Amaya-Jackson, L. (2008). Evidence-based psychosocial treatments for children and adolescents exposed to traumatic events. *Journal of Clinical Child and Adolescent Psychology, 37*, 156–183.

Stallard, P. (2002). Cognitive behaviour therapy with children and young people: A selective review of key issues. *Behavioural and Cognitive Psychotherapy, 30*, 297–309.

Stallard, P. (2006). Psychological interventions for post-traumatic reactions in children and young people: A review of randomized controlled trials. *Clinical Psychology Review, 26*(7), 895–911.

CARLA KMETT DANIELSON, PH.D.

16

Risk Reduction through Family Therapy

GENERAL CONSIDERATIONS

Susanna was 17 years old when she presented for therapy, two years after the last occasion on which an adult member of her extended family had sexually and physically abused her (abuse occurring over a several-year period). She rarely left her home any more—fearful of her anxiety symptoms and what she perceived to be a dangerous world around her. She used illicit drugs and misused prescription drugs multiple times a week, as she believed these substances exerted a powerful force in decreasing her nightmares and helping her cope with other posttraumatic stress disorder (PTSD) symptoms related to her child abuse experiences. Susanna's relationship with her mother was strained and conflictual. Susanna's mother, with her own trauma history and avoidant approach to coping with trauma-related symptoms, noted to the therapist in the first session that she had "no idea" what to do with her daughter. Susanna had quit school several months earlier, and she declaratively and hopelessly stated in her first therapy session, "I know I will never feel differently than I do today."

Unfortunately, Susanna's presentation was not atypical of teenagers who have experienced child sexual abuse (CSA) and other forms of trauma. In addition to avoidance, hyperarousal, and re-experiencing (the hallmark symptom clusters of PTSD), this population often also exhibits substance abuse and other forms of risky behavior, low distress tolerance, and family relationship problems—which have a cascading impact on everyday functioning and overall quality of life for these adolescents into adulthood. The purpose of this chapter is to describe a treatment specifically developed to help youths like Susanna—that is, to address the wide range of mental health problems extending from CSA and other forms of trauma—Risk Reduction through Family Therapy (RRFT). The chapter begins with a review of the

rationale for RRFT, and this is followed by a brief description of current research supporting the model's utility, an overview of RRFT and the theoretical underpinnings of its seven components and interventions, and a review of pretreatment conditions, including assessment. Each of the seven RRFT components is then described in greater detail. The chapter concludes with some suggestions on future directions for RRFT.

UNDERLYING RATIONALE

The journey through adolescence is bumpy for many. During this stage, individuals face various challenging developmental tasks, with puberty being among the most strenuous of undertakings. It is a time when young people straddle the roles and wishes of childhood and the responsibilities and desires of adulthood. Transitions through junior high, high school, and post-secondary education placements (e.g., college, armed forces, jobs) occur during this time. Relationships with caregivers become stressed and eventually evolve as adolescents struggle to establish their autonomy and independence. As a youth grows older, the peer group has an increasingly important role in the youth's decision making. Physiologically, many changes take place during adolescence, affecting body height and weight, hair growth, and genitalia. In addition, the adolescent brain continues to undergo change and development, which affects behavior and emotion. For example, the prefrontal cortex is the last area of the brain to complete development; change occurs in this region until a person reaches the mid-twenties. The prefrontal cortex functions as the brain's command center and governs self-regulation, such as interrupting a risky behavior, thinking before acting, and choosing among different courses of action. Changes in the prefrontal cortex during this developmental period cause decision making to shift toward brain regions that are governed more by emotional reactivity and seeking of "high reward," while behavioral inhibition is less developed. Consequently, adolescents are more likely to be impulsive and engage in risky ("high-reward") behaviors and environments.

Given that adolescents make this shift toward engagement in more high-reward-seeking behavior, it is not surprising that many young people experiment with alcohol and drugs during their adolescent years. According to the 2010 Monitoring the Future study, over 70% of adolescents had used alcohol, over 50% had been drunk, and almost 50% had used illicit drugs by the time they were in their senior year of high school (Johnston et al., 2011). Thus, the majority of youths engage in some form of substance use while in high school. Sexual activity is also normative among high school students, with approximately 40%–65% of students (varying by race/ethnicity) having sexual intercourse by their senior year (Centers for Disease Control and Prevention, 2010). Unfortunately, "normal experimentation" can cascade into engagement in problematic, risky behavior—behavior that interferes with daily tasks and overall functioning (e.g., truancy from school to get high with friends) and/or increases risk for more serious health problems (e.g., getting in a car with a drunk driver; having sex without a condom, increasing the risk for HIV and pregnancy).

Many risk and resiliency factors have been identified for substance use problems and risky sexual behaviors at each level of the ecological systems in which an adolescent exists (e.g., family activity level, peer group). Traumatic event experiences, and CSA in particular, are well-established risk factors for engagement in risky behaviors. Specifically, research clearly indicates that the estimated 2.8 million adolescents in the United States who are victims of CSA (Finkelhor et al., 2009) have an increased risk (compared with youths without CSA histories) for early initiation of substance use (e.g., Rothman et al., 2008), as well as alcohol and drug abuse disorders in adolescence (e.g., Clark & Bukstein, 1998; Kilpatrick et al., 2000) and in adulthood (e.g., Anthony & Petronis, 1995; Grant & Dawson, 1997). Risky sexual behaviors also have been strongly linked with CSA (Putnam, 2003), such as having multiple sexual partners (Randolph & Mosack, 2006) and lack of or inconsistent use of condoms (Noll, Trickett, & Putnam, 2000). Mood and anxiety symptoms and disorders (i.e., internalizing problems) among adolescents also result from CSA, with PTSD (Finkelhor et al., 2005) and major depression (Danielson et al., 2005) among the most prevalent. Comorbidity of internalizing problems and risky behaviors is common among adolescents who have experienced CSA (Danielson, Macdonald, et al., 2010). For example, epidemiological studies demonstrate that youths ages 12–17 years who have experienced CSA are over six times more likely to report comorbid PTSD and substance use disorders than those who do not report CSA (Kilpatrick et al., 2003).

The risk for CSA-related negative sequelae continues into the adult years (e.g., Danielson et al., 2009; McLean & Gallop, 2003); research with adult samples has consistently linked histories of CSA with significant mental health problems, physical health problems, and problems with everyday functioning (Noll, Trickett, & Putnam, 2000). In addition, CSA victims are at significant risk for sexual revictimization (Fergusson, Horwood, & Lynskey, 1997; Roodman & Clum, 2001). The effects of sexual revictimization are often deleterious and long-lasting because the psychological effects of interpersonal violence, including CSA, are cumulative (Messman-Moore & Long, 2003). Compared with non-revictimized individuals, revictimized individuals are more likely to meet the criteria for lifetime PTSD (Arata, 1999) and dissociative disorder (Cloitre, Scarvalone, & Difede, 1997), to experience higher levels of distress and anxiety (Messman-Moore & Long, 2000), and to demonstrate greater levels of high-risk sexual behavior and consequences, including unintended pregnancies and abortions (Wyatt, Guthrie, & Notgrass, 1992).

Alternatively, some youths report subsyndromal problems following CSA, meaning that they do not meet full diagnostic criteria (e.g., for PTSD) and/or are not yet abusing or dependent on substances. The literature suggests that these youths may be at an increased risk for delayed onset of trauma-related problems, including substance abuse, as well as sexual revictimization (as noted above). Thus, prevention and treatment efforts are still necessary to arm these youths with the skills necessary to cope with stressors in their adolescent life to reduce the risk of these problems.

Evidence-based treatments have been developed and evaluated for treating PTSD and depression among CSA victims through individual, office-based approaches (Trauma Focused-Cognitive Behavioral Therapy [TF-CBT]; Cohen et al., 2004) and among trauma-exposed immigrant youths through group, school-based approaches (Cognitive Behavioral Intervention for Trauma in Schools [CBITS]; Kataoka et al., 2003). Other evidence-based approaches were designed for reducing family violence and related aggressive behaviors and preserving in-home placement for families referred to child protective services for child physical abuse (Alternative for Families: A Cognitive Behavioral Therapy [AF-CBT; Kolko, 1996]; Multisystemic Therapy for Child Abuse and Neglect [MST-CAN; Swenson et al., 2010]). Although progress has been made in these areas—including treatment of CSA-related PTSD and depression—there are no rigorously evaluated integrated treatments for the heterogeneous and co-occurring problems extending from CSA among adolescents (e.g., substance use problems, risky sexual behaviors, low distress tolerance). Further, "risk reduction" options—approaches that bolster resiliency against these co-occurring, heterogeneous negative outcomes for subsyndromal adolescents—are needed. Research with trauma-exposed adults suggests that integrated approaches to the treatment of comorbid PTSD and substance use problems can be efficacious (Cocozza et al., 2005), particularly when they include exposure therapy (involving direct confrontation of feared memories, thoughts, feelings, situations) (Brady et al., 2001; Mills et al., 2012). Integrated intervention approaches for PTSD and substance use disorders that do not include exposure have had less robust findings (Hien et al., 2009; Najavits, Gallop, & Weiss, 2006). Prior to RRFT, no studies had been published on the efficacy of integrated approaches to risk reduction and treatment (that include exposure) for substance use problems and PTSD among adolescents. RRFT was developed as a direct result of that gap (Danielson, McCart, de Arellano, et al., 2010; Danielson, McCart, Walsh, et al., 2012).

RRFT is a risk reduction and treatment approach for adolescents with a history of CSA and other forms of trauma, integrating principles and interventions from existing empirically supported treatments (including exposure therapy) for adolescent substance use problems, PTSD, risky sexual behavior, and other negative sequelae. Preliminary data suggest that RRFT is feasibly delivered and potentially efficacious.

PRELIMINARY RESEARCH SUPPORT

Risk Reduction through Family Therapy is an integration of existing evidence-based interventions, with a primary emphasis on components of TF-CBT and principles of Multisystemic Therapy (MST; Henggeler et al., 2002). Both TF-CBT and MST have undergone rigorous evaluation (Cohen et al., 2004; Deblinger, et al., 2011; Henggeler et al., 2002). Yet, even though RRFT results from an integration of these previously evaluated interventions, it is imperative that the model go through its own rigorous evaluation (to illustrate its efficacy through multiple randomized controlled trials) for it to be designated an empirically supported treatment. The groundwork for its evaluation has been laid through the completion of two pilot clinical trials thus far (funded by the Brain and Behavior Research Foundation, through a NARSAD Young Investigator Award, and the National Institute on Drug Abuse).

As a brief overview (for details of these two studies, see Danielson, McCart, de Arellano, et al., 2010; Danielson, McCart, Walsh, et al., 2012), the feasibility of implementation and initial efficacy of RRFT were first evaluated through an open pilot trial with a small, diverse sample of 10 female adolescents (13–17 years old) who had experienced at least one memorable sexual assault (defined as unwanted/forced vaginal or anal penetration by an object, finger, or penis; oral sex; or touching of the genitalia) in their lifetime; 70% of the girls had experienced more than one incident of CSA and other forms of trauma. All participants received RRFT; symptoms were assessed at baseline, post-treatment, and at three- and six-month follow-up assessments, using psychometrically sound measures. Results from this open pilot trial showed that RRFT was feasibly implemented with adolescents and their caregivers in both office- and community-based settings. Significant treatment gains from pre- to post-treatment were found for substance use, substance use risk

(e.g., family conflict), PTSD, and depression. These improvements were maintained through the six-month post-treatment follow-up. The second study, a randomized controlled trial in which RRFT was compared with treatment as usual, was completed with a sample of 30 adolescents (12–17 years old) who had experienced a range of sexual assault events; again, 70% had experienced multi-victimizations and other forms of trauma. Assessment with psychometrically sound measures was completed at baseline, post-treatment, and three- and six-month follow-up time points. Feasibility findings from the open pilot study were replicated in this randomized controlled trial. In addition, significant within-subject treatment gains were found for substance use, substance use risk (i.e., family functioning), PTSD, depression, and risky sexual behaviors. With regard to between-group differences, RRFT outperformed treatment as usual in the following areas: substance use, substance use risk, (caregiver-reported) PTSD, depression, and general internalizing symptoms. Of note, there were no areas in which treatment as usual outperformed RRFT, and RRFT treatment gains were maintained through the six-month follow-up.

OVERVIEW AND THEORETICAL UNDERPINNINGS

As described above, RRFT includes and integrates components, skills, and principles from existing empirically supported treatments; these include TF-CBT, MST, Dialectical Behavioral Therapy (DBT; Linehan et al., 2006), Motivational Interviewing (Miller & Rollnick, 2002), and multiple psycho-education programs (e.g., SIHLE [DiClemente et al., 2004]; Sexual Revictimization Risk Reduction Program [Marx et al., 2001]). The interventions used in RRFT, then, are adapted and integrated from pragmatic, problem-focused treatments that have at least some empirical support. These typically include strategic family therapy, structural family therapy, behavioral parent training, and cognitive behavioral therapies. Through these interventions, risk factors are addressed and resiliency factors bolstered.

The seven primary treatment components of RRFT (Psychoeducation, Coping, Family Communication, Substance Abuse, PTSD, Healthy Dating and Sexual Decision Making, and Revictimization Risk Reduction) were developed from several theories. First and foremost, the treatment is based on ecological theory, which posits that each individual exists in the context of several systems (see figure 16.1). Thus, emphasis throughout the treatment is on intervening in multiple social systems, particularly the family and aspects of the youth's community (peer group, school, etc.). The treatment manual addresses how to create positive change or improvement in the family system, as well as other relevant systems, to reduce the risk for long-term problematic symptoms and behaviors. For each component of treatment, the therapist and family examine the risk and protective factors at each system level. The goal is to teach the youth and the caregivers to reduce risk factors by bol-

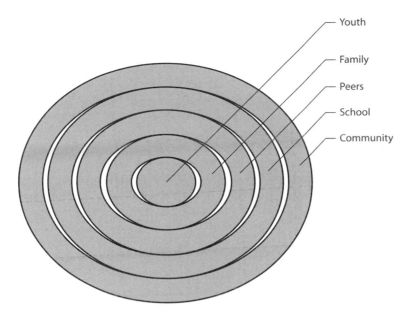

Youth
Family
Peers
School
Community

Figure 16.1. Ecological systems

stering protective factors. It is important to note here that culture cuts across all of these systems. That is, therapists are mindful of the cultural factors that may influence the treatment goals and the manner in which specific therapeutic skills are taught and learned.

Specific risk and resiliency factors for substance use problems (including initiation, use, and abuse) among adolescents are consistent with Ecological Systems Theory (Bronfenbrenner, 1979), which proposes that the individual, family, peer, school, and community environments (i.e., each level of a youth's ecology) play a role in psychological development (figure 16.1). This results in a heterogeneous array of possible risk reduction and treatment targets, such as individual maladaptive coping strategies (Carrigan et al., 2008), family conflict (Johnson & Pandina, 1991), low levels of participation in family activities (Lewis & Petry, 2005), association with substance-using peers (Guo et al., 2002), poor school attendance (Hallfors et al., 2002), and limited participation in positive, structured community activities (Mahoney & Stattin, 2000). Utilizing this ecological framework, interventions can alter or reduce these risk factors while bolstering resiliency factors.

Second, RRFT applies Mowrer's Two-Factor Theory, in which fear is thought to be acquired through a classical conditioning process by which the individual pairs a neutral stimulus (e.g., the dark) with a stimulus that invokes a fear response (e.g., sexual assault) such that the neutral stimulus elicits the fear response in the absence of the feared stimulus (being anxious in the dark when no sexual assault is occurring). Change occurs through exposure therapy in which individuals are able to diminish a fear response when they are exposed to the feared stimulus (the dark) without the feared aversive consequences (the sexual assault). Based on its adaptation from TF-CBT, RRFT includes gradual exposure therapy with adolescent sexual assault victims who have PTSD symptoms, through the de-

velopment of a detailed written or oral account of the CSA experiences and other potentially traumatic events ("trauma narrative"). As part of this exposure-based trauma narrative work, the therapist also uses cognitive behavioral therapy, helping adolescents identify and replace inaccurate and/or unhelpful beliefs they have developed and/or attributed to the CSA (e.g., "I am damaged goods"). Skills building in the area of coping (e.g., emotional reactivity) is an important preamble to the exposure work and is accomplished by teaching distress tolerance skills, relaxation, and so on. In addition to the use of exposure principles in the context of internal anxiety sensations related to PTSD, exposure can be used with emotional and somatic cues to help improve distress tolerance and to decrease potential drug use cravings as well. Thus, RRFT also involves identifying then exposing adolescents to the emotional and external cues related to their substance use behaviors, as well as trauma-related symptoms.

Third, the connection between substance use and trauma-related symptoms can be conceptualized in the context of negative reinforcement theory (Baker et al., 2004), which posits that escape and avoidance of negative affect (in this case, trauma-related distress) is the primary motive for addictive drug use. This is also referred to as the "self-medicating hypothesis." A decrease in trauma-related substance use is thought to occur with improvements in self-regulation deficits that are affected by childhood trauma (e.g., Hien, Cohen, & Campbell, 2005), such as emotional reactivity and tolerance. Thus, RRFT focuses on improving these skills through the Coping and PTSD components. Finally, psychoeducation and skills-building approaches are incorporated to address risky sexual behaviors and revictimization risk.

Extending from this theoretical framework (Ecological Theory in particular), the RRFT model follows the nine principles that guide MST, as summarized here.

1. "Finding the fit" is used to understand how identified problems "make sense" in the context of the youth's social ecology. In RRFT, the clinician works with the adolescent and family members to better understand what aspects of the youth's environment are driving problematic symptoms and behaviors (e.g., school serves as a cue for traumatic memories and hence drug cravings).

2. The "positive and strength focused" approach emphasizes the strengths and protective factors of the adolescent, family, school, peer group, and community as a strategy for making positive changes and treatment gains, and it serves to instill feelings of hope, decrease negative affect, and enhance the youth's and caregiver's confidence in themselves and in treatment. The RRFT clinician helps the adolescent and family build on existing protective factors (e.g., more consistently employing existing positive coping strategies in response to problems; increasing the number of family dinners).

3. "Increasing responsibility" emphasizes the use of interventions that encourage responsible behavior (decrease irresponsible behavior) by the youth and caregivers, rather than pathologizing the behavior. For example, in RRFT, substance use (by the adolescent and/or by the caregiver) is discussed in the context of making responsible versus irresponsible choices, rather than as unethical or immoral behavior.

4. The "present-focused, action-oriented, and well-defined" approach dictates that interventions administered in RRFT target specific and clearly defined behaviors and problems (e.g., "increase compliance with the family curfew rule" rather than "not being disrespectful at home"), which also aids the RRFT clinician in setting well-defined conditions for treatment termination.

5. "Targeting sequences" maintains that the RRFT clinician will work with the adolescent and caregivers to identify the sequence of behaviors across multiple systems that results in (or reinforces) the problematic symptoms and behaviors (e.g., the series of events and interactions that led up to and followed an episode of nonsuicidal cutting) and will work at improving the youth's interactions with his or her environment to increase healthy coping and responsible behavior.

6. A "developmentally appropriate" approach ensures that the RRFT clinician considers the developmental needs of the adolescent when selecting interventions, as well as the skills necessary to transition successfully to adulthood (e.g., ensuring that youths who have quit school identify and actively pursue alternative education or vocation options).

7. "Continuous effort" means that consistent and unremitting commitment is expected from the RRFT clinician, adolescent, and family members, to translate into more rapid progress on treatment goals and problem resolution and hence more opportunities for individual/family members to experience success. Although RRFT does not employ a 24/7 model (as in MST), the principle of continuous effort may involve going to a person's home to meet with family members, helping with case management issues (e.g., arranging for financial assistance for the family or making other appropriate referrals), engaging in more phone "check-ins" throughout the week (e.g., to determine whether a skill addressed in treatment is being employed as discussed and to provide corrective feedback as relevant), or having more than one session a week, particularly at the beginning of treatment. The latter two suggestions are particularly emphasized with adolescents and families experiencing a more severe level of problems—and are dependent on the structure and flexibility of a given clinician's treatment facility.

8. "Evaluation and accountability" means that RRFT clinicians and supervisors assume accountability for continuously evaluating the effectiveness of the implemented interventions and are ultimately responsible for positive treatment outcomes for the adolescent and the family (rather than labeling the youth as "not ready").

9. "Generalization" helps clinicians stay focused on the goal of maintaining long-term improvement by empowering the youth and family members to do most of the "work" in therapy. In other words, the adolescent and family members serve as the key to success over time.

As with TF-CBT, MST, and other evidence-based treatments, the RRFT model is meant to be flexible and to demand that each therapist use his or her own creativity in the method used to teach therapeutic skills to new clients. Overall, it is recommended that pre-treatment conditions be met before administering the main treatment components. Also, it is highly recommended that the Psychoeducation and Coping modules be administered before beginning exposure work in the PTSD component. However, certain components can be administered in a flexible order (such as Substance Abuse, Healthy Dating and Sexual Decision Making). Certainly, with youths who actively use substances, the clinician will want to deliver the Substance Abuse component early in treatment. Further, the length of treatment will vary, depending on the type and severity of symptoms and level of engagement of the adolescent and family members.

IMPORTANT PRE-TREATMENT CONDITIONS

Assessment

Baseline assessment is essential not only to understand pre-treatment functioning but also to determine which treatment components will be administered and in which order (depending on severity). Comprehensive guidelines and descriptions of trauma assessment have been published elsewhere (e.g., de Arellano & Danielson, 2008). In brief, a thorough and behaviorally specific assessment of the following should take place prior to treatment: characteristics and history of the traumatic event incident, for the adolescent and participating family members/caregivers; psychiatric symptomatology (with a specific focus on PTSD and other anxiety disorders and depression); substance use behaviors and consequences; sexual behaviors; family functioning;

school functioning; and current pleasant activities and hobbies. Special attention should be paid to developing timelines of when CSA experiences—and other forms of traumatic experiences—occurred. This information should be gathered through clinical interview, self-report measures, and caregiver report measures. Suggested measures include the UCLA PTSD Reaction Index (both adolescent and parent-report versions; Steinberg et al., 2004), the Children's Depression Inventory (Kovacs, 1983), and the Family Environment Scale (Moos & Moos, 1986). To get an accurate assessment of substance use behaviors, a Timeline Followback survey (e.g., Sobell & Sobell, 1996) is recommended (for the past ~90 days, such as Form 90), in which the youth uses a calendar to identify which specific drugs (e.g., alcohol, marijuana, cocaine) were used, on which dates, and the quantity used on those dates. Urine screens also should be gathered to corroborate self-report of substance use.

In addition to the standardized measures, RRFT clinicians complete an RRFT intake interview with each adolescent and caregiver at the beginning of treatment. This form provides a semi-structured framework for collection of information about the adolescent's sexual assault experiences, other traumatic event exposure, mental health symptoms and substance use, family constellation and history, and risk and protective factors in the youth's and family's ecology (school, community, peer group, etc.).

Socratic Approach to Enhance Engagement as Needed

Not all youths enter treatment wanting to reduce their substance use behaviors or risky sexual behaviors or wanting to engage in exposure therapy to reduce PTSD symptoms (e.g., due to avoidance). Some may be brought to treatment by caregivers, against their will, and some may be mandated to enter treatment by the Department of Social Services or the judicial system. In these instances, the first priority is to engage the adolescent and caregiver at the start of treatment. "Buy-in" from the clients will increase their adherence to treatment and decrease the likelihood of premature termination. Specific suggestions for engagement strategies are provided in the Psychoeducation component of the manual (as well as in the PTSD component, as a method of engaging the avoidant youth in exposure work). In addition to these strategies, a Socratic approach can be used (e.g., asking very specific questions to increase clients' reflection on the positive and negative aspects of their engagement in target problematic behaviors) to help motivate behavior change in these youths (see Miller & Rollnick, 2002).

The Socratic approach to increase motivation may involve the following: (1) Ask the client to rate her motivation for wanting to change a behavior or engage in treatment to improve symptoms (e.g., on a scale from 1 to 10, with 10 being the highest level of motivation and 1 being no interest in changing). (2) Based on the response to question 1, focus on any positive rating of motivation (i.e., anything rated above 1). For example, with a rating of 3, ask, "Why not a 2

or a 1?" (3) Use Socratic questioning to encourage the client to describe the pros and cons (in his own words) of engaging in a problematic behavior or maintaining a symptom versus what change would look like. For example, "Tell me more about what you like about getting high. What are the 'good parts' about it?" Following the youth's response, say, "Sounds like you feel like there are a few reasons you choose to get high. Now I would like to hear about the not-so-good parts. Tell me about some of the reasons you would consider cutting back or stopping smoking weed." Either orally repeat or reflect on the client's responses or use a large notepad or dry-erase board to write out the client's responses in two columns. Given how adolescents may learn best, keeping therapy (and pre-treatment activities) as active and interactive as possible is a useful tool. The Socratic approach to increase motivation may be used throughout RRFT as needed—when the adolescent or family members express ambivalence or resistance to the session content or previously stated treatment goals.

Stabilization Period

Adolescents who have experienced CSA may have a history of other traumatic events and may be living in a chaotic environment. For some of these adolescents and families, it may be important to have a period of stabilization before beginning the primary treatment components. This may include briefly teaching skills that will be more heavily emphasized later in treatment, such as setting family rules and/or teaching communication skills. Referrals for medication, housing, or other important areas of need may be necessary at this time. It is important that basic housing and safety needs be met before beginning RRFT. These issues are discussed and monitored throughout the treatment in conjunction with the RRFT supervisor.

TREATMENT

To summarize the description thus far, RRFT is an intervention developed to reduce the risk of substance abuse and other high-risk behaviors and of trauma-related psychopathology in adolescents who have been sexually assaulted. RRFT capitalizes on identification of empirically demonstrated risk and resiliency factors for substance abuse and trauma-related psychopathology within an ecological framework. The RRFT therapist works with each family to address risk factors (e.g., improve parental monitoring) and to bolster protective factors (e.g., increase the number of non-substance-using peers and structured, positive activities) at each level of a youth's ecology (individual, family, peer, school, and community). The culture of the adolescent and the family is assessed throughout treatment and incorporated into each intervention, as appropriate.

The manual targets seven primary, overlapping components: Psychoeducation, Coping, Family Communication, Substance Abuse, PTSD, Healthy Dating and Sexual Decision

Making, and Revictimization Risk Reduction. For the Substance Abuse and PTSD components, the therapist has the option of taking a prevention approach or a treatment approach, depending on the symptoms of the adolescent and family. The content and skills addressed in each component are derived from empirically supported interventions (e.g., contingency management for substance abuse symptoms, exposure therapy for PTSD symptoms). The goal within the components is to reduce risk factors and bolster resiliency factors that exist for each individual youth at each level of her or his ecology (figure 16.1). Table 16.1 provides a

brief overview of the content addressed in each component, including the difference between content delivered in the treatment versus prevention approach in the PTSD and Substance Abuse components. The order in which the components are administered is determined by the needs of the youth and family and is based on the severity of the problems. Exposure therapy, in the form of a written or oral trauma narrative, is implemented through the PTSD component for adolescents reporting three or more PTSD symptoms. For youths reporting minimal PTSD symptoms, prevention information is provided. On average, the RRFT

Table 16.1. Components and Content of Risk Reduction through Family Therapy

Component	Content
Psychoeducation	• Provide information about (1) prevalence of sexual assault and other forms of traumatic events; (2) reactions to such traumatic events; (3) the relation between substance use and other risky behaviors and trauma-related psychopathology. • Discuss family focus of treatment; set family rules and treatment goals. • Introduce RRFT treatment model and components. • Emphasize importance of regular attendance and consistent participation.
Family Communication	• Review/establish family rules (chores, curfews, substance use, etc.), including privileges earned for following rules and consequences for not adhering to rules. Adolescent and siblings are actively engaged in this process. • Skills building in (1) active listening; (2) effective speaking (e.g., use of "I" statements, use of nonblaming language, reduction of caregiver "over-explaining"/lecturing vs. interaction discussion). • Role-play "hotspots": reoccurring arguments in the household (what typically happens, and then replaying with new skills taught).
Coping	• Provide an overview of helpful vs. unhelpful coping. • Skills building in (1) feelings identification and expression; (2) relaxation techniques; (3) distress-tolerance skills building; (4) understanding the connection between thoughts, feelings, and behaviors; (5) thought changing; (6) problem solving.
Substance Abuse	*Treatment:* Determination of specific risk factors that appear to be motivating the youth's substance use and development of interventions surrounding these factors, with the adolescent and caregiver, such as: • Contingency management (use of rewards and consequences as tied to random drug tests and breathalyzers). • Increase in caregiver and school monitoring (e.g., helping parent modify work schedule). • Increase in participation in positive, monitored, community-based activities (e.g., YMCA, church youth group, school sports or clubs, part-time to full-time jobs), so as to increase opportunities for meeting nonusing peers and to find fun activities to replace substance-related activities. • Realistic refusal skills. • Completion of the PTSD component (e.g., when a motivating factor for substance use is related to avoidance of trauma-related memories and feelings). • Harm reduction approach for youths who are ambivalent about ceasing use, to get "foot in the door" and movement toward change. *Prevention:* Reduction of present risk factors for substance use and increase in resiliency factors (see figure 16.1 for example).
PTSD	*Treatment:* • Review of PTSD symptoms. • Exposure to trauma-related memories and cues, and addressing inaccurate and unhelpful beliefs about trauma through creation of trauma narrative. • Sharing trauma narrative with family members. *Prevention:* • Skills building in recognition of future potential PTSD symptoms, particularly avoidance. • How to address avoidance behaviors.
Healthy Dating and Sexual Decision Making	• Interactive discussion and skills building in (1) healthy vs. unhealthy relationships; (2) factors considered when engaging in sexual activity (e.g., how participant decides how far to go with a partner); (3) psychoeducation on sexually transmitted diseases, particularly HIV, and consistent condom use; (4) role-playing of assertiveness in dating (e.g., insistence on condom use); (5) importance of ongoing communication between adolescent and caregiver on these topics.
Revictimization Risk Reduction	• Psychoeducation on risk for revictimization. • Identification of risky situations, people, and places (e.g., review of scenarios of risky situations and role-playing of how to respond in these situations).

Source. Danielson, McCart, et al., 2010.

protocol is administered through weekly 60- to 90-minute sessions. However, therapists are encouraged to do phone check-ins with families between sessions, particularly when new skills have been taught, when contingency management and/or caregiver monitoring plans are first implemented for substance use or other risky behaviors (e.g., cutting), when the family is experiencing a crisis, and when a trauma narrative (i.e., exposure) has begun in session. Suggested check-outs are provided for therapists to assist in evaluating whether an adolescent and/or family member has mastered the skills taught in a specific component. For example, a suggested check-out for the Healthy Dating and Sexual Decision Making component involves demonstrating age-appropriate and adaptive decision-making skills in a scripted scenario.

The duration of treatment depends on the youth's symptom level; average length of treatment for youths who received RRFT in the randomized controlled trial described earlier was 24 sessions. When feasible and applicable, individual sessions and briefer, joint family sessions are conducted each week. However, if family members are not available for in-person sessions, phone-based check-ins are implemented. As noted earlier, therapy can be provided in either an office-based format or a community-based, outreach format.

Psychoeducation

Although the order in which the RRFT components are administered is flexible, it is generally recommended that the clinician begin with the Psychoeducation component. This is because the information shared and skills covered in this component serve as a cornerstone for the other RRFT components. Psychoeducation in RRFT parallels the psychoeducation component of TF-CBT, with an additional focus on adolescent risky behavior, engagement of the adolescent, the family system, and goal setting with the adolescent and each participating family member. As in all seven of the RRFT components, the focus is on the accomplishment of specified goals, rather than the specific procedures used to accomplish those goals. In other words, the clinician may use a range of creative strategies and approaches in this component as a method of achieving several goals.

The first goal is to ensure that the adolescent and all participating family members have an accurate and consistent understanding of how confidentiality will be handled throughout the course of treatment, including how sensitive information that does not meet the legal mandate for disclosure will be handled with regard to communication between the adolescent and caregivers. This is particularly important in RRFT, where substance use is constantly monitored and other risky behavior is discussed (e.g., sexual behavior, nonsuicidal self-injurious behavior). The objective is to have open and ongoing communication between the adolescent and caregivers on these various sensitive topics; however, this objective will probably require an evolving

process during treatment and may not always be feasible or therapeutic in all cases. Thus, suggested language in response to questions from the adolescent about the relaying of sensitive information to caregivers is as follows:

My job is to help you reach the goals you have set for us to accomplish in treatment together, as well as to help try and keep you safe. As we have discussed previously, there are some legal limits to the confidentiality of what you tell me, such as you telling me someone is hurting you or your having serious thoughts about hurting yourself. Beyond that there may be something that you tell me that would make it very difficult for me to help you reach your treatment goals *or* for me to be able to help keep you safe without discussing it with your caregiver. What I can promise you is that, if you choose to tell me—which I hope you do because it sounds like it is important to you— you and I will discuss together whether it makes sense to share this information with your [caregiver]. If after discussing it, I ultimately decide this is something important for your [caregiver] to know, I will let you be the one to tell [him or her] if you so choose and I won't disclose anything to [him or her] without telling you about it first.

The second goal of the Psychoeducation component is to achieve buy-in from the family regarding the rationale for the family focus of treatment. RRFT adopts a broad definition of "family," with the recognition that not all adolescents have parents who are able or willing to participate in treatment. Thus, beyond biological, adoptive, and step-parents, the clinician may consider extended family members, foster parents, residential treatment staff, or other champions for the youth (i.e., individuals from the adolescent's ecological systems that have the capacity to participate and be supportive) as "family members" to participate in treatment (see also the Family Communication component of the manual).

As a third goal of this component, the RRFT clinician uses data collected from the RRFT intake form and other assessment measures that may have been administered with the family (as noted earlier) to provide factual information about the youth's traumatic event experiences and trauma-related symptoms. Specifically, this includes information on the prevalence of CSA and other traumatic events experienced by the adolescent and the normalization of various incident characteristics of these events (e.g., relationship to the perpetrator; frequency of involvement of drugs and/or alcohol in abuse/assault; lack of support from peer group being more traumatic than the assault experience itself). In addition, the clinician provides a description of the specific mental health symptoms, substance use problems, risky sexual behavior, and other concerns disclosed by the adolescent and family at the intake, with an emphasis on normalizing these reactions to trauma and improving an understanding of how the CSA is related to the youth's symptoms. Unique to RRFT, the therapist reviews with the family specific risk and protective factors for substance use and other target problems identified in the ecological assessment (via the RRFT intake form), as certain environmental interventions may be implemented immediately as a result of this assessment. For example, if low parental monitoring was identified as a risk factor for a client's acute substance use problems, part of the Psychoeducation session would be used to problem-solve alternative options to improve monitoring.

Another important task to accomplish in the Psychoeducation component is providing the family with an overview of the RRFT model, including the components and skills that will be covered over the duration of treatment and the expectations for the adolescent and participating family members. This overview of the model is crucial, as it will provide an opportunity to explore barriers to treatment engagement, participation, and completion. For example, it provides an opportunity for the RRFT clinician to troubleshoot issues with a caregiver's work schedule when discussing the importance of his or her regular participation in therapy sessions and phone check-ins. Perhaps the most important goal of the Psychoeducation component in RRFT is the setting of treatment goals for the adolescent and for each participating family member—in each person's own words. These short-term goals should be described in terms of what the adolescent (and then the caregiver, etc.) would like to be different in his life following the completion of treatment (which may also include the discussion of goals 5 or 10 years down the road).

In RRFT, the adolescent completes a goal sheet, prompting him to think about areas for change in mood, behavior, family, friends, school, and so on. Goals may include increasing privileges (e.g., a later curfew) or removing punishments or may be as simple as "not having to come to therapy any more." This goal setting is imperative, as the therapist will use it as the "carrot" (i.e., incentive) to engage the adolescent and family members in each session, tying it into the rationale for each intervention implemented and each skill taught in RRFT.

Family Communication

As noted above, the definition of "family" used in RRFT is broad. Ideally, target family members will include caregivers with whom the adolescent lives and/or regularly interacts. Consistent with MST principles, the RRFT clinician adopts a "whatever it takes" approach in attempting to engage such caregivers. However, under circumstances where it is not feasible or therapeutic for the adolescent to have a primary caregiver involved in treatment, the adolescent and clinician work together to identify alternative family members or champions for the youth that exist in her ecology (e.g., extended family members, teachers, other residential treatment staff members). Even in the rare instances when no one can be identified to participate in family sessions, family work can still be completed with the adolescent, as the adolescent will benefit from learning how to effectively communicate with others in her ecology, usu-

ally including family members (and perhaps especially when family members are unsupportive or too overwhelmed to participate directly in sessions).

The goals of the Family Communication component are to assess the culture of the family environment regarding the communication of affect (positive and negative) and to provide a rationale for the importance of being able to communicate about negative feelings and stressful events; to teach effective and healthy family communication skills, such as active listening; to set clear, consistent, behaviorally specific family rules (including privileges earned or maintained for following family rules, as well as consequences for not following family rules); and to role-play problem solving of common "hotspots" for each particular family. Of note, many families entering RRFT begin treatment with strained relationships and problematic communication patterns that probably have been reinforced over time (e.g., avoidance, aggression). Thus, preparation for these family sessions includes first meeting with the adolescent and the caregiver individually and preparing them well for the joint session in which family rules and communication skills will be discussed. Ideally, the clinician aims to "set up the session for success," which means getting both parties to agree to specific and desired privileges, consequences, and compromises prior to meeting together as a family.

The Family Communication component, in particular the setting of family rules, often provides an opportunity to help work toward treatment goals set by the adolescent and the caregiver. For example, if an adolescent has identified a later curfew as a treatment goal, the clinician can suggest including this as a contingency for following other family rules, such as clean urine screens, active participation in RRFT treatment, and daily school attendance. In addition, while the family does not directly communicate about the CSA and other traumatic event experiences in this component (prior to the PTSD component and trauma narrative work), Family Communication (through role plays, family activities, etc.) provides ecologically valid scenarios to practice talking through stressful situations that may be unpleasant to address initially but become easier to discuss as communication and coping skills are taught and applied and further refined.

Coping

The Coping component, which includes and builds on the relaxation, affect regulation, and cognitive processing components of TF-CBT, focuses on building a "toolbox" of coping skills for the adolescent. Not only does the youth learn to build the toolbox by learning and experimenting with different types of coping skills in session and as part of therapy homework, but it is also imperative for the youth to recognize when and in which contexts or situations to apply various adaptive coping skills. Similarly, in the Coping component, caregivers learn the same coping skills as part of their treatment, such that they can model the use of these skills themselves and provide reminders and positive reinforcement for the youth's use of the skills outside the therapy session. Examples of the coping skills targeted are feelings identification and expression; distress tolerance (i.e., learning to "sit with" and accept negative affect that is overwhelming to the youth); and the challenging of inaccurate and unhelpful thoughts and beliefs in everyday situations and as they apply to presenting problems other than PTSD (e.g., an argument with mom; a good friend offering drugs).

Common strategies taught in this component include (1) mindfulness, so as to increase awareness of feelings and mood on a day-to-day (and hour-to-hour) basis, including potential physiological early warning signs of the onset of strong negative affect; (2) highly descriptive guided imagery of a "safe and happy" place for the adolescent to go to in his mind at any time; (3) integration of activities that the adolescent enjoys as a strategy for coping with negative feelings (e.g., listening to music, playing sports); and (4) creation of a crisis survival kit. The concept behind the crisis survival kit (often used in DBT) is that the adolescent may find it challenging to remember to employ positive coping when in an acutely distressed state. Thus, cues and reminders (and tangible items) for the application of coping strategies that have the likelihood of providing immediate acceptance and/or relief of stress—particularly strategies that use the five senses—are placed in a central, easily accessible location (e.g., a blanket that is soothing to touch; a lotion that is soothing to smell). Caregivers can then remind their child about the availability of the crisis survival kit in an escalating (emotionally distressing) situation. The Coping component can be particularly empowering when learning CBT concepts and strategies—learning that the individual has the power to change the way he feels and behaves in a given situation simply by modifying how he thinks about that situation. As in TF-CBT, RRFT clinicians are encouraged to be creative in teaching this concept, such as through books and movies enjoyable to the adolescent. RRFT clinicians also discuss maladaptive patterns of coping observed in the youth, such as substance abuse and risky sexual behavior, and review how this relates to his traumatic event experiences.

Substance Abuse

The Substance Abuse component in RRFT aims to help the adolescent and caregiver to (1) understand the potential link between the youth's substance use and her traumatic event history; (2) identify various individual and environmental (system-level) factors that are directly contributing to the substance use and to reduce these risk factors, as well as bolster protective factors within the systems accordingly; (3) identify cues for the drug use cravings and alternatives to substance use in response to those cravings; (4) enhance communication between the adolescent and caregiver regarding substance use and to aid the caregiver in providing positive reinforcements (e.g., privileges) for clean drug screens and breathalyzer tests indicating no al-

cohol use; and (5) teach the adolescent realistic drug refusal skills. This component draws heavily on the strategies used in MST, the primary one being the use of "fit circles" in determining which circumstances and variables are driving problematic behavior and symptoms. Each circumstance or variable thought to play a role in maintaining the substance-using behavior is labeled a "driver" and listed on paper. The primary one or two drivers are selected, and more detailed fit circles are drawn to determine which factors are serving to drive that particular problematic behavior or circumstance. Targeted interventions are then identified to tackle each driver. See figure 16.2 for an example.

Throughout treatment (and not solely when specifically targeting the Substance Abuse component), RRFT clinicians are encouraged to briefly assess a client's substance use over the past week or since the last session, using a Timeline Followback calendar format (as described in the Assessment section). For each using day, the clinician is also encouraged to ask the client whether or not she believes the substance use was related to her traumatic event experience. This information will help in monitoring the progress of treatment of substance abuse symptoms, as well as increase the client's awareness of the interconnectedness among comorbid symptoms, including the targeted sequence of events that may lead to poor choices with regard to substance use (i.e., marijuana use that follows exposure to a CSA cue).

PTSD

Central to the PTSD component is the development of a trauma narrative, in which the youth creates a book or other outlet to describe the details of his CSA experience(s) and his thoughts and feelings surrounding these traumatic events. The therapist works to gradually desensitize the client (and caregivers) to distress associated with these cues,

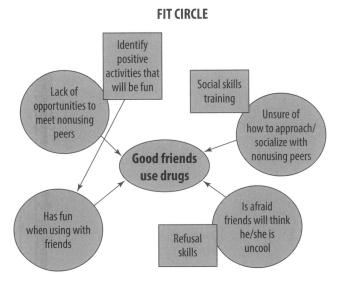

FIT CIRCLE

Figure 16.2. A sample fit circle, for a case in which a youth's peer group is determined to be a primary driver for the youth's substance abuse

memories, and feelings (i.e., gradual exposure). Once the narrative has been developed, and there is evidence that the youth has successfully managed his distress in response to writing and talking about the trauma, unhelpful and/or inaccurate beliefs developed as a result of the CSA and other traumas are discussed, with the goal of shifting these thoughts and beliefs to be more accurate and helpful. The client is then given an opportunity to make positive meaning by delineating what he has learned from the trauma event experiences. In the final stages of the trauma narrative process, the youth shares his narrative with the caregiver, when the caregiver is able to be supportive of the youth. The process for developing the trauma narrative is described elsewhere, as a major component of TF-CBT (see Cohen et al., 2006). Specific to RRFT, clinicians monitor the adolescent's substance use throughout the course of treatment—and during trauma narrative development in particular, to ensure that substance use is not being maintained or exacerbated as a means of coping through any feelings of distress related to creating the trauma narrative. Further, RRFT clinicians employ a range of creative, developmentally sensitive ideas for engaging the adolescent in gradual exposure work, as avoidance and hesitation are common among adolescent populations.

Healthy Dating and Sexual Decision Making

In this component, the therapist works with adolescents and caregivers to understand how exposure to sexual activity at an early age can affect sexual development and decision making in adolescence. The RRFT treatment goal for this component is to develop healthy sexuality and to help ensure that the youth has a healthy self-concept such that she can make the dating decisions she wants to, including keeping herself safe now and in adulthood. Body safety and self-care are important elements of this component. However, decreasing risky sexual behavior also must extend to what underlies the decision making in dating and sexual situations for these adolescents. This is accomplished in various ways in the RRFT session, including provision of corrective, healthy, age-appropriate information on sex and romantic relationships. Also, themes of inaccurate and unhelpful beliefs stemming from CSA often involve problems with trust and intimacy ("I feel alone, but having sex with this person will make me feel loved and close to him"). Thus, processing of the trauma narrative with youths who hold these inaccurate and unhelpful beliefs may indirectly address risky sexual behavior ("Having sex will not make me feel loved; there are better ways for me to feel connected with a person"). Other methods of enhancing protective factors against risky sexual behavior include providing psychoeducation about sexually transmitted diseases, HIV, and pregnancy so that the youth and caregiver are aware of the risks; discussing the youth's 5- and 10-year goals and whether current sexual decision making is consistent or inconsistent with those goals; teaching assertive negotiation skills in romantic relationships, with particular emphasis on the skills to insist on condom use; and teaching the correct method of putting on a condom (for sexually active teens). Finally, establishing open communication between youth and caregivers about sex and dating, when possible, is an important focus.

Revictimization Risk Reduction

The Revictimization component is typically administered last and can be considered a form of relapse prevention. Based on evidence-based sexual revictimization risk reduction programs (Marx et al., 2001), this component involves enhancing an adolescent's ability to recognize signals indicating risky people, places, and situations and teaching practical skills in how to handle being in these various situations. Risky scenarios are described in session, and the clinician can work with the client to improve attendance to various clues that a person or situation may not be safe. In addition, the therapist discusses the concept of sexual coercion, with a particular emphasis on how previously inaccurate and/or unhelpful core beliefs may have affected decision making in previous sexual situations—and may continue to affect decision making if the core beliefs have not been fully processed. For example, adolescents who hold core beliefs such as "I am unlovable," "I am not worthwhile," or "People won't like me unless I do what they ask" may be more susceptible to sexual coercion. In addition, the clinician discusses Internet safety (from a sexual predator standpoint) with clients and caregivers. If all RRFT components have been successfully completed, therapy typically terminates at the end of this component.

SUPERVISION

RRFT supervision aids in ensuring fidelity to the model and guides the clinician in making various treatment decisions, such as choosing the order of the seven components (e.g., whether Family Communication should be prioritized over Coping), troubleshooting engagement issues with the family, and deciding when disclosures about risky behavior should be made known to caregivers. Also, given that listening to the details of various traumatic events can weigh heavily on clinicians at times, RRFT supervision provides an opportunity for supervisors to help support clinicians in this process. Ideally, preparation for supervision is completed prior to the RRFT supervision session through completion of the RRFT supervision form. Specifically, clinicians complete a structured form in which they report which component(s) were targeted in a particular therapy session (with the adolescent and then with other participating family members); list which treatment goals were of focus; and draw fit circles to illustrate either overall case conceptualization (following the intake session) or conceptualization of a problem targeted for a particular session, including interventions being implemented in response to the various drivers identified. Finally, the supervision form provides space for the clinician to list questions for supervision. One form should be completed for each client to be discussed in supervision.

CONCLUSIONS AND FUTURE DIRECTIONS

Risk Reduction through Family Therapy is a theoretically driven, comprehensive model for the treatment and risk reduction of substance abuse problems, PTSD, risky sexual behaviors, and other adverse mental health outcomes among adolescents who have experienced child sexual abuse and other forms of trauma. Results from a small open pilot trial and a small randomized controlled trial suggest the feasibility of RRFT and resulting treatment gains in substance use, family functioning, PTSD, depression, and risky sexual behaviors (in comparison with baseline functioning), which were maintained six months after treatment was completed. In addition, contrary to clinical lore but consistent with similar findings in adult populations, there was no evidence in these trials that engaging in exposure-based therapy (i.e., direct discussion of CSA and other forms of trauma) led to iatrogenic effects with regard to substance use. Clearly, more research is needed to establish the efficacy of this treatment. A large-scale randomized controlled trial, funded by the National Institute on Drug Abuse (principal investigator C. K. Danielson), is underway to further evaluate the utility of RRFT. The hope is that RRFT will ultimately improve clinical practice by offering a more efficient alternative to the current compartmentalized approach to treatment for this population (which often involves referrals to multiple agencies; e.g., Cocozza et al., 2005), as well as providing a risk reduction option for youths who are at elevated risk for developing substance abuse and related mental health problems in the future but are not currently meeting diagnostic thresholds. This was certainly the case for Susanna (the client presented at the beginning of the chapter), who completed treatment and follow-up assessments substance-free, without clinically significant PTSD symptoms, and with a more cohesive relationship with her mother. In addition and most importantly, Susanna reported finding meaning in life again and hope for the future—a cornerstone of effective risk reduction by any standard.

Acknowledgments

The research reported in this chapter was supported by a grant (K23DA018686) from the National Institute on Drug Abuse (NIDA; PI: C. K. Danielson) and a Young Investigator Award from NARSAD (PI: Danielson). Preparation of the manuscript was supported by a grant (R01DA031285) from NIDA (PI: Danielson) and a grant (P50 AA010761) from the National Institute on Alcohol Abuse and Alcoholism (NIAAA; PI of Center: H. Becker; PI of Clinical Component 5: Danielson). The views, policies, and opinions expressed in this chapter are those of the author and do not necessarily reflect those of NIDA, NIAAA, or NARSAD.

References

Anthony, J. C., & Petronis, K. R. (1995). Early-onset drug use and risk of later drug problems. *Drug and Alcohol Dependence, 40*(1), 9–15.

Arata, C. M. (1999). Coping with rape: The roles of prior sexual abuse and attributions of blame. *Journal of Interpersonal Violence, 14*(1), 62–78.

Baker, T. B., Piper, M. E., McCarthy, D. E., Majeskie, M. R., & Fiore, M. C. (2004). Addiction motivation reformulated: An affective processing model of negative reinforcement. *Psychological Review, 111*(1), 33–51.

Brady, K. T., Dansky, B. S., Back, S. E., Foa, E. B., & Carroll, K. M. (2001). Exposure therapy in the treatment of PTSD among cocaine-dependent individuals: Preliminary findings. *Journal of Substance Abuse Treatment, 21*(1), 47–54.

Bronfenbrenner, U. (1979). *The ecology of human development: Experiments by nature and design.* Cambridge, MA: Harvard University Press.

Carrigan, M. H., Ham, L. S., Thomas, S. E., & Randall, C. L. (2008). Alcohol outcome expectancies and drinking to cope with social situations. *Addictive Behaviors, 33*(9), 1162–1166.

Centers for Disease Control and Prevention. (2010). Youth risk behavior surveillance—United States, 2009. *MMWR Morbidity and Mortality Weekly Report, 59,* 1–142.

Clark, D. B., & Bukstein, O. G. (1998). Psychopathology in adolescent alcohol abuse and dependence. *Alcohol Health and Research World, 22,* 117–121.

Cloitre, M., Scarvalone, P., & Difede, J. (1997). Posttraumatic stress disorder, self and interpersonal dysfunction among sexually re-traumatized women. *Journal of Traumatic Stress, 10,* 435–450.

Cocozza, J. J., Jackson, E. W., Hennigan, K., Morrissey, J. P., Reed, B. G., Fallot, R., et al. (2005). Outcomes for women with co-occurring disorders and trauma: Program-level effects. *Journal of Substance Abuse Treatment, 28*(2), 109–119.

Cohen, J. A., Deblinger, E., Mannarino, A. P., & Steer, R. A. (2004). A multisite, randomized controlled trial for children with sexual abuse–related PTSD symptoms. *Journal of the American Academy of Child and Adolescent Psychiatry, 43,* 393–402. doi:10.1097/00004583-200404000-00005

Cohen, J. A., Mannarino, A. P., & Deblinger, E. (2006). *Treating trauma and traumatic grief in children and adolescents.* New York, NY: Guilford Press.

Danielson, C. K., Amstadter, A. B., Dangelmaier, R. E., Resnick, H. S., Saunders, B. E., & Kilpatrick, D. G. (2009). Trauma-related risk factors for substance abuse among male versus female young adults. *Addictive Behaviors, 34,* 395–399. doi:10.1016/j.addbeh.2008.11.009

Danielson, C. K., de Arellano, M. A., Kilpatrick, D. G., Saunders, B. E., & Resnick, H. S. (2005). Child maltreatment in depressed adolescents: Differences in symptomatology based on history of abuse. *Child Maltreatment, 10,* 37–48. doi:10.1177/1077559504271630

Danielson, C. K., Macdonald, A., Amstadter, A. B., Hanson, R., de Arellano, M. A., Saunders, B. E., & Kilpatrick, D. G. (2010). Risky behaviors and depression in conjunction with—or in the absence of—lifetime history of PTSD among sexually abused adolescents. *Child Maltreatment, 15,* 101–107. doi:10.1177/1077559509350075

Danielson, C. K., McCart, M., de Arellano, M. A., Macdonald, A., Silcott, L., & Resnick, H. (2010). Risk reduction for substance use and trauma-related psychopathology in adolescent sexual assault victims: Findings from an open trial. *Child Maltreatment, 15,* 261–268.

Danielson, C. K., McCart, M. R., Walsh, K., de Arellano, M. A., White, D., & Resnick, H. S. (2012). Reducing substance use risk and mental health problems among sexually assaulted adolescents: A pilot randomized controlled trial. *Journal of Family Psychology, 26*(4), 628–635. doi:10.1037/a0028862

de Arellano, M. A., & Danielson, C. K. (2008). Assessment of trauma history and trauma-related problems in ethnic minority child populations: An INFORMED approach. *Cognitive and Behavioral Practice, 15*(1), 53–66.

Deblinger, E., Mannarino, A. P., Cohen, J. A., Runyon, M. K., & Steer, R. A. (2011). Trauma-Focused Cognitive-Behavioral Therapy for children: Impact of the trauma narrative and treatment length. *Depression and Anxiety, 28*, 67–75.

DiClemente, R. J., Wingood, G. M., Harrington, K. F., Lang, D. L., Davis, S. L., Hook, E. W., & Robillard, A. (2004). Efficacy of an HIV prevention intervention for African American adolescent girls: A randomized controlled trial. *JAMA, 292*, 171–179. doi:10.1001/jama.292.2.171

Fergusson, D. M., Horwood, L. J., & Lynskey, M. T. (1997). Childhood sexual abuse, adolescent sexual behaviors and sexual revictimization. *Child Abuse & Neglect, 21*, 789–803.

Finkelhor, D., Ormrod, R., Turner, H., & Hamby, S. L. (2005). The victimization of children and youth: A comprehensive, national survey. *Child Maltreatment, 10*, 5–25. doi:10.1177/1077559504271287

Finkelhor, D., Turner, H., Ormrod, R., & Hamby, S. L. (2009). Violence, abuse, and crime exposure in a national sample of children and youth. *Pediatrics, 124*, 1411–1423. doi:10.1542/peds.2009-0467

Grant, B. F., & Dawson, D. A. (1997). Age at onset of alcohol use and its association with DSM-IV alcohol abuse and dependence: Results from the National Longitudinal Alcohol Epidemiologic Survey. *Journal of Substance Abuse, 9*(1), 103–110.

Guo, J., Chung, I., Hill, K. G., Hawkins, D., Catalano, R. F., & Abbott, R. D. (2002). Developmental relationships between adolescent substance use and risky sexual behavior in young adulthood. *Journal of Adolescent Health, 31*(4), 354–362.

Hallfors, D., Vevea, J. L., Iritani, B., Cho, H., Khatapoush, S., & Saxe, L. (2002). Truancy, grade point average, and sexual activity: A meta-analysis of risk indicators for youth substance use. *Journal of School Health, 72*(5), 205–211.

Henggeler, S. W., Clingempeel, W. G., Brondino, M. J., & Pickrel, S. G. (2002). Four-year follow-up of multisystemic therapy with substance abusing and dependent juvenile offenders. *Journal of the American Academy of Child and Adolescent Psychiatry, 41*, 868–874.

Hien, D., Cohen, L., & Campbell, A. (2005). Is traumatic stress a vulnerability factor for women with substance use disorders? *Clinical Psychology Review, 25*(6), 813–823.

Hien, D. A., Wells, E. A., Jiang, H., Suarez-Morales, L., Campbell, A. N., Cohen, L. R., et al. (2009). Multisite randomized trial of behavioral interventions for women with co-occurring PTSD and substance use disorders. *Journal of Consulting and Clinical Psychology, 77*(4), 607.

Johnson, V., & Pandina, R. J. (1991). Effects of family environment on adolescent substance use, delinquency, and coping styles. *American Journal of Drug and Alcohol Abuse, 17*, 71–88.

Johnston, L. D., O'Malley, P. M., Bachman, J. G., & Schulenberg, J. E. (2011). *Monitoring the future national results on adolescent drug use: Overview of key findings, 2010.* Ann Arbor, MI: Institute for Social Research, University of Michigan.

Kataoka, S. H., Stein, B. D., Jaycox, L. H., Wong, M., Escudero, P., Tu, W., et al. (2003). A school-based mental health program for traumatized Latino immigrant children. *Journal of the American Academy of Child and Adolescent Psychiatry, 42*(3), 311–318.

Kilpatrick, D. G., Acierno, R., Schnurr, P. P., Saunders, B., Resnick, H. S., & Best, C. L. (2000). Risk factors for adolescent substance abuse and dependence: Data from a national sample. *Journal of Consulting and Clinical Psychology, 68*, 19–30.

Kilpatrick, D., Ruggiero, K., Acierno, R., Saunders, B., Resnick, H., & Best, C. (2003). Violence and risk of PTSD, major depression, substance abuse/dependence, and comorbidity: Results from the NSA. *Journal of Consulting and Clinical Psychology, 71*, 692–700. doi:10.1037/0022-006X.71.4.692

Kolko, D. J. (1996). Individual cognitive behavioral treatment and family therapy for physically abused children and their offending parents: A comparison of clinical outcomes. *Child Maltreatment, 1*(4), 322–342.

Kovacs, M. (1983). *The Children's Depression Inventory: A self-rated depression scale for school-aged youngsters.* Unpublished manuscript. University of Pittsburgh School of Medicine, Pittsburgh, PA.

Lewis, M. W., & Petry, N. M. (2005). Contingency management treatments that reinforce completion of goal-related activities: Participation in family activities and its association with outcomes. *Drug and Alcohol Dependence, 79*(2), 267–271.

Linehan, M. M., Comtois, K. A., Murray, A. M., Brown, M. Z. Gallop, R. J., Heard, H. L., et al. (2006). Two-year randomized controlled trial and follow-up of Dialectical Behavior Therapy vs therapy by experts for suicidal behaviors and borderline personality disorder. *Archives of General Psychiatry, 63*(7), 757–766.

Mahoney, J. L., & Stattin, H. (2000). Leisure activities and adolescent antisocial behavior: The role of structure and social context. *Journal of Adolescence, 23*(2), 113–127.

Marx, B. P., Calhoun, K. S., Wilson, A. E., & Meyerson, L. A. (2001). Sexual revictimization prevention: An outcome evaluation. *Journal of Consulting and Clinical Psychology, 69*(1), 25–32.

McLean, L. M., & Gallop, R. (2003). Implications of childhood sexual abuse for adult borderline personality disorder and complex posttraumatic stress disorder. *American Journal of Psychiatry, 160*, 369–371.

Messman-Moore, T. L., & Long, P. J. (2000). Child sexual abuse and revictimization in the form of adult sexual abuse, adult physical abuse, and adult psychological maltreatment. *Journal of Interpersonal Violence, 15*(5), 489–502.

Messman-Moore, T. L., & Long, P. J. (2003). The role of childhood sexual abuse sequelae in the sexual revictimization of women: An empirical review and theoretical reformulation. *Clinical Psychology Review, 4*, 537–571.

Miller, W. R., & Rollnick, S. P. (2002). *Motivational interviewing: Preparing people for change.* New York, NY: Guilford Press.

Mills, K. L., Teesson, M., Back, S. E., Brady, K. T., Baker, A. L., Hopwood, S., & Ewer, P. L. (2012). Integrated exposure-based therapy for co-occurring posttraumatic stress disorder and substance dependence: A randomized controlled trial. *JAMA, 308*(7), 690–699.

Moos, R., & Moos, B. (1986). *Family Environment Scale manual* (2nd ed.). Palo Alto, CA: Consulting Psychologists Press.

Mowrer, H. O. (1960). *Learning theory and behavior.* Hoboken, NJ: John Wiley & Sons.

Najavits, L. M., Gallop, R. J., & Weiss, R. D. (2006). Seeking Safety Therapy for adolescent girls with PTSD and substance use disorder: A randomized controlled trial. *Journal of Behavioral Health Services & Research, 33*(4), 453–463.

Noll, J. G., Trickett, P. K., & Putnam, F. W. (2000). Social network constellation and sexuality of sexually abused and comparison girls in childhood and adolescence. *Child Maltreatment, 5*(4), 323–337.

Putnam, F. W. (2003). Ten-year research update review: Child sexual abuse. *Journal of the American Academy of Child and Adolescent Psychiatry, 42*(3), 269–278.

Randolph, M. E., & Mosack, K. E. (2006). Factors mediating the effects of childhood sexual abuse on risky sexual behavior among college women. *Journal of Psychology & Human Sexuality, 18*(1), 23–41.

Roodman, A. A., & Clum, G. A. (2001). Revictimization rates and method variance: A meta-analysis. *Clinical Psychology Review, 21*(2), 183–204.

Rothman, E. F., Edwards, E. M., Heeren, T., & Hingson, R. W. (2008). Adverse childhood experiences predict earlier age of drinking onset: Results from a representative US sample of current or former drinkers. *Pediatrics, 122*, 298–304. doi:10.1542/peds.2007-3412

Sobell, L. C., & Sobell, M. B. (1996). *Timeline Followback user's guide: A calendar method for assessing alcohol and drug use.* Toronto, ON: Addiction Research Foundation.

Steinberg, A. M., Brymer, M. J., Decker, K. B., & Pynoos, R. S. (2004). The UCLA Posttraumatic Stress Disorder Reaction Index. *Current Psychiatry Report, 6*, 96–100. doi:10.1007/s11920-004-0048-2

Swenson, C. C., Schaeffer, C. M., Henggeler, S. W., Faldowski, R., & Mayhew, A. M. (2010). Multisystemic Therapy for Child Abuse and Neglect: A randomized effectiveness trial. *Journal of Family Psychology, 24*(4), 497.

Wyatt, G. E., Guthrie, D., & Notgrass, C. M. (1992). Differential effects of women's child sexual abuse and subsequent sexual revictimization. *Journal of Consulting and Clinical Psychology, 60*(2), 167.

17

AMANDA M. FANNIFF, PH.D.
JUDITH V. BECKER, PH.D.
AMY L. GAMBOW, M.S.

Children and Adolescents with Sexual Behavior Problems

GENERAL CONSIDERATIONS

Children and adolescents with sexual behavior problems (SBP) have become a major focus of researchers and policymakers only in relatively recent years. Attention to juveniles with SBP increased in the 1980s and 1990s subsequent to research indicating that many adult sex offenders' deviant sexual fantasies and/or behaviors began in adolescence (e.g., Abel, Mittelman, & Becker, 1985) and the realization that juveniles represent a significant proportion of arrests for sexual crime in the United States (about 17% in 2010; U.S. Department of Justice, 2011). Due to the increasing demand for treatment of juveniles with SBP, specialized assessment and treatment approaches for adult sex offenders were adapted for use with juveniles, despite minimal evidence that such approaches would be appropriate (e.g., Chaffin, 2008). In recent years, the literature on children and adolescents with SBP has grown considerably, producing substantial information on the nature of the population as well as effective interventions.

This chapter provides an overview of common characteristics, promising subtyping approaches, and empirically supported assessment and treatment for children and adolescents with SBP. The review of children with SBP is gender-neutral, as this research often includes males and females (e.g., Gray et al., 1997; Merrick et al., 2008). The section devoted to adolescents focuses on males adjudicated for sexual offenses, as this subgroup has been the subject of the majority of the research. Interested readers are referred to the small but growing literature on female adolescents with SBP (e.g., Frey, 2010; McCartan et al., 2011).

CHILDREN WITH SEXUAL BEHAVIOR PROBLEMS

Preadolescent children often engage in sexual behavior and exploration spontaneously, such as exposing and examining their genitals and those of their peers (e.g., Friedrich et al., 1991). These behaviors generally decrease with age due to socialization and increasing awareness of cultural norms as children enter middle childhood (Friedrich et al., 1991). In contrast, some children under the age of 12 have sexual behavior problems, defined as initiating "behaviors involving sexual body parts (i.e., genitals, anus, buttocks, or breasts) that are developmentally inappropriate or potentially harmful to themselves or others" (Chaffin et al., 2008, p. 200). The objective behind these behaviors may not be linked to sexual pleasure and instead may be the product of anxiety, attention seeking, or self-soothing (Chaffin et al., 2008; Chaffin, Letourneau, & Silovsky, 2002).

Common Characteristics

Children with SBP are a heterogeneous group, and there are no clear demographic, psychiatric, or social factors that differentiate children with SBP from their same-age peers (Chaffin et al., 2008; Chaffin, Letourneau, & Silovsky, 2002). Sexual behavior problems have been observed equally in both boys and girls (Friedrich et al., 1991; Friedrich & Luecke, 1988; Gray et al., 1999; Silovsky & Niec, 2002), in contrast to the large gender differences in rates of sexual offending among adolescents and adults (U.S. Department of Justice, 2011).

One of the most common characteristics of children with SBP is a history of maltreatment, including physical abuse, verbal abuse, neglect, and witnessing domestic violence, in addition to sexual abuse (e.g., Friedrich & Luecke,

1988; Gray, Busconi, et al., 1997; Gray, Pithers, et al., 1999; Letourneau, Schoenwald, & Sheidow, 2004; Lévesque, Bigras, & Pauzé, 2010; Merrick et al., 2008; Silovsky & Niec, 2002). Contrary to early expectations, nonsexual forms of maltreatment may be equally as common as or more common than sexual abuse in children with SBP (e.g., Gray et al., 1999; Lévesque, Bigras, & Pauzé, 2010; Silovsky & Niec, 2002). Although maltreatment is a common (though not universal) characteristic of children with SBP, victimization should not be considered the sole or most critical factor in the development of SBP (Chaffin et al., 2008). Many children who experience maltreatment never act out sexually; the presence of other etiological factors may distinguish child maltreatment victims who act out sexually from those who do not. The severity and timing of maltreatment may partially explain the development of the SBP (e.g., Friedrich et al., 2003; Friedrich & Luecke, 1988; Gray et al., 1997; Merrick et al., 2008). For instance, when compared with maltreated children without SBP, those with SBP were younger at the time of abuse, they experienced more victimization incidents and more forms of abuse, and their abuse more often involved sexual intercourse (Friedrich et al., 2003; Friedrich & Luecke, 1988; Gray et al., 1999).

In addition to victimization, a high percentage of children with SBP have been found to exhibit nonsexual externalizing behaviors (Friedrich et al., 2003; Gray, Busconi, et al., 1997; Gray, Pithers, et al., 1999; Lévesque, Bigras, & Pauzé, 2010; Silovsky & Niec, 2002). Bonner, Walker, and Berliner (1999) found that children with SBP reported significantly higher levels of posttraumatic stress, attention-deficit / hyperactivity disorder (ADHD), anxiety, oppositional defiant disorder (ODD), and conduct disorder (CD) than did children without SBP. One study found that 73% of their sample met criteria for CD, 41% met criteria for ADHD, and 27% met criteria for ODD (Gray et al., 1997). Other factors that may contribute to the development of SBP include family adversity and sexualized family environments (e.g., Friedrich et al., 2003; Lévesque, Bigras, & Pauzé, 2010).

Typologies

Due to the increased awareness of SBP in children and the need for appropriate treatment, clinicians and researchers have attempted to identify homogeneous subtypes of children with SBP. Only three studies have attempted to identify meaningful subgroups empirically, each through the use of cluster analysis (Bonner, Walker, & Berliner, 1999; Hall, Mathews, & Pearce, 2002; Pithers et al., 1998), with mixed results.

Bonner and colleagues' (1999) attempt to empirically derive subgroups based on clinical characteristics was unsuccessful, so the authors proposed a typology based on the nature of the SBP at the time the children entered the study: sexually inappropriate (no physical contact with others); sexually intrusive (brief sexual contact with others); and sexually aggressive (significant or prolonged contact).

This typology merely reflects the severity of the behaviors, and its clinical implications are unclear.

Pithers and colleagues (1998) identified subtypes of children with SBP through the use of hierarchical cluster analysis, using data from a variety of clinically relevant measures as well as demographics, characteristics of the SBP, and previous victimization. The resulting five subtypes were categorized as nonsymptomatic; sexually aggressive; abuse-reactive; highly traumatized; and rule-breaking. The subgroups differed in abuse history, diagnoses, and demographic variables, but for the most part, the children in these subtypes did not engage in qualitatively different sexual behaviors. The nonsymptomatic child type was described as the least severe type, including having the fewest victims, having the least aggressive behavior, and being least likely to be diagnosed with a psychiatric disorder. The sexually aggressive and abuse-reactive children were more likely than those in the other groups to engage in penetrative acts, but the sexually aggressive youths had been victimized by fewer perpetrators and demonstrated social competence, whereas the abuse-reactive youths had more perpetrators and higher rates of disruptive behavior disorders. The rule-breaking subtype had the most frequent sexualized behaviors, had a high degree of aggression, and scored higher on externalizing than any other group. The highly traumatized child type was found to have been abused by more perpetrators and to demonstrate more attachment problems than all other types. There was considerable overlap between groups on some constructs, but the clinical meaningfulness of the subgroups is somewhat supported by differential response to treatment for one group. Children in the highly traumatized group showed a better treatment response to relapse prevention than to expressive therapy and were the most likely to show clinically significant improvement in the SBP over the course of treatment.

Hall and colleagues (2002) used hierarchical cluster analysis to identify subtypes of sexually abused children who exhibited interpersonal SBP, after selecting out a group with no SBP and a group with self-focused SBP. Three subtypes of youths with interpersonal SBP were identified: unplanned; planned noncoercive; and planned coercive. The subtypes differed in their history of maltreatment, social modeling (e.g., witnessing of other children being abused), sexual and other problematic behavior, and family functioning and characteristics. There appear to be some similarities between the subtypes identified by Hall and colleagues (2002) and by Pithers and colleagues (1998)—for example, the planned coercive group has some similarities to the abuse-reactive group—but the degree to which these two analyses overlap is unclear.

As noted by Chaffin et al. (2008), children with SBP are diverse in terms of demographics, family variables, socioeconomic status, history of abuse, and mental health problems. Although there is some support for the clinical relevance of subtyping in the study by Pithers and colleagues (1998), the research to date generally identifies groups with different severity of SBP, with children at the extreme end of the SBP continuum having more comorbid mental health, social, and family issues (Chaffin et al., 2008). None of the typologies have been subject to cross-validation, and the similarities between them are difficult to discern. In summary, future research may validate existing typologies, but as yet there are no empirically supported subtyping schemes to guide the assessment or treatment of children with SBP.

Assessment

As reported by Chaffin and colleagues (2008), intervention planning and decision making for children with SBP should be driven by individualized assessment of the child, the SBP, and the ecological context. For some children, sufficient information for treatment planning can be gathered in a single session by reviewing background material, by getting a behavioral and psychosocial history from the caregivers, from a clinical interview with the child, and through the use of a few simple assessment instruments. Contextual factors to be assessed include family relationships (e.g., caregiver monitoring and warmth, disciplinary practices), peer relationships (e.g., negative peer influences), access to pornography, witnessing or being the victim of various forms of maltreatment, and cultural factors in the home and community.

Information regarding the types of sexual behaviors, their onset and frequency, changes over time, and situations or circumstances under which the problem behaviors occur should be gathered during the evaluation (Chaffin et al., 2008). As with other problem behaviors, assessments ideally should rely on multiple informants about behavior in multiple settings (Friedrich & Trane, 2002). Clinicians may also use a structured assessment such as the Child Sexual Behavior Inventory (CSBI; Friedrich, 1997) to gather detailed information about the SBP and to distinguish normative and atypical sexual behaviors.

Given that many children with SBP present with mental health problems, information regarding the child's behavioral and emotional functioning should be gathered through the history provided by the parents and the clinical interview of the child (Chaffin et al., 2008). Structured assessment measures developed for use with children may also be helpful, such as the Child Behavior Checklist, which has versions available for use with children 6–18 as well as children 1½–5 years of age (Achenbach & Rescorla, 2001). If a child has a more complicated clinical presentation, the Diagnostic Interview Schedule for Children (DISC; Shaffer et al., 1996) or other in-depth structured interviews may prove useful. Based on initial impressions, a variety of brief assessment measures can be selected, such as the Children's Depression Inventory (CDI; Kovacs, 1992) and the Trauma Symptom Checklist for Children (TSCC; Brière, 1996). These are just a few of the available options; clinicians should select instruments relevant to the presentation of the child and appropriate to his or her developmental level.

A variety of assessment techniques that are used with adolescents and adults who have committed sexual offenses

are inappropriate for children. Polygraph assessments are often used in an effort to ensure that the offender has disclosed all offenses. Such coercive techniques should not be used with children (Chaffin et al., 2008) and could lead children to endorse behaviors in which they did not engage. Additionally, it makes little sense to use an invasive procedure such as the plethysmograph to assess sexual arousal in children with SBP, given that arousal to child targets would simply indicate arousal to peers (Chaffin et al., 2008).

Treatment

There is now convincing evidence that treatment is effective in reducing SBP in children. Meta-analytical results indicated an overall treatment effect on SBP of almost a half standard deviation at post-treatment, with better outcomes for treatment programs that target parenting/behavior management skills (St. Amand, Bard, & Silovsky, 2008). Results from the same analysis also indicated that rules about sexual behavior, sex education, abuse prevention skills, self-control skills, targeting of preschool-age children, and parental involvement in treatment were each associated with larger effect sizes. The use of techniques originally designed for interventions with adult sex offenders (e.g., identifying a cycle of abuse) was not associated with reduced SBP in children. The longest follow-up study completed to date, with 10 years of follow-up data, compared children with SBP who received a structured cognitive behavioral therapy (CBT) intervention, children with SBP who received a client-centered, psychodynamic play therapy group, and children referred for outpatient treatment for problems unrelated to SBP (Carpentier, Silovsky, & Chaffin, 2006). The CBT condition included groups for children and parents that involved identifying inappropriate sexual behavior, teaching concrete sexual behavior rules, learning behavioral self-control techniques (or parent management skills), and sex education. The results indicated that children with SBP who received the CBT intervention were no more likely than the comparison group with no SBP to have committed a subsequent sexual offense, as indicated by child welfare, juvenile justice, and criminal justice records. The children with SBP who received the play therapy intervention were more likely to commit a sexual offense over the 10-year follow-up than children in the CBT group and the comparison group. The research to date therefore suggests the most effective interventions will be structured, will provide treatment to parents and children, and will focus on parent management and self-regulation skills.

ADOLESCENTS WITH SEXUAL BEHAVIOR PROBLEMS

Common Characteristics

Research on adolescents with SBP primarily focuses on juveniles formally adjudicated for sexual offenses (JSOs). As is the case for children with sexual behavior problems, JSOs are a heterogeneous group, with no single profile of characteristics fitting all or most of these youths (Becker, Harris, & Sales, 1993). Some characteristics are frequently (though not universally) present in JSOs, including sexual abuse (e.g., Zakireh, Ronis, & Knight, 2008), other forms of child maltreatment (e.g., Fanniff & Kolko, 2012), social isolation / peer relationship problems (e.g., Miner & Munns, 2005; Ronis & Borduin, 2007), family problems (e.g., Ronis & Borduin, 2007; Sigurdsson et al., 2010), substance abuse (Långström & Lindblad, 2000; Sigurdsson et al., 2010), sexual deviance (Zakireh, Ronis, & Knight, 2008), and psychopathology (including disruptive behavior disorders; e.g., Långström & Lindblad, 2000).

Early research in the field largely consisted of descriptive studies of small samples, frequently without a comparison group and sometimes lacking standardized measures. The field has advanced significantly on all of these fronts, with enough well-conducted research to support the use of meta-analysis to combine results across studies. Seto and Lalumière (2010) conducted a meta-analysis comparing JSOs with other delinquent adolescents, using 59 independent studies. Results indicated that JSOs were more likely to have sexual and other abuse histories, anxiety, low self-esteem, social isolation, atypical sexual interests, and early exposure to sex and pornography. JSOs and other delinquent juveniles have similarly elevated rates of conduct problems, antisocial personality traits, antisocial attitudes and beliefs, and family problems. JSOs had fewer previous offenses, delinquent peer associations, and substance abuse problems than other delinquent juveniles.

Typologies

Researchers have attempted to develop typologies of JSOs in an effort to identify homogeneous subgroups with unique treatment needs. Efforts to subtype JSOs by a single characteristic (e.g., victim age; Fanniff & Kolko, 2012; Ronis & Borduin, 2007) generally have not produced consistent differences between groups across studies. Subtyping adolescents adjudicated for sexual offenses into those with a prior history of nonsexual offenses and those without (e.g., Butler & Seto, 2002) may be clinically meaningful, as risk assessment measures have differential validity in these groups (Rajlic & Gretton, 2010).

In contrast to studies focused on a single characteristic, the use of cluster analysis to identify subtypes based on clinical characteristics may produce more meaningful subgroups. W. R. Smith, Monastersky, and Deisher (1987) analyzed Minnesota Multiphasic Personality Inventory profiles and identified four subgroups: shy/over-controlled; demanding/narcissistic; socially outgoing / emotionally over-controlled; and a group with poor self-control and judgment. There were some differences in the types of offenses committed across these groups but no analyses on the clinical significance of these subtypes. Worling (2001) attempted

to replicate this work using the California Personality Inventory. Cluster analysis revealed four subtypes similar to those of W. R. Smith and colleagues (1987): antisocial/impulsive; unusual/isolated; over-controlled/reserved; and confident/aggressive. Worling (2001) found that the antisocial/impulsive and unusual/isolated groups had significantly higher general and violent recidivism than the other groups. Two studies have used cluster analysis on results from the Millon Adolescent Clinical Inventory to identify subtypes of JSOs. Richardson and colleagues (2004) identified five groups (normal, antisocial, submissive, dysthymic/inhibited, and dysthymic/negativistic), whereas Oxnam and Vess (2008) identified four (inadequate, antisocial, conforming, and passive-aggressive). Offense and victim characteristics were similar across groups for both models. The similarities in the subtypes identified by these four studies using three personality assessment measures lend some convergent evidence for the validity of these distinctions, but as yet, there is limited evidence on the clinical utility of these subtyping schemes.

Hunter (2006) reported on research that clustered JSOs on personality constructs such as hostile masculinity and psychosocial deficits to produce a three-group model: adolescent-onset, nonparaphilic; early-adolescent-onset, paraphilic, and life-course persistent. These groups differed in a number of expected ways in variables reflecting victim characteristics and criminal history (Hunter, 2006), but again, the clinical implications of these subgroups for treatment have not yet been demonstrated.

In summary, the research on subtyping of JSOs is promising, but no particular typology has been cross-validated and been shown to have clinical implications. Across studies, one group that consistently emerges is a generally antisocial subtype. The identification of this group is consistent with the experience of clinicians (e.g., Becker & Kaplan, 1988) and with the considerable overlap in clinical characteristics between JSOs and other delinquent juveniles (e.g., Ronis & Borduin, 2007). Such a group probably has different treatment needs than adolescents who are socially isolated, present with internalizing problems, and/or demonstrate a persistent pattern of interest in children. Additional research on subtyping of JSOs will clarify the nature of other subgroups that may similarly have implications for assessment and treatment.

Assessment

Evaluations of adolescents with SBP for the purposes of disposition and treatment planning should include a thorough clinical interview with the child, review of documentation, and interviews with collateral sources (if possible), with the goal of gathering information on the individual juvenile as well as the multiple systems in which he or she functions, including family, peers, school, and community (e.g., Collie & Ward, 2007). The assessment process may be aided by the use of structured assessment measures tapping a variety of constructs, such as personality, psychopathology, behavior problems, family functioning, and neuropsychological functioning, depending on the presentation of the particular adolescent. A review of such measures is beyond the scope of this chapter. Instead, we focus on specialized assessment techniques for use with JSOs. These specialized techniques fall into two primary categories: assessment of sexual interest and risk assessment.

ASSESSMENT OF SEXUAL INTEREST. A number of specialized tools have been developed for determining whether adolescents with SBP have persistent deviant sexual interests. A variety of self-report measures are available, including the Adolescent Cognitions Scale (Hunter et al., 1991), the Adolescent Sexual Interest Card Sort (Hunter, Becker, & Kaplan, 1995), and the Multiphasic Sex Inventory-II (Nichols & Molinder Assessments, 2001). There is limited information in peer-reviewed publications about the psychometric properties of these measures. Clinicians may find them useful for gathering information but should be cautious in interpretation, given their lack of validity evidence.

Concerns about the validity of self-reported sexual interests in this population have contributed to the use of biologically based assessments, with the goal of obtaining more objective information. The plethysmograph measures changes in penile tumescence in response to stimuli reflecting various potential targets of interest (e.g., Seto, 2001). At least 9% of treatment programs for male adolescents in the United States and 20% of programs in Canada that responded to a recent Safer Society survey reported using this technique (McGrath et al., 2010). The construct validity of the plethysmograph is supported by research indicating greater deviant arousal in expected subgroups of juveniles (e.g., those with male child victims; Clift, Rajlic, & Gretton, 2009; Rice et al., 2012; Seto, Lalumière, & Blanchard, 2000) and by findings showing that deviant interest in children as assessed by the plethysmograph is associated with greater numbers of victims (Blanchard & Barbaree, 2005; Seto, Lalumière, & Blanchard, 2000). In contrast, research demonstrating unexpected associations between deviant arousal and individual characteristics (e.g., a history of sexual or physical victimization; Becker, Kaplan, & Tenke, 1992) raises concerns about the measure's construct validity. Also, it is difficult to determine the diagnostic accuracy of the plethysmograph, given that there is no gold standard with which results can be compared: both self-report and victim selection are imperfect proxies for deviant sexual interests (Fanniff & Becker, 2006). Perhaps unsurprisingly, research on the connection between phallometrically assessed deviant arousal and sexual recidivism is mixed (e.g., Clift, Rajlic, & Gretton, 2009; Gretton et al., 2001). There is promising new research, however, that indicates one possible way to capitalize on a potential flaw of plethysmography: the ability to suppress arousal. Arousal to child stimuli when instructed to suppress arousal has been shown to be more predictive of sexual recidivism than arousal in the absence of instructions regarding suppression (Clift, Rajlic, & Gretton, 2009). This suggests that juveniles who are unable to control their arousal response to child stimuli are the most likely to continue to engage in SBP. These results need to be replicated but offer perhaps the most convincing data thus far regarding the utility of the plethysmograph with JSOs.

Measures of viewing time provide a less invasive strategy for assessing sexual interest. These measures ask examinees to rate the attractiveness of a variety of images, while the amount of time spent looking at each image is surreptitiously recorded as the (purportedly) objective measure of interest. Two such measures have been investigated in adolescents with SBP: the Abel Assessment for Sexual Interest (AASI) and the Affinity Measure of Sexual Interest. In initial research, the test-retest reliability and sensitivity/specificity of the AASI were both found to be limited (G. Smith & Fischer, 1999). Accuracy was determined by comparing viewing time indices with victim selection, which is an imperfect proxy for deviant sexual interest (Abel, 2000; Fanniff & Becker, 2006). Subsequent research has demonstrated that adolescents with child victims viewed slides of children longer than adolescents with peer or adult victims (Abel et al., 2004). Only one study reports on the psychometric properties of the Affinity Measure of Sexual Interest when used with JSOs. Although results showed significant correlations between the ratings of attractiveness provided by the respondent and viewing time for the majority of stimulus categories, the significant negative correlation between viewing time and attractiveness ratings of adult females in this study raises significant concerns about validity (Worling, 2006).

Overall, there is some promising evidence that objective measures of sexual interest may provide some useful information for evaluators, yet it is difficult to establish the error rates of such instruments, given the lack of an appropriate standard by which to evaluate accuracy. Despite some promising research on these measures of deviant sexual interest, for now, the establishment of a strong therapeutic alliance probably enables providers to gather sufficient information for effective treatment (Becker & Harris, 2004).

RISK ASSESSMENT. The assessment of risk in adolescents with SBP has seen major advances in the past decade, yet the evidence for the predictive validity of specialized risk assessment measures designed for this population remains somewhat mixed. We focus here on the two measures that evaluators report using most frequently (Viljoen, McLachlan, & Vincent, 2010): the Juvenile Sex Offender Assessment Protocol-II (J-SOAP-II; Prentky & Righthand, 2003) and the Estimate of Risk of Adolescent Sexual Offense Recidivism (ERASOR; Worling & Curwen, 2001).

The J-SOAP-II is the most frequently studied risk assessment measure for adolescents with SBP (Viljoen, Mordell, & Beneteau, 2012), and the research on its psychometric properties is promising. It is a 28-item instrument developed to assist in assessing sexual and general recidivism risk in males 12–18 years of age who have engaged in coercive sexual behavior, whether formally adjudicated or not (Prentky & Righthand, 2003). The J-SOAP-II comprises four scales: Scale 1 (Sexual Drive/Preoccupation), Scale 2 (Impulsive/Antisocial Behavior), Scale 3 (Intervention), and Scale 4 (Community Stability/Adjustment). The measure is designed to be scored based on all available information, and scoring based on both file review and a clinical interview may be superior to file review only (Fanniff & Letourneau, 2012). While the authors of the J-SOAP-II are interested in developing it into an actuarial measure with specific risk estimates for various cut-scores (Prentky & Righthand, 2003), it currently functions as a checklist of empirically supported risk factors to consider.

There is promising evidence for the psychometric properties of the J-SOAP-II, although the variability among studies raises concerns about relying on this instrument in risk evaluations for the courts. The total score is consistently found to have good internal consistency (e.g., Aebi et al., 2011; Martinez, Flores, & Rosenfeld, 2007) and good to excellent inter-rater reliability (e.g., Aebi et al., 2011; Caldwell, Ziemke, & Vitacco, 2008; Chu et al., 2012). The internal consistencies of the individual scales are generally found to be acceptable, with a few exceptions (e.g., Aebi et al., 2011; Fanniff & Letourneau, 2012; Martinez, Flores, & Rosenfeld, 2007). The inter-rater reliability estimates for the individual scales generally fall in the good to excellent range (Aebi et al., 2011; Caldwell, Ziemke, & Vitacco, 2008; Rajlic & Gretton, 2010), although multiple studies have found unacceptably low inter-rater agreement for Scale 4 (Aebi et al., 2011; Fanniff & Letourneau, 2012; Martinez, Flores, & Rosenfeld., 2007). More concerning are the mixed results thus far regarding the ability of the J-SOAP-II to predict sexual recidivism: some studies have demonstrated a significant positive predictive relationship for the total score and/or individual scales (e.g., Chu et al., 2012; Martinez, Flores, & Rosenfeld 2007; Prentky et al., 2010; Rajlic & Gretton, 2010), others find no relationship (e.g., Caldwell, Ziemke, & Vitacco, 2008; Viljoen et al., 2008), and one found a significant negative relationship (Caldwell & Dickinson, 2009). A recent meta-analysis found a significant positive predictive relationship with sexual recidivism across studies, with the effect sizes for the individual scales and the total score falling in the medium range (Viljoen, Mordell, & Beneteau, 2012). The J-SOAP-II in its current form is not intended to stand alone but rather to inform risk judgments in combination with other information; however, clinical judgments of risk made after completing the J-SOAP-II and a violence risk measure were not associated with sexual recidivism above chance levels (Elkovitch et al., 2008).

In contrast to the J-SOAP-II's actuarial-inspired design, the ERASOR was designed to function as a structured professional judgment instrument (Worling & Curwen, 2001).

Evaluators rate each item as absent, partially present, or present and then weigh those factors according to the particulars of the case to produce an overall risk rating of low, moderate, or high. The 25 items of the ERASOR encompass both static and dynamic risk factors and fall into five categories: Sexual Interests, Attitudes, and Behaviors; Historical Sexual Assaults; Psychosocial Functioning; Family/Environmental Functioning; and Treatment. The ERASOR should be scored based on at least a clinical interview of the adolescent and official records regarding the offense, but additional sources should be used whenever possible.

As with the J-SOAP-II, there is some promising evidence for the reliability and validity of the ERASOR, but variability among studies suggests caution in relying on this instrument in disposition evaluations. To evaluate internal consistency and inter-rater reliability, numerical scores are often applied to the ERASOR items to produce item scores and a total score. The ERASOR has acceptable internal consistency (Worling, 2004). The inter-rater reliability is good to excellent for the clinical risk rating, individual item scores, and total score (Viljoen et al., 2009; Worling, 2004; Worling, Bookalam, & Litteljohn, 2012), although one study found an unacceptably low estimate for both the clinical risk rating and the total score (Chu et al., 2012). Again, evidence on predictive validity is mixed: some research shows a significant predictive relationship with sexual recidivism for both the total score and the clinical risk rating (Chu et al., 2012; Rajlic & Gretton, 2010), while others find evidence for the predictive accuracy of only one of these (Worling, Bookalam, & Litteljohn, 2012) or neither (Viljoen et al., 2009). The recent meta-analysis by Viljoen and colleagues (2012) found that both the total score and the clinical risk rating were significantly predictive of sexual recidivism across studies, with effect sizes in the medium range.

Overall, the research on the predictive validity of the J-SOAP-II and ERASOR is encouraging, and the recent meta-analysis by Viljoen and colleagues (2012) may bolster evaluators' use of these measures in legal contexts. Additional research with a variety of populations and under various assessment conditions is needed, with particular attention to the possibility that these measures may be more accurate with particular subgroups (Rajlic & Gretton, 2010) or with specific age groups (e.g., Viljoen et al., 2008). Given the severity of consequences faced by juveniles adjudicated for sexual offenses, including indefinite civil commitment as a sexually violent predator (e.g., Becker & Hicks, 2003), evaluators are urged to be cautious in presenting information about risk to legal decision-makers and to highlight the limitations of currently available strategies. Additionally, it is recommended that in their risk evaluations, evaluators highlight the low base rate of sexual recidivism, the fluidity of sexuality and ongoing cognitive development in adolescence, the success of treatment with this population, and ecological risk factors (Vitacco et al., 2009).

Treatment

There is substantial evidence that treatment for adolescents with SBP is effective in reducing recidivism rates. A significant overall effect of treatment has been found in two meta-analyses (Reitzel & Carbonell, 2006; Walker et al., 2005). Reitzel and Carbonell (2006) reported that 7.37% of juveniles who received treatment recidivated sexually, whereas 18.93% of the comparison group committed a subsequent sexual offense. Both meta-analyses indicated that CBT and Multisystemic Therapy (MST) have stronger treatment effects than other intervention strategies; our review here focuses on these two approaches.

CBT remains the dominant treatment model relied on by treatment programs for adolescents (McGrath et al., 2010). The therapy is typically offered as a multi-component intervention delivered in a group format. Cognitive restructuring is typically a major component of CBT for adolescents with SBP (e.g., Becker, 1990). Behavioral techniques designed to reduce deviant sexual interest are also often included in CBT programs, such as verbal satiation (clients rehearse deviant fantasies to the point of boredom) and covert sensitization (clients interrupt deviant fantasies with images of the negative consequences that could follow an offense). Both techniques have been shown to reduce deviant sexual arousal for at least a subset of adolescents (Hunter & Goodwin, 1992; Kaplan, Morales, & Becker, 1993; Weinrott, Riggan, & Frothingham, 1997), although a more recent examination of covert sensitization found temporary increases in deviant fantasies, with post-treatment rates being equivalent to pre-treatment rates of deviant fantasy (Aylwin, Reddon, & Burke, 2005). At least two additional studies found decreased deviant arousal after completion of multi-component CBT packages (Becker, Kaplan, & Kavoussi, 1988; Hunter & Santos, 1990).

Although these results are promising, recidivism should be examined directly, given the evidence that reductions in deviant arousal are not associated with reductions in recidivism in adults (Rice, Quinsey, & Harris, 1991). Two studies of one CBT-based intervention program found reductions in sexual, violent nonsexual, and nonviolent recidivism at average follow-ups of 6.23 years (Worling & Curwen, 2000) and 16.23 years (Worling, Litteljohn, & Bookalam, 2010). The intervention program combined CBT with relapse prevention techniques delivered across individual, group, and family treatment modalities (Worling & Curwen, 2000). The treatment also focused on nonsexual concerns, such as social skills, self-esteem, and anger. Over the longer follow-up period, recidivism rates for treated adolescents and comparison group adolescents were, respectively, 28% and 52% for nonviolent offenses, 22% and 39% for violent nonsexual offenses, and 9% and 21% for sexual offenses (Worling, Litteljohn, & Bookalam, 2010). This research program provides the most encouraging results regarding the effectiveness of CBT. However, treatment dropouts and refusers were included in the comparison group, and this limits the confidence in the results, given the nonrandom nature of group assignment (Letourneau, 2004).

MST is less commonly identified as the main theoretical orientation of treatment programs (McGrath et al., 2010), but this approach is the only treatment with randomized controlled trials demonstrating its effectiveness in reducing recidivism in JSOs (Borduin et al., 1990; Borduin, Schaeffer, & Heiblum, 2009; Letourneau et al., 2009). Originally developed for the treatment of seriously delinquent juveniles, MST is designed to create change in the youth's broader ecological context (including family, peer, school, and community systems) in addition to individual factors. Treatment is designed to leverage the natural strengths in the various interacting systems surrounding the youth to build his prosocial peer relationships and effective coping skills and to support parents in more effective supervision and discipline (Letourneau et al., 2009). Although the conclusions that could be drawn from the initial study (Borduin et al., 1990) were limited by the small sample size, subsequent evaluations have shown significant reductions in problematic sexual behaviors, general delinquency, substance use, and externalizing behaviors (Letourneau et al., 2009), as well as in sexual and nonsexual recidivism (Borduin, Schaeffer, & Heiblum, 2009). Together with evidence on the effectiveness of MST with general delinquent populations (e.g., Curtis, Ronan, & Borduin, 2004), these studies provide substantial support for the use of this intervention for adolescents with SBP.

In summary, the research on treatment for adolescents with SBP suggests that treated youths, overall, are less likely to continue sexually offending than those who do not receive treatment. The research on CBT suffers from major methodological limitations; nonetheless, meta-analyses indicate that both CBT and MST are particularly effective for this population. The intervention program evaluated in the highest-quality CBT outcomes research has an important parallel with MST: a focus on the broader ecological context of the juvenile and inclusion of non-sex-specific treatment targets. Other promising new approaches share these qualities (e.g., Hunter et al., 2004). Clinicians should broaden the scope of their interventions in this manner as much as possible to maximize positive treatment effects. Applying the principles of the risk-need-responsivity model (Andrews & Bonta, 2010), by providing more intensive interventions to higher-risk youths, targeting criminogenic needs, and attending to factors that influence individual response to treatment, is also likely to improve outcomes (Hanson et al. 2009; Vieira, Skilling, & Peterson-Badali, 2009).

CONCLUSIONS

The research on children and adolescents with SBP has advanced considerably in the past two decades, elucidating the characteristics of the populations and providing guidance on appropriate assessment and treatment. As more has been discovered, the differences between the two groups—

children and adolescents—and between both groups and adult offenders have become increasingly clear. It is also clear that treatment is effective for both populations, although the nature of effective treatment differs by developmental level. Despite low recidivism rates and the availability of effective treatments, public policy has not yet adjusted to fit the empirical evidence (e.g., Chaffin, 2008). Further research is needed, not only on the assessment and treatment of both children and adolescents with SBP, but on the impact of social control policies as well (e.g., Letourneau & Armstrong, 2008). Additionally, although this is not a topic of the chapter, psychologists and public health researchers should focus on the development of primary and secondary prevention strategies to prevent the onset of SBP in youths.

References

Abel, G. G. (2000). The importance of meeting research standards: A reply to Fischer and Smith's articles on the Abel Assessment for Sexual Interest™. *Sexual Abuse: A Journal of Research and Treatment, 12*(2), 155–161. doi:10.1177/107906320001200206

Abel, G. G., Jordan, A., Rouleau, J. L., Emerick, R., Barboza-Whitehead, S., & Osborn, C. (2004). Use of visual reaction time to assess male adolescents who molest children. *Sexual Abuse: A Journal of Research and Treatment, 16*(3), 255–265. doi:10.1177/107906320401600306

Abel, G. G., Mittelman, M., & Becker, J. V. (1985). Sexual offenders: Results of assessment and recommendations for treatment. In H. H. Ben-Aron, S. I. Huckers, & C. D. Webster (Eds.), *Clinical criminology: Current concepts* (pp. 191–205). Toronto, ON: M & M Graphics.

Achenbach, T. M., & Rescorla, L. A. (2001). *Manual for the ASEBA School-Age Forms & Profiles*. Burlington, VT: University of Vermont, Research Center for Children, Youth, & Families.

Aebi, M., Plattner, B., Steinhausen, H.-C., & Bessler, C. (2011). Predicting sexual and nonsexual recidivism in a consecutive sample of juveniles convicted of sexual offences. *Sexual Abuse: A Journal of Research and Treatment, 23*(4), 456–473. doi:10.1177/1079063210384634

Andrews, D. A., & Bonta, J. (2010). *The psychology of criminal conduct* (5th ed.). New Providence, NJ: Matthew Bender & Company.

Aylwin, A. S., Reddon, J. R., & Burke, A. R. (2005). Sexual fantasies of adolescent male sex offenders in residential treatment: A descriptive study. *Archives of Sexual Behavior, 34*(2), 231–239. doi:10.1007/s10508-005-1800-3

Becker, J. V. (1990). Treating adolescent sexual offenders. *Professional Psychology: Research and Practice, 21*(5), 362–365. doi:10.1037/0735-7028.21.5.362

Becker, J. V., & Harris, C. (2004). The psychophysiological assessment of juvenile offenders. In G. O'Reilly, W. L. Marshall, A. Carr, & R. C. Beckett (Eds.), *The handbook of clinical intervention with young people who sexually abuse* (pp. 191–202). New York, NY: Psychology Press.

Becker, J. V., Harris, C. D., & Sales, B. D. (1993). Juveniles who commit sexual offenses: A critical review of research. In G. C. Nagayama Hall, R. Hirschman, J. R. Graham, & M. S. Zaragoza (Eds.), *Sexual aggression* (pp. 215–228). Washington, DC: Taylor & Francis.

Becker, J. V., & Hicks, S. J. (2003). Juvenile sexual offenders: Characteristics, interventions, and policy issues. *Annals of the New York Academy of Sciences, 989*(1), 397–410. doi:10.1111/j.1749-6632.2003.tb07321.x

Becker, J. V., & Kaplan, M. S. (1988). The assessment of adolescent sexual offenders. In R. Prinz (Ed.), *Advances in behavioral assessment of children and families* (Vol. 4, pp. 97–118). Greenwich, CT: JAI Press.

Becker, J. V., Kaplan, M. S., & Kavoussi, R. (1988). Measuring the effectiveness of treatment for the aggressive adolescent sexual offender. *Annals of the New York Academy of Sciences, 528*(1), 215–222. doi:10.1111/j.1749-6632.1988.tb50865.x

Becker, J. V., Kaplan, M. S., & Tenke, C. E. (1992). The relationship of abuse history, denial and erectile response profiles of adolescent sexual perpetrators. *Behavior Therapy, 23*(1), 87–97. doi:10.1016/S0005-7894(05)80310-7

Blanchard, R., & Barbaree, H. E. (2005). The strength of sexual arousal as a function of the age of the sex offender: Comparisons among pedophiles, hebephiles, and teleiophiles. *Sexual Abuse: A Journal of Research and Treatment, 17*(4), 441–456. doi:10.1177/107906320501700407

Bonner, B. L., Walker, C. E., & Berliner, L. (1999). *Children with sexual behavior problems: Assessment and treatment—Final report* (Grant No. 90-CA-1469). Washington, DC: U.S. Department of Health and Human Services, National Clearinghouse on Child Abuse and Neglect.

Borduin, C. M., Henggeler, S. W., Blaske, D. M., & Stein, R. J. (1990). Multisystemic treatment of adolescent sexual offenders. *International Journal of Offender Therapy and Comparative Criminology, 34*(2), 105–113. doi:10.1177/0306624X9003400204

Borduin, C. M., Schaeffer, C. M., & Heiblum, N. (2009). A randomized clinical trial of multisystemic therapy with juvenile sexual offenders: Effects on youth social ecology and criminal activity. *Journal of Consulting and Clinical Psychology, 77*(1), 26–37. doi:10.1037/a0013035

Brière, J. (1996). *Trauma Symptom Checklist for Children: Professional manual*. Odessa, FL: Psychological Assessment Resources.

Butler, S. M., & Seto, M. C. (2002). Distinguishing two types of adolescent sex offenders. *Journal of the American Academy of Child and Adolescent Psychiatry, 41*(1), 83–90. doi:10.1097/00004583-200201000-00015

Caldwell, M. F., & Dickinson, C. (2009). Sex offender registration and recidivism risk in juvenile sexual offenders. *Behavioral Sciences & the Law, 27*, 941–956. doi:10.1002/bsl.907

Caldwell, M. F., Ziemke, M. H., & Vitacco, M. J. (2008). An examination of the Sex Offender Registration and Notification Act as applied to juveniles: Evaluating the ability to predict sexual recidivism. *Psychology, Public Policy, and Law, 14*(2), 89–114. doi:10.1037/a0013241

Carpentier, M. Y., Silovsky, J. F., & Chaffin, M. (2006). Randomized trial of treatment for children with sexual behavior problems: Ten-year follow-up. *Journal of Consulting and Clinical Psychology, 74*(3), 482–488. doi:10.1037/0022-006X.74.3.482

Chaffin, M. (2008). Our minds are made up—Don't confuse us with the facts: Commentary on policies concerning children with sexual behavior problems and juvenile sex offenders. *Child Maltreatment, 13*(2), 110–121. doi:10.1177/1077559508314510

Chaffin, M., Berliner, L., Block, R., Cavanagh Johnson, T., Friedrich, W. N., Garza Louis, D., et al. (2008). Report of the ATSA Task Force on Children with Sexual Behavior Problems. *Child Maltreatment, 13*(2), 199–218. doi:10.1177/1077559507306718

Chaffin, M., Letourneau, E., & Silovsky, J. F. (2002). Adults, adolescents, and children who sexually abuse children: A developmental perspective. In J. E. B. Myers, L. Berliner, J. Briere, C. Jenny, T. Hendrix, C. Jenny, & T. E. Reid. (Eds.),

The APSAC handbook on child maltreatment (2nd ed., pp. 205–232). Thousand Oaks, CA: Sage Publications.

Chu, C. M., Ng, K., Fong, J., & Teoh, J. (2012). Assessing youth who sexually offended: The predictive validity of the ERASOR, J-SOAP-II, and YLS/CMI in a non-Western context. *Sexual Abuse: A Journal of Research and Treatment, 24*(2), 153–174. doi:10.1177/1079063211404250

Clift, R. J. W., Rajlic, G., & Gretton, H. M. (2009). Discriminative and predictive validity of the penile plethysmograph in adolescent sex offenders. *Sexual Abuse: A Journal of Research and Treatment, 21*(3), 335–362. doi:10.1177/1079063209338491

Collie, R. M., & Ward, T. (2007). Current empirical assessment methods for adolescents and children who sexually abuse others. *Journal of Human Behavior in the Social Environment, 16*(4), 75–99. doi:10.1080/10911350802081634

Curtis, N. M., Ronan, K. R., & Borduin, C. M. (2004). Multisystemic treatment: A meta-analysis of outcome studies. *Journal of Family Psychology, 18*(3), 411–419. doi:10.1037/0893-3200.18.3.411

Elkovitch, N., Viljoen, J. L., Scalora, M. J., & Ullman, D. (2008). Assessing risk of reoffending in adolescents who have committed a sexual offense: The accuracy of clinical judgments after completion of risk assessment instruments. *Behavioral Sciences & the Law, 26*(4), 511–528. doi:10.1002/bsl.832

Fanniff, A. M., & Becker, J. V. (2006). Specialized assessment and treatment of adolescent sex offenders. *Aggression and Violent Behavior, 11*(3), 265–282. doi:10.1016/j.avb.2005.08.003

Fanniff, A. M., & Kolko, D. J. (2012). Victim age based subtypes of juveniles adjudicated for sexual offenses: Comparisons across domains in an outpatient sample. *Sexual Abuse: A Journal of Research and Treatment, 24*(3), 224–264. doi:10.1177/1079063211416516

Fanniff, A. M., & Letourneau, E. J. (2012). Another piece of the puzzle: Psychometric properties of the J-SOAP-II. *Sexual Abuse: A Journal of Research and Treatment, 24*(4), 378–408. doi:10.1177/1079063211431842

Frey, L. L. (2010). The juvenile female sexual offender: Characteristics, treatment and research. In T. A. Gannon & F. Cortoni (Eds.), *Female sexual offenders: Theory, assessment, and treatment* (pp. 53–71). New York, NY: John Wiley & Sons.

Friedrich, W. N. (1997). *Child Sexual Behavior Inventory: Professional manual.* Odessa, FL: Psychological Assessment Resources.

Friedrich, W. N., Davies, W. H., Feher, E., & Wright, J. (2003). Sexual behavior problems in preteen children: Developmental, ecological, and behavioral correlates. *Annals of the New York Academy of Sciences, 989*(1), 95–104. doi:10.1111/j.1749-6632.2003.tb07296.x

Friedrich, W. N., Grambsch, P., Broughton, D., Kuiper, J., & Beilke, R. L. (1991). Normative sexual behavior in children. *Pediatrics, 88*, 456–464.

Friedrich, W. N., & Luecke, W. (1988). Young school-age sexually aggressive children. *Professional Psychology Research and Practice, 19*(2), 155–164.

Friedrich, W. N., & Trane, S. T. (2002). Sexual behavior in children across multiple settings. *Child Abuse & Neglect, 26(3)*, 243–245. doi:10.1016/S0145-2134(01)00322-2

Gray, A., Busconi, A., Houchens, P., & Pithers, W. D. (1997). Children with sexual behavior problems and their caregivers: Demographics, functioning, and clinical patterns. *Sexual Abuse: A Journal of Research and Treatment, 9*(4), 267–290. doi:10.1177/107906329700900402

Gray, A., Pithers, W. D., Busconi, A., & Houchens, P. (1999). Developmental and etiological characteristics of children with sexual behavior problems: Treatment implications. *Child Abuse & Neglect, 23*(6), 601–621.

Gretton, H. M., McBride, M., Hare, R. D., O'Shaughnessy, R., & Kumka, G. (2001). Psychopathy and recidivism in adolescent sex offenders. *Criminal Justice and Behavior, 28*(4), 427–449. doi:10.1177/009385480102800403

Hall, D. K., Mathews, F., & Pearce, J. (2002). Sexual behavior problems in sexually abused children: A preliminary typology. *Child Abuse & Neglect, 26*(3), 289–312. doi:10.1016/S0145-2134(01)00326-X

Hanson, R. K., Bourgon, G., Helmus, L., & Hodgson, S. (2009). The principles of effective correctional treatment also apply to sexual offenders: A meta-analysis. *Criminal Justice and Behavior, 36*(9), 865–891. doi:10.1177/0093854809338545

Hunter, J. A. (2006). Understanding diversity in juvenile sexual offenders: Implications for assessment, treatment, and legal management. In R. E. Longo & D. S. Prescott (Eds.), *Current perspectives: Working with sexually aggressive youth and youth with sexual behavior problems* (pp. 63–77). Holyoke, MA: NEARI Press.

Hunter, J. A., Becker, J. V., & Kaplan, M. S. (1995). The Adolescent Sexual Interest Card Sort: Test-retest reliability and concurrent validity in relation to phallometric assessment. *Archives of Sexual Behavior, 24*(5), 555–561. doi:10.1007/BF01541834

Hunter, J. A., Becker, J. V., Kaplan, M., & Goodwin, D. W. (1991). Reliability and discriminative validity of the Adolescent Cognitions Scale for juvenile offenders. *Annals of Sex Research, 4*(3–4), 281–286. doi:10.1007/BF00850058

Hunter, J. A., Gilbertson, S. A., Vedros, D., & Morton, M. (2004). Strengthening community-based programming for juvenile sexual offenders: Key concepts and paradigm shifts. *Child Maltreatment, 9*(2), 177–189. doi:10.1177/1077559504264261

Hunter, J. A., & Goodwin, D. W. (1992). The clinical utility of satiation therapy with juvenile sexual offenders: Variations and efficacy. *Annals of Sex Research, 5*(2), 71–80. doi:10.1007/BF00849732

Hunter, J., & Santos, D. (1990). The use of specialized cognitive-behavioral therapies in the treatment of adolescent sexual offenders. *International Journal of Offender Therapy and Comparative Criminology, 34*(3), 239–247. doi:10.1177/0306624X9003400307

Kaplan, M. S., Morales, M., & Becker, J. V. (1993). The impact of verbal satiation on adolescent sex offenders: A preliminary report. *Journal of Child Sexual Abuse, 2*, 81–88. doi:10.1300/J070v02n03_06

Kovacs, M. (1992). *Children's Depression Inventory.* North Tonawanda, NY: Multi-Health Systems.

Långström, N., & Lindblad, F. (2000). Young sex offenders: Background, personality, and crime characteristics in a Swedish forensic psychiatric sample. *Nordic Journal of Psychiatry, 54*(2), 113–120.

Letourneau, E. J. (2004). A comment on the first report [Letter to the editor]. *Sexual Abuse: A Journal of Research and Treatment, 16*, 77–81.

Letourneau, E. J., & Armstrong, K. S. (2008). Recidivism rates for registered and nonregistered juvenile sexual offenders. *Sexual Abuse: A Journal of Research and Treatment, 20*(4), 393–408. doi:10.1177/1079063208324661

Letourneau, E. J., Henggeler, S. W., Borduin, C. M., Schewe, P. A., McCart, M. R., Chapman, J. E., et al. (2009). Multisystemic therapy for juvenile sexual offenders: 1-year results from a randomized effectiveness trial. *Journal of Family Psychology, 23*(1), 89–102. doi:10.1037/a0014352

Letourneau, E. J., Schoenwald, S. K., & Sheidow, A. J. (2004). Children and adolescents with sexual behavior problems. *Child Maltreatment, 9*(1), 49–61. doi:10.1177/1077559503260308

Lévesque, M., Bigras, M., & Pauzé, R. (2010). Externalizing problems and problematic sexual behaviors: Same etiology? *Aggressive Behavior, 36*(6), 358–370. doi:10.1002/ab.20362

Martinez, R., Flores, J., & Rosenfeld, B. (2007). Validity of the Juvenile Sex Offender Assessment Protocol-II (J-SOAP-II) in a sample of urban minority youth. *Criminal Justice and Behavior, 34*(10), 1284–1295. doi:10.1177/0093854807301791

McCartan, F. M., Law, H., Murphy, M., & Bailey, S. (2011). Child and adolescent females who present with sexually abusive behaviours: A 10-year UK prevalence study. *Journal of Sexual Aggression, 17*(1), 4–14. doi:10.1080/13552600.2010.488302

McGrath, R., Cumming, G., Burchard, B., Zeoli, S., & Ellerby, L. (2010). *Current practices and emerging trends in sexual abuser management: The Safer Society 2009 North American Survey.* Brandon, VT: Safer Society Press.

Merrick, M. T., Litrownik, A. J., Everson, M. D., & Cox, C. E. (2008). Beyond sexual abuse: The impact of other maltreatment experiences on sexualized behavior. *Child Maltreatment, 13*(2), 122–132. doi:10.1177/1077559507306715

Miner, M. H., & Munns, R. (2005). Isolation and normlessness: Attitudinal comparisons of adolescent sex offenders, juvenile offenders, and nondelinquents. *International Journal of Offender Therapy and Comparative Criminology, 49*(5), 491–504. doi:10.1177/0306624X04274103

Nichols & Molinder Assessments. (2001). *Multiphasic Sex Inventory-II, Adolescent Male Form.* Fircrest, WA: Author.

Oxnam, P., & Vess, J. (2008). A typology of adolescent sexual offenders: Millon Adolescent Clinical Inventory profiles, developmental factors, and offence characteristics. *Journal of Forensic Psychiatry & Psychology, 19*(2), 228–242. doi:10.1080/14789940701694452

Pithers, W. D., Gray, A., Busconi, A., & Houchens, P. (1998). Children with sexual behavior problems: Identification of five distinct child types and related treatment considerations. *Child Maltreatment, 3*(4), 384–406. doi:10.1177/1077559598003004010

Prentky, R. A., Li, N.-C., Righthand, S., Schuler, A., Cavanaugh, D., & Lee, A. F. (2010). Assessing risk of sexually abusive behavior among youth in a child welfare sample. *Behavioral Sciences & the Law, 28*(1), 24–45. doi:10.1002/bsl.920

Prentky, R., & Righthand, S. (2003). *Juvenile Sex Offender Assessment Protocol-II (J-SOAP-II) manual.* Bridgewater, MA: Justice Resource Institute.

Rajlic, G., & Gretton, H. M. (2010). An examination of two sexual recidivism risk measures in adolescent offenders: The moderating effect of offender type. *Criminal Justice and Behavior, 37*(10), 1066–1085. doi:10.1177/0093854810376354

Reitzel, L. R., & Carbonell, J. L. (2006). The effectiveness of sexual offender treatment for juveniles as measured by recidivism: A meta-analysis. *Sexual Abuse: A Journal of Research and Treatment, 18*(4), 401–421. doi:10.1177/107906320601800407

Rice, M. E., Harris, G. T., Lang, C., & Chaplin, T. C. (2012). Adolescents who have sexually offended: Is phallometry valid? *Sexual Abuse: A Journal of Research and Treatment, 24*(2), 133–152. doi:10.1177/1079063211404249

Rice, M. E., Quinsey, V. L., & Harris, G. T. (1991). Sexual recidivism among child molesters released from a maximum security psychiatric institution. *Journal of Consulting and Clinical Psychology, 59*(3), 381–386. doi:10.1037/0022-006X.59.3.381

Richardson, G., Kelly, T. P., Graham, F., & Bhate, S. R. (2004). A personality-based taxonomy of sexually abusive adolescents derived from the Millon Adolescent Clinical Inventory (MACI). *British Journal of Clinical Psychology, 43*(3), 285–298. doi:10.1348/0144665031752998

Ronis, S. T., & Borduin, C. M. (2007). Individual, family, peer, and academic characteristics of male juvenile sexual offenders. *Journal of Abnormal Child Psychology, 35*(2), 153–163. doi:10.1007/s10802-006-9058-3

Seto, M. C. (2001). The value of phallometry in the assessment of male sex offenders. *Journal of Forensic Psychology Practice, 1*(2), 65–75. doi:10.1300/J158v01n02_05

Seto, M. C., & Lalumière, M. L. (2010). What is so special about male adolescent sexual offending? A review and test of explanations through meta-analysis. *Psychological Bulletin, 136*(4), 526–575. doi:10.1037/a0019700

Seto, M. C., Lalumière, M. L., & Blanchard, R. (2000). The discriminative validity of a phallometric test for pedophilic interests among adolescent sex offenders against children. *Psychological Assessment, 12*(3), 319–327. doi:10.1037//1040-3590.12.3.319

Shaffer, D., Fisher, P., Dulcan, M. K., Davies, M., Piacentini, J., Schwab-Stone, M. E., et al. (1996). The NIMH Diagnostic Interview Schedule for Children Version 2.3 (DISC-2.3): Description, acceptability, prevalence rates, and performance in the MECA study. *Journal of the American Academy of Child and Adolescent Psychiatry, 35*(7), 865–877. doi:10.1097/00004583-199607000-00012

Sigurdsson, J. F., Gudjonsson, G., Asgeirsdottir, B. B., & Sigfusdottir, I. D. (2010). Sexually abusive youth: What are the background factors that distinguish them from other youth? *Psychology, Crime, & Law, 16*(4), 289–303. doi:10.1080/10683160802665757

Silovsky, J. F., & Niec, L. (2002). Characteristics of young children with sexual behavior problems: A pilot study. *Child Maltreatment, 7*(3), 187–197. doi:10.1177/1077559502007003002

Smith, G., & Fischer, L. (1999). Assessment of juvenile sexual offenders: Reliability and validity of the Abel Assessment for Interest in Paraphilias. *Sexual Abuse: A Journal of Research and Treatment, 11*(3), 207–216. doi:10.1177/107906329901100304

Smith, W. R., Monastersky, C., & Deisher, R. M. (1987). MMPI-based personality types among juvenile sex offenders. *Journal of Clinical Psychology, 43*(4), 422–430. doi:10.1002/1097-4679(198707)43:4<422::AID-JCLP2270430414>3.0.CO;2-3

St. Amand, A., Bard, D. E., & Silovsky, J. F. (2008). Meta-analysis of treatment for child sexual behavior problems: Practice elements and outcomes. *Child Maltreatment, 13*(2), 145–166. doi:10.1177/1077559508315353

U.S. Department of Justice, Federal Bureau of Investigation. (2011, September). *Crime in the United States, 2010.* www.fbi.gov/about-us/cjis/ucr/crime-in-the-u.s/2010/crime-in-the-u.s.-2010/index-page

Vieira, T. A., Skilling, T. A., & Peterson-Badali, M. (2009). Matching court-ordered services with treatment needs: Predicting treatment success with young offenders. *Criminal Justice and Behavior, 36*(4), 385–401. doi:10.1177/0093854808331249

Viljoen, J. L., Elkovitch, N., Scalora, M. J., & Ullman, D. (2009). Assessment of reoffense risk in adolescents who have committed sexual offenses: Predictive validity of the ERASOR, PCL:YV, YLS/CMI, and Static-99. *Criminal Justice and Behavior, 36*(10), 981–1000. doi:10.1177/0093854809340991

Viljoen, J. L., McLachlan, K., & Vincent, G. M. (2010). Assessing violence risk and psychopathy in juvenile and adult offenders: A survey of clinical practices. *Assessment 17*(3), 337–395. doi:10.1177/1073191109359587

Viljoen, J. L., Mordell, S., & Beneteau, J. L. (2012). Prediction of adolescent sexual reoffending: A meta-analysis of the J-SOAP-II, ERASOR, J-SORRAT-II, and Static-99. *Law and Human Behavior, 36*(5), 423–438. doi:10.1037/h0093938

Viljoen, J. L., Scalora, M., Cuadra, L., Bader, S., Chávez, V. N., Ullman, D., et al. (2008). Assessing risk for violence in adolescents who have sexually offended: A comparison of the

J-SOAP-II, J-SORRAT-II, and SAVRY. *Criminal Justice and Behavior, 35*(1), 5–23. doi:10.1177/0093854807307521

Vitacco, M. J., Caldwell, M., Ryba, N. L., Malesky, A., & Kurus, S. J. (2009). Assessing risk in adolescent sexual offenders: Recommendations for clinical practice. *Behavioral Sciences & the Law, 27*, 929–940. doi:10.1002/bsl.909

Walker, D. F., McGovern, S. K., Poey, E. L., & Otis, K. E. (2005). Treatment effectiveness for male adolescent sexual offenders: A meta-analysis and review. *Journal of Child Sexual Abuse, 13*(3), 281–293. doi:10.1300/J070v13n03_14

Weinrott, M. R., Riggan, M., & Frothingham, S. (1997). Reducing deviant arousal in juvenile sex offenders using vicarious sensitization. *Journal of Interpersonal Violence, 12*(5), 704–728. doi:10.1177/088626097012005007

Worling, J. R. (2001). Personality-based typology of adolescent male sexual offenders: Differences in recidivism rates, victim-selection characteristics, and personal victimization histories. *Sexual Abuse: A Journal of Research and Treatment, 13*(3), 149–166. doi:10.1177/107906320101300301

Worling, J. R. (2004). The Estimate of Risk of Adolescent Sexual Offense Recidivism (ERASOR): Preliminary psychometric data. *Sexual Abuse: A Journal of Research and Treatment, 16*(3), 235–254. doi:10.1177/107906320401600305

Worling, J. R. (2006). Assessing sexual arousal with adolescent males who have offended sexually: Self-report and unobtrusively measured viewing time. *Sexual Abuse: A Journal of Research and Treatment, 18*(4), 383–400. doi:10.1007/s11194-006-9024-1

Worling, J. R., Bookalam, D., & Litteljohn, A. (2012). Prospective validity of the Estimate of Risk of Adolescent Sexual Offense Recidivism (ERASOR). *Sexual Abuse: A Journal of Research and Treatment, 24*(3), 203–223. doi:10.1177/1079063211407080

Worling, J. R., & Curwen, T. (2000). Adolescent sexual offender recidivism: Success of specialized treatment and implications for risk prediction. *Child Abuse & Neglect, 24*(7), 965–982. doi:10.1016/S0145-2134(00)00147-2

Worling, J. R., & Curwen, T. (2001). Estimate of Risk of Adolescent Sexual Offense Recidivism (ERASOR; Version 2.0). In M. C. Calder (Ed.), *Juveniles and children who sexually abuse: Frameworks for assessment* (pp. 372–397). Lyme Regis, UK: Russell House.

Worling, J. R., Litteljohn, A., & Bookalam, D. (2010). 20-year prospective follow-up study of specialized treatment for adolescents who offend sexually. *Behavioral Sciences & the Law, 28*(1), 46–57. doi:10.1002/bsl.912

Zakireh, B., Ronis, S. T., & Knight, R. A. (2008). Individual beliefs, attitudes, and victimization histories of male juvenile sexual offenders. *Sexual Abuse: A Journal of Research and Treatment, 20*(3), 323–351. doi:10.1177/1079063208322424

PART IV Short- and Long-Term
Medical Treatment

MARTIN A. FINKEL, D.O., FAAP

18

Medical Management of Sexual Abuse

A Therapeutic Approach

GENERAL CONSIDERATIONS

This chapter focuses on the role of the medical examination of the sexually abused child and how the evaluation can be conducted to be of therapeutic value to the child and family, as well as to serve the system's need to ensure the child's protection and safety. Sexually abused children can experience physical injuries and contract sexually transmitted infections (STIs) as a result of their victimization, but fewer than 5% of these children have physical examination findings that are diagnostic of injury or an STI (Adams et al., 1994; Centers for Disease Control and Prevention, 2010; Christian et al., 2000; Heger et al., 2002; McCann & Voris, 1992). If 95% of sexually abused children present without acute trauma or an STI, then one might ask, what is the role of the medical examination and of what value is it to the child and the child protection system?

When appropriately conducted, the medical examination of a child suspected of being sexually abused can be critical to understanding the child's experience. All who work within the field of child protection have come to realize that no one discipline has the key to understanding the complete experience of a child when the suspicion of sexual abuse arises. Rather, it is the collective insights of all the disciplines that provide the best opportunity to understand the child's experience and to chart a path for optimal outcomes, whether medical, mental health, child protection, and/or law enforcement. Each professional, regardless of discipline, has a responsibility to work with objectivity and balance while understanding what to expect from colleagues in other disciplines. Each discipline may think it is first in importance, but none has absolute control over the processes by which cases are managed, because the goal is to do what is in the best interests of the child.

Providers of medical services should know what the other professionals in the child protection system expect from them. For example, the child protection reporting agency wants to know whether the medical diagnosis supports the concern about sexual abuse and what the impact of the abuse is on the child: how can the child best be protected and what are the therapeutic needs of the child and family? Law enforcement sees sexual victimization through the lens of "where's the evidence?" and how justice and society can be served and protected. The mental health professional has the responsibility to assess both the short- and long-term psychological consequences of the abuse and ensure that the child and family receive the therapeutic services they need.

Each community differs in the scope of professional expertise available to it, yet every child still needs the spectrum of expertise necessary to meet his or her needs. When an imbalance of professional expertise exists, there is the potential for a skewed intervention that ultimately will not serve the best interests of the child. Where these limitations exist, it is best to recognize them and take steps to build capacity where needed.

KEY ELEMENTS OF THE MEDICAL DIAGNOSIS OF CHILD SEXUAL ABUSE

Everyone involved in the assessment of allegations of child sexual abuse wants to know what the evidence is that supports the suspicion and whether there is enough evidence for substantiation. The medical provider has the potential to identify and collect "evidence" in any one or all of the following categories: (1) medical history/behaviors, (2) acute or healed anogenital and/or extragenital trauma, (3) pregnancy in an adolescent, (4) sexually transmitted infections, and (5) forensic evidence such as trace materials (seminal products).

Of the potential sources of "evidence," the most important will be found in the medical history details (Finkel & Alexander, 2011). This, however, may be the most difficult task for the health professional, in great part because it is not intuitively obvious how to engage children of various ages, developmental levels, and language abilities in sharing the difficult details of their experience.

The question might arise of who is best equipped to determine the details of a child's experience: the health professional, the child protective services (CPS) worker, or the law enforcement/forensic interviewer? The answer is, it depends. Each discipline has the potential to obtain discipline-specific information that helps it decide how to ensure best outcomes, whether in the realm of health care, protection from further harm, or legal protections. It is not that one source of information is better than another; it is that the details a child will share with a health professional may be quantitatively and qualitatively different from those imparted in other interviews. The reassurance that a health professional can provide to children in addressing specific concerns about their body cannot be provided by any discipline other than medicine. When children tell about their experience through CPS and law enforcement interviews or in the context of a medical history, there is always the possibility of some contradictory details, but it is more likely that the details will be consistent, further reinforcing the concern about abuse. There is nothing inherently wrong or traumatic for children in having to retell their experience, if they tell it to knowledgeable and skilled professionals. The retelling, in fact, can be therapeutic, as evidenced by the important role of the trauma narrative in healing for children who receive Trauma-Focused Cognitive Behavioral Therapy (Deblinger, Mannarino, Cohen, & Steer, 2006; Deblinger, Mannarino, Cohen, Runyon, & Steer, 2011).

INDICATIONS AND JUSTIFICATION FOR A MEDICAL EXAMINATION WHEN SEXUAL ABUSE IS SUSPECTED

A medical evaluation is indicated in cases of suspected child abuse to address two primary needs: (1) the diagnosis and treatment of "abnormality," which includes recognition and treatment of acute or healed physical findings, diagnosis and treatment of STIs, and identification, collection, and preservation of physical/forensic evidence; and (2) the diagnosis and treatment of "normality," which reflects an understanding of the need to address body image / wellness concerns that can arise as a result of sexual abuse.

Ultimately, the medical examination plays an important role that no other discipline can play in identifying and addressing the child's worries and concerns about body image and/or physical intactness. When both "abnormality and normality" are addressed, children can take an important step forward on the therapeutic road toward putting their experience behind them. The decision as to whether a medical examination is necessary is based on whether there is sufficient information to initiate an investigation by CPS and/or law enforcement—if so, this is an indication for the child to have a medical examination. The issue then becomes simply one of appropriate timing. The single most important question regarding timing is the interval since the child experienced the alleged abuse. If the physical contact occurred within 24–96 hours, it may be possible—depending on the details of the type of contact—to identify injuries and collect physical evidence (Adams et al., 2007; Christian, 2011). A child's having experienced something within that time frame, however, does not mean that positive findings will be identified. Forensic evidence is decidedly unusual, and recovering such evidence after 24 hours in prepubertal children is unlikely (Christian et al., 2000). In adolescents who have experienced vaginal penetration with ejaculation without a condom, collection of seminal products up to 96 hours after the event is possible.

The child should undergo only one physical examination whenever possible, carried out by someone who understands how to conduct a comprehensive assessment and formulate a defensible opinion. Follow-up examinations are appropriate to check for healing when injuries are present and for effective treatment of STIs if these are present.

A DETAILED MEDICAL HISTORY THAT BOTH ASSISTS IN SUBSTANTIATION AND IS THERAPEUTIC

The medical history of a child with suspected sexual abuse differs from the forensic interview in both its purpose and its approach. The medical professional knows that the single most important source of information critical to the formulation of any diagnosis is the medical history. The history guides the physical examination, directs testing decisions, and assists in creating a differential diagnosis and, ultimately, in formulating a diagnosis. This proven medical model is aptly applied to making the diagnosis of child sexual abuse. There are unique challenges when obtaining a medical history for children suspected of being sexually abused, and the examining medical professional needs knowledge and skill to obtain the medical history of the alleged abuse from the child. There is nothing intuitive about asking questions regarding a child's sexual victimization (Deblinger et al., 2011). It is difficult for both the clinician and the child, given the emotionally charged nature of the content. The potential for success is directly related to the historian's understanding the "disease of sexual victimization," for without this understanding, it is unlikely that the right questions will be asked or will be asked in a manner that helps facilitate the child's sharing the details of his experience (Finkelhor & Browne, 1985, 1986; Finkelhor et al., 1990).

All diseases have a natural timeline over which they become clinically evident, with a common set of signs and symptoms associated with that particular disease. If we consider sexual victimization as a disease and look at the unique characteristics of this as a disease, we quickly become aware that it is not a random, capricious experience for each child but an experience that has many common elements for all sexually abused children. With an understanding of these common elements, the clinician has the opportunity to obtain a structured history that may provide details that support making the diagnosis. What makes this history unique and challenging is that the child may find it very difficult to talk about, for a variety of reasons but commonly including embarrassment, shame, stigmatization, fear of not being believed, and/or fear of the consequences of disclosure (Browne & Finkelhor, 1986; Finkelhor et al., 1990; Summit, 1983). If the historian understands these unique concerns, the questions can be crafted in a way that is nonjudgmental, facilitating, and empathic.

The two-way dialogue that should be occurring during the medical history is approached in a different manner than is used in a forensic interview by law enforcement and/or in fact-finding questioning by CPS. The medical history is for the purpose of diagnosis and treatment, whereas the forensic interview is a law enforcement tool and the CPS questioning is focused on safety and risk.

The historian must convey, in introductory interactions with the child, an ability to understand the child's experience and to address his worries and concerns. If the child has a sense that he will benefit from sharing details, he is more likely to do so. An opening comment by the clinician, "What today is about is for me to learn some things from you, but also an opportunity for you to learn some things from me," or something similar, can set the stage for the two-way dialogue. Another type of comment that emphasizes the value of the physical examination is, "One of the things I'd like you to do is to think about any worries, questions, or concerns you have about your body, because once we finish talking, I'll do a physical exam to address any concerns about your body and to make sure you're physically fine and provide treatment if it's needed." Experience shows that when the health professional interacts in an understanding and respectful manner, the child will relax and be more likely to share previously withheld information (Finkel, 2008).

RAPPORT-BUILDING BEGINS

Rapport-building provides an opportunity for the health professional to explain the purpose of the examination, address any fears concerning the examination, and assess the child's ability to provide a narrative. Under most circumstances, the historian has some preliminary information about the presenting concerns, which helps inform the approach to beginning the medical history. For example, if the historian knows the circumstances under which the disclosure occurred and that it was a purposeful disclosure, the following comments and questions could help with rapport-building: "Most kids don't tell about things that are so difficult. Why did you decide to tell?" "What do you

want to happen now that you have told?" "Most kids find it difficult to tell. Did you find it difficult?" "What made it so difficult for you to tell?" (Alaggia, 2004; Goodman et al., 2003).

It is not uncommon for a child to think she is the only person in the world to whom this has happened. A comment that addresses this concern might be, "I talk to kids everyday, just like you, some older, some younger. When they have been able to tell about something that was done to them by someone they know and trust, that can be confusing and difficult to understand. That happens to a lot of kids. Did something like that happen to you?" Many children believe that what they experienced was their fault. Asking the child whose fault she thinks it was will provide an opportunity to determine whether she thinks it was hers. If she feels that she was at fault, then asking the question "Why do you think it was your fault?" allows her to articulate her feelings of guilt and gives the clinician an opportunity to address the child's sense of being culpable in situations in which she had no choice. By asking "Did the person who did this want you to tell?" the interviewer can explore the dynamic of secrecy that allows continuation of the activities over time. If the child answers no, the follow-up question is, "How do you know they didn't want you to tell?" In response, the child may explain the things she was told that led her to maintain secrecy and/or may express her fears concerning the consequences of disclosure. Another question that serves to empower children who have experienced abuse is, "If you could ask the person who did this a question or tell them something, what would you want them to hear?" Along the same line, the question "What do you want to happen now that you've told?" can also be empowering.

All of the suggested questions open up the opportunity to begin a dialogue that includes "therapeutic messages" that begin to address misperceptions and communicate to the child that she is speaking with someone who can understand her experience and can help. Regardless of age, if the child believes she is talking with someone who understands her, she is more likely to share details not previously shared with others. There is an inherent trust that patients of all ages have in their health care professional that increases the probability of sharing information. As one child said, "I can tell you because you're a doctor" (Finkel, 2008).

MEDICAL HISTORY TO ELICIT DETAILS OF THE ALLEGED EXPERIENCE

Taking the medical history in these cases is not just asking a series of random questions but follows a structure that elicits details common to sexual victimization. Since most sexual abuse is not a single event but a series of interactions that evolve over time, the historian, to the degree that is possible, must approach the history of abuse chronologically. The specifics of the questions will be determined in part by the child's age, cognitive/developmental capabilities, and language abilities. When young children are given an opportunity to talk about a positive experience during the rapport-building component, the historian can determine whether or not the child can provide a logical narrative (Lyon, 2010).

The types of questions can be divided into three broad categories: (1) the what, when, where, and why questions to elicit contextual details; (2) questions that assist the health professional in understanding the medical consequences of the contact for diagnosis and treatment purposes; and (3) questions that elicit information about body image and mental health consequences.

The What, When, Where, and Why

Questions should be asked about each of the following aspects of the disease of sexual victimization:

1. Who was the perpetrator and what was the access, opportunity, and frequency of contact?
2. How was the activity represented to the child? How was the child initially engaged in the sexual activity (or activities)? Was the child tricked, coerced, deceived, or forced?
3. What was the first thing the child experienced that seemed confusing, difficult to understand, or uncomfortable? How did the activities progress over time? What were the details of the sexual interactions? What was done to the child and what was he made to do? Were videos or images of pornographic acts involved?
4. Did the child maintain secrecy? If so, what were the things the child was told or perceived that led to maintaining secrecy?
5. How did the disclosure occur—purposeful, accidental, or elicited? Why did the child tell? What was the time interval between disclosure and the last contact?
6. Was the response to telling or the disclosure supportive or one of disbelief?
7. Were there any efforts to undermine the child's credibility by the offending individual or others? Was there a recantation, and if so, what were the contributing circumstances? (Finkel & Alexander, 2011).

Understanding the Medical Consequences for Diagnosis and Treatment Purposes

After obtaining contextual details about the specifics of the sexual contact, the historian should seek information about possible health consequences, such as injuries, sexually transmitted infections, or risk of pregnancy. The simple question that follows a child's description of a specific act is, "How did that feel?" Even the response "It hurt" will require asking for clarification: "Are you talking about hurting your feelings, your body, or both?" The potential for physical residua is greater if the child complains of physical discomfort, but most of the injuries children experience as a result of sexual contact are superficial and will have healed completely, depending on the time interval between the last contact and the examination. Other follow-up questions to "It hurt" may be "Tell me more" or "Did you see anything that made you know you were hurt?" In response, the child may disclose that she had bleeding, prompting additional questions about where the bleeding was seen, how much was seen, and how long it lasted. It is also important to ask whether the child experienced pain just while the contact was occurring, or after, or both. In studies, dysuria was described by 37% of girls who reported genital contact and whose dysuria was not attributed to a preexisting condition, thus confirming genital trauma with certainty (DeLago, Deblinger, et al., 2008; DeLago, Finkel, et al., 2012; Ellsworth, Mergurerian, & Copening, 1995).

When children describe genital contact, whether oral, vaginal or anal, there may be details to suggest the child came in contact with potentially infected genital secretions, placing her at risk for an STI. The manner in which this information is provided is frequently idiosyncratic, reflecting something children would have had no way of knowing unless they had experienced it. A 6-year-old boy described a teenage boy "rubbing his privates on the young boy's hiney" and then described the older boy as "sprinkling on his back," reflecting an age-appropriate description of ejaculation.

When a child discloses "penetration," it is important to understand what the child means before conducting the examination. To a young child, the word *in* may mean "between" or "on," but to an adolescent, who may have a more mature understanding of her body, it could mean true vaginal and/or anal penetration. A helpful tool for clarifying *in* is the Ortho anatomical model of the female genitalia. With this model, the child can demonstrate her perception of "in" and/or may demonstrate uncertainty. When prepubertal children experience true penetration into the vagina, there is likely to be a history of pain and, potentially, bleeding; this provides the opportunity to diagnose either acute or healed trauma, depending on when the child presents in relation to the time of contact. In the pubertal child the estrogenized hymen has great elasticity, and determining whether vaginal penetration occurred can be difficult. Whitley (1978) found that 54% of women denied any bleeding associated with their first consensual intercourse. Kellogg, Menard, and Santos (2004) noted that only 2 of 36 pregnant adolescents had genital examination findings that, on their own, were diagnostic of vaginal penetration. When a child experiences anal penetration, there is the potential for trauma to the anal verge tissues and the mucocutaneous tissue. Trauma to the mucocutaneous junction can result in complaints about a burning sensation with passage of a bowel movement. This is a corollary to the experience of dysuria that follows trauma to the urethra and surrounding tissue during vulvar coitus or vaginal penetration.

Body Image and Mental Health Consequences

One of the most important therapeutic aspects of the child's interaction with the health professional is a discussion of worries or concerns about his body (Byram, Wagner, & Waller, 1995; Harter, Alexander, & Neimyer, 1988; Waller, Hamilton, & Rose, 1993). The child should be given an opportunity to express any such worries or concerns when the medical history is being obtained. This may be the first time the child has had an opportunity to voice concerns and/or reveal distortions of thinking about his body integrity. Knowing about these concerns before proceeding with the examination is essential and is an important component of diagnosing and treating the residual trauma of the sexual victimization.

The literature supports the clinical observation that sexually abused children may view themselves differently following the abusive experience (Byram, Wagner, & Waller, 1995). The stigmatization and shame experienced by most victims contribute to the feeling of being "damaged goods" (Finkelhor & Browne, 1985). There is also an association between eating disorders, body image, and sexual victimization (Waller, Hamilton, & Rose, 1993).

In great part, concerns about body intactness may stem from children's incorrect perception about the degree of physical intrusiveness they have experienced. Some girls, even those for whom it is developmentally impossible to become pregnant, think they could be pregnant with penetration limited to the vaginal vestibule (vulvar coitus). Adolescents who experience penetration limited to the vaginal vestibule might think that, as a result, they are no longer a virgin. There is value in addressing such discrepancies between a child's perception of her experience and what she has actually experienced. When adolescents have experienced vaginal penetration, a thorough physical examination can let them know that their body is still fine, that they will be able to engage in normal, healthy, consensual sexual activities in the future, that their potential to have children is unaffected, and that no one will be able to tell that they have been sexually abused. Each and every one of these messages can be reassuring and of great therapeutic value as young people begin to put these experiences behind them.

The health professional should assume that any sexually inappropriate contact has the potential for significant psychological sequelae. Simply stated, there is no direct correlation between the degree of physical intrusiveness and psychological intrusiveness. Assessment of the impact of the victimization is most often made by a psychologist and/or psychiatrist. It is appropriate, however, to note any observations that reflect distress or alterations of mood during the medical examination. The health professional should ask about cutting, suicidal ideation, and use of alcohol and illicit drugs.

Victims of sexual abuse may have unusual fears, usually having to do with the effect of the sexual abuse on their bodies. One 8-year-old girl asked if it were true that you could get breast cancer if someone put his mouth on your breast. A 9-year-old girl, following the perpetrator's ejaculation onto her genitalia, worried for months that sperm were still inside her. A 6-year-old girl was convinced she was pregnant because when she sat on the potty and looked in the mirror, she saw that her "tummy puffed out." A 10-year-old boy was worried that he was going to get the "dying disease"—AIDS—because of the sexual abuse he had experienced. Each of these children had these worries successfully addressed when the health professional identified their concerns and addressed them within the context of a complete, head-to-toe examination. Even children who do not express concerns about their body during the medical history are relieved after being told by the physician, after the examination, that they are normal. Nonoffending parents also are reassured that their child is normal after the examination. Some children may require continued reassurance in the postdiagnostic period.

After the examination, the physician must decide what information to share with the child and the nonoffending parent. The extent of that information will depend on the child's age, emotional stability, and expressed concerns. It is important to remember that an overly paternalistic attitude in withholding information to "protect the child" may inadvertently represent a further betrayal of trust. In most cases, it is sufficient to tell the child that any injuries he had have healed, that he is fine, and that nobody could ever tell he had been injured. Older children may need appropriate reassurance that their experience will not directly interfere with their ability to have children when they are adults. Boys may worry that their experience might make them become homosexual, and a discussion should address this, as well as other potential concerns.

CONDUCTING THE MEDICAL EXAMINATION

As a result of the medical history, the examining health professional will have a much better understanding of the potential for identifying physical residua and the need to collect evidence and/or test for STIs, as well as an estimate of the child's fear and anxiety regarding the examination. The anogenital examination should be conducted within the context of a head-to-toe examination. By conducting a head-to-toe examination, the clinician is giving the message that all parts of the child's body are important and that this exam will look at the child, in totality, for her well-being. The examiner should take time to explain what the exam entails, in a developmentally appropriate manner. The accompanying adult may be fearful that the prepubertal child will have a speculum examination and that this will be physically intrusive and painful. Explaining what to expect can make the adult more relaxed and supportive of the child throughout the examination. If there is a need to use a speculum in a pubertal child, the clinician should explain how that decision will be made and what to expect.

The factors that can enhance children's or adolescents' cooperativeness are anticipating and addressing their fears and anxiety, demystifying the examination, giving them a sense of control throughout the exam, and providing choices. Choices might include whom they want in the room as a support person throughout the examination. Young children might prefer sitting in their mother's lap and having an opportunity to feel a Q-tip and/or a gloved hand before being touched, and then watching the examination on a video monitor. Video colposcopy is an excellent tool that can demystify the examination by giving the child a choice as to whether she wants to watch the exam, providing a greater sense of participation and control (Mears et al., 2003; Palusci & Cyrus, 2001). The video colposcope is simply an excellent light source with magnification capabilities that enhances the visualization of genital and anal anatomy. This instrument does not touch the child, and there is no discomfort associated with its use. Video colposcopy allows recording of the examination, reducing the need for a repeat exam if the examiner's interpretation is challenged, and serves as a baseline reference for concerns in the future (Ricci, 1994). Younger children might want to see their finger nails or belly button on TV to demonstrate that this instrument just magnifies and helps the health professional take a better look.

The examination room should be child friendly, and the examiner should be patient and empathic and take whatever time is necessary for the child to be comfortable. Under no circumstances should the child be forcibly restrained to conduct the examination. Some patients may not be emotionally ready to cooperate. If that is the case, the clinician should explain why the examination can help the child and that he or she will be pleased to do it when the child is emotionally ready. If the child will not cooperate and there is a need to conduct an examination to assess the extent of trauma, the child can receive either conscious sedation or anesthesia.

UNDERSTANDING AND INTERPRETING PHYSICAL EVIDENCE

Two of the most significant challenges for the examining physician are (1) interpreting healed changes in anogenital anatomy without knowledge of the premorbid state and (2) differentiating accidental from nonaccidental patterns of injury (Christian, 2011; Clayden, 1987; Heger-Heppenstall et al., 2003; McCann & Voris, 1992).

Acute injuries to the genitalia are infrequent because most children are engaged in sexually inappropriate activities with a person they know and who does not intend physical harm. When injuries do occur, they are generally superficial, and most heal without posttraumatic residua. Most children do not disclose abuse until they feel safe, sometimes long after the last contact. Consequently, at the time of disclosure, they may have no acute signs of trauma. Only a small percentage of children (<5%) sustain signifi-

cant injuries that heal with distinct and diagnostic posttraumatic findings (Heger-Heppenstall et al., 2003). Observations indicate that when acute injuries are significant and heal through the repair process resulting in formation of granulation tissue, the chronic, healed posttraumatic findings may appear different than might be anticipated from the appearance of the acute injury. Consequently, the retrospective interpretation of healed posttraumatic findings can be difficult (Finkel, 1989).

Acutely injured children should undergo an immediate examination to assess the extent of the injuries and a follow-up examination to ensure complete healing and document the resolution of the injury. The frequency of reexamination will depend on the extent of the injury. Superficial injuries generally heal within 96 hours, if not complicated by an infection. Thus, one follow-up examination is generally sufficient to document the somewhat predictable healing of the most acute superficial injuries. More extensive injuries heal with the development of scar tissue, so examinations over a longer period (up to a year) may be required. The stages of healing progression associated with fibrin clot formation, proliferation of neovascularized granulation tissue, and eventual wound retraction each give a distinctly different appearance to the injury and should be visualized and documented (Finkel, 1989).

Differentiating accidental from inflicted trauma is best done by considering the history of the event given by the caregiver, child, and witness(es); the presenting circumstances for medical care; the scene investigation, if needed; and the pattern of injuries. Straddle injuries have a classic unilateral crush-injury pattern. Impaling injuries that are accidental vary in the pattern of trauma, primarily based on the type of object. As a general rule, impaling injuries such as a child falling onto a bicycle seat-post create a distinct pattern and present emergently with little question as to the mechanism of injury.

Just as genital injuries are most likely to be superficial, so are anal injuries, whether in boys or girls, following sodomy (Clayden, 1987). In sodomy, there are many variables that mitigate or exacerbate the potential for injury and thus the diagnostic findings. Extragenital signs of trauma are infrequent, but when observed, they can usually be correlated with a history of the use of force and restraint.

The initial examination must include an assessment for the risk of an STI, and if at risk, the child should be appropriately tested and treated. If any examination findings suggest the presence of "forensic evidence," this should be collected and preserved.

Longitudinal studies reflect the difficulty in predicting the healed appearance of acute injuries when those injuries heal by the repair process that forms scar tissue, which can distort the appearance of the tissues (Finkel, 1989; Heger-Heppenstall et al., 2003; Myers, 2009). Most genital and anal injuries that children incur are superficial and heal by the process of regeneration of labile cells, and as a result, unless the injury is observed acutely, the examination will find no residua from the acute injuries and the findings could be described as "normal."

Another variable in interpreting residua is the time differential between the sexual contact and disclosure. If a child incurred significant trauma when prepubertal and delays disclosure until puberty, the effect of puberty in girls complicates the recognition of scar tissue due to estrogen's effect on the tissues. Estrogen causes changes to the thin mucosal appearance of the prepubertal hymen and vestibular structures. As pubertal development progresses, the hymen becomes thickened, redundant, and elastic and changes in color from the un-estrogenized erythematous vascularized appearance to a pinkish white coloration. In puberty, if no knowledge of the premorbid state exists, only the most obvious nonacute changes to the hymeneal membrane can be said to be residual to sexual contact. Acute signs of trauma are readily visualized, whether prepubertal or pubertal. Longitudinal studies demonstrating developmental changes in genital structures will assist in differentiating between the residua from sexual trauma and changes in the appearance of the hymen as a result of normal development.

FORMULATING A DIAGNOSTIC OPINION

One of the most important tasks in cases of suspected child sexual abuse is the formulation of a medical record that clearly states the health professional's diagnostic assessment and the basis for it (Finkel, 2009). The report should be written in a clear, objective, and non-editorial style. It should have a consistent format to ensure that it includes all necessary information utilized to reach the diagnosis and recommend a treatment plan.

When articulating a diagnosis, it is not sufficient to conclude that a physical examination is consistent with the history and neither confirms nor denies the allegations. Conclusions such as these are easily challenged. Examination findings may be categorized as follows: (1) medical findings that can be stated to confirm the allegations with diagnostic certainty; (2) nonspecific findings temporally related to specific events that can be corroborated by the history or by other investigative details and thus support an association between the findings/history and the alleged contact; (3) findings that are nonspecific and thus are seen in both abused and nonabused children; and (4) findings that have no relevance to the allegations.

When there are no physical findings but clear historical details reflective of sexual contact, the clinician must explain the factors that account for such circumstances. If there are no residua to the alleged contact, the report should state why this can be the case. If a child provides a history that reflects his perception of penetration but the physical examination does not confirm such, the report should explain why this discrepancy can exist. A report that is factual and educates its reader is invaluable to CPS, law enforcement, courts, defense attorneys, and the report author. A complete medical report will ultimately play an important role should the case proceed to either civil or criminal proceedings and may reduce the need for court testimony. Reports that are illegible, lacking in detail, and/or biased serve little purpose and are a disservice to the child.

Supplemental reports will be necessary to summarize the outcome of follow-up examinations, test results, and additional recommendations emanating from multidisciplinary review. A routine recommendation too often overlooked by physicians is a referral for a mental health assessment of the impact of the abuse and treatment recommendations. This recommendation may influence the decision of CPS and law enforcement to provide mental health services. Increasingly, CPS is limiting its involvement to "protection," and once the child no longer appears at risk, agencies are closing cases.

No matter how thorough and thoughtful the medical professional has been in obtaining the medical history and interpreting the examination results, there will always be the potential for a challenge to one's opinion. The best preparation for legal proceedings is to be meticulous in recording information in the medical record and review of accompanying reports (McCann & Voris, 1992; Mears et al., 2003; Myers, 1986). Any attempt to rehabilitate an ill-prepared report long after the initial examination is fraught with many challenges.

Although only a relatively small percentage of cases proceed to prosecution and to trial, those that do test the reliability of the examining physician's conclusions and the basis that supports them. Cases usually come to court action long after the medical encounter, often more than a year later. Because of the significant time delay between prosecution and trial, a medical record that is well crafted and complete is invaluable to the physician when preparing for either civil or criminal proceedings.

RECOMMENDATIONS FOR THE POSTDIAGNOSTIC NEEDS OF THE CHILD AND FAMILY

Once a diagnosis of child sexual abuse is made and the concern is substantiated, the medical professional plays an important role in emphasizing the value of and facilitating referrals for appropriate mental health services for the child and family. If there is a lack of certainty about whether sexual abuse occurred but concerns remain, a referral for further assessment by a psychologist or psychiatrist is appropriate. Fortunately, children can be resilient and are encouragingly responsive to evidenced-based treatment approaches, such as Trauma-Focused Cognitive Behavioral Therapy (TF-CBT; Deblinger et al., 2006).

Although some children and families would prefer to simply forget about the sexual abuse, the most effective way for all to recover from this kind of experience is for the child to talk with a mental health professional. Before children receive therapy, they should undergo an initial battery of psychological measures that help understand the impact of the abuse. A few representative examples of such measures are the Child Sexual Behavior Inventory–Revised, the Trauma Symptom Checklist for Children, the Children's Impact of Traumatic Events Scale–Revised, and the Children's Attributions and Perceptions Scale. About 40%–50% of children who experience sexual abuse will have symptoms of posttraumatic stress disorder. Sexually abused children are at risk for developing sexualized behavior problems, which may increase their vulnerability to further abuse (Friedrich et al., 1998; Kellogg & Committee on Child Abuse and Neglect, 2009). There are many factors that can mediate for or against a successful outcome for the child. One of the most significant factors that fosters a positive outcome is the belief and support of a nonoffending caregiver(s). Mothers and fathers of sexually abused children require therapeutic and educational interventions, as they are often secondary victims. When mothers and fathers receive appropriate support, they are in a better position to be supportive of their child and others affected by the abuse.

CONCLUSIONS

The objective of the medical examination when child sexual abuse is alleged is much more than simply diagnosing physical signs of trauma and sexually transmitted infections and collecting forensic evidence. If the medical evaluation, history, and physical are conducted with an understanding of the "disease" of sexual victimization, there is the potential both to glean a more complete understanding of the child's experience than might be obtained by other professional disciplines and, simultaneously, to be one of the first steps toward therapeutic intervention.

References

Adams, J. A., Harper, K., Knudson, S., & Revilla, J. (1994). Examination findings in legally confirmed child sexual abuse: It's normal to be normal. *Pediatrics, 94*, 148–150.

Adams, J. A., Kaplan, R. A., Starling, S. P., Mehta, N. H., Finkel, M. A., Botash, A. S., et al. (2007). Guidelines for medical care of children who may have been sexually abused. *Journal of Pediatric and Adolescent Gynecology, 20*(3), 163–172.

Alaggia, R. (2004). Many ways of telling: Expanding conceptualizations of child sexual abuse disclosure. *Child Abuse & Neglect, 28*(11), 1213–1227.

Browne, A., & Finkelhor, D. (1986). Initial and long-term effects: A review of the research. In D. Finkelhor (Ed.), *A sourcebook on child sexual abuse* (pp. 143–179). Beverly Hills, CA: Sage Publications.

Byram, V., Wagner, H., & Waller, G. (1995). Sexual abuse and body image distortion. *Child Abuse & Neglect, 19*, 507–510.

Centers for Disease Control and Prevention. (2010). Sexual assault and STDs. In *Sexually transmitted diseases treatment guidelines, 2010.* www.cdc.gov/std/treatment/2010/sexual-assault.htm#a2

Christian, C. W. (2011). Timing of the medical examination. *Journal of Child Sexual Abuse, 20*(5), 505–520.

Christian, C. W., Lavelle, J. M., De Jong, A. R., Loiselle, J., Brenner, L., & Joffe, M. (2000). Forensic evidence findings in prepubertal victims of sexual assault. *Pediatrics, 106*(1, Pt. 1), 100–104.

Clayden, G. S. (1987). Anal appearance and child sexual abuse. *Lancet, 1*, 620.

Deblinger, E., Mannarino, A. P., Cohen, J. A., Runyon, M. K., & Steer, R. A. (2011). Trauma-Focused Cognitive Behavioral Therapy for children: Impact of the trauma narrative and treatment length. *Depression and Anxiety, 28*(1), 67–75.

Deblinger, E., Mannarino, A. P., Cohen, J. A., & Steer, R. A. (2006). A follow-up study of a multisite, randomized, controlled trial for children with sexual abuse–related PTSD symptoms. *Journal of the American Academy of Child and Adolescent Psychiatry, 45*(12), 1474–1484.

DeLago, C., Deblinger, E., Schroeder, C., & Finkel, M. A. (2008). Girls who disclose sexual abuse: Urogenital symptoms and signs after genital contact. *Pediatrics, 122*(2), e281–286.

DeLago, C., Finkel, M. A., Clarke, C., & Deblinger, E. D. (2012). Urogenital symptoms after sexual abuse vs. irritant contacts. *Journal of Pediatric and Adolescent Gynecology, 25*, 334–339.

Ellsworth, P. I., Mergurerian, P. A., & Copening, M. E. (1995). Sexual abuse: Another causative factor in dysfunctional voiding. *Journal of Urology, 153*, 773–776.

Finkel, M. A. (1989). Anogenital trauma in sexually abused children. *Pediatrics, 84*, 317.

Finkel, M. A. (2008). "I can tell you because you're a doctor" *Pediatrics, 122*(8), 422.

Finkel, M. A. (2009). Documentation, report formulation and conclusions. In M. A. Finkel & A. P. Giardino (Eds.), *Medical evaluation of child sexual abuse: A practical guide* (3rd ed., pp. 357–370). Elk Grove Village, IL: American Academy of Pediatrics.

Finkel, M. A., & Alexander, R. A. (2011). Conducting the medical history. *Journal of Child Sexual Abuse, 20*(5), 486–504.

Finkelhor, D., & Browne, A. (1985). The traumatic impact of child sexual abuse: A conceptualization. *American Journal of Orthopsychiatry, 55*(4), 530–541.

Finkelhor, D., & Browne, A. (1986). Impact of child sexual abuse: A review of the research. *Psychological Bulletin, 99*, 66–77.

Finkelhor, D., Hotaling, G., Lewis, I. A., & Smith, C. (1990). Sexual abuse in a national survey of adult men and women: Prevalence, characteristics, and risk factors. *Child Abuse & Neglect, 14*(1), 19–28.

Friedrich, W. N., Fisher, J., Broughton, D., Houston, M., & Shafram, C. R. (1998). Normative sexual behavior in children: A contemporary sample. *Pediatrics, 101*, e9.

Goodman, T. B., Edelstein, R. S., Goodman, G. S., Jones, D. P., & Gordon, D. S. (2003). Why children tell: A model of children's disclosure of child sexual abuse. *Child Abuse & Neglect, 27*, 525–540.

Harter, S., Alexander, P. C., & Neimyer, R. A. (1988). Long-term effects of incestuous child abuse in college women: Social adjustment, social cognition, and family characteristics. *Journal of Consulting and Clinical Psychology, 58*, 5–8.

Heger, A., Ticson, L., Velasquez, O., & Bernier, R. (2002). Children referred for possible sexual abuse: Medical findings in 2384 children. *Child Abuse & Neglect, 26*, 645–659.

Heger-Heppenstall, G., McConnell, G., Ticson, L., Guerra, L., Lister, J., & Zaragoza, T. (2003). Healing patterns in anogenital injuries: A longitudinal study of injuries associated with sexual abuse, accidental injuries, or genital surgery in the preadolescent child. *Pediatrics, 112*(4), 829–837.

Kellogg, N. D., & Committee on Child Abuse and Neglect, American Academy of Pediatrics. (2009). Clinical report: The evaluation of sexual behaviors in children. *Pediatrics, 124*, 992–998. doi:10.1542/peds.2009-1692

Kellogg, N. D., Menard, S. W., & Santos, A. (2004). Genital anatomy in pregnant adolescents: "Normal" does not mean "nothing happened." *Pediatrics, 113*(1), e67–69.

Lyon, T. D. (2010). Investigative interviewing of the child. In D. N. Duquette & A. M. Haralambie (Eds.), *Child welfare law and practice* (2nd ed., pp. 87–109). Denver, CO: Bradford Publishing.

McCann, J., & Voris, J. (1992). Genital injuries resulting from sexual abuse: A longitudinal study. *Pediatrics, 89*, 307.

Mears, C. J., Heflin, A. H., Finkel, M. A., Deblinger, E., & Steer, R. A. (2003). Adolescents' responses to sexual abuse evaluation including the use of video colposcopy. *Journal of Adolescent Health, 33*(1), 18–34.

Myers, J. E. B. (1986). The role of the physician in preserving verbal evidence of child abuse. *Journal of Pediatrics, 109*, 409.

Myers, J. E. B. (2009). Legal issues in the medical evaluation of child sexual abuse. In M. A. Finkel & A. P. Giardino (Eds.), *Medical evaluation of child sexual abuse: A practical guide* (3rd ed., pp. 313–340). Elk Grove Village, IL: American Academy of Pediatrics.

Palusci, V. J., & Cyrus, T. A. (2001). Reaction to videocolposcopy in the assessment of child sexual abuse. *Child Abuse & Neglect, 25*(11), 1135–1146.

Ricci, L. R. (1994). Photodocumentation of the abused child. In R. M. Reece (Ed.), *Child abuse: Medical diagnosis and management* (pp. 248–265). Philadelphia, PA: Lea & Febiger.

Summit, R. C. (1983). The child sexual abuse accommodation syndrome. *Child Abuse & Neglect, 7*(2), 177–193.

Waller, G., Hamilton, K., & Rose, N. (1993). Sexual abuse and body image distortion in the eating disorders. *British Journal of Clinical Psychology, 32*, 350–352.

Whitley, N. (1978). The first coital experience of one hundred women. *JOGNN, 7*(4), 41–45.

19

ROBERT M. REECE, M.D.
RONALD C. SAVAGE, ED.D.
NAOMI SUGAR, M.D.

Treatment of Physical Child Abuse

GENERAL CONSIDERATIONS

The medical literature on the treatment of physical child abuse beyond the acute phase of injury is sparse. This derives from fragmentation of the medical care of these children: one set of physicians sees the child in the emergency department, another set cares for the child on the hospital inpatient services, then, after the child's discharge from the acute care setting, and in the best case scenario, still another group of medical personnel assumes control of the child's medical care. Too often, however, unless there are serious identifiable medical conditions, children who have been physically abused get little or no coordinated medical follow-up, and they have no "medical home" where comprehensive attention can be paid to their medical needs.

Physical child abuse can be categorized by organ system involvement or by severity of impairment. Children have been physically abused by suffering injuries to their skin, their skeletal structures, or their internal or visceral organs, or traumatic injuries to their skull and/or intracranial structures. A smaller number of children are victims of medical child abuse, otherwise known as Munchausen syndrome by proxy, or of intentional immersions (drowning or near-drowning). Bizarre forms of physical abuse include microwave burning, fatal pepper aspiration, perforations of the hypopharynx, scarification and tattooing, insertions of needles into various parts of the body, intentional eye, ear, and dental injuries, intentional poisonings or intoxications, and religious or cult practices resulting in withholding of medical care or extreme paddling that results in rhabdomyolysis and renal failure.

The most severe and long-lasting physical injuries usually involve the skin, intra-abdominal or intra-thoracic organ damage, or, most seriously, brain damage—which is where we begin our discussion.

ABUSIVE HEAD TRAUMA (INFLICTED TRAUMATIC BRAIN INJURY)

Treatment in the Acute Phase

The lesions of brain injury are caused by an array of insults to the brain. This cascade of events begins with traumatic contusions, sometimes accompanied by hemorrhage into the brain parenchyma and shearing of tissue planes. The damaged brain cells react with a characteristic cell response, causing cerebral edema and resulting in rising pressure within the cranial vault. Hypoxia, due both to respiratory impairments secondary to brainstem damage and to the brain swelling that compresses blood vessels carrying oxygenated blood to the brain cells, contributes to the destruction of brain tissue. Hypercarbia, seizures, and variations in blood pressure add to the metabolic chaos in the brain substance. As brain cells die, they release excitatory enzymes that exert a toxic influence on neurons adjacent to the traumatic and hypoxic-ischemic zones.

The cornerstone of effective initial treatment of all head-injured children, whether inflicted or accidental injury, is accurate assessment of the elements of the injuries. This assignment often falls to the first responders and the medical care team in the receiving hospital, usually in the emergency department. All head-injured children need the "ABCs"—the fundamentals of airway, breathing, and circulation—immobilization of the cervical spine, and securing of intravenous (IV) access. Once these have been accomplished, other treatment priorities can be established, taking into account what information is available about the general medical history of the child, diseases or conditions known to exist in the child's family, a description of how the injury occurred, the timing of the injury, and the time of appearance of the first signs and symptoms. A key question is when the child was last observed performing normal activities. Close attention should be paid to the caretakers' proffered mechanism of injury, which can suggest the kinds of injuries to suspect. Further valuable history includes the kinds of resuscitation measures that were required and used. Then the obvious clinical evaluations must be carried out: the physical and neurological examination, the assignment of severity scores, using a variety of scales—Glasgow Coma Scale (GCS; Teasdale and Jennett, 1974), Children's Coma Scale (CCS; Reilly et al., 1988), and the CHOP Infant Coma Scale, also called the Infant Face Scale (IFS; Durham et al., 2000) (see tables 19.1, 19.2, and 19.3)—followed by deciding which radiological and laboratory evaluations are necessary. The authors of the CHOP Infant Coma Scale found that the face scale alone may be sufficient to "provide the best prognostic indicator of cortical damage in infants with severe traumatic brain injury . . . and may prove to be a simple and practical bedside index of brain injury severity in children under 2 years of age" (Durham et al., 2000, p. 737).

Deterioration after a head injury is estimated by this variety of scales, none of which is perfect. It is particularly important in this initial evaluation to perform a thorough, complete general physical examination to avoid missing injuries in other parts of the body, which could be life-threatening in their own right. The status of the head-injured child is a continuously evolving one and needs repeated observations to ensure proper medical responses. Initial signs and symptoms may be mild and nonspecific, such as breathing difficulties, alterations in vital signs because of disruption of centers in the brainstem, irritability,

Table 19.1. Glasgow Coma Scale (GCS)

Score	Motor	Verbal	Eye Opening
6	Obeys commands	—	—
5	Localizes	Oriented	—
4	Withdraws	Confused	Spontaneous
3	Flexor posturing	Inappropriate words	To voice
2	Extensor posturing	Incomprehensible	To pain
1	None/flaccid	None	None

Note. Scores range from 3 to 15: 13-15 = mild injury; 9-12 = moderate injury; 3-8 = severe injury.
— = Not applicable

Table 19.2. Children's Coma Score (CCS)

Score	Motor	Verbal	Eye Opening
6	Spontaneous	—	—
5	Purposeful/localizes	Coos, babbles	—
4	Withdraws	Irritable, cries	Spontaneous
3	Flexor posturing	Cries to pain	To voice
2	Extensor posturing	Moans to pain	To pain
1	None/flaccid	None	None

Note. Scores range from 3 to 15: 13-15 = mild injury; 9-12 = moderate injury; 3-8 = severe injury.
— = Not applicable

Table 19.3. Infant Face Scale (IFS)

Score	Motor	Verbal/Face	Eye Opening
6	Spontaneous normal movements	—	—
5	Hypoactive	Cries (grimaces with crying sounds and/or tears) spontaneously, with handling or to minor pain	—
4	Nonspecific movement to deep pain only (trapezius pinch)	Same as above, alternating with sleep only	Spontaneous
3	Abnormal rhythmic spontaneous movements; seizure-like activity	Cries to deep pain only (trapezius pinch)	Verbal stimulation or to touch
2	Extension, either spontaneous or to painful stimuli	Grimaces only to pain	Painful stimulation
1	Flaccid	No facial expression to pain	None

Note. Scores range from 3 to 15: 13–15 = mild injury; 9–12 = moderate injury; 3–8 = severe injury.
— = Not applicable

lethargy, or simple feeding refusal. More serious symptoms include vomiting, seizures, enlarging head size, apnea, unresponsiveness, or coma.

Delayed development of lethargy, irritability, and behavioral changes may be seen after seemingly minor head injuries in children, usually within 10–30 minutes, with progression of symptoms over the next 1–2 hours; gradually, the child recovers, usually within 12 hours (Adelson et al., 2003). These children need close observation, and sometimes a CT scan is performed to rule out cerebral edema or bleeding. Postconcussive frequent vomiting may prompt a CT scan, but these patients recover with expectant management (Adelson et al., 2003). In approximately 10% of pediatric head injuries, posttraumatic seizures occur, the vast majority (90%) within 24 hours (Hahn et al., 1988; Jennett, 1976).

The critical questions are whether the infant or young child has suffered a mild, moderate, or severe head injury; whether the patient needs imaging by CT or MRI head scans; and whether the child needs to be admitted to the hospital. One study examined pediatric patients with normal neurological findings in the emergency department, and although 28% had abnormal CT findings, only 4% had evidence of intracranial injuries (Shunk, Rodgerson, & Woodward, 1996). But other studies found a higher incidence of intracranial injuries (Dietrich et al., 1993; Hahn & McLone, 1993). A more recent large, multicenter prospective study in the United Kingdom involving 10 hospitals derived a "Children's Head Injury Algorithm for the Prediction of Important Clinical Events" (CHALICE) decision rule for head injury in children (Dunning et al., 2006). The study included 22,772 children with any severity of head injury, and all participating institutions used a protocol that collected 40 clinical variables for each child. All children who had a clinically significant head injury (death, or need for neurosurgical intervention, or abnormality on a CT scan) were identified. Of the original cohort, 281 showed an abnormality on CT, 137 had a neurosurgical operation, and 15 died. The CHALICE rule was derived with a sensitivity of 98% and a specificity of 87%. Dunning et al. (2006) state the CHALICE rule as follows:

A computed tomography scan is required if any of the following criteria are present:
➤ History
• Witnessed loss of consciousness of >5 minutes duration
• History of amnesia (either retrograde or antegrade) of >5 minutes duration
• Abnormal drowsiness (defined as drowsiness in excess of that expected by the examining doctor)
• >3 vomits after head injury
• Suspicion of non-accidental injury (NAI, defined as any suspicion of NAI by the examining doctor)
• Seizure after head injury in a patient who has no history of epilepsy
➤ Examination
• GCS <14, or GCS of <15 if <1 year old
• Suspicion of penetrating or depressed skull fracture or tense fontanel
• Signs of a basilar skull fracture (defined as evidence of blood or cerebrospinal fluid from ear or nose, panda eyes, Battles sign, hemotympanum, facial crepitus or serious facial injury)
• Positive focal neurology (defined as any focal neurology, including motor, sensory, coordination or reflex abnormality)
• Presence of bruise, swelling or laceration >5 cm if <1 year old
➤ Mechanism
• High speed road traffic accident either as a pedestrian, cyclist or occupant (defined as accident with speed >40 miles/hour)
• Fall of >3 meters (10 feet)
• High-speed injury from a projectile or an object
• If none of the above variables are present, the patient is at low risk of intracranial pathology.

A study from 2003 developed a decision rule involving 2,043 children with blunt head trauma seen in a pediatric trauma center, using an observational cohort study (Palchak et al., 2003). The authors concluded that important factors for identifying children at low risk for traumatic brain injury (TBI) after blunt head trauma included the absence of the following: abnormal mental status, clinical signs of skull fracture, a history of vomiting, scalp hematoma, and headache In 2012, a systematic review of eight clinical prediction rules found that no study validated a rule in a separate population or assessed its impact in actual practice (Maguire et al., 2012). The two studies thought to be of high quality were the two mentioned above, but Maguire and colleagues believe these rules need to be prospectively validated in different populations before they can be recommended for adoption. They also state that no high-quality and high-performing rule has been derived for very young children.

Recently, another approach to assessing children with mild head injury has emerged. This employs measurement of a serum and cerebrospinal fluid (CSF) marker to assist in screening infants who are at high risk for inflicted traumatic brain injury (iTBI) and whose injuries could be missed by other conventional diagnostic approaches. Berger and colleagues (2006) did a prospective case-control study of 98 well-appearing infants who presented with nonspecific symptoms and no history of trauma. Serum or CSF was collected, and the markers neuron-specific enolase (NSE), S100B, and myelin-basic protein (MBP) were measured. Fourteen of these patients were diagnosed as having iTBI. The marker S100B was neither sensitive nor specific for iTBI, but five patients who were not identified as having iTBI at the time of enrollment were identified at follow-up as being possible victims of abuse. Four had increased NSE at enrollment. The authors concluded that NSE and MBP may be useful as a screening test to identify infants who are at increased risk for iTBI and could benefit from evaluation with a CT scan. In a subsequent study, Berger et al. (2008) compared the concentrations of 44 serum biomarkers in 16 infants with mild iTBI and 20 infants without brain injury. There were significant group differences in the concentrations of 9 of the 44 markers. Vascular cellular adhesion molecule showed the most significant group differences. The authors believe these results suggest that significant changes occur in the serum biomarker profile after mild iTBI. Another study showed that MBP increased markedly in the CSF after severe TBI (Su et al., 2012). The use of such biomarkers to help identify head injuries holds much promise but needs further research to clarify how these markers should be used.

In children with moderate or severe head injury, the first consideration remains maintenance of the ABCs (airway, breathing, circulation). Endotracheal intubation is usually performed, the cervical spine stabilized, and IV access established for circulation and the administration of drugs. Hypothermia should be suspected and body temperature maintained. Plane radiographs of the head and neck and upper thorax should be complemented by CT and/or MRI scans of the head. The aforementioned attention to a complete physical and neurological examination applies in these cases as well.

Cerebral edema and a rise in intracranial pressure are consequences of TBI and need close observation. Intracranial monitoring is often accomplished with a fiberoptic sensor inserted into the subdural space. Sometimes a ventricular catheter is used instead, offering the additional advantage of withdrawing CSF to help lower intracranial pressure (Dias, 2004). Adequate oxygenation, head elevation, and maintenance of euvolemia are the current goals for the management of intracranial pressure (Adelson et al., 2003). Decompressive craniotomy is done in the most extreme cases. Steroids, hyperventilation, and restriction of fluids are no longer thought to be of any value. Pain control, fever control, seizure prophylaxis or treatment, bladder drainage, and nonrestrictive cervical collars are adjuncts. Mannitol, as an osmotic diuretic, is considered to be useful, as is the use of inotropic drugs such as dopamine (Adelson et al., 2003). Close attention needs to be paid to water and electrolyte balance in the general circulation, and vigilance with regard to infection, particularly meningitis, is essential. Prophylactic antibiotics are controversial, but if meningitis is diagnosed through CSF examination and culture, broad-spectrum antibiotics such as vancomycin and cephalosporins are used first, while awaiting the results of culture and sensitivity testing. Most small subdural hematomas are managed nonoperatively. Large subdural hematomas producing a mass effect are usually evacuated surgically (Adelson et al., 2003).

In 2007, Dean and colleagues surveyed 194 U.S. physicians to determine the degree of agreement on the evidence-based recommendations for the treatment of severe TBI in children. Of those surveyed, 36 were neurosurgeons and 158 were nonsurgeons, most of these (155) intensivists. There was only 60% agreement on all recommendations. For some treatments, however, more than 90% agreed with the recommendations: use of sedation, monitoring cerebral perfusion pressure, and avoiding the use of hyperthermia and steroids. More than two-thirds followed treatment recommendations for intracranial pressure, using hyperosmolar therapy, using mild and aggressive hyperventilation as second-line therapy, and considering the use of barbiturates and decompressive craniotomy as second-line therapies. Dean et al. opined that the low percentages of agreement were based on the perception that supporting evidence for certain therapies was not strong: neuromuscular blockade, CSF drainage, 3% saline, or a serum osmolality of 360 mOsm/L as the threshold to withhold mannitol. As in many areas of medical practice, there are certain areas of agreement but other areas where the science has not been convincing enough for some physicians to adopt a therapy.

Long-Term Sequelae and Treatment

Although it is true that mortality is significantly higher for children with inflicted TBI than for those with accidental TBI (16.8% vs. 10.7%) and that more children with iTBI die in the hospital than in the pre-hospital setting compared with children with accidental trauma (Rorke-Adams et al., 2009; Sills, Libby, & Orton, 2005), TBI, whether from abuse or from accidental causes, has similar long-term outcomes. The treatment strategies are also similar. Some of the long-term neurological and psychological consequences of these lesions include posttraumatic seizure disorders, spasticity, cognitive impairments, attention deficit disorders, and disinhibition. Other outcomes include poor executive functioning, memory deficit, wake-sleep cycle disturbances, abnormal responses to external and internal stimuli, communication disorders, focal paralyses, quadriplegia (paralysis in all four extremities), and spastic quadriparesis (weakness in all four extremities.)

A variety of other conditions may complicate the long-term care of the brain-injured individual. Psychiatric disorders are not uncommon. Some patients have insight into their problems, but some are depressed, and mood and behavior problems are common. Some of these conditions are treated with drugs such as fluoxetine (Prozac), which is in a class of medications called selective serotonin reuptake inhibitors. They work by increasing the amount and availability of serotonin. Sleep disorders can be treated with melatonin, which helps to choreograph sleep cycles. Various orthopedic problems need attention, such as contractures and scoliosis and kyphosis. Osteopenia and osteoporosis secondary to immobility and exacerbated by the use of anticonvulsants can lead to fractures. Some patients experience gastroesophageal reflux due to their restricted mobility, and in extreme cases, surgical fundoplication is required. In patients with tracheostomies, special attention must be paid to the management of the stoma. Similar diligence has to be directed toward care of gastrostomy feeding tubes and colostomy, cystostomy, and nephrostomy appliances. Skin infections around these stomas are challenges, and urinary tract infection is a constant threat. If total parenteral nutrition is required, all of the attendant problems that come with this delivery of nutrients need attention.

Immobility itself brings a range of special issues. Breakdown of skin over bony prominences can lead to chronic bedsores. Recurrent pneumonia is an ongoing threat due to the inability of some patients to handle secretions of the respiratory tract, or due to aspiration of materials from the mouth, nose, and throat, or simply due to the gravitational forces of the pendent segments of the lung resulting from immobility. Nosocomial infections are likewise a challenge. Drug-resistant organisms are more common in institutional settings, so these patients are at increased risk not only because of their physical vulnerability but also because they are in a closed population.

Body temperature regulation is often hampered because of neurological damage to the brainstem. Dysautonomia, a severe, debilitating result of TBI, is characterized by temperature dysregulation, disturbances in hemodynamics, and dystonic muscle contractions (Kirk et al., 2012). The signs of this disorder include fever, tachypnea, hypertension, tachycardia, diaphoresis, and dystonia. Kirk et al. (2012), in a study of 249 children with TBI and a variety of other conditions, found evidence of dysautonomia in 10% of the children with TBI and in 31% of the children with cardiac arrest. An earlier study reported a similar prevalence of dysautonomia in children after TBI, at 12% (Krach et al., 1997).

A substantial number of patients with TBI have endocrinopathies involving the hypothalamic-pituitary-adrenal axis. Norwood and colleagues (2010) reported growth hormone deficiencies in 6 of 32 patients with TBI. Kaulfers et al. (2010) found an overall incidence of endocrine abnormality of 15% at 1 month after injury, 75% at 6 months, and 29% at 12 months. A year after the injury, 14% of the patients had precocious puberty, 9% exhibited hypothyroidism, and 5% had growth hormone deficiency. Park and colleagues (2010) studied 45 adults who had sustained TBI and found pituitary hormone deficiency in 31% (growth hormone, adrenocorticotropic hormone, thyroid-stimulating hormone, luteinizing hormone, and follicle-stimulating hormone). Krahulik et al. (2010), in a study of 89 adults with TBI who were observed prospectively from the time of injury to one year post-injury, found that 21% had primary hormonal dysfunction of the pituitary gland. The major deficits included growth hormone dysfunction, hypogonadism, and diabetes insipidus. These abnormalities were seen mostly in patients who had worse GCS outcome scores and whose MRI scans demonstrated empty sella syndrome.

Eye lesions can also present problems. Some of these patients have suffered retinal hemorrhages, most of which resolve in the acute phase of brain injury, but those with retinal detachment or retinoschisis may have longer-term visual impairment, and some patients have cortical blindness due to their brain injury. Such patients may experience ophthalmic inflammations or infections, dry eye syndrome, or corneal pathology.

SPASTICITY. The physical manifestations of spasticity are pain, involuntary movements, abnormal postures, and resistance to movement (Richardson, 2002). Increasing muscle length is attempted through splinting, casting, positioning, and seating. Increasing muscle strength through exercises and weight training is another goal, although the evidence for this treatment is slim (Richardson, 2002). Motor relearning programs that engage the individual in practice, emphasizing and encouraging the use of the nonfunctioning limbs, have shown promise. There are electrical modalities, such as the functional electrical stimulator, but again, the evidence for efficacy is slight. The use of electromyography allows the therapist to quantify muscle problems and gauge improvement. By far the most important function of the therapist is that of educator and facilitator (Richardson, 2002).

Baclofen, a drug that can be taken orally, acts on the spinal cord nerves to decrease spasticity. Baclofen blocks pre- and postsynaptic gamma aminobutyric acid beta receptors. Some patients benefit from direct delivery of baclofen into the spinal canal. The Medtronic SynchroMed II programmable infusion system can be used for this purpose. The pump, nicknamed "the hockey pump" because of its resemblance to a hockey puck in size and shape, consists of an infusion device implanted into the abdomen, with an attached intraspinal catheter. An external programmer operates the pump. The Medtronic company (www.medtronic.com) states that this system provides precise drug delivery for chronic intrathecal baclofen therapy (ITB Therapy). Diazepam, a benzodiazepine, relieves spasticity by central blockade of gamma aminobutyric acid alpha receptors (Chou & Peterson, 2005). Another approach to the spasticity seen in adductor muscle groups is to inject botulinum toxin (Botox) into the affected muscles. The obvious disadvantage to this is the need for repeated injections.

SEIZURES. The drugs of first choice for the treatment of seizures are gabapentin (Neurontin) or levetiracetum (Keppra) because of the paucity of side effects. Broad-spectrum drugs such as divalproex sodium (Depakote) or topiramate (Topamax) are used in certain circumstances. Focal seizures are treated with carbamazepine (Tegretol), and sometimes the older drug phenobarbital is still used. Other approaches for treating refractory seizures include the use of a ketogenic diet and implanted vagus nerve stimulators (cyberonics.com).

Outcomes

Minns, Jones, and Barlow (2005) performed the most comprehensive analysis of outcome studies on children with nonaccidental head injury. They examined all peer-reviewed retrospective and prospective studies on outcomes published between 1970 and 2004 and concluded that the results for mortality and neurodevelopmental sequelae were universally poor. They conceded, however, that these studies comprised selective hospital cases that may not reflect the broad picture. And there was great heterogeneity in the studies: the studies differed in design; some lacked comparison groups; the duration of follow-up was variable; injury severity was not uniform; and the outcome scales used to judge the level of function were different in the early studies and the later ones. The mortality rate in these studies was 7%, but for children under 2 years of age the mortality rate was 20%. Fatalities due to accidental head injury in children are rare, somewhere between 2% and 4%, with younger children at higher risk. There is a high incidence (34%) of severely disabled children with gross developmental delay among survivors of nonaccidental head injury during infancy. Minns and colleagues note that "these severely disabled children are frequently blind, nonverbal and cognitively impaired, have epilepsy and behavioral problems, are wheelchair dependent and rely on adults for their daily care throughout their life." Twenty-five percent of survivors had moderate disability. Even those children with a "good outcome" frequently functioned "in the normal education stream but may require remedial help and may display behavioural problems." A "good outcome" in survivors of nonaccidental head injury was seen in around 11% of children.

One constant refrain in the studies on children with iTBI is that even if there was an initial period of apparently complete recovery, nearly all of the children became disabled after an interval of 6 months to 5 years (Bonnier, Nassogne, & Evrard, 1995; Catroppa et al., 2008; Ewing-Cobbs et al., 1999; Haviland & Russell, 1997). Interruption of brain growth took 4 months to appear; long track signs, 6–12 months; epilepsy, 2 years; and behavioral and neuropsychological signs, such as pervasive developmental disorders, hyperkinetic behavior, and anxiety, 3–6 years. Motor deficits were seen in 38% of survivors of nonaccidental head injury, and cranial nerve deficits in 20% (Barlow et al 2004; Ewing-Cobbs et al., 1998). Haviland and Russell (1997) claimed that motor and cranial nerve deficits were the most common presenting complaints. The overall incidence of posttraumatic seizures in nonaccidental head injury is 30%, derived from the studies analyzed by Minns et al. (2005).

Anderson and colleagues have regularly reported on outcomes in samples of children aged 2–7 years with TBI (Anderson, Catroppa, et al., 2005, 2009; Anderson, Godfrey, et al., 2012; Anderson, Spencer-Smith, et al., 2009; Hessen, Nestvold, & Anderson, 2007), but unfortunately, all of their studies excluded patients with nonaccidental (inflicted) TBI, so their results are not applicable to the population we are attempting to describe. Makaroff and Putnam (2003) and Koskiniemi et al. (1995) reviewed the literature on outcomes of iTBI from 1975 to 2002 and found that the majority of these children had poor outcomes, with roughly one-fifth of the children dying and only 22% of survivors in the aggregate studies having no impairment. Ewing-Cobbs and colleagues showed that nearly one-half of victims of iTBI had impaired scores for emotional regulation and motor quality (Ewing-Cobbs, Kramer, et al., 1998; Ewing-Cobbs, Prasad, et al., 1999). Lind et al. (2012) assessed the long-term outcomes of victims of severe shaken baby syndrome. These were patients who had been admitted to one rehabilitation hospital in France between 1996 and 2005. Forty-seven patients were included in this study, with a median length of follow-up of 8 years (range 44–144 months); only seven children (15%) had returned to a normal life (Glasgow Outcome Scale [GOS] I). Nineteen patients (40%) suffered severe neurological impairment (GOS III and IV). Children had motor deficits in 45% of cases, epilepsy in 38%, visual deficit in 45%, sleep disorders in 17%, language abnormalities in 49%, attention deficits in 79%, and behavioral disorders in 53%. Eighty-three percent of the children continued to need rehabilitation services.

Most outcome studies have not followed up on these children for long periods of time. This is due to the difficulty in tracking the whereabouts of these children and the reluctance of caretakers to participate in follow-up studies; in addition, some children have been removed from their parents' care and are in the custody of government agencies, which are disinclined to make the children available for follow-up studies. But it is clear that children who survive iTBI have poor outcomes, based mainly on the extreme severity of this form of brain injury, the hypoxic-ischemic damage secondary to apnea after the inflicted injury, and the very young age of the infants who comprise the vast majority of these cases.

Treatment Models and Programs for Children with Residual Deficits

Specialized medical attention can help reduce the impact of assault on young children, but many children are still left with permanent brain damage and residual deficits that often worsen over time. These young survivors of physical assault and resulting brain damage most often require specialized post-acute medical services for a variety of neurodevelopmental disabilities, including cognitive impairments, social and behavior problems, physical movement deficits, partial or complete loss of vision, hearing impairments, seizure disorders, cerebral palsy, and sucking and swallowing disorders. Unfortunately, some of these children also end up in permanent states of minimal consciousness and require very complex services and supports.

From a medical perspective, these are clearly children and youths with special health care needs. The Maternal and Child Health Bureau of the U.S. Department of Health and Human Services, Health Resources and Services Administration, defines this population as "those who have or are at increased risk for a chronic physical, development, behavioral, or emotional condition and who also require health and related services of a type or amount beyond that required by children generally" (Maternal and Child Health Bureau, 2012).

Treatment programs that are successful in helping this population of children make functional gains are those that uniquely combine therapies from best practices in rehabilitation medicine (e.g., developmental pediatrics, pediatric physiatry, pediatric neurology, pediatric psychiatry), best practices in therapeutic interventions (e.g., speech and language therapy [SLP], physical therapy [PT], occupational therapy [OT], neuropsychology, developmental psychology), and best practices in special education (direct instruction, integrated therapies, vocational training, transition planning) (see figure 19.1).

For the most part, however, schools and homes, not hospitals, are the largest providers of post-acute services for these children. In addition, how such children are defined from a medical perspective (i.e., children with abusive head trauma) does not necessarily match the special education classification categories under IDEA, the Individuals with Disabilities Education Act, the nation's special education law.

Congress originally enacted IDEA in 1975 to ensure that children with disabilities have the opportunity to receive a free, appropriate public education, just like other children. The law has been revised many times over the years. Congress amended the law in December 2004, with final regulations published in August 2006 (Part B, for school-age children) and September 2011 (Part C, for babies and toddlers).

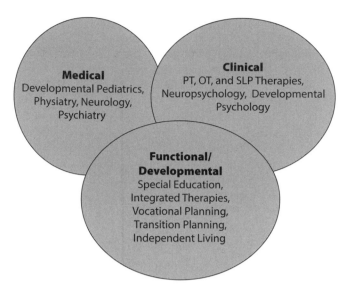

Figure 19.1. Successful treatment programs combine best practices in rehabilitation medicine, therapeutic interventions, and special education.

IDEA has 14 categories of disability, including 2 categories that better define children with TBI so that they may qualify for special education services and supports. Traumatic brain injury is defined in IDEA as

> an acquired injury to the brain caused by an external physical force, resulting in total or partial functional disability or psychosocial impairment, or both, that adversely affects a child's educational performance. The term applies to open or closed head injuries resulting in impairments in one or more areas, such as cognition; language; memory; attention; reasoning; abstract thinking; judgment; problem-solving; sensory, perceptual, and motor abilities; psycho-social behavior; physical functions; information processing; and speech. The term does not apply to brain injuries that are congenital or degenerative, or to brain injuries induced by birth trauma. (34 C.F.R. Part 300/A/300/B(c)(12))

A second category under IDEA that may be used to qualify children with TBI for special education services is "other health impairment" (OHI). OHI refers to children who have limited strength, vitality, or alertness, including a heightened alertness to environmental stimuli, that result in limited alertness with respect to the educational environment. OHI is defined in IDEA as an impairment that is

> due to chronic or acute health problems such as asthma, attention deficit disorder or attention deficit hyperactivity disorder, diabetes, epilepsy, a heart condition, hemophilia, lead poisoning, leukemia, nephritis, rheumatic fever, sickle cell anemia, and Tourette syndrome; and adversely affects a child's educational performance. (34 C.F.R. Part 300/300.7/C/9)

Hence, for many children who survive abusive head trauma with brain damage, residual deficits, and related medical prob-

lems, it may be beneficial to have both TBI and OHI listed as categories of disability to get them qualified for special services and to ensure that all the child's needs are identified.

Unfortunately, schools are not required to provide medical services to children, only those services that are educationally relevant—that is, a child may be in a wheelchair and not receive physical therapy services if his or her movement deficits do not impede learning. This often presents parents, foster parents, and/or guardians with a complex dilemma, since insurance companies are also not required to provide therapy services "beyond the school house door." While some children may continue to receive much-needed outpatient therapies (after school, on weekends) to maintain and/or improve their functioning, many, because of funding issues, do not. Therefore, even though these children have multiple and intertwined medical, clinical, and special education needs, they may not receive the services they require unless private funding is available.

Over the years, parents and guardians have advocated for these children, and many schools and hospitals have responded by developing different models to serve such children. First and foremost, it is important to get these children identified and qualified for special education services in order to start the process, and physicians can play a key role in advocating for such.

Special Education Services for Children with Disabilities

The Individuals with Disabilities Education Act governs how states and public agencies provide early intervention, special education, and related services to more than 6.5 million eligible infants, toddlers, children, and youths with disabilities. Infants and toddlers with disabilities (ages 0–2 years) and their families receive early intervention services under IDEA Part C. Children and youths (ages 3–21) receive special education and related services under IDEA Part B.

Each public school child who receives special education and related services must have an Individualized Education Program (IEP). Each IEP must be designed for one student and must be a truly *individualized* document. The IEP creates an opportunity for teachers, parents, school administrators, related services personnel, and students (when appropriate) to work together to improve educational results for children with disabilities. The IEP also identifies vocational training, independent living, and transition services (after high school) that need to be part of the child's special education program. The IEP is the cornerstone of a quality education for each child with a disability.

For example, early intervention services are designed to meet the needs of infants and toddlers who have a developmental delay or disability. Such programs are concerned with all the basic and new skills that babies typically develop during the first three years of life, including the following:

- *Physical* (reaching, rolling, crawling, walking)
- *Cognitive* (thinking, learning, solving problems)

- *Communication* (talking, listening, understanding)
- *Social/emotional* (playing, feeling secure and happy)
- *Self-help* (eating, dressing)

There are also several resources that can be very helpful to families, childcare providers, and educators:

- Division for Early Childhood, through the Council for Exceptional Children (www.dec-sped.org)
- National Association for the Education of Young Children (www.naeyc.org)
- National Early Childhood Technical Assistance Center (www.nectac.org)
- Services for babies and toddlers to the third birthday (Part C of IDEA; see the website of the National Dissemination Center for Children with Disabilities, www.nichcy.org/babies)

Sample Programs and Treatment Models

While the special education system defines *what* and *how* we teach children, the *where* we teach children may include a number of different settings, depending on parents' choice, medical needs, available resources, and/or available funding. Some of these settings include special education programs within the public schools, private special education schools, schools within hospitals, schools within skilled nursing facilities, schools within long-term residential programs, home-based school programs, and/or a hybrid of these places. The selection of "placement" is obviously best determined by the child's strengths, needs, and preferences; however, in many areas there is a profound lack of resources for these children, especially in rural areas.

HOSPITAL SCHOOLS. Many children's hospitals over the years have developed hospital schools. These are designed for children with complex medical needs who require long periods of inpatient hospital stay for chronic illness or inpatient rehabilitation. Hospital school programs focus on school-age children who can continue to achieve academic goals and interact with peers. Certified teachers collaborate with the student's classroom and/or homebound teacher and other health care professionals involved in the patient's care to provide appropriate educational services. For example, the Children's Hospital of Philadelphia school program helps children develop and maintain academic skills, as well as participating in familiar and "normal" activities to reduce the stress of hospitalization. Medical and clinical staff and hospital-based teachers also support parents/guardians in navigating the educational system and accessing appropriate services for their child.

SKILLED NURSING FACILITIES OR MEDICAL RESIDENTIAL FACILITIES. Some children require long-term placement in a skilled nursing facility or medical residential facility because of their complex medical needs and/or the lack of parents or guardians to care for them in a home environment. For example, the Hattie Larlham Program (medical residential facility) in Ohio offers long-term medical care for very complex, low-functioning children, who also have an opportunity to attend a private charter school program within the facility. The children receive medical services, therapy services, creative arts, and special education services all within one coordinated system of care.

A similar program at New England Pediatric Care (skilled nursing facility) in Massachusetts provides highly skilled care for medically fragile children from birth to 22 years old by combining skilled nursing, functional rehabilitation therapies (PT, OT, SLP, recreation), and special education services. These combined therapies help improve the children's overall health status, as well as maintaining their cognitive and social functioning.

The Bancroft School at Voorhees Pediatric Facility (skilled nursing and pediatric ventilator program) in New Jersey is an innovative collaboration between two private institutions. The Bancroft School is an on-site private school that provides special education services to the children at Voorhees Pediatric Facility who are medically fragile and dependent on technology and who require continuous skilled nursing care. Teachers, rehabilitation therapists, and other medical professionals work with the family or guardian to establish short- and long-term objectives to maximize the student's educational, emotional, rehabilitative, and physical development. which can facilitate, when possible, the child's re-entry into the home and community.

PRIVATE SPECIAL EDUCATION SCHOOLS. The May Center for Education and NeuroRehabilitation and the Ivy Street School in Boston are private special education schools with residential services for children with acquired brain injuries or neurological diseases. Because of their private status, the schools are able to provide the children with additional therapy support (PT, OT, SLP, psychology), nursing services, and intensive special education instruction. Children may complete their entire education there or, after a period of time, may transfer back to their community school.

HOSPITAL-TO-SCHOOL MODEL. In San Diego, the city's school district and Rady Children's Hospital joined forces and developed a hospital-to-school brain injury program with shared staffing so that children can receive special education services in the hospital, as well as medical rehabilitation services, and on discharge they can reenter school through the school's Brain Injury Service team. Children who need intense intervention are referred to the Brain Injury Learning Center for a diagnostic placement. This sequential process allows time for the brain to heal before integrating the child into a noisy, busy school environment. In a one-to-one setting, students have the opportunity to regain knowledge/skills lost and to build new learning. Those not placed at the Brain Injury Learning Center, Special Day Class, Transition Skills class, or other specialized settings are placed in their neighborhood school, with support as needed. This coordinated case management model provides children with a treatment pathway, and children are reevaluated, as necessary, by Rady specialists (physicians, neuropsychologists, therapists) as part of their ongoing care and special education services.

HOMEBOUND INSTRUCTION. Other children, because of parental choice and/or complex medical needs, may be home-schooled. Homebound instruction is governed by federal and state laws, but implementation may vary not only from state to state but also from one school district to another. Under IDEA, homebound instruction is meant for acute or catastrophic health problems that confine a child to home or hospital for a prolonged but defined period of time. The primary care physician, in collaboration with the school district's homebound education team, must specify the anticipated duration of the homebound instruction. The school identifies a team to review the pertinent data for the child with the family and to develop an IEP. In addition, the decision for non-school-based instruction must be reviewed yearly by the school team, with the goal of maintaining academic progress and returning the child to school as soon as possible. However, there are circumstances where educating the child at home for long periods of time is the best choice from a medical perspective (e.g., risk of disease, risk of emergencies, amount of skilled medical care needed).

TRAINING/CONSULTATION PROGRAMS. Other treatment models for children with disabilities include best practice treatment models for public school teachers and special educators that identify the unique needs of this population and offer training and consultation supports to the schools through an outside resource. For example, BrainSTARS in Colorado is a program that provides education, information, and consultation related to brain injury (traumatic and acquired) for families and school personnel. The BrainSTARS Manual is a comprehensive, practical manual for parents and teachers that includes background information about brain injury, child and adolescent development, and ways to create positive change, a comprehensive list of problems associated with brain injury, recommended interventions, and worksheets. The BrainSTARS model program includes ongoing supportive consultation to families and schools, along with the BrainSTARS Manual, to fine-tune interventions for a particular child's needs.

The Brain Injury Association of Pennsylvania, under a grant from the Pennsylvania Department of Health and partnered with the Pennsylvania Department of Education, created the Child & Adolescent Brain Injury School Re-Entry Program called BrainSTEPS (Strategies Teaching Educators, Parents, and Students). BrainSTEPS is a Brain Injury School Re-Entry model that is being established across Pennsylvania, and the BrainSTEPS Consulting Teams consist of professionals from a variety of disciplines who have received extensive training on educating students with TBI and are available to provide basic training and resources to schools and families.

MEDICAL CLASSROOMS. Lastly, many public schools have developed "medical classrooms" for groups of children who require specialized medical services, including nursing care and therapies (PT, OT, SLP). These schools provide intensive special education as the foundation of the program but also integrate medical supports to maintain the child's health status (medications, management of seizures, feeding, etc.).

. . .

In summary, various models and best practices exist for children who have sustained brain damage and other complications as the result of abusive head trauma. Crucial to providing these children with specialized services is to have them identified and qualified for special education services under IDEA. The choice of where to serve these children will depend on multiple factors, including medical needs, special education needs, therapy and psychological needs, available resources and funding, and parent/guardian choice.

BURNS

The majority of burns in young children are due to a failure in supervision; this neglect may be momentary or chronic. The medical features of the burn cannot distinguish types of neglect. Burns caused by deliberate infliction of injury are less common (Chester et al., 2006). Most burns in children, whether accidental or abusive, are scalds or contact burns. Chemical burns, caused by application of a caustic substance to a child's skin or mouth, are rare causes of abusive burns, although neglect is a definite contributor to many chemical burns in children. Electrical burns, caused by forcing a live electrical conduit to contact a child's mouth or skin, are even less common but have been reported.

The initial emergency assessment of an infant or child with a burn consists of attending to basic trauma ABCs—airway, breathing, and circulation—then assessing neurological disability and the type of exposure. Inhalation burns and ingestion of hot or caustic liquids can cause airway edema or swelling. Evaluating the burn itself is part of the secondary survey. The physiological status and the extent and depth of the burn determine the character of further care (Sheridan, 2005).

Full evaluation of the injury includes a detailed history of the mechanism and timing of the burn and any treatment used before presentation or during transport. A screen for associated trauma should be done even when the burns are small. For children with large burns who require fluid resuscitation, intravenous access with two large-bore IV lines and catheterization to monitor urine output are needed. When there is airway involvement due to either smoke inhalation or burns, or when pain medication depresses respiration, intubation and ventilation are necessary.

The *extent of the burn* is assessed as percentage of total body surface area (TBSA; Mlcak & Buffalo, 2007). Three different methods may be used for this estimation. The pediatric modified "Rule of 9's" is easiest, but because infants' and young children's body proportions differ from adults', care must be taken to use the appropriate infant or child chart. For infants and children, head and neck surface is 18% TBSA; each lower limb, 15%; each upper extremity, 10%; and the anterior and posterior torsos, each 16%. The Lund & Browder diagram is more accurate because the charts are more specific for age (infant, 5 years, 10 years), but it is somewhat more difficult to use. For small areas, estimation based on the patient's palm size (palm surface = 0.5% TBSA) is most straightforward (Sheridan et al., 1995). Erythema only, which indicates a superficial burn, is not included in determining the size of the burn.

The *depth of the burn* can be determined only after adequate debridement of devitalized tissue. Most burns have mixed depths, so a patient with predominately third-degree burns may have marked pain caused by more superficial burn areas. Burn injury is a dynamic process that peaks at three days. Many burns require several days of observation and debridement to determine the depth of the burn.

First-degree burns affect the epidermis only and are characterized by pain, redness, and blanching with pressure. Most sunburns are first-degree burns. These burns heal in several days without specific treatment.

Superficial second-degree burns are characterized by blisters, pain, and moist, red, weeping skin. These burns blanch with pressure. *Deep second-degree burns* extend to the dermis, and pain sensation is reduced. The color is variable, white to red; the burn may be wet or dry and does not blanch with pressure. *Third-degree burns* are full-thickness burns that involve the entire dermis and extend into the subcutaneous tissue. Their appearance is charred, leathery, firm, and depressed, and these burns can be mottled in appearance. *Fourth-degree burns* extend to the fascia, bone, joint, or muscle (Duffy, McLaughlin, & Eichelberger, 2006; Pham, Gibran, & Heimbach, 2007).

Circumferential burns are burns that encircle a body part, and these require admission to the hospital and special monitoring. Constriction can lead to a decrease in blood flow to an extremity, which, if untreated, can necessitate amputation. Circumferential burns around the torso can interfere with ventilation. Such burns require emergency escharotomy, an incision through the entire wound to release pressure. Escharotomy is usually performed 12–24 hours after injury and requires anesthesia or sedation, especially in young children (Sheridan, 2005). Escharotomy may be performed in the intensive care unit at the bedside.

Minor burns are defined by the American Burn Association as partial-thickness burns involving less than 5% TBSA in children or 10% in adolescents and with no cosmetic or functional risk to the eyes, ears, face, hands, feet, or perineum. Additional criteria are that the burn is an isolated injury (no risk of inhalation injury), does not cross major joints, and is not circumferential (Morgan, 2012). Minor burns can often be cared for in the outpatient setting. However, when there is a concern for abuse, there should be a low threshold for hospital admission to address the social situation and to train care providers in proper wound care.

Initial gentle debridement is necessary to determine the depth of the burn and reduce the risk of infection. Ruptured and large expanding blisters should be debrided, but small blisters can be left intact. Superficial burns do not require a topical antimicrobial agent. Partial-thickness burns require daily gentle cleansing with a mild soap and application of topical silver sulfadiazine cream or bacitracin ointment (with or without neomycin and polymyxin). These creams and ointments decrease bacterial contamination and maintain a moist environment that enhances re-epithelialization. Simple dressing with fine gauze maintains some protection and decreases pain (Pham, Gibran, & Heimbach, 2007; Sheridan, 2005). The wound must be monitored for infection.

Tetanus immunization should be updated. A child who has not had the primary tetanus series should, in addition to the vaccine, receive tetanus immune globulin.

Pain control for children in the outpatient setting usually requires no more than acetaminophen or a nonsteroidal anti-inflammatory medication. Oral narcotics (oxycodone or codeine) may be needed for wound care for a short period of time.

Major burns are characterized by any of the following: partial-thickness burns involving more than 10% TBSA in children under age 10 (20% TBSA in adolescents); full-thickness burns involving more than 5% TBSA; any significant burn to the face, eyes, ears, genitalia, or joints; any inhalational injuries (Hartford & Kealy, 2007). These burns are best managed in burn centers with highly experienced burn teams. Burn centers can provide the surgical, nursing, critical care, medical, nutritional, physical, and occupational therapy services that are not possible to maintain at local hospitals. Burns that are midway between minor and major require admission to a general hospital or burn center for further assessment.

Emergency resuscitation requires an assessment of airway and breathing. Intubation is required if there is smoke inhalation or respiratory depression from any cause, most commonly from pain medication. In large burns, fluid loss through open skin and edema can lead to shock, and fluid resuscitation using the Parkland (Baxter) or similar formula is critical. The initial calculation is $4\,mg/kg \times \%TBSA$ of lactated Ringer's solution, giving half in the first 8 hours and half in the next 16 hours. Children under 20 kg must have maintenance fluid and 5% dextrose added. This formula is only a starting point, since volume status must be carefully monitored with urine output and heart rate, and fluid rate must be appropriately modified (Warden, 2007).

Large burns lead to major physiological derangements. Complications include shock, pulmonary failure due to fluid overload or acute respiratory distress syndrome, and renal failure. Children with greater than 15% TBSA involvement require initial management in an intensive care setting.

Infection of burn wounds is a significant complication. Meticulous wound care is essential in the early stages. A variety of silver-containing and biological dressings are employed to decrease infection and promote healing. Daily wound cleansing and debridement are required.

Early excision and grafting leads to a significant decrease in mortality, shorter hospital stays, and lower costs of treatment, and this is standard practice for burns that are not likely to heal within 3 weeks, including many deep partial-thickness and all large full-thickness burns. Early wound closure decreases the frequency of infection, decreases the severity of contractures and hypertrophic scarring, and allows more rapid rehabilitation. Grafts are typically taken as split-thickness harvests from unburned skin, from the thighs or buttocks when possible. Sheet or meshed grafts are chosen on the basis of wound site and extent. The donor sites heal within 10–14 days. Full-thickness grafts may be used for facial burns (Pham, Gibran, & Heimbach., 2007).

Modern burn care has greatly increased survival for children with major burns. In a recent review of pediatric patients with burns involving greater than 30% TBSA admitted to a major burn center, burn size was the major predictor of mortality (Kraft et al., 2012). Children with burns of less than 50% TBSA had a mortality rate of 3%. Mortality rate increased rapidly when the burn size exceeded 60% TBSA: 16% mortality at 60%–69% TBSA; 35% mortality at 80%–89% TBSA; and 55% mortality at 90%–100% TBSA.

Chemical burns are caused by contact of the skin with caustic substances. The depth of the burn depends on the composition of the substance and the duration of contact. Early removal of contaminated clothing and copious lavage decrease the depth of burn by diluting the agent in contact with the skin. Irrigation may take 30 minutes to 2 hours. Household cleaning agents are commonly strong alkalis, and these are the most frequent cause of childhood chemical burns. Strong alkalis require much longer lavage, since without complete removal, the chemical continues to destroy skin and deeper tissues (Leonard, Scheulen, & Munster, 1982). The severity of the burn may be difficult to assess initially. After initial management, the treatment course is the same as that for thermal burns.

Children can swallow or be forced to swallow caustic chemical agents. Burns to the mouth and esophagus from household cleaners can be severe. Severe gastric injuries may also result from caustic ingestion. Early assessment by endoscopy is needed to determine the severity of the burn (Temiz et al., 2012). Gastrostomy or jejunostomy placement may be necessary to allow nutrition while bypassing the burned esophagus. If strictures form in the healing esophagus, repeated dilatation procedures can be successful in restoring esophageal function (Kay & Wyllie, 2009). More severe burns may require resection and bypass of the esophagus.

Pain Management

Pain is a major issue in burn care. Background pain is managed with acetaminophen and oral or IV opiates, which initially should be given on a schedule, not "as needed." Procedural pain associated with wound care and washing requires higher doses of opiates. In addition, in the inpatient setting, benzodiazepines are used to provide anxiolysis during procedures. When background pain is severe, long-acting opiates may be needed. Nonpharmacological management of pain includes massage, distraction, music, play, relaxation techniques, and guided imagery (Hanson et al., 2008; Martin-Herz, Thurber, & Patterson, 2000). Nonpharmacological techniques are used to augment, not replace, pain medication. Parents and caregivers frequently benefit from these techniques as well and can learn the techniques to help their children.

Itching is a common complication of initial burn healing and healing at graft donor sites. Moderate to severe itching can persist long after burns have healed. In the short term, scratching can interfere with wound healing and graft adherence and also interferes with sleep. In the longer term, persistent itching is intensely annoying and distracting. Heat, physical activity, and stress are triggers for itching. Antihistamines, cool compresses, and lotions are the cornerstones of treatment. Antihistamines such as diphenhydramine, hydroxyzine, and cyproheptadine all can be tried. Gabapentin has been used for adults and shows some promise in this situation. Local infection with *Staphylococcus aureus* may worsen itching, and antibiotics may be useful in these instances.

Hypertrophic Scars and Contractures

Wounds that heal within two to three weeks do not tend to form scars. Slower-healing wounds normally heal by scar formation and skin contracture. Scars that are elevated, thickened, and irregular are hypertrophic scars. When scars are anticipated, custom-fit pressure garments are often used to reduce scar formation. When used on the face, these garments hide the wound but appear highly abnormal to others.

Contractures of joints have serious functional consequences. Physical therapy for range of motion is a critical early treatment. Stretching is required several times a day, and children may protest because of pain. Early mobilization by walking is needed, even for foot burns. Splints are used in the acute phase to maintain the joint in extension and decrease development of contractures (Serghiou et al., 2007).

Late scar revisions may be needed to resect hypertrophic scars and to release contractures for functional and cosmetic reasons. Repeated surgical procedures may be required in some cases (Huang, 2007).

Psychological Reactions and Sequelae

Acute stress reaction, occurring within one month after exposure to a traumatic event, is common in children with burns. Symptoms of acute stress disorder include arousal symptoms, avoidance, and re-experiencing the traumatic event. One study followed up on 130 young children with relatively small (mean TBSA 3.24%), nonintentional burns (De Young et al., 2012). In the initial weeks, these children manifested excessive clinginess (58%), tantrums (50%), avoidance or distress around trauma reminders (52%), sleep disturbances (40%), nightmares (30%), and aggression (27%). At the six-month follow-up, most of these children appeared to be psychologically recovered (72%), but a high proportion (27%) continued to manifest significant symptoms of a psychological disorder.

For children who have major burns, the traumatic events, including dressing changes, surgical grafts, and hospitalizations, may be repeated and prolonged. The severity of injury alone does not reliably predict posttraumatic symptoms (Brosbe, Hoefling, & Faust, 2011). A high proportion of children admitted to the intensive care unit and their parents develop acute stress reaction (Nelson & Gold, 2012). Stoddard et al. (2006) found that in a group of 52 nonabused children 12–48 months of age who were hospitalized with burns (mean TBSA 14.1%), acute stress symptoms were related to the magnitude of the burn and to parents' acute stress symptoms. For victims of physical abuse, the experience of injury by a loved caregiver and then separation from that person may be additional severe compounding traumas.

Long-Term Outcomes

There are no studies of psychological outcomes specifically for children with abusive burns. Several studies of pediatric survivors of major nonabusive burns demonstrate positive psychological and quality-of-life outcomes. Surprisingly, the severity of the burn has little relationship to psychological outcome. In several studies, outcome was highly related to family factors. Blakeney et al. (1993) studied 60 children with major burns (>15% TBSA) at least one year after their burn injury. Rating scales completed by parents showed concerns for problematic child behaviors and diminished competence compared with norms, although all children were within the standardized normal range. Teachers reported fewer problems than parents. The burn severity did not correlate with psychological outcomes. A recent study of parents of 94 children age 6 months to 15 years who had been hospitalized with burns found that parents reported more overall psychological difficulties in the children compared with normed peer samples (Willebrand et al., 2011). Analyses indicated that parents' psychological symptoms and other family variables were more influential than injury-related variables in parental reports of child psychological problems after burns.

Psychological and quality-of-life outcomes have repeatedly been shown to be closely related to family factors (Landolt, Grubenmann, & Meuli, 2002). Families that were "cohesive"—that pulled together as a unit and were committed and supportive to each other as well as to the child—were associated with better psychological outcomes for the child. This family cohesion may not have existed previously but may have developed after the burn event (LeDoux et al., 1998).

In a study of 101 young adults who experienced severe burns (>30% TBSA) in childhood or adolescence, Meyer et al. (2004) found that the majority were comparable to peers in developmental achievements such as employment and interpersonal relationships. Young women endorsed significantly more somatic complaints, thought problems, withdrawal, and aggressive and delinquent behavior than peers. Good outcomes appeared to be related to acceptance by family, friends, and community.

ABDOMINAL TRAUMA

Significant force is required to cause injury to the abdominal organs. Abdominal trauma is conventionally divided into *penetrating trauma*, typically caused by stabs or bullets, and *blunt trauma*, caused by a blow to the abdomen. Accidental blunt abdominal trauma is caused by motor vehicle crashes, automobile-on-pedestrian impacts, falls from a height, bicycle crashes, or similar events. In the absence of such a witnessed history, intentional trauma must be suspected. Abusive abdominal injury is usually caused by an adult's kick or punch to the child's abdomen, sometimes multiple blows. Abusive abdominal trauma is second only to head trauma as a cause of fatality in child abuse.

In an analysis of a national hospitalization database, Lane et al. (2012) found that in 2006, 203 children were hospitalized in the United States for abusive abdominal trauma—5.9% of all pediatric abdominal trauma admissions in that year. For infants under 1 year, abusive injury caused more than a quarter of all abdominal trauma admissions. However, children with abdominal injury comprise only a small proportion of those hospitalized with abusive injury. In Lane et al.'s (2012) study of children ages 0–9 years hospitalized for abuse, about 4% had abdominal trauma.

Blunt injury can damage solid organs, including the liver, spleen, pancreas, and kidney, or hollow viscus organs, including the stomach, duodenum, and large and small intestines. Wounds to solid organs cause lacerations and bleeding of varying severity. Pancreatic injuries are less common but may be severe. Hollow organs may form hematomas or may rupture; spillage of stomach or intestinal contents leads to an intense and life-threatening inflammatory response. The mesentery, the tissue that attaches the intestine in the abdomen, can also be injured.

In a cross-sectional comparison study of children with abusive abdominal injury versus accidental injury in the United Kingdom, Barnes et al. (2005) found significant differences in age and injury patterns. Abused children were much younger than children whose injury resulted from road-traffic accidents or falls (abuse: mean age 3.73 years; road-traffic accidents: mean age 9.7 years; falls: mean age

10.39 years). Fifty-five percent of the abused children had gut (hollow viscus) injury, compared with 21% of those hurt in road-traffic accidents and 10% of those injured in falls. Trokel et al. (2006) reviewed the U.S. Pediatric National Trauma Registry for children under 5 years with blunt abdominal injury, excluding those who had been injured in a motor vehicle accident. They found that hollow viscus injury and pancreatic injury were much more frequent in the abused children (hollow viscus injury: 35.1% vs. 6.1%; pancreatic injury: 14.1% vs. 4.8%).

Wood et al. (2005) compared 121 children with inflicted abdominal injury and a comparison group with unintentional injury. The abused children were significantly younger and had more severe injury. Children in the abused group had more frequent hollow organ (bowel) injury, and combined solid organ and bowel injury was found only in this group. The abused children presented later after injury than the accidentally injured children, but delay to care alone was not an accurate predictor of abuse.

In a retrospective review of abnormal abdominal CT findings in 35 young abused children, Hilmes et al. (2011) found that the most common solid organ injury was to the liver (42.9%), followed by the spleen and kidney (17.1% each). Bowel and mesenteric injuries occurred in 40% of these children, and bowel perforation in 11.4%. Liver, bowel, and mesenteric injuries were frequently found in combination.

Mortality following abdominal trauma is much higher in abused children than in those with accidental injury. This may be due to the younger age of abuse victims, delay in care, or associated head injury (Canty, Canty, & Brown, 1999; Lane et al., 2011; Ledbetter et al., 1988; Trokel et al., 2004, 2006).

Although there are multiple identifiable risk factors, including patient age, bowel injury, pancreatic injury, and delay in care, the diagnosis of abusive trauma depends on (1) the absence of a compatible history, and (2) the presence of other abuse-related findings, such as bruises, burns, fractures, and head trauma. As in all medical evaluations, a thorough evaluation for alternative diagnoses and contributing preexisting pathology is mandatory.

Diagnosis

In accidental injury, the mechanism of injury often raises concern about abdominal trauma. A motor vehicle crash with a child wearing only an auto lap belt, a fall from a height, or a fall onto bicycle handlebars are all indicators that abdominal trauma should be ruled out. For abused children, there may be a false history of a short fall, or no history at all. Abdominal wall bruising, tenderness, and distension are signs of possible organ injury. The absence of these signs cannot be reassuring, however, since significant injury can be present despite an apparently normal exam. In a prospective multicenter observational study of children who were evaluated for abuse, 3.2% (54 of 1,676) had abdominal injuries, and 31% of these (17 of 54) had clinically "occult" injury, without abdominal tenderness, bruising, or distension (Lindberg et al., 2009).

Abdominal CT with intravenous contrast is the preferred diagnostic test for abdominal solid organ injury (Bixby, Callahan, & Taylor, 2008). Ultrasound FAST scan is a noninvasive and rapid limited ultrasound examination directed solely at identifying the presence of free intraperitoneal fluid. In the context of traumatic injury, free fluid is usually due to hemorrhage. However, the FAST scan is not sensitive in children and may miss a significant number of serious injuries (Bixby, Callahan, & Taylor, 2008).

Lab tests show elevated liver enzymes (aspartate aminotransferase [AST], alanine aminotransferase [ALT]) in many gastrointestinal conditions, including abdominal trauma. In a prospective study of abused children, Lindberg et al. (2009) concluded that AST or ALT above 80 IU indicated the need for abdominal CT (sensitivity 77%, specificity 82%, positive predictive value 16%). Serum amylase and lipase are preferred tests for pancreatic injury, although these are not highly sensitive or specific. Injury to the kidney results from a direct blow to the flank. Urinalysis usually shows red blood cells or frank blood. Renal imaging by IV contrast CT with delayed sequences is the standard imaging modality.

Bowel (hollow viscus) injury is less common than solid organ injury after blunt trauma. Although CT is highly sensitive for the detection of solid organ injury, it is not as accurate in detecting bowel injury (Bixby, Callahan, & Taylor, 2008; Peters et al., 2006) Adjunctive imaging includes ultrasound and an upper gastrointestinal series with oral contrast. When a CT is not performed or imaging results are equivocal, a child may be admitted to the hospital for serial abdominal exams (Schonfeld & Lee, 2012).

In abusive injury, dating of the injury may be significant in determining who was with the child at the time of the abuse. CT scan is not reliable in dating abdominal injury, since resolution depends on the type and severity of the damage (Raissaki et al., 2011). There is preliminary evidence that the timing of the rise and fall of AST and ALT may be useful in timing injury (Baxter et al., 2008). When operative repair of the bowel is performed, the pathology of the resected tissue can be assessed for tissue response to injury, and this may assist in timing the injury.

Principles of Care

Initial stabilization should follow the Advance Trauma Life Support protocol, with evaluation of and support for airway, breathing, and circulation addressed first. Assessment for abdominal injury is part of the secondary survey (American College of Surgeons, 2011).

When the child presents with shock and acute abdominal injury and does not respond to fluid resuscitation, emergency laparotomy is indicated. Likewise, when bowel perforation is recognized, urgent operative repair is needed. In selected cases, hemorrhage can be treated with nonoperative angiographic embolization (Kiankhooy et al., 2010). In severe abdominal injury, surgical repair may be staged— that is, completed in several partial operations (Shapiro et al., 2000). This strategy, known as damage control surgery, abbreviates the initial surgery after control of bleeding and contamination. The patient is then returned to the intensive care unit for ongoing resuscitation. The abdomen may be left open for several days until the final surgery is completed.

Solid Organ Injury

The large majority of patients of all ages with solid organ trauma are treated nonoperatively. Nonoperative care results in more rapid recovery and fewer complications. Trauma to the liver, spleen, and kidney is graded by CT findings, from subcapsular hematoma (grade 1) to complete disruption from the vascular stem or shattering of the organ (spleen and kidney: grade 5; liver: grade 5 or 6. However, the decision to operate is based on hemodynamic stability, not on CT findings. Cases of even high-grade trauma can often be managed nonoperatively (Croce et al., 1995; Malhotra et al., 2000). After stabilization, patients are admitted to the hospital for monitoring. Those with higher-grade injuries are admitted to intensive care. If the patient continues to actively bleed into the abdomen, nonoperative management has failed and surgery is required. In selected cases, angiographic embolization is an option, although this modality has not been extensively used in children (Kiankhooy et al., 2010).

When the spleen is absent or surgically removed, children are at risk for overwhelming bacterial infection by encapsulated organisms. The optimal time for immunizations is 14 days before or 14 days after spleen removal. Immunizations for pneumococcus, *Haemophilus influenzae*, and meningococcus should be given according to recommendations by the Centers for Disease Control and Prevention (2011).

PANCREAS INJURY. A forceful blow to the upper abdomen can crush the pancreas against the spinal column. A well-known accidental mechanism is when a child falls onto the end of a bicycle handlebar. The pancreas does not bleed extensively, but the injury causes contusions and release of pancreatic digestive enzymes, leading to intense local inflammation. The treatment is complete bowel rest by restriction of oral intake, IV hydration, and parenteral nutrition. When a major pancreatic duct is disrupted distally, operative removal of the distal pancreas is usually indicated. When the ductal disruption is proximal, stent placement may be an option (Mattix et al., 2007). Prolonged parenteral nutrition is often required to allow healing. Pancreatic pseudocysts may form in the healing process, and these require subsequent drainage.

KIDNEY TRAUMA. Nonoperative management has become the mainstay of treatment of renal trauma in children. In a prospective study of children with accidental kidney injury admitted to a level 1 trauma center, although 13% (5 of 39) required blood transfusions, 97% (38 of 39) were managed nonsurgically (Fitzgerald et al., 2011). A meta-analysis of high-grade renal injuries in children concluded that conservative management is highly successful (Umbreit, Routh, & Husmann, 2009).

Hollow Organ Injury

The diagnosis of hollow viscus injury may be delayed because these injuries are not always apparent on initial abdominal CT (Peters et al., 2006). When there is clear evidence of rupture, with free air in the abdomen, surgical intervention is urgently indicated. When diagnosis is not clear, hospital admission and serial abdominal examinations may be required.

Injury to the duodenum, the outlet of the stomach to the small intestine, most frequently results in a hematoma of the duodenal wall (Bensard et al., 1996; Desai et al., 2003). This hematoma may lead to obstruction. Bowel rest and pain control are the mainstays of treatment, along with IV fluids and parenteral nutrition. Duodenal perforation requires surgical repair.

The jejunum is the most common site of intestinal rupture. Stomach rupture is rare but can occur if the stomach is distended after a meal and there is a severe blow to the abdomen. Open laparotomy is standard management for all hollow viscus perforations, but laparoscopic intervention may be an option in some situations.

Mesenteric hematomas can compromise blood flow to the bowel, resulting in late perforations and peritonitis. Pain and tenderness may appear 12–24 hours after the injury. Other late complications of bowel trauma and surgery include obstruction, sepsis, wound infection, and abscess formation. With these complications, the hospital stay may last weeks.

Outcomes

The long-term outcome of abdominal trauma depends on the nature and severity of the injury. There are no standard guidelines for a child's return to active play, and considerable variation exists in recommendations. Most children are restricted from bicycle or tricycle riding or climbing for a minimum of two weeks, although children with more severe injuries will be restricted for a longer time. Abused children have longer hospital stays, incur higher costs, and have higher mortality than children with accidental abdominal injury (Lane et al., 2011). The outcome for the child with abdominal trauma who does not have serious head injury, whether treated with observation or surgical intervention, is generally excellent.

In Memoriam

Dr. Naomi Sugar contributed the sections in this chapter on burns and abdominal trauma. Sadly, she died on July 21, 2013. She was a colleague of Dr. Kenneth Feldman at the University of Washington in Seattle. Dr. Feldman said of her: "Naomi was a superb colleague in child abuse pediatrics. Her low-key, down-to-earth, and caring approach to cases was excellent. She was always respectful of and compassionate with families. She contributed greatly to our Seattle studies of what is and what is not abuse."

Naomi graduated from the Medical College of Wisconsin in Milwaukee in 1979 and did her residency at Children's Hospital of Pittsburgh, followed by a fellowship in behavioral pediatrics at the University of Washington. She also had a master's degree in English literature. She was medical director of the Harborview Center for Sexual Assault and Traumatic Stress in Seattle. Naomi will be missed.

References

Adelson, P. D., Bratton, S. L., Carney, N. A., Chestnut, R. M., du Cordray, H. E., Goldstein, B., et al. (2003). Guidelines for the acute medical management of severe traumatic brain injury in infants, children, and adolescents. *Pediatric Critical Care Medicine, 4*(3, Suppl.), S1–75.

American College of Surgeons. (2011). *The ATLS program: Advanced Trauma Life Support.* www.facs.org/trauma/atls/program.html

Anderson, V., Catroppa, C., Morse, S., Haritou, F., & Rosenfeld, J. (2005). Functional plasticity or vulnerability after early brain injury? *Pediatrics, 116,* 1374–1382.

Anderson, V., Catroppa, C., Morse, S., Haritou, F., & Rosenfeld, J. V. (2009). Intellectual outcome from preschool traumatic brain injury: A 5-year prospective, longitudinal study. *Pediatrics, 124,* e1064–1071.

Anderson, V., Godfrey, C., Rosenfeld, J. V., & Catroppa, C. (2012). 10 years outcome from childhood traumatic brain injury. *International Journal of Developmental Neuroscience, 30,* 217–224.

Anderson, V., Spencer-Smith, M., Leventer, R., Coleman, L., Anderson, P., Williams, J., et al. (2009). Childhood brain insult: Can age at insult help us predict outcome? *Brain, 132,* 45–56.

Barlow, K. M., Thompson, E., Johnson, D., & Minns, R. A. (2004). The neurological outcome of non-accidental head injury. *Pediatric Rehabilitation, 7,* 195–203.

Barnes, P. M., Norton, C. M., Dunstan, F. D., Kemp, A. M., Yates, D. W., & Sibert, J. R. (2005). Abdominal injury due to child abuse. *Lancet, 366*(9481), 234–235. doi:10.1016/s0140-6736(05)66913-9

Baxter, A. L., Lindberg, D. M., Burke, B. L., Shults, J., & Holmes, J. F. (2008). Hepatic enzyme decline after pediatric blunt trauma: A tool for timing child abuse? *Child Abuse & Neglect, 32*(9), 838–845. doi:10.1016/j.chiabu.2007.09.013

Bensard, D. D., Beaver, B. L., Besner, G. E., & Cooney, D. R. (1996). Small bowel injury in children after blunt abdominal trauma: Is diagnostic delay important? *Journal of Trauma, 41*(3), 476–483.

Berger, R. P., Dulani, T., Adelson, D., Leventhal, J. M., Richichi, R., & Kochanek, P. M. (2006). Identification of inflicted traumatic brain injury in well-appearing infants using serum

and cerebrospinal markers: A possible screening tool. *Pediatrics, 117,* 325–332.

Berger, R. P., Ta'asan, S., Rand, A., Lokshin, A., & Kochanek, P. (2008). Multiplex assessment of serum biomarker concentrations in well-appearing children with inflicted traumatic brain injury. *Pediatric Research, 65,* 97–102.

Bixby, S. D., Callahan, M. J., & Taylor, G. A. (2008). Imaging in pediatric blunt abdominal trauma. *Seminars in Roentgenology, 43*(1), 72–82. doi:10.1053/j.ro.2007.08.009

Blakeney, P., Meyer, W., Moore, P., Broemeling, L., Hunt, R., Robson, M., & Herndon, D. (1993). Social competence and behavioral problems of pediatric survivors of burns. *Journal of Burn Care and Rehabilitation, 14*(1), 65–72.

Bonnier, C., Nassogne, M.-C., & Evrard, P. (1995). Outcome and prognosis of whiplash shaken infant syndrome: Late consequences after a symptom-free interval. *Developmental Medicine and Child Neurology, 37,* 943–956.

Brosbe, M. S., Hoefling, K., & Faust, J. (2011). Predicting posttraumatic stress following pediatric injury: A systematic review. *Journal of Pediatric Psychology, 36*(6), 718–729. doi:10.1093/jpepsy/jsq115

Canty, T. G., Sr., Canty, T. G., Jr., & Brown, C. (1999). Injuries of the gastrointestinal tract from blunt trauma in children: A 12-year experience at a designated pediatric trauma center. *Journal of Trauma, 46*(2), 234–240.

Catroppa, C., Anderson, V. A., Morse, S. A., Haritou, F., & Rosenfeld, J. V. (2008). Outcome and predictors of functional recovery 5 years following pediatric traumatic brain injury (TBI). *Journal of Pediatric Psychology, 33,* 707–718.

Centers for Disease Control and Prevention. (2011). Recommended immunization schedules for persons aged 0 through 18 years—United States, 2012. *MMWR Morbidity and Mortality Weekly Report, 61*(5), 1–4.

Chester, D. L., Jose, R. M., Aldyami, E., King, H., & Moiemen, N. S. (2006) Non-accidental burns in children—Are we neglecting neglect? *Burns, 32,* 222–228.

Chou, R., & Peterson, K. (2005). *Drug class review: Skeletal muscle relaxants—Final report* [Internet]. Portland, OR: Oregon Health & Science University.

Croce, M. A., Fabian, T. C., Menke, P. G., Waddle-Smith, L., Minard, G., Kudsk, K. A., & Pritchard, F. E. (1995). Nonoperative management of blunt hepatic trauma is the treatment of choice for hemodynamically stable patients: Results of a prospective trial. *Annals of Surgery, 221*(6), 744–753; discussion 753–745.

Dean, N. P., Boslaugh, S., Adelson, P. D., Pineda, J. A., & Leonard, J. R. (2007). Physician agreement with evidence-based recommendations for the treatment of severe traumatic brain injury in children. *Journal of Neurosurgery, 107*(5, Suppl.), 387–391.

Desai, K. M., Dorward, I. G., Minkes, R. K., & Dillon, P. A. (2003). Blunt duodenal injuries in children. *Journal of Trauma, 54*(4), 640–645; discussion 645–646. doi:10.1097/01.ta.0000056184.80706.9b

De Young, A. C., Kenardy, J. A., Cobham, V. E., & Kimble, R. (2012). Prevalence, comorbidity and course of trauma reactions in young burn-injured children. *Journal of Child Psychology and Psychiatry, 53*(1), 56–63. doi:10.1111/j.1469-7610.2011.02431.x

Dias, M. S. (2004). Traumatic brain and spinal cord injury. *Pediatric Clinics of North America, 51,* 271–303.

Dietrich, A. M., Bowman, M. J., Ginn-Pease, M. E., Kosnik, E., & King, D. (1993). Pediatric head injuries: Can clinical factors reliably predict an abnormality on computed tomography? *Annals of Emergency Medicine, 22*(10), 1535–1540.

Duffy, B. J., McLaughlin, P. M., & Eichelberger, M. R. (2006). Assessment, triage, and early management of burns in children. *Clinical Pediatric Emergency Medicine, 7*(2), 82–93. doi:10.1016/j.cpem.2006.04.001

Dunning, J., Daly, J. P., Lomas, J.-P., Lecky, F., Batchelor, J., & Mackway-Jones, K., Children's Head Injury Algorithm for the Prediction of Important Clinical Events Study Group. (2006). Derivation of the children's head injury algorithm for the prediction of important clinical events decision rule for head injury in children. *Archives of Disease in Childhood, 91*, 885–891.

Durham, S., Clancy, R. R., Leuthhardt, E., Sun, P., Kamerling, S., Dominguez, T., & Duhaine, A. (2000). CHOP Infant Coma Scale ("Infant Face Scale"): A novel coma scale for children less than two years of age. *Journal of Neurotrauma, 17*, 729–737.

Ewing-Cobbs, L., Kramer, L., Prasad, M., Canales, D. N., Louis, P.T., Fletcher, J. M., et al. (1998). Neuroimaging, physical and developmental findings after inflicted and non-inflicted traumatic brain injury in young children. *Pediatrics, 102*, 300–307.

Ewing-Cobbs, L., Prasad, M., Kramer, L., & Landry, S. (1999). Inflicted traumatic brain injury: Relationship of developmental outcome to severity of injury. *Pediatric Neurosurgery, 31*, 251–258.

Fitzgerald, C. L., Tran, P., Burnell, J., Broghammer, J. A., & Santucci, R. (2011). Instituting a conservative management protocol for pediatric blunt renal trauma: Evaluation of a prospectively maintained patient registry. *Journal of Urology, 185*(3), 1058–1064. doi:10.1016/j.juro.2010.10.045

Hahn, Y. S., Fuchs, S., Flannery, A. M., Barthel, M. J., & McLane, D. G. (1988). Factors influencing post-traumatic seizures in children. *Neurosurgery, 22*, 864–867.

Hahn, Y. S., & McLone, D. G. (1993). Risk factors in the outcome of children with minor head injury. *Pediatric Neurosurgery, 19*, 135–142.

Hanson, M. D., Gauld, M., Wathen, C. N., & Macmillan, H. L. (2008). Nonpharmacological interventions for acute wound care distress in pediatric patients with burn injury: A systematic review. *Journal of Burn Care & Research, 29*(5), 730–741. doi:10.1097/BCR.0b013e318184812e

Hartford, C. E., & Kealy, G. P. (2007). Care of outpatient burns. In D. N. Herndon (Ed.), *Total burn care* (3rd ed., pp. 67–80). Edinburgh, UK: W. B. Saunders.

Haviland, J., & Russell, R. I. R. (1997). Outcome after severe non-accidental head injury. *Archives of Disease in Childhood, 77*, 504–507.

Hessen, E., Nestvold, K., & Anderson, V. (2007). Neuropsychological function 23 years after mild traumatic brain injury: A comparison of outcome after paediatric and adult head injuries. *Brain Injury, 21*, 963–979.

Hilmes, M. A., Hernanz-Schulman, M., Greeley, C. S., Piercey, L. M., Yu, C., & Kan, J. H. (2011). CT identification of abdominal injuries in abused pre-school-age children. *Pediatric Radiology, 41*(5), 643–651. doi:10.1007/s00247-010-1899-9

Huang, T. (2007). Overview of burn reconstruction. In D. N. Herndon (Ed.), *Total burn care* (3rd ed., pp. 674–686). Edinburgh, UK: W. B. Saunders.

Jennett, B. (1976). Posttraumatic epilepsy. In P. J. Vinken & G. W. Bruyn (Eds.), *Handbook of clinical neurology* (Vol. 24, pp. 445–454). New York, NY: American Elsevier Publishing.

Kaulfers, A.-M. D., Backeljauw, P. F., Reifschneider, K., Blum, S., Michaud, L., Weiss, M., & Rose, S. (2010). Endocrine dysfunction following traumatic brain injury in children. *Journal of Pediatrics, 157*, 894–899.

Kay, M., & Wyllie, R. (2009). Caustic ingestions in children. *Current Opinions in Pediatrics, 21*(5), 651–654. doi:10.1097/MOP.0b013e32832e2764

Kiankhooy, A., Sartorelli, K. H., Vane, D. W., & Bhave, A. D. (2010). Angiographic embolization is safe and effective therapy for blunt abdominal solid organ injury in children. *Journal of Trauma, 68*(3), 526–531. doi:10.1097/TA.0b013e3181d3e5b7

Kirk, K. A., Shoyket, M., Jeong, J. H., Tyler-Kabara, E. C., Henderson, M. J., Bell, M. J., & Fink, E. L. (2008). Dysautonomia after pediatric brain injury. *Developmental Medicine and Child Neurology, 54*, 759–764.

Koskiniemi, M., Kyykka, T., Nybo, T., & Jarho, L. (1995). Long-term outcome after severe brain injury in preschoolers is worse than expected. *Archives of Pediatrics & Adolescent Medicine, 149*, 249–254.

Krach, L. E., Kriel, R. L., Morris, W. F., Warhol, B. L., & Luxenberg, M. G. (1997). Central autonomic dysfunction following acquired brain injury in children. *Neurorehabilitation and Neural Repair, 11*, 41–45.

Kraft, R., Herndon, D. N., Al-Mousawi, A. M., Williams, F. N., Finnerty, C. C., & Jeschke, M. G. (2012). Burn size and survival probability in paediatric patients in modern burn care: A prospective observational cohort study. *Lancet, 379*(9820), 1013–1021. doi:10.1016/S0140-6736(11)61345-7

Krahulik, D., Zapletalova, J., Frysak, Z., & Vaverka, M. (2010). Dysfunction of hypothalamic-hypophysial axis after traumatic brain injury in adults. *Journal of Neurosurgery, 113*, 581–584.

Landolt, M. A., Grubenmann, S., & Meuli, M. (2002). Family impact greatest: Predictors of quality of life and psychological adjustment in pediatric burn survivors. *Journal of Trauma, 53*(6), 1146–1151. doi:10.1097/01.ta.0000033763.65011.89

Lane, W. G., Dubowitz, H., Langenberg, P., & Dischinger, P. (2012). Epidemiology of abusive abdominal trauma hospitalizations in United States children. *Child Abuse & Neglect, 36*(2), 142–148. doi:10.1016/j.chiabu.2011.09.010

Lane, W. G., Lotwin, I., Dubowitz, H., Langenberg, P., & Dischinger, P. (2011). Outcomes for children hospitalized with abusive versus noninflicted abdominal trauma. *Pediatrics, 127*(6), e1400–1405. doi:10.1542/peds.2010-2096

Ledbetter, D. J., Hatch, E. I., Jr., Feldman, K. W., Fligner, C. L., & Tapper, D. (1988). Diagnostic and surgical implications of child abuse. *Archives of Surgery, 123*(9), 1101–1105.

LeDoux, J., Meyer, W. J., 3rd, Blakeney, P. E., & Herndon, D. N. (1998). Relationship between parental emotional states, family environment and the behavioural adjustment of pediatric burn survivors. *Burns, 24*(5), 425–432.

Leonard, L. G., Scheulen, J. J., & Munster, A. M. (1982). Chemical burns: Effect of prompt first aid. *Journal of Trauma, 22*(5), 420–423.

Lind, K., Toure, H., Brugel, D., Laurent-Vannier, A., & Chevignard, M. (2012). Long-term outcome after severe shaken baby syndrome. *Annals of Physical and Rehabilitation Medicine, 55*(Suppl. 1), e233.

Lindberg, D., Makoroff, K., Harper, N., Laskey, A., Bechtel, K., Deye, K., & Shapiro, R. (2009). Utility of hepatic transaminases to recognize abuse in children. *Pediatrics, 124*(2), 509–516. doi:10.1542/peds.2008-2348

Maguire, J. L., Boutis, K., Uleryk, E. M., Laupacis, A., & Parkin, P. C. (2012). Should a head-injured child receive a head CT scan? A systematic review of clinical prediction rules. *Pediatrics, 124*, e145–154.

Makaroff, K. L., & Putnam, F. W. (2003). Outcomes of infants and children with inflicted traumatic brain injury. *Developmental Medicine and Child Neurology, 45*, 497–502.

Malhotra, A. K., Fabian, T. C., Croce, M. A., Gavin, T. J., Kudsk, K. A., Minard, G., & Pritchard, F. E. (2000). Blunt hepatic injury: A paradigm shift from operative to nonoperative management in the 1990s. *Annals of Surgery, 231*(6), 804–813.

Martin-Herz, S. P., Thurber, C. A., & Patterson, D. R. (2000). Psychological principles of burn wound pain in children: II. Treatment applications. *Journal of Burn Care and Rehabilitation, 21*(5), 458–472; discussion 457.

Maternal and Child Health Bureau, U.S. Department of Health and Human Services, Health Resources and Services Administration. 2012. *National survey of children with special healthcare needs.* www.childhealthdata.org

Mattix, K. D., Tataria, M., Holmes, J., Kristoffersen, K., Brown, R., Groner, J., et al. (2007). Pediatric pancreatic trauma: Predictors of nonoperative management failure and associated outcomes. *Journal of Pediatric Surgery, 42*(2), 340–344. doi:10.1016/j.jpedsurg.2006.10.006

Meyer, W. J., 3rd, Blakeney, P., Russell, W., Thomas, C., Robert, R., Berniger, F., & Holzer, C., 3rd. (2004). Psychological problems reported by young adults who were burned as children. *Journal of Burn Care and Rehabilitation, 25*(1), 98–106. doi:10.1097/01.BCR.0000107203.48726.67

Minns, R. A., Jones, P. A., & Barlow, K. M. (2005). Outcome and prognosis of nonaccidental head injury in infants. In R. A. Minns & J. K. Brown (Eds.), *Shaking and other non-accidental head injuries in children* (pp. 364–414). London, UK: MacKeith Press.

Mlcak, R. P., & Buffalo, M. C. (2007). Pre-hospital managment, transportation, and emergency care. In D. N. Herndon (Ed.), *Total burn care* (3rd ed., pp. 81–92). Edinburgh, UK: W. B. Saunders.

Morgan, W. F. (2012). Treatment of minor thermal burns. *UpToDate.* www.uptodateonline.com

Nelson, L. P., & Gold, J. I. (2012). Posttraumatic stress disorder in children and their parents following admission to the pediatric intensive care unit: A review. *Pediatric Critical Care Medicine, 13*(3), 338–347. doi:10.1097/PCC.0b013e3182196a8f

Norwood, K. W., DeBoer, M. D., Gurka, M. J., Kuperminc, M. N., Rogol, A. D., Blackman, J. A., et al. (2010). Traumatic brain injury in children and adolescents: Surveillance for pituitary dysfunction. *Clinical Pediatrics, 49*, 1044–1049.

Palchak, M. J., Holmes, J. F., Vance, C. W., Gelber, R. E., Schauer, B. A., Harrison, M. J., et al. (2003). A decision rule for identifying children at low risk for brain injuries after blunt head trauma. *Annals of Emergency Medicine, 42*, 492–508.

Park, K. D., Kim, D. Y., Lee, J. K., Nam, H., & Park, Y. (2010). Anterior pituitary dysfunction in moderate-to-severe chronic traumatic brain injury and the influence on functional outcome. *Brain Injury, 24*, 1330–1335.

Peters, E., LoSasso, B., Foley, J., Rodarte, A., Duthie, S., & Senac, M. O., Jr. (2006). Blunt bowel and mesenteric injuries in children: Do nonspecific computed tomography findings reliably identify these injuries? *Pediatric Critical Care Medicine, 7*(6), 551–556. doi:10.1097/01.pcc.0000244428.31624.ab

Pham, T. N., Gibran, N. S., & Heimbach, D. M. (2007). Evaluation of the burn wound: Management decisions. In D. N. Herndon (Ed.), *Total burn care* (3rd ed., pp. 119–126). Edinburgh, UK: W. B. Saunders.

Raissaki, M., Veyrac, C., Blondiaux, E., & Hadjigeorgi, C. (2011). Abdominal imaging in child abuse [Review]. *Pediatric Radiology, 41*(1), 4–16; quiz 137–138. doi:10.1007/s00247-010-1882-5

Reilly, P. L., Simpson, D. A., Sprod, R., & Thomas, L. (1988). Assessing the conscious level in infants and young children: A pediatric version of the Glasgow Coma Scale. *Child's Nervous System, 4*, 30–33.

Richardson, D. (2002). Physical therapy in spasticity. *European Journal of Neurology, 9*(Suppl. 1), 17–22.

Rorke-Adams, L., Duhaime, C.-A., Jenny, C., & Smith, W. L. (2009). Head trauma. In R. M. Reece & C. W. Christian (Eds.), *Child abuse: Medical diagnosis and treatment* (3rd ed.). Elk Grove Village, IL: American Academy of Pediatrics.

Schonfeld, D., & Lee, L. K. (2012). Blunt abdominal trauma in children. *Current Opinions in Pediatrics, 24*(3), 314–318. doi:10.1097/MOP.0b013e328352de97

Serghiou, M. A., Ott, S., Farmer, S., Morgan, D., Gibson, P., & Suman, O. E. (2007). Comprehensive rehabilitation of the burn patient. In D. N. Herndon (Ed.), *Total burn care* (3rd ed., pp. 620–651). Edinburgh, UK: W. B. Saunders.

Shapiro, M. B., Jenkins, D. H., Schwab, C. W., & Rotondo, M. F. (2000). Damage control: Collective review. *Journal of Trauma, 49*(5), 969–978.

Sheridan, R. (2005). Outpatient burn care in the emergency department [Review]. *Pediatric Emergency Care, 21*(7), 449–456; quiz 457–449.

Sheridan, R., Petras, L., Basha, G., Salvo, P., Cifrino, C., Hinson, M., et al. (1995). Planimetry study of the percent of body surface represented by the hand and palm: Sizing irregular burns is more accurately done with the palm. *Journal of Burn Care and Rehabilitation, 16*(6), 605–606.

Shunk, J. E., Rodgerson, J. D., & Woodward, G. A. (1996). The utility of head computed tomographic scanning in pediatric patients with normal neurologic examination in the emergency department. *Pediatric Emergency Care, 12*, 160–165.

Sills, M. R., Libby, A. M., & Orton, H. D. (2005). Prehospital and in-hospital mortality: A comparison of intentional and unintentional traumatic brain injuries in Colorado children. *Archives of Pediatrics & Adolescent Medicine, 159*, 665–670.

Stoddard, F. J., Saxe, G., Ronfeldt, H., Drake, J. E., Burns, J., Edgren, C., & Sheridan, R. (2006). Acute stress symptoms in young children with burns. *Journal of the American Academy of Child and Adolescent Psychiatry, 45*(1), 87–93. doi:10.1097/01.chi.0000184934.71917.3a

Su, E., Bell, M. J., Kochanek, P. M., Wisniewski, S. R., Bayir, H., Clark, R. S., et al. (2012). Increased CSF concentrations of myelin basic protein after TBI in infants and children: Absence of significant effect of therapeutic hypothermia. *Neurocritical Care.* Advance online publication.

Teasdale, G., & Jennett, B. (1974). Assessment of coma and impaired consciousness: A practical scale. *Lancet, 2*, 337–347.

Temiz, A., Oguzkurt, P., Ezer, S. S., Ince, E., & Hicsonmez, A. (2012). Predictability of outcome of caustic ingestion by esophagogastroduodenoscopy in children. *World Journal of Gastroenterology, 18*(10), 1098–1103. doi:10.3748/wjg.v18.i10.1098

Trokel, M., DiScala, C., Terrin, N. C., & Sege, R. D. (2004). Blunt abdominal injury in the young pediatric patient: Child abuse and patient outcomes. *Child Maltreatment, 9*(1), 111–117. doi:10.1177/1077559503260310

Trokel, M., Discala, C., Terrin, N. C., & Sege, R. D. (2006). Patient and injury characteristics in abusive abdominal injuries. *Pediatric Emergency Care, 22*(10), 700–704. doi:10.1097/01.pec.0000238734.76413.d0

Umbreit, E. C., Routh, J. C., & Husmann, D. A. (2009). Nonoperative management of nonvascular grade IV blunt renal trauma in children: Meta-analysis and systematic review. *Urology, 74*(3), 579–582. doi:10.1016/j.urology.2009.04.049

Warden, G. D. (2007). Fluid resuscitation and early management. In D. N. Herndon (Ed.), *Total burn care* (3rd ed., pp. 107–118). Edinburgh, UK: W. B. Saunders.

Willebrand, M., Sveen, J., Ramklint, M. D., Bergquist, R. N., Huss, M. D., & Sjoberg, M. D. (2011). Psychological problems in children with burns: Parents' reports on the Strengths and Difficulties Questionnaire. *Burns, 37*(8), 1309–1316. doi:10.1016/j.burns.2011.08.003

Wood, J., Rubin, D. M., Nance, M. L., & Christian, C. W. (2005). Distinguishing inflicted versus accidental abdominal injuries in young children. *Journal of Trauma, 59*(5), 1203–1208.

20

Intervening with Families When Children Are Neglected

Child neglect is the most common and the least understood form of child maltreatment. The purpose of this chapter is to synthesize what we know about promising approaches to help families meet the basic needs of their children. This is not to suggest that neglect is only the result of omissions by caregivers but acknowledges the primary role of the family in nurturing children. This chapter will integrate knowledge that has been previously generated through recent efforts to review the limited research on effective interventions (DePanfilis, 1996; Gaudin, 1988, 1993b; Gaudin, Wodarski, Arkinson, & Avery, 1990/91; Howing, Wodarski, Gaudin, & Kurtz, 1989; Smokowski & Wodarski, 1996) and propose intervention strategies based on the field's best collective knowledge and experience.

DEFINITIONS

For the purposes of this chapter, neglect (1) refers to acts of omission of care to meet a child's basic needs that (2) result in harm or a threat of harm to children (Dubowitz, Black, Starr, & Zuravin, 1993). This definition infers that neglectful conditions are not always due to omissions by caregivers alone but may also be due to other factors beyond the control of impoverished families. This author concurs with a very early paper (Lewis, 1969) that underscored the importance of the social context of neglect. Lewis defined *parental neglect* as insufficient child care and guidance by a responsible adult and *community neglect* as insufficient provision of resources to support parents in their efforts to provide children with adequate care and guidance. In both instances, the responsible persons (parents or community authorities) are not likely to provide adequate care without outside intervention.

Going beyond this definition, a child's basic needs may not be met in many different ways. Using a combination of definitions (American Professional Society on the Abuse of Children [APSAC], 1995; Magura & Moses, 1986; U.S. Department of Health and Human Services [U.S. DHHS], 1988; Zuravin & DePanfilis, 1996), intervention may need to address the following circumstances when children's basic needs are not met: inadequate supervision, inappropriate substitute child care, abandonment, instability of living arrangements, failure to receive needed health care, inattention to personal hygiene, inattention to household sanitary conditions, inattention to household safety, presence of hazardous physical conditions in the home, inattention to nutritional needs, inadequacy of clothing, witnessing violence, permitting drug or alcohol use (or both), permitting other maladaptive behavior, inadequate nurturance or affection, isolation, inattention to mental health care needs, and inattention to educational needs.

PRINCIPLES FOR EFFECTIVE INTERVENTION

Considering the multiple pathways that can lead to neglect (see Crittenden, 1999) and the many ways in which a child's basic needs may not be met, it is not surprising that there is little empirical research that provides clear support for one intervention approach versus another. However, although there may be much more that we need to learn, findings from recent reviews (DePanfilis, 1996; Gaudin, 1988, 1993b; Gaudin et al., 1990/91; Howing et al., 1989; Smokowski & Wodarski, 1996) do suggest some basic principles for practitioners who intervene with families when children's basic needs are not met.

Reprinted from D. DePanfilis (1999), Intervening with Families When Children Are Neglected. In H. Dubowitz (Ed.), *Neglected Children: Research, Practice, and Policy.* Thousand Oaks, CA: Sage Publications, Inc.

Ecological-Developmental Framework

Intervention is more likely to be effective if it operates from a conceptual framework that views neglect within a system of risk and protective factors interacting across four levels: (1) the individual or ontogenic level, (2) the family microsystems, (3) the exosystem, and (4) the social macro system (Belsky, 1980). The National Research Council (1993) succinctly describes this model as follows:

> The ontogenic level involves individual characteristics and the changing developmental status of family members. The family microsystem includes the family environment, parenting styles, and interactions among family members. The exosystem consists of the community in which the family lives, the work place of the parents, school and peer groups of the family members, formal and informal social supports and services available to the family, and other factors such as family income, employment, and job availability. Finally, the social macro system consists of the overarching values and beliefs of the culture. (p. 110)

To be most effective, intervention should be directed at multiple levels (ontogenic, family microsystem, and exosystem) depending on the specific needs of the family. In addition, over the long term, programs should consider strategies to also address the social macro system. Policy initiatives must be targeted at social conditions that continue to oppress large segments of the population, especially the poorest of the poor, including families who are unable to provide minimally adequate care for their children (Nelson, Saunders, & Landsman, 1993). Examples suggested by Nelson and colleagues include the availability of affordable child care, increased education and employment opportunities, adequate low-income housing and rent subsidies, and large-scale drug prevention and treatment initiatives. Policies further need to ensure that both family preservation and support services are integrated into community institutions, such as schools, churches, and recreational organizations serving families (Thomlison, 1997). Thomlison suggests that risk-focused programing should prevent the accumulation of risk factors; establish and maintain prosocial situations and opportunities; focus on resilience and adaptation; facilitate active involvement of parents, children, and others in planning; ensure that services to at-risk populations are both necessary and sufficient; provide timely, careful, and expert evaluation, assessment, and follow-up services throughout the formative childhood years; and build safe, stable environments to permit families to establish structure, routines, rituals, and organization. Because this chapter is geared to intervention with families, the reader is encouraged to refer to Gelles (1999) for further discussion of these and other macro-level interventions.

Importance of Outreach and Community

Families with children whose basic needs may not be met are typically poor and lack access to resources (Gaudin, 1993b; Smale, 1995). Furthermore, these families are more likely to be socially isolated, experience loneliness, and lack social support in both rural and urban areas than non-neglecting comparison groups (DePanfilis, 1996). Last, traditional, in-office, one-to-one counseling by professionals has proven to be ineffective with neglect (Cohn & Daro, 1987). Intervention therefore must include aggressive outreach and advocacy and be designed to mobilize concrete formal and informal helping resources.

Services provided in the home and within the neighborhood and community are therefore essential. The helper is in a much better position to understand the family in their daily environment and to break down and manage the natural resistance of the family to change (Anderson & Stewart, 1983). To be most effective, interventions must be a collaborative process between the family and the community. Strategies should encourage an inclusive process that allows people from schools, churches, health centers, businesses, child care facilities, and other sectors to come together to plan and carry out goals for strengthening their neighborhood (Zuravin & Shay, 1992). In turn, people will be linked to people, and informal helping relationships will be built.

Importance of Family Assessment

Effective intervention to remedy child neglect must be based on a comprehensive assessment of the family, with attention to the *type* of neglect that may be apparent and to the *specific contributing causes* at the individual, family, neighborhood, and community levels (Gaudin, 1988, 1993b). When available, this assessment should be undertaken in conjunction with other service providers to form a comprehensive picture of the individual, interpersonal, and societal pressures on the family members—individually and as a group. For both practice accountability and usefulness, practitioners should consider using standardized clinical measures of risk and protective factors as well as parenting attitudes, knowledge, and skills for assessment and recording information (Smokowski & Wodarski, 1996). Examples of clinical measures and recording formats that may be useful are provided in several texts (Bloom, Fischer, & Orme, 1995; Dunst, Trivette, & Deal, 1988; Fischer & Corcoran, 1994a, 1994b; Hudson, 1982; Karls & Wandrei, 1994; Magura & Moses, 1986; Magura, Moses, & Jones, 1987; McCubbin, Thompson, & McCubbin, 1996; Walmyr Publishing Co., 1990, 1992).

Because each family is unique and families with neglect problems are heterogeneous, no single intervention will be effective in all situations (National Research Council, 1993; Wolfe, 1993). Interventions must be tailored to the specific needs of individual families, and programs must be flexible to accommodate differences. There are significant differences between families who have experienced chronic multiple problems that led to neglect compared with families who may have experienced a recent crisis—for example, homelessness or unemployment—that has led to a child's basic needs being unmet (Nelson et al., 1993). Furthermore, because of the many different types of family systems, it is important that intervention be geared to the family's own definition of family and to culturally based differences and strengths (Lloyd & Sallee, 1994). In the past, mainstream efforts with families have focused too heavily on mothers without enough attention to fathers and other primary caregivers.

Importance of a Helping Alliance and Partnership with the Family

Many families at risk for neglect may not have had positive experiences with formal systems. A key component of many effective programs is to create a helping alliance and partnership with the family (Bean, 1994; Dore & Alexander, 1996; Kenemore, 1993). This requirement is especially challenging because some caregivers with neglect problems have difficulty forming and sustaining mutually supportive interpersonal relationships (Dore & Alexander, 1996; Gaudin & Polansky 1986; Gaudin, Polansky, Kilpatrick, & Shilton, 1993). One of the key challenges for practitioners is to form positive connections and partnerships with families so that they will have an opportunity to tackle the difficult challenges in their lives (McCurdy, Hurvis, & Clark, 1996). Successful engagement with families who may be resistant to intervention requires an ability to feel and demonstrate empathy with caregivers (Siu & Hogan, 1989) despite their initial resistance to intervention. Building relationships with caregivers models conflict resolution for building harmonious relationships that nurture the development of vulnerable family members (Bowlby, 1988; Crittenden, 1991). Crittenden suggests that when the practitioner sensitively attends to the affective communication of family members, a pattern of feedback loops leading to mutual accommodation and assimilation is established. These dialogues acknowledge and support caregiver strengths and provide family members with a secure base for developing communicative skills (Bowlby, 1988). Through this process, practitioners can create interventions tailor-made to each family's needs and competencies (Crittenden, 1991). To be effective over time, the intervention must help families develop more sustaining relationships with others. If intervention is neighborhood based, then these relationships are more likely to continue after intervention ends.

Importance of Empowerment-Based Practice

Several neglect-focused demonstration projects have reported on the importance of using empowerment approaches (Lee, 1994; Solomon, 1976) in their work with families (DiLeonardi, 1993; Landsman, Nelson, Allen, & Tyler, 1992; Mugridge, 1991; U.S. DHHS, 1993; Witt, Dayton, & Sheinvald, 1992; Zuravin & Shay, 1992). "Empowering families means carrying out interventions in a manner in which family members acquire a sense of control over

their lives as a result of their efforts to meet their needs" (Dunst et al., 1988, p. 88). To decrease the risk of neglect, interventions must help families learn to effectively manage the multiple stresses and conditions within the family and in their neighborhoods. Family members should be empowered to resolve their own problems and avoid dependence on the social service system (Lloyd & Sallee, 1994). Empowerment denotes a partnership between the practitioner and the family and involves the development and use of the capacities of the individual, family, organization, and community (Fraser & Galinsky, 1997). Drawing on these capacities helps families fully realize their own abilities and goals (Cowger, 1994; Gutierrez, 1990; Gutierrez, Glen Maye, & DeLois, 1995; Simon, 1994). The role of the helper becomes one of partner, guide, mediator, advocate, coach, and enabler.

Importance of Emphasizing Strengths

The strengths perspective is being increasingly applied with diverse populations (Saleebey, 1996, 1997; Trivette, Dunst, Deal, Hamer, & Prompst, 1990) and has particular relevance to families at risk for neglect and other forms of maltreatment (DePanfilis & Wilson, 1996). A strengths-based orientation helps build on a family's existing competencies and resources to respond to crises and stress; to meet needs; and to promote, enhance, and strengthen the functioning of the family system. Strengths-based practice involves a paradigmatic shift from a deficit approach, which emphasizes problems and pathology, to a positive partnership with the family. The focus of assessments (described earlier) is therefore on the complex interplay of both risks and strengths related to individual family members, the family as a unit, and the broader neighborhood and environment.

When a child's basic needs are unmet, we must understand what conditions within and outside the family may be contributing as well as what resources exist within and outside the family to help the family address the problem. The intervention, however, may not correct the problem but instead enable caregivers to meet the needs of family members who will be better able to have the time, energy, and resources for enhancing the well-being and development of the family (Dunst et al., 1988). As emphasized by Hobbs et al. (1984),

> Families are the critical element in the rearing of healthy, competent, and caring children. We suggest however that families—all families—cannot perform this function as well as they might unless they are supported by a caring and strong community, for it is community [support] that provides the informal and formal supplements to families' own resources. Just as a child needs nurturance, stimulation, and the resources that caring adults bring to his or her life, so too, do parents—as individuals and as adults filling socially valued roles (for example, parent, worker)—need the

resources made possible by a caring community if they are to fulfill their roles well. (p. 46)

Importance of Culturally Competent Intervention

Risk and protective factors for child neglect may differ according to race and ethnicity. It is well established that families of color, and especially African American families, are disproportionately represented in the child welfare system (Children's Defense Fund, 1990; Leashore, Chipungu, & Everett, 1991; National Black Child Development Institute, 1990). Most often these families are poor and poorly educated (Brissett-Chapman, 1997). Furthermore, it is well documented that "children from African American, Hispanic, and other racial and ethnic backgrounds are subject to the direct and indirect effects of discrimination, compounding and exacerbating their risk for many kinds of problems" (Fraser & Galinsky, 1997, p. 272).

The need to increase cultural competency among helping professionals is a response to three factors in the United States: (1) increasing cultural diversity (Sue, Arrendondo, & McDavis, 1992), (2) the underrepresentation of professionals from diverse backgrounds in our helping institutions (McPhatter, 1997), and (3) inadequate delivery of social and mental health services to maltreated children and families of color (Gould, 1991). In particular, Gould suggests that families of color have received inadequate and often inappropriate and damaging child welfare services. There is compelling evidence to support this argument. For example, African American families and children have been denied access to many of the services of the child welfare system (Close, 1983), or they have received differential treatment within that system (Albers, Reilly, & Rittner, 1993; Stehno, 1982). Furthermore, minority children enter the foster care system disproportionately, partially influenced by poverty and by conversion of informal kinship arrangements to formal foster placements (Danzy & Jackson, 1997), and once in the system, they remain longer than Caucasian children, do not receive as many in-home support services as Caucasian children, and have a disproportionate number of undesirable experiences (Billingsley & Giovannoni, 1972; Gould, 1991; Mech, 1985). For example, African American children are more likely to be placed in transracial foster and adoptive homes than are Caucasian children and more likely to enter care as young children (Fein, 1991). Gould (1991) also suggests that African American children fare worse than white children or any other minority children on all measures of service delivery, such as recommended versus actual length of placement, number of services, adoption services, and worker contact with child and principal caregivers.

Because neglected children and their families continue to represent more than half of the caseload of our child welfare agencies (U.S. DHHS, 1996), it is imperative that we work to increase the cultural competence of service providers. Basic cultural competence is achieved when organizations and practitioners accept and respect difference; engage in ongoing cultural self-assessment; expand their diversity knowledge and skills; and adapt service models to fit the target population's culture, situation, and perceived needs (Rauch, North, Rowe, & Risley-Curtiss, 1993). Culture is a set of beliefs, attitudes, values, and standards of behavior that are passed from one generation to the next. It includes language, worldview, dress, food, styles of communication, notions of wellness, healing techniques, child-drearing patterns, and self-identity (Abney 1996). Human beings create culture, and each group develops its own over time. Culture is dynamic and changing, not static; it evolves as conditions change. Every culture has a set of assumptions made up of beliefs that are so completely accepted by the group that they do not need to be stated, questioned, or defended. In brief, cultural competency is the ability to understand, to the best of one's ability, the worldview of our culturally different clients (or peers) and adapt our practice accordingly. To best meet the needs of families, practitioners must understand the world from the clients' points of view and help in a constructive manner.

At a symposium on neglect, Abney (U.S. DHHS, 1993) outlined needs of neglectful families that a culturally competent system should address. At the micro level, families need opportunities to build empowerment skills and to be involved in the advocacy process and peer support groups. At the macro level, families need financial assistance; housing; training focused on job retention; income augmentation to promote economic self-sufficiency; child care and health care; culturally sensitive research; substance abuse prevention and treatment programs; services that are geographically accessible, bilingual, and culturally sensitive; and greater participation in program planning and implementation by professionals of color and community representatives (U.S. DHHS, 1993).

Developmental Appropriateness of Interventions

It is critical that practitioners consider the developmental levels of children, caregivers, and the family as a system in their assessments and intervention strategies. For example, a child whose basic physical and emotional needs have been neglected will often suffer significant developmental delays (see Gaudin, 1999). Interventions may need to offer opportunities for developmental remediation (e.g., therapeutic day care) while at the same time working on the attachment relationships between caregivers and children. Caregivers may bring a host of developmental issues to the family (e.g., unresolved losses, abuse, or deprivation during childhood) or may have difficulty assuming parental roles and responsibilities in adolescence. Described by Polansky, Chalmers, Williams, and Buttenwieser (1981) as "apathy-futility syndrome" or "psychological complexity" by Pianta, Egeland, and Erickson (1989), neglectful caregiving may be related to a failure of caregivers to have received nurturing as children. Cognitive interventions can help these caregivers change dysfunctional self-perceptions resulting from early

Table 20.1. Interventions When Children Are Neglected

Ecological (Concrete)	Ecological (Social Support)	Developmental	Cognitive-Behavioral	Individual	Family System
Housing assistance	Individual social support	Therapeutic day care	Social skills training	Alcohol or other drug in-patient and out-patient counseling, detoxification	Home-based family-centered counseling regarding family functioning, communication skills, home management, roles, and responsibilities
Emergency financial, food, or other assistance	Connections to church activities	Individual assistance with developmental role achievement (e.g., parenting)	Communication skill building		
Clothing, household items	Mentor involvement	Public health visiting, with focus on developmental interventions, including attachment needs of family members	Teaching home management, parent-child interaction, meal preparation skills, and other life skills	12-Step programs	
Advocacy for availability or accessibility to community resources	Social support groups			Mental health in-patient and out-patient counseling	Center-based family therapy
Hands-on assistance to increase safety and sanitation of home (home management aides)	Development of neighborhood child care co-op		Teach new thought processes (e.g., regarding childhood history)	Crisis intervention	Mobilizing family strengths
	Neighborhood center activities	Peer groups (often at schools) geared to developmental tasks (e.g., adolescence)		Stress management counseling	Nurturing family camps
Transportation	Social networking		Parenting education	Play therapy	Family sculpting
Free or low-cost medical care	Recreation programs	Mentors to provide nurturing, cultural enrichment, recreation, role modeling	Employment counseling or training (or both)		
Low-cost but quality child care (parent aide, volunteer)	Cultural festivals and other activities		Financial management counseling		
			Problem-solving training		

neglect or abuse and break the intergenerational cycle of maltreatment (Egeland & Erickson, 1990). Last, the family may be stressed due to its developmental stage as a system (e.g., blended, young) or due to conflict in roles when the family is composed of caregivers across generations. As the drug epidemic has grown, we increasingly see grandparents raising their grandchildren due to neglect by drug-addicted parents. These newly constituted families often lack security due to informal arrangements and inadequate resources (financial and physical) to provide adequately for children (Kelley, 1996). Furthermore, the life cycle stages through which families evolve (Carter & McGoldrick, 1988) are interrupted; caregivers who thought that their childrearing days were over are unexpectedly unable to look forward to fewer demands during their retirement. In sum, it is essential that our interventions target the developmental needs of children, caregivers, and the family as a system.

INTERVENTIONS

The goal of intervention, to help families within communities meet the basic needs of their children, is to provide the mix and intensity of services appropriate to each family's need. Interventions are geared to increase the ability of families to successfully nurture their children by enabling families to use resources and opportunities in the community that will help them alleviate stress, overcome knowledge and skill deficits, and build and maintain caregiving

competencies. Because the contributors to neglect are varied, interventions may be directed to developing or providing (or both) (1) concrete resources, (2) social support, (3) developmental remediation, (4) cognitive or behavioral interventions, (5) individually oriented interventions, (6) family-focused interventions, or (7) some combination of these (see table 20.1).

Provision of Concrete Resources

Several types of neglect (e.g., household sanitation and safety, personal hygiene, nutritional neglect, and lack of supervision) may be the results of deficits in concrete resources. Furthermore, the stress of poverty and its many consequences (e.g., living in inadequate housing within crime-ridden neighborhoods) can contribute to a sense of powerlessness that further affects caregiving capacity to meet children's basic needs. Helping families access concrete resources supports adequate care of their children and is often crucial *before* families can address other factors in their lives that may affect care of their children. Examples include housing assistance; emergency financial, food, and energy assistance; affordable and quality child care; transportation; home management assistance; and free or low-cost medical care. These concrete resources are needed to help families move beyond mere survival to more optimal functioning, including improved care of their children (Nelson et al., 1993).

Social Support Interventions

Sufficient evidence exists that families who are socially isolated, experience loneliness, and lack social support in both rural and urban settings may be more prone to neglect than matched comparison groups (DePanfilis, 1996). A social network among a group of people serves to provide nurturance and reinforcement for efforts to cope with life on a day-to-day basis (Whittaker & Garbarino, 1983). Interventions are geared to provide or mobilize the personal social network of a family to serve one or more social support functions, including emotional, and material support, knowledge information, appraisal support (information pertinent to self-evaluation), and companionship. Studies on the stress-buffering role of social support and from intervention programs involving mobilization of social support suggest that both a confidant and a network help protect families against stress (Gottlieb, 1985).

To evaluate the meaningfulness of available social support, one must assess the *actual* network (accessibility, frequency of interaction, and closeness) and the *perceived* social support—from friends and from family (DePanfilis, 1996). Models for assessing the quantity and quality of a family's linkages with formal and informal supportive resources include (1) the Eco Map (Hartman, 1978); (2) the Social Network Map (Tracy, 1990; Tracy & Whittaker, 1990); (3) the Social Network Assessment Guide (Gaudin et al., 1990/91); (4) the Index of Social Network Strengths (Gaudin, 1979); (5) the Pattison Psychosocial Inventory (Hurd, Pattison, & Smith, 1981); (6) the Social Network Form (Wellman, 1981; Wolf, 1983); and (7) three instruments developed by Dunst et al. (1988): the Family Support Scale, the Inventory of Social Support, and the Personal Network Matrix. Each of these has its strengths and may be used in varied situations to enable families to identify individuals and systems in their lives that help them negotiate their often difficult life circumstances.

Once specific needs have been assessed, interventions vary from individual support by a paraprofessional or volunteer to parent groups geared to connect parents to each other within a neighborhood and community. Opportunities for helping families build the social supports they need are varied and multiple and offer hope that someone will "be there" for them, long after formal intervention has been discontinued. These services are crucial to an empowerment philosophy (DiLeonardi, 1993; U.S. DHHS, 1993; Witt et al., 1992; Zuravin & Shay, 1992).

There are advantages and disadvantages to both group and individual support intervention models. Because neglectful caregivers may lack basic verbal-social interaction skills (Gaudin, 1993a, p. 76; Gaudin et al., 1990/91), they may not easily develop positive social connections with others in a group setting. As a result, Gaudin (1993b) suggests that because neglectful caregivers may be ill at ease in groups, extra efforts must be made to engage these parents by providing child care, transportation, refreshments, and social activities; structuring group meetings; and limiting group size to 8 to 12 members. With these ingredients, caregivers are more likely to attend and to develop relationships with others in the group.

Intervention strategies that include lay services, such as parent aide counseling, have been shown to be more effective than traditional services in reducing the propensity for future maltreatment by neglectful parents (Cohn, 1979). Intensive contact with a volunteer, lay therapist, or parent aide helps expand and enrich impoverished networks and provides new information, positive norms, and helpful suggestions about child care. One of the advantages of this intervention is that services can be individualized, which is less likely in group interventions. However, when these services are delivered by paraprofessionals or volunteers, training, clear definitions of roles and tasks, and close supervision are critical (Videka-Sherman, 1988).

Developmental Remediation

Families with neglect problems have often experienced all types of loss in their lives. The developmental perspective provides a frame of reference for understanding the growth and functioning of human beings in the context of their families and their families' transactions with their environments (Pecora, Whittaker, & Maluccio, 1992). This perspective views human behavior and social functioning within an environmental context. It goes beyond ecology by including the stages and tasks of the family's life cycle, the biopsychosocial principles of individual growth and development, and goals and needs that are common to all human beings and families. In addition, a developmental perspective considers the particular aspirations, needs, and qualities of each person and each family in light of diversity in such areas as culture, ethnicity, race, class, and sexual orientation.

Intervention with families who have experienced difficulty meeting the basic needs of their children should be guided by an optimistic view of the capacity of children and adults to overcome early deprivation through nurturing experiences throughout the life cycle. This optimistic view should guide intervention but be balanced by a realistic appraisal of the capacity of caregivers to eventually meet the needs of their children.

Although few programs that offer therapeutic services geared to developmental issues have been evaluated, there are some promising approaches for helping children and their caregivers overcome serious caregiving deficits that may have evolved over generations. For children, preschool programs, such as Head Start, have demonstrated value in enhancing self-esteem and skills in disadvantaged children (Daro, 1988; Howing et al., 1989). Programs with therapeutic activities to provide cognitive stimulation, cultural enrichment, and development of motor skills and social skills were found to significantly improve children's functioning and the prevention of repeated maltreatment (Daro, 1988). Many therapeutic day care programs recognize that their interventions need to include the family. They may provide both child-oriented services, such as health, developmental, and psychological services, and involve caregivers in parent education and support groups (Miller & Whittaker, 1988).

Cognitive-Behavioral Interventions

Numerous studies support the effectiveness of using behavioral techniques in individual therapy with caregivers who have neglect or physical-abuse problems (Crimmins, Bradlyn, St. Lawrence, & Kelly, 1984; Crozier & Katz, 1979; Eyberg & Matarazzo, 1980; Reavley & Gilbert, 1979; Szykula & Fleischman, 1985; Wolfe et al., 1982; Wolfe, Sandler, & Kaufman, 1981). Specific techniques are selected after individual assessment and may include the following:

- Verbal instruction (e.g., about basic child care), often in combination with other techniques
- Social skills training, such as modeling, role-play, and behavior rehearsal (e.g., for preparation in handling specific child care tasks)
- Stress management, such as relaxation techniques and stress inoculation training, which involves relaxation training, cognitive coping skills, and behavioral rehearsal skills when caregivers are depressed or experience other negative effects of life stressors
- Cognitive restructuring, a process to assist clients to gain awareness of dysfunctional and self-defeating thoughts and misconceptions that impair functioning and to replace them with beliefs and behaviors that lead to enhanced functioning used when caregivers are feeling overwhelmed and powerless

These techniques are especially useful with neglectful families if they target both the environment and the individual. Project 12-Ways is one such program that uses an ecobehavioral approach (Lutzker, 1990; Lutzker & Rice, 1984, 1987) and reports success in reducing safety hazards in the home (Tertinger, Greene, & Lutzker, 1984). Using a home accident prevention inventory, practitioners formally assess the injury hazards that may be present in homes and then use several behavioral-educational treatment strategies to help families make their homes safer for children. Other improvements with such intervention strategies have been noted in the areas of nutrition, home cleanliness and personal hygiene, affective skills, and identification and reporting of children's illnesses (Lutzker, 1990). Azar (1986) agrees that a cognitive-behavioral and developmental framework can focus not only on person-based deficits, such as parent-child interaction, impulse control, or parental cognitive dysfunctions, but also on environmentally based problems, such as stress level of a family and the social support network.

Other cognitive-behavioral interventions are geared to enable caregivers to modify negative, dysfunctional self-images incorporated as a result of early experiences of neglect and abuse. Project STEEP is an example of an intensive, individual, in-home counseling and group intervention program that seeks to change negative self-perceptions and break the intergenerational cycle of maltreatment (Egeland & Erickson, 1990). The effectiveness of this approach, however, has yet to be conclusively established.

Last, there are promising examples of group interventions (Daro, 1988; Gaudin et al., 1990/91) that provide information on basic child care and skills, problem solving, home management, and social interaction skills. An example of a program that is designed to be offered in groups or in the home is the Nurturing Program (Bavolek, 1988). Implemented extensively throughout the United States and in parts of Europe and South America, the Nurturing Program evaluations show significant increases in knowledge of appropriate parenting skills and techniques; increased empathic awareness of children's needs; and decreased use of corporal punishment, inappropriate expectations, and parent-child role reversals (Bavolek, Comstock, & McLaughlin, 1983).

Interventions Focused on the Individual

Neglect often results due to multiple factors. Individually oriented intervention is sometimes needed to address problems that interfere with caregiving (e.g., mental health or drug problems) as well as child-specific interventions to help children overcome the consequences of neglect.

The needs of some children are neglected because their caregivers suffer from emotional and mental health problems. For example, Gaines, Sandgrund, Green, and Power (1978) found that mothers with neglect problems were functioning more poorly than abusive mothers relative to coping with stress and meeting their children's emotional needs. Similarly, in a study of low-income mothers in Baltimore, Zuravin (1988) found that as depression of mothers increased from mild to moderate to severe, the probability of neglect increased. Such findings suggest that following a comprehensive assessment of the family's needs and strengths, some caregivers require a mix of individual therapy and supports to help them overcome depression and other mental health problems that impair their ability to adequately care for their children.

Many professionals have also called attention to the fact that children from families with alcohol or other drug problems are overwhelming the service delivery capacities of the child protective services system (Besharov, 1994; Curtis & McCullough, 1993; Dore, Doris, & Wright, 1995). It is crucial that the comprehensive assessment evaluate the possibility of substance abuse (Olson, Allen, & Azzi-Lessing, 1996) and facilitate a treatment approach to help caregivers recover from their addiction and improve their abilities to provide care for their children. Olson et al. (1996) suggest that the risk of child maltreatment problems among families whose caregivers have a substance abuse problem is affected by eight dimensions: (1) commitment to recovery, (2) patterns of use, (3) effect on child caring, (4) effect on lifestyle, (5) supports for recovery, (6) parent's self-efficacy, (7) parent's self-care, and (8) quality of neighborhood.

Following the assessment, effective service to substance-abusing families requires the expertise of health care providers, substance abuse counselors, and child welfare workers. Collaboration among these service providers enhances interventions by increasing the family's access to services in the community. Major barriers to collaboration, such as interagency biases, differing philosophies, and control issues, may be overcome by joint planning and joint ownership of the service delivery program (Azzi-Lessing & Olsen, 1996; Denton, 1992; Kropenske & Howard, 1994).

Neglected children may require individual attention to help them overcome serious deficits in cognitive, academic, and social skills. For school-age children and adolescents, Gaudin (1993a) suggests that the following interventions may help: (1) special education programs to remedy deficits in cognitive stimulation and motivation to learn, (2) school- or community-based tutorial programs using professional teachers or volunteers to provide academic help and encourage relationships with nurturing adults, and (3) personal-skills-development classes for older children and adolescents to develop life skills appropriate to their ages and developmental levels.

Family-Focused, Home-Based Interventions

After a review of 19 demonstration programs, Daro (1988) concluded that interventions that included family members, rather than focusing on the primary caregiver, were more successful. Her findings further suggested that traditional, in-office, one-to-one counseling by professionals was ineffective with neglect. Polansky et al. (1981) drew similar conclusions and suggested that intervention is necessary with families to disturb the dysfunctional family balance to achieve a more functional family system that does not sacrifice the needs of the children. Gaudin (1993a) suggested that family interventions may "seek to reallocate family role tasks, establish clear intergenerational boundaries, clarify communication among family members, reframe parents' dysfunctional perceptions of themselves and their children, and enable parents to assume a strong leadership role in the family" (pp. 36–37).

Often, family-focused interventions are combined with the provision of concrete services, including the range of emergency and concrete resources previously discussed. Thus, a major part of family-focused intervention includes helping the family obtain concrete services, such as transportation, recreational opportunities, employment, financial assistance, housework assistance, child care, food assistance, medical care, toys and educational resources, utility assistance, and clothing assistance (Pecora et al., 1992). Family interventions are geared to empower the family to improve the safety of their environment and access resources needed to provide adequate child care. Homemaker services are an important support because primary caregivers may lack knowledge about basic household skills and homemakers can be effective role models. It is important that families learn more effective ways to manage their limited resources to avoid crises such as evictions, loss of food, and shortages of other resources to meet the basic needs of children.

CONCLUSIONS

Although strong empirical support for specific interventions is lacking, our combined practice wisdom does suggest some valuable principles for helping families provide adequate care for their children. These principles are rooted in an ecological developmental framework that targets intervention at the individual, family, and community system levels. Interventions must reach out to families in their communities and neighborhoods and include an individualized family assessment. Child neglect results from a complex interplay of both risk and protective factors; intervention should be tailored to meet the unique needs and strengths of each family. Integral ingredients in all interventions, however, are the development of a helping alliance and partnership with the family and empowering families to develop and use their strengths. Furthermore, practitioners must accept and respect differences and adapt service models to meet the needs of each family, its culture, situation, and perceived needs.

Following a comprehensive family assessment, promising interventions are directed to developing or providing concrete resources, social support, developmental remediation, cognitive or behavioral interventions, individually oriented interventions, and family-focused interventions. Services are geared to empower families to access the resources needed to manage the multiple stresses and strains in their lives so that they may provide children with adequate care and guidance. It is also essential that services are available to help children overcome developmental deficits that may have resulted from chronic inattention to their needs.

Because progress with families may be slow, programs should be designed flexibly, routinely (at least every 3 months) assess progress, and adjust treatment plans when necessary. In addition, there is evidence that addressing neglect takes more time compared with other types of child maltreatment (Cohn & Daro, 1987; Miller & Whittaker, 1988), particularly in cases involving chronic neglect and substance abuse (Nelson et al., 1993; Nelson, Landsman, Tyler, & Richards, 1996).

It must further be recognized that even under the best of circumstances, individual family-oriented intervention can only be expected to partially address the widespread problem of child neglect. There is an urgent need for policies to be targeted at social conditions that increase the risk of neglect. For example, we are currently at a crossroads as states implement welfare reform. These changes could lead to either improvement or deterioration in the economic circumstances of poor families and children, contributing to changes in the demand for child welfare services (Courtney, 1997). Because neglect is so directly linked to economic conditions and the availability of resources, states are challenged to implement plans that truly will lift families out of poverty and shift child care for children from daily supervision by ineffective parents to government-subsidized child care settings. On the other hand, families could also see a significant deterioration in their economic well-being as parents are forced to take low-paying jobs and settle for substandard child care. We are challenged to make the best of this hastily crafted reform to avoid increased societal neglect of our children.

Last, with respect to the family-level interventions that we do provide, it is imperative that we further efforts to evaluate outcomes toward learning what specific interventions are most effective in working with whom. In particular, our knowledge base is not refined to the level that we know what form(s) of intervention are best to meet the needs of families who are unmotivated to access needed services or specifically for what length of time services are needed. Although our models and evaluations are becoming more sophisticated, there is also a clear need to design programs that examine the cost-effectiveness of programs so that we have a better understanding of what types of interventions are best for addressing specific needs. At a minimum, our studies need to clearly describe the population that is being served (situational neglect, chronic neglect, specific subtypes of neglect), including differences between treatment and comparison groups, the intervention model (including specifically what types of services are provided to whom), the length and intensity of interventions, the treatment outcomes being targeted, and the standardized measures that are used for evaluating outcomes.

References

Abney, V. D. (1996). Cultural competency in the field of child maltreatment. In J. Briere, L. Berliner, J. A. Bulkely, C. Jenny, & T. Reid (Eds.), The APSAC handbook on child maltreatment (pp. 409–419). Thousand Oaks, CA: Sage.

Albers, E. C., Reilly, T., & Rittner, B. (1993). Children in foster care: Possible factors affecting permanency planning. Child and Adolescent Social Work Journal, 10, 329–333.

American Professional Society on the Abuse of Children. (1995). Psychosocial evaluation of suspected psychological maltreatment in children and adolescents. Chicago: Author.

Anderson, C. M., & Stewart, S. (1983). Mastering resistance: A practical guide to family therapy. New York: Guilford.

Azar, S. T. (1986). A framework for understanding child maltreatment: An integration of cognitive behavioural and developmental perspectives. Canadian Journal of Behavioural Science, 18, 340–355.

Azzi-Lessing, L., & Olsen, L. J. (1996). Substance abuse–affected families in the child welfare system: New challenges, new alliances. Social Work, 41, 15–23.

Bavolek, S. J. (1988). The nurturing programs for parents and children. Park City, UT: Family Development Resources.

Bavolek, S. J., Comstock, C. M., & McLaughlin, J. A. (1983). The nurturing programs: A validated approach for reducing dysfunc-

tional family interaction (Final report, Program No. 1R01MA 34862). Rockville, MD: National Institutes of Health.

Bean, N. M. (1994). Stranger in our home: Rural families talk about the experience of having received in-home family services. Unpublished doctoral dissertation, Case Western Reserve University, Mandel School of Applied Social Sciences, Cleveland, OH.

Belsky, J. (1980). Child maltreatment: An ecological integration. American Psychologist, 35, 320–335.

Besharov, D. J. (1994). When drug addicts have children. Washington, DC: Child Welfare League of America.

Billingsley, A., & Giovannoni, J. M. (1972). Children of the storm. New York: Harcourt, Brace & Jovanovich.

Bloom, M., Fischer, J., & Orme, J. (1995). Evaluating practice: Guidelines for the accountable professional (2nd ed.). Boston: Allyn & Bacon.

Bowlby, J. (1988). A secure base: Clinical applications of attachment theory. London: Tavistock/Routledge.

Brissett-Chapman, S. (1997). Child protection risk assessment and African American children: Cultural ramifications for families and communities. Child Welfare, 76, 45–63.

Carter, B., & McGoldrick, M. (Eds.). (1988). The changing life cycle—A framework for family therapy (2nd ed.). New York: Gardner.

Children's Defense Fund. (1990). A report card briefing book and action primer. Washington, DC: Author.

Close, M. (1983). Child welfare and people of color: Denial of equal access. Social Work Research and Abstracts, 19(4), 576–577.

Cohn, A. H. (1979). Effective treatment of child abuse and neglect. Social Work, 24, 513–519.

Cohn, A. H., & Daro, D. (1987). Is treatment too late: What ten years of evaluative research tell us. Child Abuse and Neglect, 11, 433–442.

Courtney, M. E. (1997). Welfare reform and child welfare services. In S. B. Kamerman & S. J. Kahn (Eds.), Child welfare in the context of welfare "reform." New York: Columbia University School of Social Work.

Cowger, C. D. (1994). Assessing client strengths: Clinical assessment for client empowerment. Social Work, 39, 262–268.

Crimmins, D. B., Bradlyn, A. S., St. Lawrence, J. S., & Kelly, J. A. (1984). A training technique for improving the parent-child interaction skills of an abusive neglectful mother. Child Abuse and Neglect, 8, 533–539.

Crittenden, P. M. (1991). Treatment of child abuse and neglect. Human Systems: The Journal of Systemic Consultation & Management, 2, 161–179.

Crittenden, P. M. (1999). Child neglect: Causes and contributors. In H. Dubowitz (Ed.), Neglected children: Research, practice, and policy (pp. 47–68). Thousand Oaks, CA: Sage.

Crozier, J., & Katz, R. C. (1979). Social learning treatment of child abuse. Journal of Behavior Therapy and Psychiatry, 10, 213–220.

Curtis, P. A., & McCullough, C. (1993). The impact of alcohol and other drugs on the child welfare system. Child Welfare, 62, 533–542.

Danzy, J., & Jackson, S. M. (1997). Family preservation and support services: A missed opportunity for kinship care. Child Welfare, 76, 31–44.

Daro, D. (1988). Confronting child abuse. New York: Free Press.

Denton, I. (1992). Challenges of collaborating to serve substance-abusing mothers and their children. Paper presented at the conference Working Together: Linkages for Preserving Families Affected by Alcohol and Other Drugs, Richmond, VA.

DePanfilis, D. (1996). Social isolation of neglectful families: A review of social support assessment and intervention models. Child Maltreatment, 1, 37–52.

DePanfilis, D., & Wilson, C. (1996). Applying the strengths perspective with maltreating families. *The APSAC Advisor, 9*(3), 15–20.

DiLeonardi, J. W (1993). Families in poverty and chronic neglect of children. *Families in Society, 74*, 557–562.

Dore, M. M., & Alexander, L. B. (1996). Preserving families at risk of child abuse and neglect: The role of the helping alliance. *Child Abuse and Neglect, 20*, 349–361.

Dore, M. M., Doris, J. M., & Wright, P. (1995). Identifying substance abuse in maltreating families: A child welfare challenge. *Child Abuse and Neglect, 19*, 531–543.

Dubowitz, H., Black, M., Starr, R. H., & Zuravin, S. J. (1993). A conceptual definition of child neglect. *Criminal Justice and Behavior, 20*, 8–26.

Dunst, C., Trivette, C., & Deal, A. (1988). *Enabling and empowering families*. Cambridge, MA: Brookline.

Egeland, F., & Erickson, M. F. (1990). Rising above the past: Strategies for helping new mothers break the cycle of abuse and neglect. *Zero to Three, 10*, 29–35.

Eyberg, S. M., & Matarazzo, R. G. (1980). Training parents as therapists: A comparison between individual parent-child interaction training and parent group didactic training. *Journal of Clinical Psychology, 36*, 492–499.

Fein, E. (1991). The elusive search for certainty in child welfare: Introduction. *American Journal of Orthopsychiatry, 61*(4), 576–577.

Fischer, J., & Corcoran, K. (1994a). *Measures for clinical practice: Vol. 1. Couples, families and children* (2nd ed.). New York: Free Press.

Fischer, J., & Corcoran, K. (1994b). *Measures for clinical practice: Vol. 2. Adults* (2nd ed.). New York: Free Press.

Fraser, M. W., & Galinsky, M. J. (1997). Toward a resilience-based model of practice. In M. W. Fraser (Ed.), *Risk and resilience in childhood: An ecological perspective*. Washington, DC: NASW Press.

Gaines, R., Sandgrund, A., Green, A., & Power, E. (1978). Etiological factors in child maltreatment: A multivariate study of abusing, neglecting, and normal mothers. *Journal of Abnormal Psychology, 87*, 531–540.

Gaudin, J. M., Jr. (1979). *Mothers' perceived strength of primary group networks and maternal child abuse*. Unpublished doctoral dissertation, Florida State University, Tallahassee.

Gaudin, J. M., Jr. (1988). Treatment of families who neglect their children. In E. M. Nunnally, C. S. Chilman, & F. M. Cox (Eds.), *Mental illness, delinquency, addictions, and neglect* (pp. 167–249). Newbury Park, CA: Sage.

Gaudin, J. M., Jr. (1993a). *Child neglect: A guide for intervention*. Washington, DC: National Center on Child Abuse and Neglect.

Gaudin, J. M., Jr. (1993b). Effective intervention with neglectful families. *Criminal Justice and Behavior, 20*, 66–89.

Gaudin, J. M., Jr. (1999). Child neglect: Short-term and long-term outcomes. In H. Dubowitz (Ed.), *Neglected children: Research, practice, and policy* (pp. 89–108). Thousand Oaks, CA: Sage.

Gaudin, J. M., Jr., & Polansky, N. A. (1986). Social distances and the neglectful family: Sex, race, and social class influences. *Children and Youth Services Review, 8*, 1–12.

Gaudin, J. M., Jr., Polansky, N. A., Kilpatrick, A. C., & Shilton, P. (1993). Loneliness, depression, stress, and social supports in neglectful families. *American Journal of Orthopsychiatry, 63*, 597–605.

Gaudin, J. M., Jr., Wodarski, J. S., Arkinson, M. K., & Avery, L. S. (1990/91). Remedying child neglect: Effectiveness of social network interventions. *The Journal of Applied Social Sciences, 15*, 97–123.

Gelles, R. J. (1999). Policy issues in child neglect. In H. Dubowitz (Ed.), *Neglected children: Research, practice, and policy* (pp. 278–298). Thousand Oaks, CA: Sage.

Gottlieb, B. (1985). Theory into practice: Issues that surface in planning interventions that mobilize support. In I. G. Sarason & B. R. Sarason (Eds.), *Social support: Theory, research, and applications* (pp. 417–437). Dordrecht, Holland: Martinus Nijhof.

Gould, K. H. (1991). Limiting damage is not enough: A minority perspective on child welfare issues. In J. E. Everett, S. S. Chipungu, & B. R. Leashore (Eds.), *Child welfare: An Africentric perspective* (pp. 58–78). New Brunswick, NJ: Rutgers University Press.

Gutierrez, L. M. (1990). Working with women of color: An empowerment perspective. *Social Work, 35*, 149–154.

Gutierrez, L., Glen Maye, L., & DeLois, K. (1995). The organizational context of empowerment practice: Implications for social work administration. *Social Work, 40*, 249–258.

Hartman, A. (1978). Diagrammatic assessments of family relationships. *Social Casework, 59*, 465–476.

Hill, R. B. (1971). *The strengths of black families*. New York: National Urban League.

Hobbs, N., Dokecki, P. R., Hoover-Dempsey, K. V., Moroney, R. M., Shayne, M. W., & Weeks, K. H. (1984). *Strengthening families*. San Francisco: Jossey-Bass.

Howing, P., Wodarski, J., Gaudin, J., & Kurtz, P. D. (1989). Effective interventions to ameliorate the incidence of child maltreatment: The empirical base. *Social Work, 34*, 330–338.

Hudson, W. (1982). *The clinical measurement package: A field manual*. Homewood, IL: Dorsey.

Hurd, G., Pattison, E. M., & Smith, J. E. (1981, February). *Test-re-test reliability of social network self reports: The Pattison Psychosocial Inventory (PPI)*. Paper presented to Sun Belt Social Networks Conference, Tampa, FL.

Karls, J. M., & Wandrei, K. E. (Eds.). (1994). *Pie manual: Person-in-environment system*. Washington, DC: National Association of Social Workers.

Kelley, S. J. (1996). *Neglected children in intergenerational kinship care* (Neglect demonstration project proposal submitted by Georgia State University to the National Center on Child Abuse and Neglect). Available from Dr. Susan Kelley, Georgia State University, Office of Research, College of Health Sciences, University Plaza, Atlanta, GA 30303.

Kenemore, T. K. (1993). The helping relationship: Getting in touch with the client's experience. In *National Center on Child Abuse and Neglect Chronic Neglect Symposium Proceedings, June 1993* (pp. 51–53). Chicago: National Center on Child Abuse and Neglect.

Kropenske, V., & Howard, J. (1994). *Protecting children in substance-abusing families*. Washington, DC: National Center on Child Abuse and Neglect.

Landsman, M. J., Nelson, K., Allen, M., & Tyler, M. (1992). *The self-sufficiency project: Final report*. Iowa City, IA: National Resource Center in Family Based Services.

Leashore, B. R., Chipungu, S. S., & Everett, J. E. (1991). *Child welfare: An Africentric perspective*. New Brunswick, NJ: Rutgers University Press.

Lee, J. A. B. (1994). *The empowerment approach to social work practice*. New York: Columbia University Press.

Lewis, H. (1969). Parental and community neglect: Twin responsibilities of protective services. *Children, 16*, 114–118.

Lewis, J. M., & Looney, J. G. (1983). *The long struggle: Well-functioning working class black families*. New York: Brunner-Mazel.

Lloyd, J. C., & Sallee, A. L. (1994). The challenge and potential of family preservation services in the public child welfare system. *Protecting Children, 10*(3), 3–6.

Lutzker, J. R. (1990). Behavioral treatment of child neglect. *Behavior Modification, 14*, 301–315.

Lutzker, J. R., & Rice, J. M. (1984). Project 12-Ways: Measuring outcome of a large in-home service for treatment and prevention of child abuse and neglect. *Child Abuse and Neglect, 8*, 519–524.

Lutzker, J. R., & Rice, J. M. (1987). Using recidivism data to evaluate Project 12-Ways: An ecobehavioral approach to the treatment and prevention of child abuse and neglect. *Journal of Family Violence, 2*, 283–290.

Magura, S., & Moses, B. S. (1986). *Outcome measures for child welfare services.* Washington, DC: Child Welfare League of America.

Magura, S., Moses, B. S., & Jones, M. A. (1987). *Assessing risk and measuring change in families: The family risk scales.* Washington, DC: Child Welfare League of America.

McCubbin, H., Thompson, A., & McCubbin, M. (1996). *Family assessment: Resiliency, coping and adaptation, inventories for research and practice.* Madison: University of Wisconsin Systems.

McCurdy, K., Hurvis, S., & Clark, J. (1996). Engaging and retaining families in child abuse prevention programs. *The APSAC Advisor, 9*(3), 1, 3–9.

McPhatter, A. R. (1997). Cultural competence in child welfare: What is it? How do we achieve it? What happens without it? *Child Welfare, 76*, 255–278.

Mech, E. V. (1985). Public social services to minority children and their families. In R. O. Washington & J. Boros-Hull (Eds.), *Children in need of roots* (pp. 133–186). Davis, CA: International Dialogue Press.

Miller, J. L., & Whittaker, J. K. (1988). Social services and social support: Blended programs for families at risk of child maltreatment. *Child Welfare, 67*, 161–174.

Mugridge, G. B. (1991, September). *Reducing chronic neglect.* Paper presented at the Ninth National Conference on Child Abuse and Neglect, Denver, CO.

National Black Child Development Institute. (1990). *The status of African-American children.* Washington, DC: Author.

National Research Council. (1993). *Understanding child abuse and neglect.* Washington, DC: National Academy Press.

Nelson, K., Landsman, M., Tyler, M., & Richardson, B. (1996, fall). Examining the length of service and cost-effectiveness of intensive family service. *The Prevention Report, 2*, 13–17.

Nelson, K. E., Saunders, E. J., & Landsman, M. J. (1993). Chronic neglect in perspective. *Social Work, 38*, 661–671.

Olson, L. J., Allen, D., & Azzi-Lessing, L. (1996). Assessing risk in families affected by substance abuse. *Child Abuse and Neglect, 20*, 833–842.

Pecora, P., Whittaker, J., & Maluccio, A. (1992). *The child welfare challenge: Policy, practice, and research.* New York: Aldine.

Pianta, R., Egeland, B., & Erickson, M. F. (1989). The antecedents of maltreatment: Results of the mother-child interaction research project. In D. Cicchetti & V. Carlson (Eds.), *Child maltreatment: Theory and research on the causes of child abuse and neglect* (pp. 203–253). New York: Cambridge University Press.

Polansky, N. A., Chalmers, M. A., Williams, D. P., & Buttenwieser, E. W. (1981). *Damaged parents: An anatomy of child neglect.* Chicago: University of Chicago Press.

Rauch, J. B., North, C., Rowe, C., & Risley-Curtiss, C. (1993). *Diversity competence: A learning guide.* Baltimore: University of Maryland at Baltimore, School of Social Work.

Reavley, W., & Gilbert, M. T. (1979). The analysis and treatment of child abuse by behavioral psychotherapy. *Child Abuse and Neglect, 3*, 509–514.

Saleebey, D. (1996). The strengths perspective in social work practice: Extensions and cautions. *Social Work, 41*, 296–305.

Saleebey, D. (Ed.). (1997). *The strengths perspective in social work practice* (2nd ed.). New York: Longman.

Simon, B. L. (1994). *The empowerment tradition in American social work: A history.* New York: Columbia University Press.

Siu, S. F., & Hogan, P. T. (1989). Public child welfare: The need for clinical social work. *Social Work, 34*, 423–428.

Smale, G. G. (1995). Integrating community and individual practice: A new paradigm for practice. In P. Adams & K. Nelson (Eds.), *Reinventing human services community- and family-centered practice* (pp. 59–80). New York: Aldine de Gruyter.

Smokowski, P. R., & Wodarski, J. S. (1996). The effectiveness of child welfare services for poor, neglected children: A review of the empirical evidence. *Research on Social Work Practice, 6*, 504–523.

Solomon, B. B. (1976). *Black empowerment: Social work in oppressed communities.* New York: Columbia University Press.

Stehno, S. M. (1982). Differential treatment of minority children in service systems. *Social Work, 27*, 39–45.

Sue, D. W., Arrendondo, P., & McDavis, R. J. (1992). Multicultural counseling competencies and standards: A call to the profession. *Journal of Multicultural Counseling, 20*, 64–88.

Szykula, S. A., & Fleischman, M. J. (1985). Reducing out-of-home placements of abused children: Two controlled field studies. *Child Abuse and Neglect, 9*, 277–283.

Tertinger, D., Greene, B., & Lutzker, J. (1984). Home safety: Development and validation of one component of an ecobehavioral treatment program for abused and neglected children. *Journal of Applied Behavior Analysis, 17*, 159–174.

Thomlison, B. (1997). Risk and protective factors in child maltreatment. In M. W. Fraser (Ed.), *Risk and resilience in childhood: An ecological perspective.* Washington, DC: NASW Press.

Tracy, E. M. (1990). Identifying social support resources of at-risk families. *Social Work, 38*, 252–258.

Tracy, E. M., & Whittaker, J. K. (1990). The social network map: Assessing social support in clinical practice. *Families in Society, 7*, 461–470.

Trivette, C. M., Dunst, C. J., Deal, A. G., Hamer, A. W., & Prompst, S. (1990). Assessing family strengths and family functioning style. *Topics in Early Childhood Special Education, 10*(1), 16–35.

U.S. Department of Health and Human Services, National Center on Child Abuse and Neglect. (1988). *Study findings: Study of national incidence and prevalence of child abuse and neglect: 1988.* Washington, DC: Government Printing Office.

U.S. Department of Health and Human Services, National Center on Child Abuse and Neglect. (1993). *Chronic neglect symposium proceedings.* Washington, DC: Author.

U.S. Department of Health and Human Services, National Center on Child Abuse and Neglect. (1996). *Child maltreatment, 1994: Reports from the states to the National Center on Child Abuse and Neglect.* Washington, DC: Government Printing Office.

Videka-Sherman, L. (1988). Intervention for child neglect: The empirical knowledge base. In *Child neglect monograph: Proceedings from a symposium* (pp. 46–63). Washington, DC: National Center on Child Abuse and Neglect.

Walmyr Publishing Co. (1990). *MPSI technical manual.* Tempe, AZ: Author.

Walmyr Publishing Co. (1992). *Walmyr assessment scales scoring manual.* Tempe, AZ: Author.

Wellman, B. (1981). Applying network analysis to the study of support. In B. H. Gottlieb (Ed.), *Social networks and social support* (pp. 171–200). Beverly Hills, CA: Sage.

Whittaker, J., & Garbarino, J. (1983). *Social support networks: Informal helping in the human services.* New York: Aldine.

Witt, C., Dayton, C., & Sheinvald, J. K. (1992). *The family empowerment program: A social group work model of long term, intensive, and innovative strategies to reduce the incidence of chronic neglect for at risk parents* (National Center on Child Abuse and Neglect, Grant # 90CA1392). Pontiac, MI: Oakland Family Services.

Wolf, B. M. (1983). *Social network form: Information and scoring instructions.* Unpublished monograph, Temple University, Philadelphia, PA.

Wolfe, D. A. (1993). Prevention of child neglect: Emerging issues. *Criminal Justice and Behavior, 20,* 90–111.

Wolfe, D. A., Sandler, J., & Kaufman, K. (1981). A competency-based parent training program for child abusers. *Journal of Consulting and Clinical Psychology, 49,* 633–640.

Wolfe, D. A., St. Lawrence, J., Graves, K., Brehony, K., Bradlyn, D., & Kelly, J. A. (1982). Intensive behavioral parent training for a child abusive mother. *Behavior Therapy, 13,* 438–451.

Zuravin, S. J. (1988). Child abuse, child neglect, and maternal depression: Is there a connection? In *Child neglect monograph: Proceedings from a symposium* (pp. 40–45). Washington, DC: National Center on Child Abuse and Neglect.

Zuravin, S. J., & DePanfilis, D. (1996). *Child maltreatment recurrences among families served by Child Protective Services: Final report* (National Center on Child Abuse and Neglect Grant # 90CA1497). Baltimore: University of Maryland at Baltimore, School of Social Work.

Zuravin, S., & Shay, S. (1992). Preventing child neglect. In D. DePanfilis & T. Birch (Eds.), *Proceedings: National Child Maltreatment Prevention Symposium, June 1991.* Washington, DC: National Center on Child Abuse and Neglect.

HANS B. KERSTEN, M.D.
DAVID S. BENNETT, PH.D.

21

Failure to Thrive and Maltreatment

GENERAL CONSIDERATIONS

Failure to thrive (FTT) refers to faltering weight, typically in early childhood. It is a common problem seen by pediatricians today and has been a concern for physicians for more than a hundred years. FTT occurs when there is a deceleration in growth velocity, and it is an important physical sign (Zenel, 1997) or manifestation of childhood disease (Shaheen et al., 1968) that may be caused by almost any type of chronic disease (English, 1978). The approach to diagnosis of FTT is known to most physicians and can become expensive and frustrating.

One of the first cases in the literature was in the first edition of *The Diseases of Infancy and Childhood* by L. Emmett Holt, published in 1897. Holt described a child who "ceased to thrive" and recognized that FTT could occur in a variety of clinical scenarios (Schwartz, 2000; Stanga et al., 2008). Chaplan later described how FTT in orphans could be caused by the "institution" in which they lived. These children had poor diets, atrophy, and a "downward trend" to death if they returned from the hospital to the same environment (orphanage) from which they came. Widdowson (1951) described the deleterious effects of psychosocial deprivation on the growth of orphans in occupied Germany in the late 1940s. Others believed that children with FTT were emotionally deprived by their caregivers, leading to growth retardation. The term *maternal deprivation syndrome* was used, because mothers were usually the primary caretaker (Patton, 1963; Skuse, 1985). Such early observations led to the understanding that FTT was closely associated with neglect or maltreatment. This perspective, however, was challenged by research demonstrating that maternally deprived infants were underweight because of "undereating" resulting from being offered too little food or not accepting it, not because of the psychological effects of mater-

nal deprivation (Whitten, Pettit, & Fischhoff, 1969). This and subsequent research led to our current understanding of the multifactorial nature of FTT, with some suggesting that the emphasis on parental culpability in FTT in the absence of direct evidence of neglect is wrong (Skuse, 1985) and that FTT is "distinct" from neglect (Black et al., 2006).

As described in this chapter, it is now recognized that medical, dietary, psychosocial, and behavioral factors all need to be considered when assessing children for FTT. Consistent with FTT's diverse etiologies, a multidisciplinary approach to treatment is necessary to address ways to enhance caloric intake in each of these domains. The chapter presents some specific recommendations for the assessment and treatment of FTT.

EPIDEMIOLOGY

Despite the lack of current data on the prevalence of FTT, older published data are available from a variety of clinical settings. Historically, children with FTT were often admitted for an extensive workup to determine the etiology. In a retrospective review of charts, FTT accounted for 1%–5% of admissions to tertiary care hospitals (Berwick, Levy, & Kleinerman, 1982; English, 1978; Shaheen et al., 1968). A more recent review found that anywhere between 2% and 24% of patients admitted to the hospital have symptoms of FTT (Joosten & Hulst, 2008). There are limited epidemiological data from outpatient settings, but the incidence of FTT in primary care clinics was found to be as much as 10% of outpatient visits (Frank & Zeisel, 1998; Mitchell, Gorrell, & Greenberg, 1980; Zenel, 1997). In addition, as many as 30% of visits to some emergency departments are for children with FTT (Frank & Zeisel, 1998; Zenel, 1997). Some studies suggest that one-third to one-half of cases of FTT may go unrecognized (Batchelor, 1996; C. M. Wright,

2000). So, it is conceivable that these numbers could be even higher.

An understanding of the definition of FTT, the factors that place particular infants and maternal-infant dyads at risk, and the pathophysiology of FTT is fundamental to the approach to treatment of this condition.

DEFINITION

The use of growth charts to plot children's growth over time is critically important for physicians and provides an essential indicator of children's overall health and wellness. They have been used in this way for at least a century (T. Cole, 2003; Grummer-Strawn, Reinold, & Krebs, 2010); they provide valuable information to health care providers about children who may be undernourished and are considered the gold standard in pediatrics (Phillips & Shulman, 2013). The growth parameters provide an objective measure of a child's growth and show how far from the statistical norm these measures are (Jaffe, 2011). Although there are no universally recognized criteria for FTT, specific criteria for children less than 2 years old can be identified by plotting children's weight on a standardized growth chart (Bithoney, Dubowitz, & Egan, 1992; Jaffe, 2011; Kirkland & Motil, 2011; Zenel, 1997). Weight and length may both be affected, but weight is more affected than length (Gahagan & Holmes, 1998).

The criteria are as follows: weight is below the 3rd or 5th percentile for age on more than one occasion; weight falls across two major percentiles (e.g., from 50% to less than 10%) on the standardized growth chart, using the 90th, 75th, 50th, 25th, 10th, and 5th percentiles; weight is less than 80% of ideal weight for age; and weight/length is less than 5%, which suggests malnutrition (Gahagan & Holmes, 1998; Jaffe, 2011). These definitions signify that weight is the primary measure of concern, although height and head circumference may be affected if FTT persists. Use of these criteria will capture most cases of children with growth failure, but there are exceptions to these criteria when all growth parameters are affected; these exceptions include familial short stature, infants who were small for gestational age, preterm infants, normally "lean" infants, overweight infants whose height gain increases while weight gain decreases, and children with genetic syndromes (Kirkland & Motil, 2011). Although these are well-recognized criteria to help the clinician identify FTT, the definition should not be based solely on growth charts. Careful measurement and plotting of growth parameters is essential but must be combined with critical thinking or judgment for each patient to assess whether FTT is present.

The Centers for Disease Control and Prevention (CDC) growth charts provide a well-recognized standard for plotting growth parameters in the United States. The CDC charts are based on samples of children from around the United States at particular times and places (Grummer-Strawn, Reinold, & Krebs, 2010). The primary sample is from 1963–1994, from various U.S. cities. In an effort to improve the accuracy of the charts for children less than 2 months of age, the charts were updated in 2000 with data from large samples of children. As a result, these charts provide a *reference* of how children grew at a specific point in time. However, based on the premise that children's weight should be compared with that of *children with ideal growth standards*, the World Health Organization (WHO) developed growth charts to provide international standards of growth for children 0–59 months of age (Grummer-Strawn, Reinold, & Krebs, 2010).

The CDC convened an expert panel from the American Academy of Pediatrics and the National Institutes of Health to review the evidence and provide guidance for health care providers on which growth charts to use (Grummer-Strawn, Reinold, & Krebs, 2010). The panel recommended that clinicians should use the 2006 WHO growth charts for children under 24 months of age but should continue to use the CDC growth charts for children 2–19 years of age.

"ORGANIC" VERSUS "NONORGANIC"

Failure to thrive is better thought of as a sign of a disease than as an actual disease. This is highlighted by the fact that so many diseases in pediatrics can cause FTT. The differential diagnosis is enormous and beyond the scope of this chapter. Historically, these children were often admitted for extensive workups that were expensive and time-consuming. A useful way to approach these cases was to separate the etiology into "organic" versus "nonorganic" causes. Organic causes have a medical etiology, and nonorganic causes are related to the environment. This division helped physicians organize their approach to evaluation and treatment of these children. This led to the concept that children who were admitted for FTT, were given adequate nutrition and nursing care, and did not gain weight must have an organic cause of FTT. Conversely, if a child gained weight in the hospital, there must be a nonorganic cause. In the late 1960s, Glaser et al. (1968) noted that an organic cause of FTT could not be established in a majority of cases in spite of repeated and detailed clinical investigations. Essentially, the home environment was often determined to be the cause, through nutritional, emotional, or stimulatory deprivation (Zenel, 1997).

Over the next few decades, research helped us understand more about the etiology of nonorganic FTT and all the psychosocial influences on children with this condition. The role of the mother was described in cases of children with nonorganic FTT. The mother was anecdotally described as having character problems, depression, anxiety, social isolation, or low intelligence (Zenel, 1997). These characteristics ostensibly resulted in inadequate maternal-child interactions with possible emotional deprivation. The children were underweight because they were not offered adequate food by their mother or did not accept it. It was also believed that the "inherent behavior" or temperament of a child could cause poor feeding and undernutrition, if this was not understood or was missed by the parents (Chatoor et al., 1998). However, by the mid-1980s, Skuse (1985) recognized that for children with nonorganic FTT, multiple etiologies were often needed to explain all the factors at play in their FTT or undernutrition. The FTT or undernutrition was thought to be due to both inadequate provision of food and inadequate intake. As a result, the dichotomizing of FTT into organic versus nonorganic became less useful and oversimplified the etiology of this common problem. Therefore, the approach to children with FTT should include assessment of organic, behavioral, and environmental factors to adequately address the multifactorial etiology.

RISK FACTORS

Early studies of institutionalized children led to the belief that maltreatment, particularly neglect, was a primary cause of FTT. Maltreatment, however, is only one of the many causes of FTT and is present in only a small minority of cases (C. M. Wright, 2000). While FTT and maltreatment share some common risk factors, including poverty, insecure child attachment, and maternal depression (Chatoor et al., 1998; Dubowitz, Kim, et al., 2011; Dubowitz, Zuckerman, et al., 1989; O'Brien et al., 2004), other risk factors are somewhat specific to FTT. Medical risk factors include prematurity and/or intrauterine growth retardation, developmental delay, congenital anomalies (e.g., cleft lip and palate), intrauterine exposures to infections or toxins, lead poisoning, anemia, and a host of other conditions that result in inadequate caloric intake, increased metabolic rate, inadequate digestion, or malabsorption (Kirkland & Motil, 2011).

Dietary risk factors for FTT include excessive juice intake, delayed weaning from breastfeeding, and delayed introduction of solid foods (Smith & Lifshitz, 1994; C. M. Wright, 2000). Child factors include poor appetite, being a "picky" eater, oral-sensory difficulties, and behavior problems (Kerr, Black, & Krishnakumar, 2000; Ramsay, Gisel, & Boutry, 1993; C. M. Wright, 2000). Other risk factors are irregular feeding and sleep schedules, excessively brief or long meal times, and failure to use a high chair for young children (Mathiesen et al., 1989; Ramsay, Gisel, & Boutry, 1993; Stewart & Meyer, 2004). Parent-child interaction during feeding may also contribute to FTT, as parents who use less affectionate touch, more negative touch, and more arbitrary termination of feedings may increase children's risk for feeding problems and FTT (Drotar et al., 1990; Feldman et al., 2004). More broadly, psychosocial factors such as maternal depression, poverty, and food insecurity may contribute to FTT (Kersten & Bennett, 2012; O'Brien et al., 2004). Thus, there are many different factors that might cause a child to have faltering weight and that need to be assessed and considered when developing a treatment plan.

DEVELOPMENTAL EFFECTS

There have been concerns about the effects of failure to thrive on children since it was first described by Holt in 1897. Severe FTT has been shown to adversely affect the immune system and lead to vitamin deficiencies (Perrin et al., 2003). However, FTT exerts its greatest effect on the developing brain. In children from a developing country, malnourishment was shown to adversely affect future growth and cognitive development (Rudolf & Logan, 2005; Waterflow, 1974); nonorganic FTT was not as severe as in developed countries, and the resultant effects on development also appeared to be less severe, though still significant. Children previously hospitalized for nonorganic FTT were found to have lower height, weight, and verbal intelligence and poorer language development than a comparison group, when followed up more than a decade later (Oates, Peacock, & Forrest, 1985). These results prompted close follow-up and ongoing treatment for children with FTT. An extensive body of evidence has since accumulated on the effects on cognitive development in children with nonorganic FTT.

A meta-analysis by Corbett and Drewett (2004) supported the notion that FTT can have significant long-term effects on cognitive development. The effect of FTT on IQ was smaller when children were older, but the overall effect was still equivalent to losing 4.2 points in IQ. While this might represent a small difference between two individual children, it is more significant for a population, particularly if it leads to increased use of special education services. The 4.2 IQ point difference is comparable to or greater than the effects of other recognized environmental variables such as prenatal cocaine exposure and bottle feeding (Corbett & Drewett, 2004). In a systematic review that included children with weight less than the 10th percentile, Rudolf and Logan (2005) found a difference of about 3 IQ points. They concluded that FTT is not important at a population level and that the aggressive approach to treatment needed reassessing. However, this review included children with weight up to the 10th percentile who probably would not have met the criteria for FTT, which was likely to diminish the overall effect.

Other longitudinal studies of children with FTT have reported long-term measurable deficits in learning and behavioral difficulties, as well as changes in IQ (Black et al., 2007; Drotar & Sturm, 1988; Emond et al., 2007). While the effects may be fairly subtle for most children, there is individual variability in response to FTT. At present, we are largely unable to identify those particular children who are at greatest risk for the most severe developmental impairment, although the severity of faltering weight and perhaps the presence of maltreatment history may place children at greater risk (Perrin et al., 2003). Collectively, these studies support the aggressive approach to treatment of children with FTT taken by many practitioners today.

PATHOPHYSIOLOGY

While maltreatment is present in a small minority of cases of FTT (C. M. Wright, 2000), there are many other factors that may contribute to the onset of this condition. The resulting undernutrition associated with FTT was argued to be due to both inadequate provision of food and inadequate intake (Skuse, 1985). This has resulted in a "transactional model" to evaluate FTT and recognizes that economic factors, social networks, health beliefs, parental/familial health, and family psychosocial dynamics may each play a role in the etiology of FTT (Kirkland & Motil, 2011), but for an individual case, not all of these factors may come into play. Therefore, many authors have described a practical approach (see table 21.1) to determine the source of the undernutrition (Zenel, 1997). The most common cause of FTT is inadequate caloric intake due to a variety of medical, environmental, and psychosocial factors.

Table 21.1. Causes of Failure to Thrive, Physical Findings, and Diagnostic Workup Considerations

Pathological Mechanism	Associated Symptoms	Physical Examination Findings	Diagnostic Considerations
Inadequate caloric intake / appetite	*Poor food intake:* • Chronic illness • Excess juice/water intake • Factitious food allergy • Food fads • Gastroesophageal reflux (GER) • Inadequate formula preparation • Inadequate quantity of food • Inadequate parental knowledge of appropriate diet • Inappropriate feeding technique • Insufficient lactation in mother • Maternal/infant dysfunction • Mechanical problems (e.g., cleft palate, nasal obstruction, adenoidal hypertrophy, dental lesions) • Sucking or swallowing dysfunction (e.g. CNS, neuromuscular, esophageal motility problems) *Food not available:* • Child abuse/neglect • Poverty, food insecurity • Psychosocial problems	• Weight <5% • Signs of abuse or neglect • Minimal subcutaneous fat • Oral or nasal abnormalities • Protuberant abdomen • Hypotonia	• Complete dietary history and psychosocial evaluation • Complete blood count (CBC) • Basic metabolic panel • Blood lead level • Consider extensive laboratory and radiological workup in suspected child abuse
Inadequate caloric absorption / increased losses	• Malabsorption (e.g., lactose intolerance, cystic fibrosis, cardiac disease, malrotation, inflammatory bowel disease, milk allergy, parasites, celiac disease) • Biliary atresia, cirrhosis • Chronic GER • Chronic vomiting (e.g., gastroenteritis, increased intracranial pressure, adrenal insufficiency, drugs) • Chronic renal disease • Necrotizing enterocolitis, short bowel syndrome • Pancreatic insufficiency	• Weight <5% • Dysmorphism suggestive of chronic disease • Minimal subcutaneous fat • Organomegaly • Protuberant abdomen • Skin/mucosal changes	• Stool pathogens • Stool fat • Cystic fibrosis screening • CBC / erythrocyte sedimentation rate (ESR) • Basic metabolic profile • Urinalysis
Excessive caloric expenditure / ineffective utilization	• Hyperthyroidism • Malignancy • Chronic disease (e.g., cardiac, renal, endocrine, hepatic) • Chronic metabolic problems (e.g., hypercalcemia, storage diseases, inborn errors of metabolism, galactosemia, diabetes mellitus, adrenal insufficiency) • Chronic respiratory insufficiency (e.g., bronchopulmonary dysplasia, congenital heart disease) • Chronic systemic infection (e.g., urinary tract infection, tuberculosis, HIV)	• Weight <5% • Cardiac or lung findings • Dysmorphism • Lymphadenopathy • Minimal subcutaneous fat • Organomegaly • Thyroid goiter • Skin dysmorphology	• CBC • Chemistry panel, BUN, creatinine • ESR/C-reactive protein • Liver function tests • PPD • TSH • HIV

Source. Adapted from Frank & Zeisel, 1998; Kirkland & Motil, 2011; Stephens et al., 2008.

In infants less than 2 months old, feeding problems are the most common factor in FTT (S. Cole & Lanham, 2011; Emond et al., 2007); these include poor sucking and/or swallowing and breastfeeding problems. Older infants or toddlers with FTT may have a history of difficulty transitioning to solid foods, delayed weaning from breastfeeding (C. M. Wright, 2000), inadequate intake of formula or breast milk (Emond et al., 2007), or too great an intake of juices (Dennison, 1996; Smith & Lifshitz, 1994), or parents' overconcern with healthy eating (S. Cole & Lanham, 2011; Schwartz, 2000) may lead them to avoid high-calorie foods.

Children with inadequate caloric intake often have a lack of appetite, are picky eaters, and have persistent emesis, difficulty chewing or swallowing, or shortness of breath with feeding, and they may be more likely to have behavior problems that can interfere with eating (Kerr, Black, & Krishnakumar, 2000; Nutzenadel, 2011; Ramsay, Gisel, & Boutry, 1993; C. Wright, Loughridge, & Moore, 2000). Intake can also be affected by poor structural factors, as children with FTT may have irregular feeding and sleep schedules and/or excessively brief or long meal times (Mathiesen et al., 1989; Ramsay, Gisel, & Boutry, 1993) and may not use a high chair or booster seat (Mathiesen et al., 1989; Ramsay, Gisel, & Boutry, 1993; Stewart & Meyer, 2004). Parent-child interactions during feeding are also important, as parents who use less affectionate touch, more negative touch, and more arbitrary termination of feedings may increase risk for feeding problems and FTT (Drotar et al., 1990; Feldman et al., 2004). Psychosocial factors play a large role in this dynamic as well. FTT can occur in any socioeconomic group but is more common in families in poverty, in families with mental health issues, and where there is inadequate understanding of nutrition. More broadly, psychosocial factors such as maternal depression, poverty, and food insecurity may also be associated with FTT (Kersten & Bennett, 2012; O'Brien et al., 2004).

Children may also have inadequate caloric absorption due to food sensitivities such as cow's milk protein allergy or celiac disease. Children may have persistent emesis (e.g., due to metabolic disorders, gastroesophageal reflux) leading to inadequate caloric intake. A meticulous history and physical examination is essential to pick up these types of FTT (S. Cole & Lanham, 2011; Kirkland & Motil, 2011; Stephens et al., 2008; Zenel, 1997).

Another category of FTT is excessive caloric expenditure. These types of conditions are associated with underlying medical conditions such as congenital heart disease, chronic hypoxia (e.g., chronic lung disease with prematurity), metabolic disease (e.g., hyperthyroidism, diabetes), chronic immunodeficiency, or recurrent infections or malignancies that increase the basal metabolic rate (Zenel, 1997). Typically, FTT develops within the first few months of life, since this is when infants typically have exponential growth and cannot get enough calories to meet the high demand (S. Cole & Lanham, 2011).

MALTREATMENT

Identifying "direct evidence" of maltreatment may be a challenging task (Skuse, 1985). Several correlates of maltreatment were identified in a retrospective study that compared 17 children whose FTT may have involved maltreatment with 68 whose FTT did not (Mash et al., 2011). Parents of children referred for possible maltreatment, not surprisingly, were more likely to exhibit noncompliance with medical recommendations. This included refusing recommended services, changing formula or nutritional supplement drinks without consulting the medical team, and not following the recommended feeding regimen. Children with FTT who were referred for maltreatment also were more likely to have been preterm, received care at multiple institutions, received subspecialty evaluation for reported problems in multiple organ systems, been evaluated for mitochondrial disorder, and been reported by parents to have allergies, and they were more likely to have a sibling with similar symptoms. Potentially maltreated children also were more likely to have had a nasogastric or gastrostomy tube. While children with FTT may certainly present with such a medical history without having been maltreated, the more of these characteristics present in the history, the greater the concern about possible maltreatment. In addition, Mash and colleagues (2011) state that inconsistencies observed by the treatment team and a clinical course that fails to suggest a clear etiology may also be suggestive of maltreatment contributing to FTT.

There are many questionnaires that can be used to screen for child maltreatment, although they do not focus primarily on FTT. These include measures that directly assess neglectful or abusive behavior, such as the Parent-Child Conflict Tactics Scale (Straus et al., 1998) and the Mother-Child Neglect Scale (Lounds, Borkowski, & Whitman, 2006), as well as those that assess child-rearing beliefs and other parental characteristics associated with elevated risk for maltreatment, such as the Adult-Adolescent Parenting Inventory (Bavolek & Keene, 1999) and the Child Abuse Potential Inventory (Milner et al., 1984). Child reports also may be a useful supplement to parent reports for children beyond the toddler age, although preschool-age children are more vulnerable to suggestion and their self-reports are less consistent than those of older children (Bruck & Ceci, 1999; Crossman, Scullin, & Melnyk, 2004). Likewise, while directly observing parent-child interaction can be useful, observed differences in parenting behaviors between maltreating and nonmaltreating parents may be relatively small (Wilson et al., 2010).

Several notable limitations are relevant to our ability to identify maltreatment. First, socially desirable responding or behavior can confound our efforts. For example, about one-third of parents with a history of child protective services (CPS) involvement with their child were found to deny this history when enrolling in a study (Bennett, Sullivan, & Lewis, 2006; Bennett et al., 2012). The parents who denied CPS involvement were less likely to report neglectful or harsh parenting on self-report measures than were parents who acknowledged their CPS history. Similarly, 21% of parents with a likely or definite history of abuse were found to completely deny (and 47% to partially deny) allegations of abuse when interviewed by CPS staff (Lanyon, Dannenbaum, & Brown, 1991). Second, many child maltreatment assessment measures lack well-developed norms and fail to report norms separately by age group. Third, and perhaps most important for FTT, self-report measures used to screen for maltreatment do not necessarily identify those indicators of maltreatment that are most common in children with FTT, such as those identified by Mash and colleagues (2011).

Supplementing direct assessment of maltreatment with screening for family and child factors related to maltreatment may enhance our ability to identify at-risk families. Parental substance use and depression, for example, are consistently associated with increased rates of child maltreatment (Chaffin, Kelleher, & Hollenberg, 1996; Dubowitz et al., 2011). Maternal depression, in particular, may be associated with FTT. In a community study of children 2 years old and younger, those with FTT were 50% (or more) more likely to have a mother who screened positive for depression (O'Brien et al., 2004). In our own clinic, we have found that 24% of mothers and 13% of fathers screen positive for significant depressive symptoms on the Center for Epidemiological Studies Depression scale (Dubowitz et al., 2011; Radloff, 1977). In addition to parents' emotional adjustment, low maternal education level, a greater number of children in the family, and poor child performance on a developmental assessment in early childhood also predict future child maltreatment (Dubowitz et al., 2011). Identifying risk factors such as parental depression and providing appropriate supports may help to strengthen families and prevent future maltreatment, as well as improve adherence to treatment recommendations for FTT.

EVALUATION

The goal of evaluating children with FTT is to systematically identify any contributing factors so that they can be addressed with the caregivers. This includes reviewing all the growth charts, completing a thorough and meticulous history and physical examination, and ordering appropriate laboratory testing. Once this is complete, a plan can be developed to increase the child's caloric intake. This process can be long and difficult. The health care provider must show concern and try to avoid placing blame on the caregivers (Zenel, 1997). The approach must be "nonaccusatory" to get all of the important information contributing to the FTT and to establish a therapeutic relationship with the family that will improve treatment outcomes (English, 1978). The evaluation begins with a careful history, since many of the problems that cause FTT may be revealed with a thorough history.

The perinatal and birth history provide important details on factors that may compromise growth and affect the interaction between parent and child (S. Cole & Lanham, 2011; Kirkland & Motil, 2011; Nutzenadel, 2011; Zenel, 1997). Maternal infections during pregnancy, exposure to toxic substances (e.g., smoking, drugs, alcohol) or medications (e.g., anticonvulsants), and the mother's reaction to the pregnancy may contribute to a child's low birth weight or be predisposing factors for FTT (Bithoney, Dubowitz, & Egan, 1992; Kirkland & Motil, 2011).

A detailed medical history is also needed to determine the effect of any chronic diseases on the child's growth. Many different types of diseases (e.g., celiac disease, infectious diarrhea, gastroesophageal reflux) may adversely affect nutritional intake, absorption, or energy needs. Frequent minor illness (e.g., recurrent acute otitis media, upper respiratory illnesses) could also decrease a child's appetite or be a sign of immunodeficiency. A detailed review of systems is needed to look for subtle symptoms of medical conditions that can cause FTT (e.g., steatorrhea as a sign of malabsorption). Recurrent injuries may indicate neglect, while caring for a child with multiple medical problems could negatively affect a family's functioning.

A thorough family history may reveal diseases that could affect growth. Any medical or mental health problems should be reviewed, and parental height should be determined to assess its role in slow growth or constitutional growth delay or short stature.

The dietary history is extremely important. Detailed information on nutritional intake can assist in identifying problem areas, including feeding, mealtime length, place, and structure, who feeds the child, methods of feeding, volumes, and formula and food preparation (e.g., mixing the correct amount of water to formula, adding butter or oil to food) A three-day dietary history is a standard way of assessing children's typical intake. In addition, calorie counts can be done and may reveal diluted formula or insufficient calories. Many children consume too much juice. Caregivers may provide too much juice (Dennison, 1996; Smith & Lifshitz, 1994), have misconceptions about their child's caloric needs, or restrict food that they perceive is unhealthy (Schwartz, 2000). Finally, questions assessing food intake out of the home, such as at daycare or school, can provide insight into eating behaviors (S. Cole & Lanham, 2011).

Juice intake is of particular concern in the evaluation of FTT. There is some evidence that fruit juice consumption may contribute to a healthy diet in children (O'Neil et al., 2012) since it can provide some vitamins or minerals, but fruit juice consumption among U.S. children has recently shown significant increases (Fulgoni & Quann, 2012). Over 50% of U.S. children consume fruit juice daily, and it accounts for more than 50% of children's fruit servings (Fulgoni & Quann, 2012). Excessive juice intake is associated with a number of health concerns in children (Dennison, 1996; Schwartz, 2000), extremes in growth (Dennison et al., 1999), and nonorganic FTT (Dennison, 1996; Smith & Lifshitz, 1994). In one study of juice consumption, 35% of parents reported that their 1- to 5-year-old children consumed two or more cups of juice per day. More specifically, 49% of parents in families whose household income was less than $30,000 and 23% of parents in families earning more than $100,000 reported that their children drank two or more cups of juice each day (United Press International, 2012). In a small study of juice intake by children referred for FTT, fruit juice accounted for up to 60% of daily intake and was thought to be a contributing factor in FTT by displacing foods that are more calorie- and nutrient-dense (Smith & Lifshitz, 1994). In our database of more than five hundred children referred for evaluation of FTT, the average amount of liquids consumed (in addition to milk) was 18 ounces per day. So, asking specific questions about the amount of juice consumption is an important part of the dietary history.

The last part of the dietary history is observation of feeding. Feeding aversions, subtle oromotor dysfunction, signs of neglect, or mealtime feeding behaviors of the child or caregiver can be picked up during these observations (Kirkland & Motil, 2011).

The psychosocial history is extremely important for any child being evaluated for FTT because psychosocial stressors are the most common cause of insufficient caloric intake in children (Kirkland & Motil, 2011). The psychosocial history should include the family composition, caregivers' employment status, family's financial state, family stressors, degree of social isolation, and any indicators of poverty. Screening for WIC (Women, Infants, and Children) eligibility, SNAP (Supplemental Nutrition Assistance Program) benefits, and food insecurity is important (Kersten & Bennett, 2012; Kirkland & Motil, 2011). The strengths and weaknesses of the parents' skills, the support systems for the family, and the emotional adjustment of the caregivers are all important parts of the assessment.

Developmental milestones should also be assessed, since children with FTT are at increased risk for developmental and behavior problems (Jaffe, 2011; Kirkland & Motil, 2011; Schwartz, 2000; Zenel, 1997). This is a prime reason to be concerned about young children with FTT because they are at a critical period of brain growth. Insufficient calories can affect brain growth and have persistent effects on development and IQ. In addition, developmental and behavior problems can contribute to the child's feeding difficulties or the interaction between the caregiver and child. Subtle neurological defects can interfere with feeding and lead to inadequate caloric intake. Evaluation of these milestones can give valuable clues to the etiology of the FTT and provide critical information to help formulate a treatment plan.

The complete physical examination should focus on any concerns raised during the history and on identifying signs of genetic or medical diseases that may be contributing to the FTT (Bithoney, Dubowitz, & Egan., 1992; Frank &

Zeisel, 1998; Jaffe, 2011; Nutzenadel, 2011; Schwartz, 2000; Zenel, 1997). The examination should begin with accurate growth measurements of weight, length, and head circumference, which are sequentially plotted on growth charts to evaluate growth over time. Most examinations of children with FTT show normal findings, but the examiner should look for subtle signs of dysmorphology that are clues to genetic disorders or signs of pulmonary, cardiac, or gastrointestinal disorders, or even subtle signs of neglect or abuse such as poor hygiene, extensive bruising, or inappropriate behavior (S. Cole & Lanham, 2011; Kirkland & Motil, 2011; Schwartz, 2000; Zenel, 1997).

The child's nutritional status should be assessed during the physical examination. Various methods have been used to assess the severity of malnutrition (Phillips & Shulman, 2013). These methods assess the extent to which a child is underweight by using percentage of median weight for age or percentage of age-appropriate weight for length. Measurements of skinfold thickness using calipers are not routinely done since the results are not very reproducible (Nutzenadel, 2011).

Historically, extensive laboratory testing was done to rule out medical or organic causes of FTT (Jaffe, 2011; Schwartz, 2000; Sills, 1978; Zenel, 1997). As it has become clear that FTT itself is not a disease, that it is multifactorial, and that the overwhelming majority of cases are nonorganic, the laboratory workup has become more focused. Laboratory tests and diagnostic procedures should be based only on signs and symptoms evident in the history or physical examination. Sills (1978) reviewed the charts of almost two hundred children hospitalized with FTT and found that they had had 2,607 laboratory tests during the hospitalization. Although 18% of the children were determined to have "organic" causes for their FTT, only 1.4% of all laboratory studies provided positive diagnostic assistance. Every single case of organic FTT had a positive finding in the history or physical examination that suggested the diagnosis. This study confirmed the importance of the history and physical examination and helped change the thinking about extensive laboratory evaluation of children with FTT. Although Still's study was done more than 30 years ago, there still is no evidence to support extensive laboratory workup for children with FTT.

TREATMENT

The primary goal of treatment is to increase the number of calories to improve weight gain. Since the etiology of FTT has been shown to be multifactorial and children are likely to have symptoms over a period of time, it is important that health care providers have a clear understanding of all the factors that have contributed to the child's FTT. A treatment plan should address as many factors as possible to improve outcomes. The treatment may be as simple as learning to mix formula correctly, or it may involve addressing many different contributing factors. Treatment is most likely to be effective if a rapport has been established with the family (English, 1978) and if the parent-child dyad is treated as a unit (Bithoney, Dubowitz, & Egan, 1992). Given the common social, psychological, medical, and dietary considerations in children evaluated for FTT, the primary provider should work very closely with other professionals such as social workers, dietitians, psychologists, nurses, and occupational or physical therapists. A multidisciplinary approach is optimal for the treatment of FTT (Bithoney et al., 1991; Hampton, 1996; Hobbs & Hanks, 1996; Kesler & Dawson, 1999). Some primary care providers will be able to do this in their own office, but multidisciplinary teams have been shown to be a very effective way to care for these children.

The major focus for children with FTT should be on nutritional management. The caloric intake must be increased to 1.5× normal (Jaffe, 2011; Schwartz, 2000; Zenel, 1997). This may be accomplished by providing ad lib feedings, increasing the caloric density of foods or liquids, and limiting foods (e.g., juice) that have minimal nutritional value. The dietary beliefs of families also should be addressed. The amount of juice must be decreased, and some vegetarian families may need to add eggs to their mealtimes. Lastly, the family's access to food may need to be addressed. Determining whether eligible families are getting WIC or SNAP benefits is very important. Also, families might need information about food banks in their region. Each of these things will help to increase the calories the child is consuming.

Nonmedical Treatment

Given that FTT is multiply determined, multiple etiological factors may need to be addressed in treatment. Children with nonorganic FTT, compared with those with organic FTT, are more likely to experience abnormal parental feeding practices and food refusal, food fixation, and anticipatory gagging (Levy et al., 2009). Assessment of parental feeding practices begins with a review of foods and beverages that the child is offered. As a group, parents of children with FTT, like neglectful parents, tend to be relatively young (Stier et al., 1993) and, as such, may not have adequate knowledge of children's diet. Children with FTT, for example, may have excessive liquid intake (Smith & Lifshitz, 1994). Parents may give low-calorie, low-fat foods in an attempt to provide a healthy diet (McCann et al., 1994), although we also see families who are not as health conscious but who offer relatively low-calorie "junk foods" such as chips and crackers, perhaps in part due to their relatively low cost. Educating families to replace low-calorie liquids with milk or supplemental drinks (e.g., PediaSure), reduce overall liquid intake, and offer a variety of foods that include high-calorie options is often a primary intervention to boost a child's caloric intake.

Behavioral interventions for poor feeding among children with FTT focus on increasing or improving (1) the structure and routine of meals, (2) the intake of a variety of foods, (3) positive child behaviors at mealtime (e.g., self-feeding), and (4) pleasant parent-child interactions at meals. In addition, behavioral interventions attempt to decrease negative child behaviors (e.g., throwing food) and parents' mealtime stress (Fisher & Silverman, 2007). Structural changes might include using a high chair or booster seat to help keep the child seated, having meals of adequate but not excessive length (e.g., 30 minutes), having a set schedule of meal and snack times to promote eating when hungry as opposed to grazing throughout the day, and reducing potential distractions such as TV at mealtimes.

Food refusal and picky eating, common among young children, may contribute to FTT (Ekstein, Laniado, & Glick, 2010; Equit et al., 2012). Encouraging parents and siblings to eat with the child can lead to increased intake of both novel and familiar foods (Birch, 1999; Salvy et al., 2008). More intense interventions, however, may be needed for children with severe food refusal. When a child refuses food, some parents offer another, more preferred food, which may inadvertently reinforce the child's initial refusal behavior. Parents also may allow their child to discontinue a meal after refusing to eat, particularly if the child begins to cry, throw food, or otherwise have a tantrum. While ending the mealtime may decrease the child's tantrum, it may also reinforce food refusal, particularly if such escape is followed by access to a preferred activity such as playing or watching TV. Escape-prevention techniques such as repeatedly returning a child who has left the table to his or her chair or keeping a spoon at the child's lips until it is accepted into the mouth (Kerwin, 1999; O'Reilly & Lancioni, 2001) are effective in increasing food acceptance, particularly when combined with reinforcement (Piazza et al., 2003). Nonetheless, practitioners should assess medical factors such as food allergies, constipation, and gastroesophageal reflux that may contribute to increased food refusal. While the clinician can work with parents to try to develop interventions following these principles, doing so may be difficult in a traditional outpatient model, as children with severe food refusal may benefit from more frequent treatment that is focused on feeding therapy (Williams et al., 2007).

Changing dietary patterns, be it asking a family to reduce the child's liquid intake or begin to use a high chair, may initially increase the likelihood of noncompliance and temper tantrums. In general, behavior problems appear to be more common among children with FTT, although findings are not consistent, and most studies have examined such problems at follow-up as opposed to at the time of diagnosis (Black et al., 2007; Drotar & Sturm, 1992; Dykman et al., 2001; Kerr, Black, & Krishnakumar, 2000). Children with a history of both FTT and maltreatment, in particular, exhibit more behavior problems than children who have only FTT or a history of maltreatment (Kerr, Black, & Krishnakumar, 2000). Parents of children with FTT may have limited problem-solving abilities (Robinson, Drotar, & Boutry, 2001) and greater difficulty in dealing with the parenting challenges brought on by FTT. Teaching general parenting skills, such as consistently ignoring tantrums whose function may be to escape eating and providing warnings and consequences such as time-out or response cost (e.g., not being able to watch a TV show) for inappropriate behaviors (such as getting a juice box out of the refrigerator without asking), is often an important part of treatment for parents of children with FTT. This is particularly true for children whose FTT may be related to a developmental disorder such as autism, which may be more common among children with FTT (Keen, 2008).

Excessive parental worry over a child's being underweight can lead to more negative parent-child interactions at mealtime (Gueron-Sela et al., 2011). Parental pressure to eat may result in increased food avoidance or refusal (C. M. Wright, Parkinson, & Drewett, 2006). More generally, parental depression should be assessed and treatment referrals made when indicated, because, as noted earlier, mothers of children with FTT exhibit increased depressive symptoms in some studies (O'Brien et al., 2004; C. M. Wright, Parkinson, & Drewett, 2006). Parents with depression may have greater difficulty implementing treatment recommendations to address their child's FTT (DiMatteo, Lepper, & Croghan, 2000).

Sleeping patterns should also be considered, as parents of children with feeding problems report their child's shorter sleep duration and delayed sleep onset (Tauman et al., 2011). While there are many potential reasons for sleep problems, initiating a consistent bedtime routine can enhance sleep (Mindell et al., 2009) and help lead to a more regular eating schedule. For example, improved nighttime sleep may allow children to wake earlier, providing greater opportunity for breakfast. In addition, meals and snacks can be better spaced throughout the day as opposed to condensed into a relatively tight schedule in which children may eat less due to lack of hunger following their most recent meal or snack.

Home Visitation

Home visits can be useful to further assess feeding in the home environment, to provide additional support around feeding and parenting issues, and for observation of the home environment if there are concerns about neglect. Several randomized controlled studies have examined home visitation as an intervention for FTT. In one study, infants with FTT who received weekly home visits gained skills in interactive competence, and their parents became more controlling during feeding—although these changes were not associated with improved weight (Black et al., 1995). However, at the age 8 follow-up, children who received home visits as infants did have a body mass index 8% greater than that of children who did not receive visits (Black et al., 2007). A second trial of 2-year-olds found that families who received home visits had children whose weight, height, and appetite were greater than those of comparison children at the age 3 follow-up (C. M. Wright et al., 1998), although a third trial did not find home visits to be associated with improved weights (Raynor et al., 1999). In lieu of home visits, asking parents to bring a videotape of mealtimes to the clinic or conducting feeding observations in the clinic can provide additional opportunities to directly assess parent and child skills and behaviors during feeding.

Inpatient versus Outpatient Management

Admission to the hospital was the standard practice of physicians evaluating FTT until relatively recently. A two-week admission would help the physician complete the workup, observe the interaction of the family with the patient, allow subspecialists to weigh in on the evaluation, and monitor proper weight gain. Record reviews of hospitalized children with FTT showed that less than 2% of laboratory studies aided in the diagnosis of FTT (Berwick, Levy, & Kleinerman, 1982; Sills, 1978), and the positive cases could be predicted based on a thorough history and physical examination. The reviews found that the history and physical examination are the most important tools in diagnosing FTT in children. The hospitalization workup does not usually aid in the case workup or establish a diagnosis and has become cost prohibitive. Also, patients and their families are best served by keeping them out of the hospital. In short, hospitalization has little impact on the evaluation of children with FTT (Berwick, Levy, & Kleinerman, 1982; S. Cole & Lanham, 2011; Jaffe, 2011; Schwartz, 2000; Sills, 1978; Zenel, 1997). Evaluation by the primary doctor or subspecialist and management by the primary doctor or multidisciplinary team are best done on an outpatient basis. The inclusion of home visits and multidisciplinary teams can improve the child's weight gain and further decrease the need for hospitalization.

Still, there are some indications for admitting children with FTT. First, a child who does not respond to outpatient management may be admitted to document weight gain or provide a controlled environment to assess caloric intake and overall and mealtime interaction with the caregivers (Jaffe, 2011; Schwartz, 2000). However, weight gain may fluctuate in the hospital, even when children are being fed an appropriate number of calories. Assessment of proper weight gain is best done on an outpatient basis, when growth parameters can be tracked over several weeks or months. Hospitalization should be considered if the child shows significant signs of malnutrition or neglect. When receiving lots of calories after malnutrition, the child should be observed for signs of electrolyte disturbance. Low phosphate levels have been described in these situations (Stanga et al., 2008). If there is any suspicion of neglect or signs of physical abuse during the evaluation or treatment of children with FTT, an admission can be warranted because that child is at risk of harm. Weight gain during an admission may also support the notion of neglect if there is a significant increase in caloric intake and weight gain (Block & Krebs, 2005). Finally, if the caregiver has severe psychosocial impairment, hospitalization should be considered to protect the child and obtain an evaluation from CPS (T. Cole, 2003; Zenel, 1997).

Gastrostomy Tubes

The focus of treatment of FTT to increase caloric intake may lead to the placement of a gastrostomy or enteral tube for supplemental feedings. Some advocate the early use of tubes to accelerate weight gain, since children show significant catch-up growth following tube placement (Schwartz, 2000). However, this decision must be balanced against the decreased appetite and worsening of feeding behaviors that inevitably happen when a nasogastric or percutaneous gastrostomy tube is placed. Gastrostomy tubes should be considered when children fail to take adequate caloric intake for proper weight gain in spite of continued attempts to change their behavior.

CONCLUSIONS

Failure to thrive is a syndrome that causes a deceleration in weight gain that has a multifactorial origin. Although this condition was thought to be commonly associated with neglect and child abuse, these are not common causes of FTT. Accurate growth parameters plotted on a growth chart should be combined with a thorough and meticulous history and physical examination to determine the multifactorial etiology of the child's FTT. The primary goal of treatment is to increase the caloric intake. A multidisciplinary team approach is an optimal way to reach this goal.

References

Batchelor, J. A. (1996). Has recognition of failure to thrive changed? *Child: Care, Health and Development, 22*(4), 235–240.

Bavolek, S., & Keene, R. (1999). *Adult-Adolescent Parenting Inventory—AAPI-2: Administration and development handbook.* Park City, UT: Family Development Practice.

Bennett, D. S., Sullivan, M. W., & Lewis, M. (2006). Relations of parental report and observation of parenting to maltreatment history. *Child Maltreatment, 11*(1), 63–75. doi:10.1177/1077559505283589

Bennett, D. S., Sullivan, M. W., McVey, A., & Lewis, M. (2012). *Are parenting scales able to identify mothers with a history of neglect? A comparison of the CAP, CTSPC, and PSI-SF.* Paper presented at the Translational Research on Child Neglect Consortium Meeting, Bethesda, MD.

Berwick, D. M., Levy, J. C., & Kleinerman, R. (1982). Failure to thrive: Diagnostic yield of hospitalisation. *Archives of Disease in Childhood, 57*(5), 347–351.

Birch, L. L. (1999). Development of food preferences. *Annual Review of Nutrition, 19*, 41–62. doi:10.1146/annurev.nutr.19.1.41

Bithoney, W. G., Dubowitz, H., & Egan, H. (1992). Failure to thrive / growth deficiency. *Pediatrics in Review, 13*(12), 453–460.

Bithoney, W. G., McJunkin, J., Michalek, J., Snyder, J., Egan, H., & Epstein, D. (1991). The effect of a multidisciplinary team approach on weight gain in nonorganic failure-to-thrive children. *Journal of Developmental and Behavioral Pediatrics, 12*(4), 254–258.

Black, M. M., Dubowitz, H., Casey, P. H., Cutts, D., Drewett, R. F., Drotar, D., et al. (2006). Failure to thrive as distinct from child neglect. *Pediatrics, 117*(4), 1456–1458; author reply 1458–1459. doi:10.1542/peds.2005-3043

Black, M. M., Dubowitz, H., Hutcheson, J., Berenson-Howard, J., & Starr, R. H., Jr. (1995). A randomized clinical trial of home intervention for children with failure to thrive. *Pediatrics, 95*(6), 807–814.

Black, M. M., Dubowitz, H., Krishnakumar, A., & Starr, R. H., Jr. (2007). Early intervention and recovery among children with failure to thrive: Follow-up at age 8. *Pediatrics, 120*(1), 59–69. doi:10.1542/peds.2006-1657

Block, R. W., & Krebs, N. F. (2005). Failure to thrive as a manifestation of child neglect. *Pediatrics, 116*(5), 1234–1237. doi:10.1542/peds.2005-2032

Bruck, M., & Ceci, S. J. (1999). The suggestibility of children's memory. *Annual Reviews of Psychology, 50*, 419–439. doi:10.1146/annurev.psych.50.1.419

Chaffin, M., Kelleher, K., & Hollenberg, J. (1996). Onset of physical abuse and neglect: Psychiatric, substance abuse, and social risk factors from prospective community data. *Child Abuse & Neglect, 20*(3), 191–203.

Chatoor, I., Ganiban, J., Colin, V., Plummer, N., & Harmon, R. J. (1998). Attachment and feeding problems: A reexamination of nonorganic failure to thrive and attachment insecurity. *Journal of the American Academy of Child and Adolescent Psychiatry, 37*(11), 1217–1224. doi:10.1097/00004583-199811000-00023

Cole, S. Z., & Lanham, J. S. (2011). Failure to thrive: An update. *American Family Physician, 83*(7), 829–834.

Cole, T. J. (2003). The secular trend in human physical growth: A biological view. *Economics and Human Biology, 1*(2), 161–168. doi:10.1016/S1570-677X(02)00033-3

Corbett, S. S., & Drewett, R. F. (2004). To what extent is failure to thrive in infancy associated with poorer cognitive development? A review and meta-analysis. *Journal of Child Psychology and Psychiatry, 45*(3), 641–654.

Crossman, A. M., Scullin, H., & Melnyk, L. (2004). Individual and developmental differences in suggestibility. *Applied Cognitive Psychology, 18*(8), 941–945.

Dennison, B. A. (1996). Fruit juice consumption by infants and children: A review. *Journal of the American College of Nutrition, 15*(5, Suppl.), 4–11S.

Dennison, B. A., Rockwell, H. L., Nichols, M. J., & Jenkins, P. (1999). Children's growth parameters vary by type of fruit juice consumed. *Journal of the American College of Nutrition, 18*(4), 346–352.

DiMatteo, M. R., Lepper, H. S., & Croghan, T. W. (2000). Depression is a risk factor for noncompliance with medical treatment: Meta-analysis of the effects of anxiety and depression on patient adherence. *Archives of Internal Medicine, 160*(14), 2101–2107.

Drotar, D., Eckerle, D., Satola, J., Pallotta, J., & Wyatt, B. (1990). Maternal interactional behavior with nonorganic failure-to-thrive infants: A case comparison study. *Child Abuse & Neglect, 14*(1), 41–51.

Drotar, D., & Sturm, L. (1988). Prediction of intellectual development in young children with early histories of nonorganic failure-to-thrive. *Journal of Pediatric Psychology, 13*(2), 281–296.

Drotar, D., & Sturm, L. (1992). Personality development, problem solving, and behavior problems among preschool children with early histories of nonorganic failure-to-thrive: A controlled study. *Journal of Developmental and Behavioral Pediatrics, 13*(4), 266–273.

Dubowitz, H., Kim, J., Black, M. M., Weisbart, C., Semiatin, J., & Magder, L. S. (2011). Identifying children at high risk for a child maltreatment report. *Child Abuse & Neglect, 35*(2), 96–104. doi:10.1016/j.chiabu.2010.09.003

Dubowitz, H., Zuckerman, D. M., Bithoney, W. G., & Newberger, E. H. (1989). Child abuse and failure to thrive: Individual, familial, and environmental characteristics. *Violence and Victims, 4*(3), 191–201.

Dykman, R. A., Casey, P. H., Ackerman, P. T., & McPherson, W. B. (2001). Behavioral and cognitive status in school-aged children with a history of failure to thrive during early childhood. *Clinical Pediatrics, 40*(2), 63–70.

Ekstein, S., Laniado, D., & Glick, B. (2010). Does picky eating affect weight-for-length measurements in young children? *Clinical Pediatrics, 49*(3), 217–220. doi:10.1177/0009922809337331

Emond, A., Drewett, R., Blair, P., & Emmett, P. (2007). Postnatal factors associated with failure to thrive in term infants in the Avon Longitudinal Study of Parents and Children. *Archives of Disease in Childhood, 92*(2), 115–119. doi:10.1136/adc.2005.091496

English, P. C. (1978). Failure to thrive without organic reason. *Pediatric Annals, 7*(11), 774–781.

Equit, M., Palmke, M., Becker, N., Moritz, A. M., Becker, S., & von Gontard, A. (2012). Eating problems in young children—A population-based study. *Acta Paediatrica.* doi:10.1111/apa.12078

Feldman, R., Keren, M., Gross-Rozval, O., & Tyano, S. (2004). Mother-child touch patterns in infant feeding disorders: Relation to maternal, child, and environmental factors. *Journal of the American Academy of Child and Adolescent Psychiatry, 43*(9), 1089–1097. doi:10.1097/01.chi.0000132810.98922.83

Fisher, E., & Silverman, A. (2007). Behavioral conceptualization, assessment, and treatment of pediatric feeding disorders. *Seminars in Speech and Language, 36*(7), 223–231.

Frank, D., & Zeisel, S. H. (1998). Failure to thrive. *Pediatric Clinics of North America, 35*(6), 1187–1206.

Fulgoni, V. L., 3rd, & Quann, E. E. (2012). National trends in beverage consumption in children from birth to 5 years: Analysis of NHANES across three decades. *Nutrition Journal, 11*(1), 92. doi:10.1186/1475-2891-11-92

Gahagan, S., & Holmes, R. (1998). A stepwise approach to evaluation of undernutrition and failure to thrive. *Pediatric Clinics of North America, 45*(1), 169–187.

Glaser, H. H., Heagarty, M. C., Bullard, D. M., Jr., & Pivchik, E. C. (1968). Physical and psychological development of children with early failure to thrive. *Journal of Pediatrics, 73*(5), 690–698.

Grummer-Strawn, L. M., Reinold, C., & Krebs, N. F. (2010). Use of World Health Organization and CDC growth charts for children aged 0–59 months in the United States. *MMWR Morbidity and Mortality Weekly Report: Recommendations and Reports, 59*(RR-9), 1–15.

Gueron-Sela, N., Atzaba-Poria, N., Meiri, G., & Yerushalmi, B. (2011). Maternal worries about child underweight mediate and moderate the relationship between child feeding disorders and mother-child feeding interactions. *Journal of Pediatric Psychology, 36*(7), 827–836. doi:10.1093/jpepsy/jsr001

Hampton, D. (1996). Resolving the feeding difficulties associated with non-organic failure to thrive. *Child: Care, Health and Development, 22*(4), 261–271.

Hobbs, C., & Hanks, H. G. (1996). A multidisciplinary approach for the treatment of children with failure to thrive. *Child: Care, Health and Development, 22*(4), 273–284.

Jaffe, A. C. (2011). Failure to thrive: Current clinical concepts. *Pediatrics in Review, 32*(3), 100–107; quiz 108. doi:10.1542/pir.32-3-100

Joosten, K. F., & Hulst, J. M. (2008). Prevalence of malnutrition in pediatric hospital patients. *Current Opinion in Pediatrics, 20*(5), 590–596. doi:10.1097/MOP.0b013e32830c6ede

Keen, D. V. (2008). Childhood autism, feeding problems and failure to thrive in early infancy: Seven case studies. *European Child & Adolescent Psychiatry, 17*(4), 209–216. doi:10.1007/s00787-007-0655-7

Kerr, M. A., Black, M. M., & Krishnakumar, A. (2000). Failure-to-thrive, maltreatment and the behavior and development of 6-year-old children from low-income, urban families: A cumulative risk model. *Child Abuse & Neglect, 24*(5), 587–598.

Kersten, H. B., & Bennett, D. (2012). A multidisciplinary team experience with food insecurity and failure to thrive. *Journal of Applied Research on Children: Informing Policy for Children at Risk, 3*(1), 1–21.

Kerwin, M. L. (1999). Empirically supported treatments in pediatric psychology: Severe feeding problems. *Journal of Pediatric Psychology, 24*, 193–214.

Kesler, D. B., & Dawson, P. (1999). *Failure to thrive and pediatric undernutrition: A transdisciplinary approach.* Baltimore, MD: Paul H. Brookes Publishing.

Kirkland, R. T., & Motil, K. J. (2011). Etiology and evaluation of failure to thrive (undernutrition) in children younger than two years. *UpToDate.* www.uptodate.com/contents/etiology-and-evaluation-of-failure-to-thrive-undernutrition-in-children-younger-than-two-years

Lanyon, R. I., Dannenbaum, S. E., & Brown, A. R. (1991). Detection of deliberate denial in child abusers. *Journal of Interpersonal Violence, 6*, 301–309.

Levy, Y., Levy, A., Zangen, T., Kornfeld, L., Dalal, I., Samuel, E., et al. (2009). Diagnostic clues for identification of nonorganic vs organic causes of food refusal and poor feeding. *Journal of Pediatric Gastroenterology and Nutrition, 48*(3), 355–362.

Lounds, J. J., Borkowski, J. G., & Whitman, T. L. (2006). The potential for child neglect: The case of adolescent mothers and their children. *Child Maltreatment, 11*(3), 281–294. doi:10.1177/1077559506289864

Mash, C., Frazier, T., Nowacki, A., Worley, S., & Goldfarb, J. (2011). Development of a risk-stratification tool for medical child abuse in failure to thrive. *Pediatrics, 128*(6), e1467–1473. doi:10.1542/peds.2011-1080

Mathiesen, B., Skuse, D. H., Wolke, D., & Reilly, S. (1989). Oral-motor dysfunction and failure to thrive among inner-city infants. *Developmental Medicine and Child Neurology, 31*, 293–302.

McCann, J. B., Stein, A., Fairburn, C. G., & Dunger, D. B. (1994). Eating habits and attitudes of mothers of children with non-organic failure to thrive. *Archives of Disease in Childhood, 70*(3), 234–236.

Milner, J. S., Gold, R. G., Ayoub, C., & Jacewitz, M. M. (1984). Predictive validity of the Child Abuse Potential Inventory. *Journal of Consulting and Clinical Psychology, 52*(5), 879–884.

Mindell, J. A., Telofski, L. S., Wiegand, B., & Kurtz, E. S. (2009). A nightly bedtime routine: Impact on sleep in young children and maternal mood. *Sleep, 32*(5), 599–606.

Mitchell, W. G., Gorrell, R. W., & Greenberg, R. A. (1980). Failure-to-thrive: A study in a primary care setting—Epidemiology and follow-up. *Pediatrics, 65*(5), 971–977.

Nutzenadel, W. (2011). Failure to thrive in childhood. *Deutsches Ärzteblatt International, 108*(38), 642–649. doi:10.3238/arztebl.2011.0642

Oates, R. K., Peacock, A., & Forrest, D. (1985). Long-term effects of nonorganic failure to thrive. *Pediatrics, 75*(1), 36–40.

O'Brien, L. M., Heycock, E. G., Hanna, M., Jones, P. W., & Cox, J. L. (2004). Postnatal depression and faltering growth: A community study. *Pediatrics, 113*(5), 1242–1247.

O'Neil, C. E., Nicklas, T. A., Zanovec, M., Kleinman, R. E., & Fulgoni, V. L. (2012). Fruit juice consumption is associated with improved nutrient adequacy in children and adolescents: The National Health and Nutrition Examination Survey (NHANES) 2003–2006. *Public Health Nutrition, 15*(10), 1871–1878. doi:10.1017/S1368980012000031

O'Reilly, M. F., & Lancioni, G. E. (2001). Treating food refusal in a child with Williams syndrome using the parent as therapist in the home setting. *Journal of Intellectual Disability Research, 45*(Pt. 1), 41–46.

Patton, R. G. (1963). *Growth failure in maternal deprivation.* Springfield, OH: Charles C. Thomas.

Perrin, E. C., Cole, C. H., Frank, D. A., Glicken, S. R., Guerina, N., Petit, K., et al. (2003). Criteria for determining disability in infants and children: Failure to thrive. *Evidence Report / Technology Assessment (Summary), 72,* 1–5.

Phillips, S. M., & Shulman, R. J. (2013). Measurement of growth in children. *UpToDate.* www.uptodate.com/contents/measurement-of-growth-in-children

Piazza, C. C., Patel, M. R., Gulotta, C. S., Sevin, B. M., & Layer, S. A. (2003). On the relative contributions of positive reinforcement and escape extinction in the treatment of food refusal. *Journal of Applied Behavior Analysis, 36*(3), 309–324.

Radloff, L. S. (1977). The CES-D Scale: A self-report depression scale for research in the general population. *Applied Psychological Measurement, 1,* 385–401.

Ramsay, M., Gisel, E. G., & Boutry, M. (1993). Non-organic failure to thrive: Growth failure secondary to feeding-skills disorder. *Developmental Medicine and Child Neurology, 35*(4), 285–297.

Raynor, P., Rudolf, M. C., Cooper, K., Marchant, P., & Cottrell, D. (1999). A randomised controlled trial of specialist health visitor intervention for failure to thrive. *Archives of Disease in Childhood, 80*(6), 500–506.

Robinson, J. R., Drotar, D., & Boutry, M. (2001). Problem-solving abilities among mothers of infants with failure to thrive. *Journal of Pediatric Psychology, 26*(1), 21–32.

Rudolf, M. C., & Logan, S. (2005). What is the long term outcome for children who fail to thrive? A systematic review. *Archives of Disease in Childhood, 90*(9), 925–931. doi:10.1136/adc.2004.050179

Salvy, S. J., Vartanian, L. R., Coelho, J. S., Jarrin, D., & Pliner, P. P. (2008). The role of familiarity on modeling of eating and food consumption in children. *Appetite, 50*(2–3), 514–518. doi:10.1016/j.appet.2007.10.009

Schwartz, I. D. (2000). Failure to thrive: An old nemesis in the new millennium. *Pediatrics in Review, 21*(8), 257–264; quiz 264.

Shaheen, E., Alexander, D., Truskowsky, M., & Barbero, G. J. (1968). Failure to thrive—A retrospective profile. *Clinical Pediatrics, 7*(5), 255–261.

Sills, R. H. (1978). Failure to thrive. The role of clinical and laboratory evaluation. *American Journal of Diseases of Children, 132*(10), 967–969.

Skuse, D. H. (1985). Non-organic failure to thrive: A reappraisal. *Archives of Disease in Childhood, 60*(2), 173–178.

Smith, M. M., & Lifshitz, F. (1994). Excess fruit juice consumption as a contributing factor in nonorganic failure to thrive. *Pediatrics, 93*(3), 438–443.

Stanga, Z., Brunner, A., Leuenberger, M., Grimble, R. F., Shenkin, A., Allison, S. P., & Lobo, D. N. (2008). Nutrition in clinical practice—The refeeding syndrome: Illustrative cases and guidelines for prevention and treatment. *European Journal of Clinical Nutrition, 62*(6), 687–694. doi:10.1038/sj.ejcn.1602854

Stephens, M. B., Gentry, B. C., Michener, M. D., Kendall, S. K., & Gauer, R. (2008). Clinical inquiries: What is the clinical workup for failure to thrive? *Journal of Family Practice, 57*(4), 264–266.

Stewart, K. B., & Meyer, L. (2004). Parent-child interactions and everyday routines in young children with failure to thrive. *American Journal of Occupational Therapy, 58*(3), 342–346.

Stier, D. M., Leventhal, J. M., Berg, A. T., Johnson, L., & Mezger, J. (1993). Are children born to young mothers at increased risk of maltreatment? *Pediatrics, 91*(3), 642–648.

Straus, M. A., Hamby, S. L., Finkelhor, D., Moore, D. W., & Runyan, D. (1998). Identification of child maltreatment with the Parent-Child Conflict Tactics Scales: Development and psychometric data for a national sample of American parents. *Child Abuse & Neglect, 22*(4), 249–270.

Tauman, R., Levine, A., Avni, H., Nehama, H., Greenfeld, M., & Sivan, Y. (2011). Coexistence of sleep and feeding disturbances in young children. *Pediatrics, 127*(3), e615–621. doi:10.1542/peds.2010-2309

United Press International. (2012, December 11). *Study: Kids drink too much fruit juice.* www.upi.com/Health_News/2012/02/22/Study-Kids-drink-too-much-fruit-juice/UPI-13121329968185

Waterflow, J. C. (1974). Some aspects of childhood malnutrition as a public health problem. *BMJ, 4*(5936), 88–90.

Whitten, C. F., Pettit, M. G., & Fischhoff, J. (1969). Evidence that growth failure from maternal deprivation is secondary to undereating. *JAMA, 209*(11), 1675–1682.

Widdowson, E. M. (1951). Mental contentment and physical growth. *Lancet, 1*(6668), 1316–1318.

Williams, K. E., Riegel, K., Gibbons, B., & Field, D. G. (2007). Intensive behavioral treatment for severe feeding problems: A cost-effective alternative to tube feeding? *Journal of Developmental and Physical Disabilities, 19,* 227–235.

Wilson, R., Norris, A. M., Shi, X., & Rack, J. J. (2010). Comparing physically abused, neglected, and nonmaltreated children during interactions with their parents: A meta-analysis of observational studies. *Communication Monographs, 77,* 540–575.

Wright, C., Loughridge, J., & Moore, G. (2000). Failure to thrive in a population context: Two contrasting studies of feeding and nutritional status. *Proceedings of the Nutrition Society, 59*(1), 37–45.

Wright, C. M. (2000). Identification and management of failure to thrive: A community perspective. *Archives of Disease in Childhood, 82*(1), 5–9.

Wright, C. M., Callum, J., Birks, E., & Jarvis, S. (1998). Effect of community based management in failure to thrive: Randomised controlled trial. *BMJ, 317*(7158), 571–574.

Wright, C. M., Parkinson, K. N., & Drewett, R. F. (2006). How does maternal and child feeding behavior relate to weight gain and failure to thrive? Data from a prospective birth cohort. *Pediatrics, 117*(4), 1262–1269. doi: 10.1542/peds.2005-1215

Zenel, J. A. (1997). Failure to thrive: A general pediatrician's perspective. *Pediatrics in Review, 18*(11), 371–378.

PART V Education, Training, Dissemination, and Implementation in Communities

BENJAMIN E. SAUNDERS, PH.D.
ROCHELLE F. HANSON, PH.D.

22

Innovative Methods for Implementing Evidence-Supported Interventions for Mental Health Treatment of Child and Adolescent Victims of Violence

GENERAL CONSIDERATIONS

A large body of research has found that violence is pervasive in the lives of American children and adolescents and is associated with the development of serious mental health disorders and problems. The 2009 National Survey of Children's Exposure to violence found that 61% of American children and youths had experienced or witnessed at least one incident of violent victimization within the past year (Finkelhor, Turner, et al., 2009). Research also has found that most children and adolescents exposed to violence have experienced or witnessed more than one type of interpersonal violence (Finkelhor, Ormrod, & Turner, 2009; Saunders, 2003). Exposure to violence, particularly multiple forms of violence, is found to be a chief risk factor for the development of serious psychiatric disorders and problems such as posttraumatic stress disorder (PTSD), major depression, substance abuse, delinquent behavior, and a host of other emotional and behavioral difficulties (Berliner, 2010; Hanson et al., 2008; McLaughlin et al., 2012; Rheingold et al., 2012; Walsh et al., 2012). Psychological trauma resulting from violence exposure has been identified as a key component in the relationship between violence exposure and functional problems (Hall, 2000).

In response to the growing awareness of the extent of violence in the lives of children and its connection to serious mental health difficulties, interventions targeting violence and trauma-related mental health problems have been developed, empirically tested, and found to be effective in substantially reducing the emotional and behavioral impact of violence exposure among children and youths. There are now a large number of evidence-supported interventions (ESIs; treatment approaches and programs that have met a high threshold of empirical research support for their therapeutic efficacy) that can be of benefit to abused and traumatized children. Saunders, Berliner, and Hanson (2004) found that 16 of the 25 reviewed mental health treatments often used with sexually or physically abused children had at least some empirical evidence for their efficacy. Silverman and colleagues (2008) reviewed 21 efficacious child trauma treatments. The National Registry of Evidence-based Programs and Practices (Substance Abuse and Mental Health Services Administration, 2013) lists 12 treatments that have proved effective for children who have experienced violence or trauma. The California Evidence-Based Clearinghouse for Child Welfare (Chadwick Center for Children and Families, 2013) identifies 4 programs rated as either "supported" or "well-supported" by research evidence for efficacy in reducing psychological trauma. CrimeSolutions.gov, maintained by the U.S. Department of Justice, describes 20 interventions or programs with enough research support to be deemed "effective" for children exposed to violence (Office of Justice Programs, 2013).

Many of these programs have been found to be effective for a wide diversity of populations (Huey & Polo, 2008). Several of these evidence-supported treatment approaches and programs have large numbers of randomized clinical trials and systematic reviews indicating that they produce moderate to large treatment effect sizes, far exceeding the minimum requirements for being classified as an ESI by reputable review sources (Cary & McMillian, 2012; Macdonald et al., 2012). Therefore, though some gaps remain, the good news for the child abuse field is that while violence exposure can result in serious mental health problems for many children and youths, mental health treatments have been developed, repeatedly tested, and found to be effective in reducing these problems.

Moreover, both clinical efficacy trials, effectiveness studies, and services research studies find that, in general, ESIs outperform treatment as usual in community service settings (Chaffin & Friedrich, 2004; Weisz, Jensen-Doss, & Hawley, 2006). One review of studies of children's mental health services in community agencies found no discernible impact on the usual course of presenting problems (Weisz et al., 1995). This finding compares with the moderate to large treatment effects commonly found with ESIs. Therefore, ESIs produce substantially better outcomes than the typical services delivered by many community service agencies and providers to children exposed to violence.

LOFTY GOALS FOR EVIDENCE-SUPPORTED INTERVENTIONS

The persuasiveness of these findings about ESIs was reflected in several influential reports describing the large "chasm" between what is known scientifically about effective health and mental health treatments and services and the challenge to service professionals, administrators, and policymakers to rapidly deploy ESIs in frontline agencies (Chadwick Center for Children and Families, 2004; Institute of Medicine, 2001; Saunders, Berliner, & Hanson, 2004). In the past decade, many organizations, government agencies, and professionals have called for ESIs and evidence-based practices to become the national standard (American Psychological Association, 2005; Chadwick Center for Children and Families, 2004; Saunders, Berliner, & Hanson, 2004), as a means of bridging the gap between science and practice. Some commentators have suggested that, with the overwhelming scientific evidence now available, not using ESIs as first-choice treatments in daily practice could be considered an ethical issue for practitioners working with victimized children (Saunders, 2012a).

This national dialogue and the developing consensus on the value of evidence-based practice have spawned lofty goals for the dissemination and implementation of ESIs. Professional organizations, policymakers, researchers, government officials, service agency networks such as the National Child Traumatic Stress Network (www.nctsn.org), and many practitioners have called for (1) widespread and universal availability of ESIs for all victimized children who need them; (2) high penetration of the use of ESIs with appropriate clients within service systems helping victimized children; (3) use of ESIs with reasonable fidelity; and (4) sustained use of ESIs as a regular part of everyday service delivery. The challenge, of course, is how to make these goals a reality.

BUILD IT AND THEY WILL COME

At face value, this set of goals seems rather simple and straightforward and essentially means that mental health professionals working with victimized children should provide the best practice available on a regular basis. When asked how this result might be achieved, groups of community service professionals, agency administrators, and policymakers nearly always respond, "Train therapists." This response is logical because it is based on the beliefs that (1) if an adequate supply of therapists are trained in an ESI, they will use it, and the children who need effective treatment will receive it; and (2) standard continuing professional education approaches are adequate to train community service providers in an ESI and enable them to use it, with adherence to and competence in the model, within their current service settings. Getting therapists trained means simply offering training in the ESIs through the existing continuing education system. Practically speaking, this means that several therapists from a service organization would attend a one- to two-day training workshop conducted by an approved trainer in the ESI, after which they would implement the intervention in their daily work.

Studies have found that this sort of "train therapists" approach does increase knowledge of the intervention and result in more positive attitudes about using it. Unfortunately, it generally does not result in sufficient competence in the clinical skills needed to deliver the treatment with adherence and proficiency, nor does it promote therapists' behavior change (i.e., therapists now using the ESI regularly with the children they treat) (Beidas & Kendall, 2010). Therapists often pick and choose new treatment techniques that they find interesting, but they are not likely to implement the new ESI with fidelity with large numbers of children who need it. And over time, if no support is available from the treatment setting, use of the new approach tends to diminish and is often dropped.

To remedy these problems, therapist training plans were extended and improved. Longer and more intense training, up to four and five days, was offered. Training used active learning approaches and better training materials and incorporated adult learning principles to increase skills development. Basic training was supplemented with ongoing expert case consultation for therapists as they began to use the new treatment in their work. Research has found that this training-plus-consultation approach does result in better knowledge of the treatment on the part of therapists, better clinical skills, better fidelity, and a greater likelihood that therapists will use the intervention (Beidas et al., 2012). It is probably not surprising that more sophisticated approaches to clinical training result in better learning and that ongoing consultation or "coaching" by expert trainers is associated with greater ESI use with fidelity.

While engaging therapists in good training will result in more well-trained therapists who are willing to use the intervention, other challenges often emerge as agencies attempt to implement an ESI as part of their standard program. Therapists frequently find that they run into organizational and administrative obstacles when trying to conduct a new treatment with fidelity. Administrators may not provide the instrumental, interpersonal, and administrative support necessary to fully implement the intervention. Clinical supervisors often are not adequately trained in the intervention and consequently cannot provide effective and supportive supervision, particularly as therapists engage in initial implementation of the ESI. Some supervisors may discourage the use of the new treatment because they are not familiar with it and are more comfortable with current treatment approaches. Charting and billing systems may not accommodate to the new intervention, and funding sources may not pay for some of its components. Typical service delivery standards used at the agency (e.g., seeing clients once every two weeks or once a month) may not fit with fidelity to the new treatment model.

Client-related problems may present challenges as well. There may be cultural, familial, logistical, or other aspects of the client population that make it difficult for them to accept, engage in, or benefit from the new treatment. Common service problems such as high client no-show rates for appointments, sporadic attendance, and a lack of willingness to do therapy assignments outside the treatment sessions may make it difficult to deliver the new treatment with fidelity. Even if solutions for these initial implementation problems are found, normal staff turnover patterns often mean that therapists who were trained in the ESI—and have served as champions for it within the agency—leave the organization over time, threatening the ability of the agency to mentor new hires and to continue delivering the treatment.

Clearly, well-trained and motivated therapists are necessary to implementing a new ESI within a mental health service agency. But the sorts of challenges described above suggest that the simple response of training therapists usually is not sufficient to establish and maintain a new treatment within a service organization.

IMPLEMENTATION SCIENCE: THE SUPPORTIVE IMPLEMENTATION MODEL

The emerging (and complex) field of implementation science (Proctor et al., 2009) has much to say about the chal-lenges of achieving the "simple" task of providing the most appropriate ESIs to abused and traumatized children within a mental health service agency. Significant research has examined the roles of multilevel system constructs such as public policy supports for ESIs, organizational characteristics and climate, administrative characteristics and support, community acceptance, supervisory support, therapists' attitudes, and methods of clinical training in the implementation process (Fixsen et al., 2005). It turns out that while the goal is simple, implementing a new practice within a service agency can be a complex operation if it is to be done well and with the intention of sustaining the new practice over time.

The implementation science literature cannot be adequately reviewed here, but figure 22.1 summarizes, in an oversimplified but illustrative way, some of its main findings related to the purpose of this chapter. The elements of the Supportive Implementation Model, as depicted in the figure, have been found to be important for achieving implementation of an ESI.

Training

Therapists require effective training in the new treatment model. The training approach should include sufficient hours of training to adequately learn the model and to develop some level of skill in its procedures and techniques. Training techniques should be based on adult learning principles and include procedures for practicing clinical skills. Training may be delivered through multiple training sessions—that is, an initial training session followed by more advanced training or "booster training," as therapists have time to gain experience using the model in their organizational setting with their client population.

Supportive Implementation Model

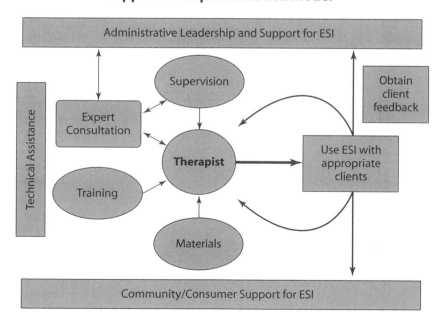

Figure 22.1. The Supportive Implementation Model for implementing an evidence-supported intervention (ESI)

Materials

More sophisticated training materials result in better learning. While traditional printed treatment manuals that cover the treatment in great detail may be necessary for initial learning, adult learning principles suggest that more condensed materials can aid in putting the treatment into practice. Simple, more condensed materials such as desk cards listing fundamental principles and components and providing outlines of clinical procedures can serve as quick reminders as therapists enter therapy sessions. Easily accessed online multimedia resources can be developed and used as an adjunct to more traditional training or to prepare therapists for their initial in-person training. For example, TF-CBTWeb (www.musc.edu/tfcbt) is a 10-hour online training course for Trauma-Focused Cognitive Behavioral Therapy (TF-CBT). It provides basic descriptions and video demonstrations of the components, procedures, and techniques of TF-CBT. Learners who complete the online course show significant gains in knowledge of TF-CBT (Saunders, Smith, & Best, 2010). This tool has been used widely as a precursor to in-person TF-CBT training, to maximize the face-to-face training time. Trainees come into the training with the basic knowledge of the treatment model and its main techniques, and in-person training can be more advanced.

Online resources also can aid consultation. TF-CBTConsult (www.musc.edu/tfcbtconsult) is an online multimedia automated consultation resource for TF-CBT. It provides text answers, videotaped "mini-lectures" by the treatment developers, and clinical demonstrations, when appropriate, that respond to more than 60 of the most commonly asked questions by therapists learning TF-CBT. Therapists can access this resource at any time to investigate their consultation questions. These sorts of materials can greatly enhance learning and implementation.

Expert Consultation and Technical Assistance

As noted above, research has found that regular, ongoing consultation or "coaching" from treatment experts greatly enhances therapists' learning of the treatment model and encourages them to implement it with fidelity and to use it with appropriate clients. Therapy requires knowledge and skills, and learning a new approach requires practice with real clients to develop these skills. Expert consultation provides reinforcement and proper corrective feedback for doing the treatment correctly. It also provides support to therapists who may be uneasy about trying to begin a new and unfamiliar therapy.

Clinical Supervision

Therapists also need regular clinical supervision in the treatment model from their regular clinical supervisors within the agency. Expert consultation cannot replace a supervisory relationship within an organization. Supervisors can provide organizational approval, encouragement, and support that an outside expert consultant cannot. Also, expert consultation is usually time-limited. When it ends, if knowledgeable and supportive supervision is not available in the therapist's agency, it will be more difficult for the therapist to sustain use of the new treatment with fidelity. This need for supervision suggests that within agencies, clinical supervisors also must be trained in the ESI and be knowledgeable and skilled in its use. Moreover, they must have the skills to provide clinical supervision in the treatment. This means that supervisors need to learn the treatment through the same mechanisms as therapists, and they also need training and ongoing expert consultation in providing supervision in the treatment.

Administrative Leadership and Support

Research shows that one of the most important factors promoting successful adoption, learning, and implementation of a new ESI in mental health service organizations is administrative transformational leadership and support (Aarons & Sommerfeld, 2012). Senior leaders in organizations need to communicate their dedication to making the new treatment a part of their program and must provide the tangible and intangible supports that are required. As noted above, therapists are likely to encounter many obstacles and challenges as they learn and begin to use a new therapeutic model. Productivity will be affected for a period of time. Administrative, billing, charting, supervisory, and outcome assessment procedures may need to be changed to support implementation. Senior leaders need to be highly involved in the implementation process so they can learn the obstacles firsthand. They should expect these challenges to emerge, understand that administrative and organizational changes are likely to be required, and work diligently with the clinical staff to identify ways to overcome these challenges. Expert consultation can help senior leaders anticipate common challenges and identify solutions that have worked with other organizations. In sum, without effective administrative leadership and support, implementation is not likely to be successful.

Community and Consumer Support

Mental health service organizations can successfully implement a new ESI and be extraordinarily well-prepared to deliver it, but if the community and target consumers do not understand it, accept it, and seek it, consistent use of the treatment will not occur. In single organization-based implementation efforts, agencies sometimes have been surprised that other community professionals do not share their enthusiasm for the new ESI. In these situations, referral patterns do not change and there is little demand for the new intervention. Without a steady stream of referrals and cooperation from other professionals, motivation to continue the new treatment often wanes. Similar results can happen with target client populations. If consumers do not accept the new intervention and see its value, there will be little support to continue its use.

Client Feedback

Perhaps the most critical element of the Supportive Implementation Model is client feedback. Ultimately, therapists, supervisors, senior leaders, community professionals, and consumers are more likely to embrace and be supportive of a new treatment that has demonstrable positive outcomes. In cases of child victimization and trauma, meaningful improvement in the symptoms, problems, and functioning of abused and traumatized children is a great convincer. Therapists like to see children and youths get better, as do others. When this happens regularly, they tend to continue to use the treatment. Similarly, if children receiving the new ESI do not improve in greater numbers, to a greater degree, and/or more rapidly, those involved will ask why they should continue to use it. This element means that measuring treatment outcomes and reporting findings to critical stakeholders is essential to successful sustainment of a new intervention.

THE LEARNING COLLABORATIVE APPROACH

Findings from the implementation literature summarized in the Supportive Implementation Model make it clear that the "train therapists" approach to ESI implementation is unlikely to be successful. Implementation efforts for mental health interventions need to incorporate many different organizational levels and roles, in addition to training therapists. Using this information, Markiewicz and colleagues, at the National Center for Child Traumatic Stress, adapted elements of the Breakthrough Series Collaborative (Institute for Healthcare Improvement, 2003) to develop the learning collaborative approach as a model of training and implementation specifically for ESIs for cases of child traumatic stress (Ebert et al., 2012; Markiewicz et al., 2006). The learning collaborative (LC) model targets a mental health service agency as the target unit. Each agency involved in an LC sends a team of participants, including senior leaders, supervisors, and sometimes consumers, as well as therapists, to take part in the training and implementation project. The goals of the LC are to learn, implement, and sustain the use of the ESI of interest within participants' respective service agencies. LCs usually involve agency teams from different geographic areas who come together to form the collaborative. In addition to involving multiple agency roles, LCs have several important elements that follow the ideas of the Supportive Implementation Model, which we summarize here.

Multiple Training Events over Time

Participants in an LC engage in a series of training events over a 9- to 12-month period. They first complete a series of "pre-work" learning activities prior to any in-person training. Then, usually two to three in-person, multiday "learning sessions" (i.e., workshops) take place over a matter of months. These multiple learning sessions provide basic training followed by advanced training. Learning sessions are separated by periods of time during which participants return to their work settings and put the new treatment into practice. As a result, subsequent training events can deal with real-world clinical and implementation problems that arise.

Use of Adult Learning Principles and Active Learning

A variety of training methods are used that focus on learning the treatment and applying it in daily practice. Participants are encouraged to consider what they can do immediately to begin to use the treatment. Training methods include active and collaborative clinical skill-building exercises, role plays, demonstrations, and practicing of skills, with a minimal level of didactic presentation.

Multiple Tracks of Training

Learning collaboratives include specific training tracks for senior leaders and clinical supervisors, in addition to training in the ESI for clinicians. Senior leaders learn to provide leadership and support for therapists as they implement the new treatment model. Clinical supervisors not only learn the treatment model but also learn how to provide effective supervision in the treatment. Senior leaders and supervisors are charged with exposing administrative, organizational, and other challenges to implementation, then problem solving and finding solutions to support the therapists.

Promotion of Team Building and Collaboration

Agency teams are encouraged to engage in problem solving as implementation challenges are discovered. Participants are also encouraged to "share relentlessly" with and "steal shamelessly" from each other in the areas of learning and implementation. An LC seeks to build a learning community whose members support one another's efforts.

Action Periods for Implementation

Action periods are the times between and following the learning sessions, typically lasting two to three months. Participants immediately put into practice what they have learned during the training, with specific training cases in which they are using the ESI. Training cases are registered with the LC organizers, and the therapy process and clinical outcomes are tracked over the course of the collaborative.

Expert Consultation

During action periods, participants receive regular expert consultation from the LC faculty, typically through affinity group conference calls for therapists, supervisors, and senior leaders. Therapists and supervisors can describe clinical challenges and receive expert clinical feedback and guidance, as well as suggestions from other participants. Senior leaders can collaborate with one another on problem solving and receive expert technical assistance. Supervisors receive help in providing supervision and working with senior leaders to overcome implementation challenges. Consultation calls run throughout the duration of the LC.

Metrics

A key element of learning collaboratives is monitoring the training impact, implementation process, and client outcomes and regularly feeding back this information to participants by providing metrics dashboards and incorporating metrics into the learning sessions. The purpose of metrics is to identify problems quickly so they can be resolved. Metrics are used to monitor participation in the LC, such as completion of the pre-work learning activities, participation in the learning sessions, and engagement in the consultation calls. Training impact (e.g., knowledge gained, attitudes changed) and satisfaction are constantly assessed, and training approaches may be changed in response to findings. Implementation factors such as the number of training cases registered, weekly assessment of the use of treatment components, fidelity monitoring, and extension of the treatment to nontraining cases are also measured. Individual LCs may measure other constructs that are particular to a service setting or a treatment. This information can be used for evaluation of the LC process, but its most important use is to provide regular feedback to participants. In this way, obstacles and challenges to learning and implementation are rapidly exposed and problem solving can begin.

Advantages of the Learning Collaborative

A key benefit of the Learning Collaborative model is the collaborative approach to learning and the development of a learning community among participants. Going through an intense and rigorous training and implementation experience with colleagues from one's workplace and from other agencies and areas, all of whom have the same goals, can produce a certain peer pressure to adopt and comply with the goals of the LC. Active learning methods that are interesting and fun also increase the excitement of the process. In essence, doing the treatment correctly, solving implementation challenges, and expanding the use of the intervention become the expected norm within the group. The use of multiple trainings over time allows participants to work through their cognitive dissonance (or even resistance) in response to doing treatment differently and permits new organizational structures or processes to be developed, take hold, and become the everyday way business is done.

The clinical LC involving multiple mental health service agency teams from often dispersed geographic areas has become a common method of training in and implementation of ESIs for abused and traumatized children. Many states and state mental health agencies have adopted the clinical LC as their standard approach to dissemination and implementation of ESIs (see chapter 23).

THE COMMUNITY-BASED LEARNING COLLABORATIVE MODEL

Child abuse cases nearly always involve multiple human service agencies. In addition to perhaps several mental health service providers and agencies, the involved organizations and professionals frequently include law enforcement, child welfare, children's advocacy centers, victims' advocates, guardians ad litem, medical service providers, drug and alcohol treatment providers, school systems, juvenile justice, domestic violence programs, rape crisis centers, the family or juvenile court, and the criminal court system. Each of these providers and service systems has particular roles and mandates in a child abuse case. Some of the agencies make determinations about whether or not an abused child is likely to need mental health services and to which therapist or agency the child and family will be referred. Many are charged with developing treatment or service plans that may include mental health therapy. Like therapists, who often have usual ways of doing practice and may be suspicious of change, communities also have well-established patterns—how the myriad systems and professionals interact around child abuse cases; the degree to which they cooperate with one another, or not; the mechanisms for screening, assessing, and referring children and families to treatment; the therapist or agency to which they frequently refer families; and routines for interacting with therapists, doing case management, assisting the treatment, monitoring the treatment, and evaluating the outcomes of treatment. These community patterns of service delivery involve many professionals and organizations, are usually reasonably ingrained in the respective communities, and are difficult to change.

Consequently, when a single mental health provider organization within a community implements a new ESI, perhaps through a clinical LC, the larger community service system and its patterns of service are probably not affected. Assume, for example, that a mental health center within a community sends six child therapists, their clinical supervisor, and their program manager to a clinical LC to learn and implement the very best ESI for child traumatic stress. Assume that the training and implementation of the new ESI by this center are successful and the center is now well-equipped to deliver the ESI, with fidelity and competence, through its six well-trained therapists. Will this change, in just one part of one of the many service agencies involved in child abuse cases in that community, meaningfully improve the community service delivery system by dramatically increasing the number of abused children that complete the ESI and have reduced symptoms and improved functioning?

This is a critical question that currently does not have a definitive answer and requires more careful research. Some studies indicate that clinical LCs do result in more referred children receiving and completing the ESI within that participating agency (e.g., Ebert et al., 2012). In other words, the newly trained clinicians and that agency are doing their jobs. This is a good outcome for the abused children within that community who are lucky enough to be referred to the implementing agency. What is unclear is whether having an ESI available at one community agency does much to change the community service patterns. Does the rest of the system become more knowledgeable about and attuned to the new ESI, understand for whom it is appropriate, understand what problems it treats, make proper referrals, increase demand for the new ESI, change case management strategies to aid ESI delivery, and help monitor treatment and treatment outcomes? Or do community service patterns remain pretty much the same?

Demand for the ESI from the rest of the service agencies in the community may be somewhat elevated for a while due to the enthusiasm of the implementing agency, but fundamental community service patterns are not likely to change based solely on a few therapists being trained at one agency. If demand for the ESI from the community is less than desired, will the mental health service agency continue to maintain the intervention as part of its program, particularly when the natural forces against sustainment (attrition of trained staff, declining administrative and supervisory support over time, newer programs being implemented, etc.) come into play?

A second issue is capacity. Training a few therapists within a community will increase the capacity to deliver an ESI somewhat, but is this capacity sufficient, given the number of children in the community who may need the intervention? Will this one change have a meaningful reach into the problem? These are all questions that need further research. Experience with LCs and anecdotal reports from implementing agencies do suggest that these are real problems in many situations. And, as indicated in the Supportive Implementation Model, without a context of community acceptance and support, implementation is less likely to last.

The Community-Based Learning Collaborative (CBLC; Project BEST, 2007) model was developed to respond to the issue of the community service pattern context for ESI implementation. A CBLC retains all of the characteristics of a clinical LC described above—including frontline workers, supervisors, and senior leaders, multiple training events over time, action periods, expert case consultation, and careful monitoring—but expands on these elements. The primary differences are that in a CBLC, (1) the unit of focus

for training and implementation is a community rather than a single agency or program, and (2) "brokers" of mental health services for abused and traumatized children within a community are included in the learning collaborative, along with the mental health clinicians. In a CBLC, clinicians *and* brokers work together through a CBLC process to implement the new ESI in their community and to change the community service patterns, involving many agencies and professionals, to support the intervention.

A *community* is self-defined by the participants. In large cities, a community may comprise a borough or several neighborhoods. In more rural areas, a community may include several counties. A *Community-Based Learning Collaborative* includes a multidisciplinary group of professionals across agencies that are regularly involved in the same cases of child abuse. *Brokers* of mental health services are defined as professionals involved in child abuse cases who (1) identify or come into contact with abused children, (2) make a determination that an abused child probably requires mental health treatment for abuse or trauma-related problems, (3) develop a treatment or service plan for the child, (4) refer the child to a mental health service provider for evaluation and treatment, (5) provide case management services, (6) monitor treatment process and treatment outcomes, and (7) often take action based on the outcome of mental health treatment and therefore have a stake in its success. Common brokers include child welfare workers, guardians ad litem, victim advocates, rape crisis center caseworkers, and juvenile justice caseworkers, as well as others.

The CBLC is based on a social-economic model of supply and demand for evidence-based mental health services. Brokers often are the gateway for abused children moving into mental health services. Therefore, as brokers come to understand the critical importance of children receiving an ESI and their role and responsibility in obtaining this for their clients, demand for the ESI within the community will increase. Therapists trained in the ESI represent the supply side. As demand increases, so does supply, resulting in a convergence within the community.

A CBLC brings these two sides together—brokers and clinicians from multiple community service organizations involved in child abuse cases—to participate in a 12- to 14-month training and implementation project with the goals of establishing the ESI of interest within the community and ensuring that all children in the community who need the ESI receive it. Each community forms a Community Change Team (CCT) consisting of broker and clinical professionals committed to these goals. Agency senior leaders, supervisors, and frontline therapists and caseworkers form the CCT and participate together in the collaborative. The CCT works throughout the CBLC, not only to learn and use new skills, but also to change the patterns of service system delivery within the community so that all children who can benefit from the ESI are identified, are routed to trained therapists, and complete the treatment. A CBLC may include CCTs from several different communities, capitalizing on collaborative learning, implementation, problem solving, and mutual support.

Because of the addition of brokers, the CBLC adds a broker track to the clinical, supervisor, and senior leader tracks of the learning collaborative. In this track, broker professionals learn about the ESI, including what problems it treats, who it is for, its treatment components and techniques, and the evidence supporting its efficacy. Brokers and clinicians learn Evidence-Based Treatment Planning, a framework for developing, following, and monitoring community consensus treatment plans that include ESIs, particularly the target ESI (Project BEST, 2008). Brokers also learn a series of case management skills for promoting treatment success; these are procedures that brokers can use to help children and families engage in treatment, participate regularly, and complete treatment. Brokers also learn how to monitor the ESI, what questions to ask therapists about treatment process and progress, and how to understand treatment outcomes. This training occurs at the same learning sessions as the clinical training. Brokers also participate in expert consultation calls in the action periods, as they put these new skills into practice.

Most important, brokers and clinicians (including senior leaders from both tracks) develop effective working relationships with each other and build inter-organizational relationships that have a common goal: making sure all abused children and their families in their community who need it receive the ESI with fidelity and complete the treatment successfully. Broker and clinical professionals work together to change the community service patterns, identify implementation challenges, and problem-solve and overcome these challenges to meet the goal for their community. Senior leaders from both broker and clinical agencies meet together regularly, participate in expert consultation calls, and work to support implementation of the ESI and expand its reach to all the children that need it in their community.

Research shows that greater intensity of inter-organizational relationships between broker and clinical agencies is associated with a higher likelihood of mental health service use by children and better mental health improvements (Bai, Wells, & Hillemeier, 2009). The CBLC is based on this notion and postulates several advantages over the clinical LC model.

- Increasing the demand for an ESI through brokers while simultaneously increasing the supply of well-trained therapists and implementing mental health agencies will result in more children receiving the treatment within a community.
- Increasing the inter-organizational relationships and cooperation between broker and provider agencies and professionals will result in more children receiving the treatment within a community.
- The ESI has greater reach—that is, a much larger proportion of abused and traumatized children within a community who need the ESI will receive it.

- A balance between high broker demand and adequate therapist supply will result in sustained use of the ESI over time within a community.

Each of these putative advantages of the CBLC approach remains to be tested empirically.

Project BEST

Project BEST (Bringing Evidence-Supported Treatments to South Carolina Children and Their Families) is a statewide effort to establish TF-CBT throughout South Carolina, using the CBLC implementation model (www.musc.edu/projectbest). To date, Project BEST has completed five CBLCs. Experience with these CBLCs and the quality improvement and metrics information from three of them are encouraging, but some challenges have also been identified (Saunders, 2012b).

The most encouraging finding is that children treated by community-based therapists participating in Project BEST had significant pre- to post-treatment declines in PTSD symptoms, equal to or better than those reported in clinical trials of TF-CBT. For 188 children treated by 91 community therapists, the pre- to post-treatment PTSD symptom decline was $d = 92$. This change compares favorably with pre- to post-treatment changes in PTSD symptoms found in the TF-CBT treatment groups in two recent clinical trials: $d = 0.64$ (Cohen, Mannarino, & Iyengar, 2011) and $d = 0.94$ (Deblinger et al., 2011). Using a standard of one-half a standard deviation (½ SD) to indicate meaningful change in symptom level, the outcome matrix for the children with initial PTSD symptom levels equal to the commonly used inclusion criteria for TF-CBT clinical trials was also encouraging. Of these children (n = 171), 73% had substantially improved PTSD symptoms; for 19%, their symptoms remained approximately the same (within ±½ SD), and 8% had an increase in PTSD symptoms greater than ½ SD. At initial assessment, 36% of these children scored at or above the clinical threshold on the UCLA PTSD Index for *DSM-IV* (Steinberg et al., 2004), indicating that they probably met PTSD diagnostic criteria. This proportion fell to 11% after treatment. Similar improvement results were found for depression symptoms. This information supports the idea that community-based therapists can use TF-CBT and achieve clinical results comparable to those found in clinical trials.

Lessons Learned

Many lessons have been learned about the CBLC process through Project BEST, and we cannot review all of these here. However, we should highlight three critical lessons. First, committed, creative, multiagency, local community leadership is very likely the most critical component of a successful CBLC. This lesson is consistent with the findings of Aarons and Sommerfeld (2012), described above, concerning implementation in general. Community implementation does require some alteration of the community service system. In some communities, changes have been minimal; in others, massive changes have been required. It is clear that without transformational leadership from the critical organizations involved in child abuse cases, these changes are unlikely to happen.

Second, the inclusion and training of brokers has proved to be an even more important element than anticipated. Brokers usually are unclear and unsure about the extent of their role and responsibilities in obtaining effective mental health treatment for their clients. They are concerned about "telling the doctor what to do." They frequently do not understand differences between treatment models. And they do not know how to monitor treatment process and outcomes. However, when brokers learn about ESIs, learn that all counseling is not the same, come to understand that all therapists are not necessarily trained in and will not automatically use the best-practice treatment, and, most important, fully understand their responsibility to seek the best treatment for their child clients, they very often become passionate and driven in their quest for the best intervention for these children. They become very active in monitoring how the treatment is going and in seeking information about treatment outcomes. So much so, that a single trained broker can quickly fill several trained therapists' caseloads to capacity. When conducting a CBLC, organizers and senior leaders must ensure that a sufficient number of therapists participate to meet the demand created by trained brokers.

Finally, the value of continuously collecting and regularly feeding back implementation, clinical, and outcome metrics to CBLC participants cannot be overemphasized. Most community practitioners, both broker and clinical, have general ideas about what is going on in their community. Metrics bring a certain empirical reality to these perspectives and can be used to motivate and direct change. When CBLC participants see how they are performing, how implementation is actually happening (or not), and how children are improving, they are rewarded for their success and quickly identify the gaps and remaining challenges. This information spawns creative and effective problem solving for real, not speculative, challenges.

Overall, the lessons learned and information generated through Project BEST have supported the conceptual framework underlying the CBLC approach. It is complicated and has a good many moving parts. It requires a significant level of community organization, preparation, and readiness assessment to engage and educate the multi-agency senior leadership needed for success. And all elements of the Supportive Implementation Model and the clinical LC approach need to be applied to both the broker and the clinical components. However, though initial results are encouraging, research is needed to test the ideas underlying the CBLC, the expected improvement results, and the components of the method.

CONCLUSIONS

Exposure to violence and abuse in childhood is widely recognized as a significant risk factor for serious social, emotional, and behavior problems among children. Evidence-supported interventions do exist to prevent and/or reduce these negative effects, but limited access means that many children, particularly those involved with the child welfare system, do not receive these interventions. Furthermore, trauma-focused ESIs are still neither well-integrated nor the standard practice of care across the multiple providers and service agencies involved in child abuse/trauma cases. As discussed in this chapter, the use of a community-based implementation model (the Community-Based Learning Collaborative), which includes both direct treatment providers and brokers (those whose primary responsibility is to identify, refer, and monitor children to ensure they receive needed services), is an innovative approach that may provide a key step in addressing this public health priority and may bring the field a step closer to meeting the needs of abused/traumatized children—particularly those involved in the child welfare system.

The CBLC is based on a social-economic model of supply and demand for evidence-based mental health services, with the overarching goals being to increase community capacity for and promote the sustained use of, availability of, and access to targeted ESIs. Although preliminary, our efforts to date suggest that the following elements are critical to this type of long-term sustained change in community service patterns: committed community leadership across multiple agencies; co-training and collaboration of clinical and broker professionals; and ongoing evaluation and provision of consistent feedback to community professionals. While preliminary findings are promising, research is needed to further test the feasibility and key components of the CBLC implementation model. To date, this approach seems to offer a means of promoting long-term change in community service patterns to increase the likelihood that all abused children and their families will receive the evidence-supported interventions they need.

References

Aarons, G. A., & Sommerfeld, D. H. (2012). Leadership, innovation climate, and attitudes toward evidence-based practice during a statewide implementation. *Journal of the American Academy of Child and Adolescent Psychiatry, 51*(4), 423–431.

American Psychological Association. (2005). *American Psychological Association policy statement on evidence-based practice in psychology.* Washington, DC: Author.

Bai, Y., Wells, R., & Hillemeier, M. M. (2009). Coordination between child welfare agencies and mental health service providers, children's service use, and outcomes. *Child Abuse & Neglect, 33,* 372–381.

Beidas, R. S., Edmunds, J. E., Marcus, S. C., & Kendall, P. C. (2012). Training and consultation to promote implementation of an empirically supported treatment: A randomized trial. *Psychiatric Services, 63,* 660–665.

Beidas, R. S., & Kendall, P. C. (2010). Training therapists in evidence-based practice: A critical review of studies from a systems-contextual perspective. *Clinical Psychology: Science and Practice, 17*(1), 1–30.

Berliner, L. (2010). Child sexual abuse: Definitions, prevalence, and consequences. In J. E. B. Myers (Ed.), *The APSAC handbook on child maltreatment* (3rd ed.). Los Angeles, CA: Sage Publications.

Cary, C. E., & McMillian, C. (2012). The data behind the dissemination: A systematic review of Trauma-Focused Cognitive Behavioral Therapy for use with children and youth. *Children and Youth Service Review, 34,* 748–757.

Chadwick Center for Children and Families. (2004). *Closing the quality chasm in child abuse treatment: Identifying and disseminating best practices.* San Diego, CA: Author.

Chadwick Center for Children and Families. (2013). *California Evidence-Based Clearinghouse for Child Welfare.* San Diego, CA: Author. www.cebc4cw.org

Chaffin, M., & Friedrich, B. (2004). Evidence-based treatments in child abuse and neglect. *Children and Youth Services Review, 26,* 1097–1113.

Cohen, J. A., Mannarino, A. P., & Iyengar, S. (2011). Community treatment of posttraumatic stress disorder for children exposed to intimate partner violence: A randomized controlled trial. *Archives of Pediatric & Adolescent Medicine, 165*(1), 16–21.

Deblinger, E., Mannarino, A. P., Cohen, J. A., Runyon, M. K., & Steer, R. A. (2011). Trauma-Focused Cognitive-Behavioral Therapy for children: Impact of the trauma narrative and treatment length. *Depression and Anxiety, 28,* 67–75.

Ebert, L., Amaya-Jackson, L., Markiewicz, J. M., Kisel, C., & Fairbank, J. A. (2012). Use of the Breakthrough Series Collaborative to support broad and sustained use of evidence-based trauma treatment for children in community practice settings. *Administration and Policy in Mental Health and Mental Health Services Research, 39*(3), 187–199.

Finkelhor, D., Ormrod, R. K., & Turner, H. A. (2009). Lifetime assessment of poly-victimization in a national sample of children and youth. *Child Abuse & Neglect, 33,* 403–411.

Finkelhor, D., Turner, H., Ormrod, R., & Hamby, S. L. (2009). Violence, abuse, and crime exposure in a national sample of children and youth. *Pediatrics, 124,* 1411–1423.

Fixsen, D. L., Naoom, S. F., Blase, K. A., Friedman, R. M., & Wallace, F. (2005). *Implementation research: A synthesis of the literature.* Tampa, FL: University of South Florida, Louis de la Parte Florida Mental Health Institute, National Implementation Research Network.

Hall, J. M. (2000). Women survivors of childhood abuse: The impact of traumatic stress on education and work. *Issues in Mental Health Nursing, 21*(5), 443–471.

Hanson, R. F., Borntrager, C. F., Self-Brown, S., Kilpatrick, D. G., Saunders, B. E., Resnick, H. S., & Amstadter, A. B. (2008). Relations among gender, violence exposure, and mental health: The National Survey of Adolescents. *American Journal of Orthopsychiatry, 78*(3), 313–321.

Huey, S. J., & Polo, A. J. (2008). Evidence-based psychosocial treatments for ethnic minority youth. *Journal of Clinical Child and Adolescent Psychology, 37*(1), 262–301.

Institute for Healthcare Improvement. (2003). *The Breakthrough Series: IHI's collaborative model for achieving breakthrough improvement* (IHI Innovation Series white paper). Boston, MA: Author. www.IHI.org

Institute of Medicine. (2001). *Crossing the quality chasm: A new health system for the 21st century.* Washington, DC: National Academy Press.

Macdonald, G., Higgins, J. P. T., Ramchandani, P., Valentine, J. C., Bronger, L. P., Klein, P., et al. (2012). Cognitive-behavioural interventions for children who have been sexually abused. *Cochrane Database of Systematic Reviews, 5,* CD001930.

Markiewicz, J., Ebert, L., Ling, D., Amaya-Jackson, L., & Kisiel, C. (2006). *Learning collaborative toolkit.* Los Angeles, CA, and Durham, NC: National Center for Child Traumatic Stress.

McLaughlin, K. A., Green, J. G., Gruber, M. J., Sampson, N. A., Zaslavsky, A. M., & Kessler, R. C. (2012). Childhood adversities and first onset of psychiatric disorders in a national sample of US adolescents. *Archives of General Psychiatry, 69*(11), 1151–1160.

Office of Justice Programs, U.S. Department of Justice. (2013). *CrimeSolutions.org.* Washington, DC: Author. http://crime solutions.gov/TopicDetails.aspx?ID=60

Proctor, E. K., Landsverk, J., Aarons, G., Chambers, D., Glisson, C., & Mittman, C. (2009). Implementation research in mental health services: An emerging science with conceptual, methodological, and training challenges. *Administration and Policy in Mental Health and Mental Health Services Research, 36*(1), 24–34.

Project BEST. (2007). *What is a Community-Based Learning Collaborative?* Charleston, SC: Author. http://academic departments.musc.edu/projectbest/collaborative/collaborate.htm

Project BEST. (2008). *What is Evidence-Based Treatment Planning?* Charleston, SC: Author. http://academicdepartments.musc.edu/projectbest/planning/ebtplanning.htm

Rheingold, A. A., Zinzow, H., Hawkins, A., Saunders, B., & Kilpatrick, D. G. (2012). Prevalence and mental health outcomes of homicide survivors in a representative sample of adolescents: Data from the 2005 National Survey of Adolescents. *Journal of Child Psychology and Psychiatry, 53,* 687–694.

Saunders, B. E. (2003). Understanding children exposed to violence: Toward an integration of overlapping fields. *Journal of Interpersonal Violence, 18*(4), 356–376.

Saunders, B. E. (2012a). Determining the best practice for treating sexually victimized children. In P. Goodyear-Brown (Ed.), *Handbook of child sexual abuse* (pp. 173–197). Hoboken, NJ: John Wiley & Sons.

Saunders, B. E. (2012b, September 10). *Project BEST: A social-economic, community-based approach to implementing evidence-based trauma treatment for abused children.* Paper presented at the 19th ISPCAN International Congress on Child Abuse and Neglect, Istanbul, Turkey.

Saunders, B. E., Berliner, L., & Hanson, R. F. (Eds.). (2004, April 26). *Child physical and sexual abuse: Guidelines for treatment* (Revised report). Charleston, SC: National Crime Victims Research and Treatment Center. http://academic departments.musc.edu/ncvc/resources_prof/reports_prof.htm

Saunders, B. E., Smith, D. W., & Best, C. L. (2010, November 4). *Effectiveness of Web-based training in disseminating evidence-based trauma interventions.* Paper presented at the 26th annual meeting of the International Society on Traumatic Stress Studies, Montreal, QC.

Silverman, W. K., Ortiz, C. D., Viswesvaran, C., Burns, B. J., Kolko, D. J., Putnam, F. W., & Amaya-Jackson, L. (2008). Evidence-based psychosocial treatment for children and adolescents exposed to traumatic events. *Journal of Clinical Child and Adolescent Psychology, 37,* 156–183.

Steinberg, A., Brymer, M., Decker, K., & Pynoos, R. S. (2004). The UCLA PTSD Reaction Index. *Current Psychiatry Reports, 6,* 96–100.

Substance Abuse and Mental Health Services Administration. (2013). *National Registry of Evidence-based Programs and*

Practices. Washington, DC: U.S. Department of Health and Human Services. www.nrepp.samhsa.gov

Walsh, K., Danielson, C. K., McCauley, J. L., Saunders, B. E., Kilpatrick, D. G., & Resnick, H. S. (2012). National prevalence of posttraumatic stress disorder among sexually revictimized adolescent, college, and adult household-residing women. *Archives of General Psychiatry, 69*(9), 935–942.

Weisz, J. R., Jensen-Doss, A., & Hawley, K. M. (2006). Evidence-based youth psychotherapies versus usual clinical care: A meta-analysis of direct comparisons. *American Psychologist, 61*(7), 671–689.

Weisz, J. R., Weiss, B., Han, S. S., Granger, D. A., & Morton, T. (1995). Effects of psychotherapy with children and adolescents revisited: A meta-analysis of treatment outcome studies. *Psychological Bulletin, 117,* 450–468.

JASON M. LANG, PH.D.
LUCY BERLINER, M.S.W.
MONICA M. FITZGERALD, PH.D.
ROBERT P. FRANKS, PH.D.

23

Statewide Efforts for Implementation of Evidence-Based Programs

GENERAL CONSIDERATIONS

A number of evidence-based programs (EBPs) have been developed to treat children who are victims of abuse, neglect, and other forms of trauma exposure. The availability of these programs in community-based mental health settings remains limited, however, and the potential public health impact of EBPs has not been realized. The goals of this chapter are to summarize the current state of implementation science and to describe three statewide approaches to EBP implementation, in Connecticut, Washington State, and Colorado. We summarize common themes and challenges from these initiatives and make some recommendations for future statewide EBP implementation efforts.

IMPLEMENTATION OF EVIDENCE-BASED PROGRAMS IN CHILD-SERVING SYSTEMS

Over the past two decades, a great deal has been learned about developing more effective programs in mental health, juvenile justice, child welfare, and other child-serving systems. This has led to an increasing emphasis on evidence-based practice, defined as "integration of the best available research with clinical expertise in the context of patient characteristics, culture, and preferences" (American Psychological Association, 2005, p. 1). Development of a range of evidence-based programs, or specific models of practice supported by research, has followed. In fact, there is now a national registry of more than 250 EBPs—including more than 160 intended for children and adolescents (www .nrepp.samhsa.gov). These EBPs are sought after to prevent or treat a variety of mental health and substance abuse concerns, including child abuse and neglect. However, the Institute of Medicine (2004) reports that it takes an average of 17 years for the implications of research on effective health care treatments to make their way to community populations. Despite the development of so many child behavioral health EBPs, there has been a limited impact on public health (DeAngelis, 2010).

Although EBPs exist for child victims of abuse and other forms of trauma exposure, few children and families receive these treatments (Chadwick Center for Children and Families, 2004; Landsverk et al., 2006; Stahmer et al., 2005). In fact, 75% of children in the child welfare system who need mental health treatment do not receive it (Burns et al., 2004). Children who do receive services rarely receive targeted EBPs (Landsverk et al., 2009). This is a cause of concern, given the scarcity of evidence that treatment traditionally delivered in community agencies is effective (McLennan et al., 2006; Weiss, Catton, & Harris, 2000). Several reasons for the limited availability of EBPs are therapists' lack of exposure to the models, resistance to changes in practice, lack of funding and resources, and lack of leadership and administrative support to overcome implementation challenges (Chadwick Center for Children and Families, 2004).

Increasingly, systems of care at the local, regional, and state levels have attempted to broadly disseminate EBPs in order to increase access to quality care and improve child, family, and public health outcomes. These efforts are well underway despite our limited knowledge about the most effective methods of EBP dissemination in public settings (McHugh & Barlow, 2010). Common implementation challenges include organizational, policy, and staffing barriers (Ganju, 2003) and the limitations of traditional didactic training methods, which have been minimally effective at creating sustainable changes in practice (Beidas & Kendall, 2010; Jensen-Doss, Cusack, & de Arellano, 2008).

Implementation within a statewide system of care presents a unique set of challenges. Typically, decisions to disseminate an EBP statewide are made by key champions, stakeholders, and policymakers because of an identified need for improved practices in a given area. State agencies responsible for major systems of care, including child welfare, mental health, juvenile justice, and education, are often confronted with the challenge of wanting to improve practice or install EBPs but lacking the internal capacity to do so. States confronted with such challenges may turn to external organizations that have this expertise to bring model programs to scale and provide the necessary training, coaching, and quality assurance required to disseminate an EBP. These organizations are often referred to as "purveyor" or "intermediary" organizations (Fixsen et al., 2005; Franks, 2011) and include academic centers, nonprofit agencies, and for-profit companies.

Purveyor and intermediary organizations have emerged within the developing field of "implementation science," which examines this process of bringing EBPs into practice (Fixsen et al., 2005). In their seminal monograph on implementation, Fixsen and colleagues define implementation science as "a specified set of activities designed to put into practice an activity or program of known dimensions" (p. 5). Implementation involves a range of processes and activities, including direct training and workforce development, coaching, technical assistance, quality assurance, and fidelity monitoring. Fixsen and colleagues identify six core stages of successful implementation: exploration, installation, initial implementation, full implementation, innovation, and sustainability. Several other reviews have also explored the processes of dissemination, diffusion, and implementation of EBPs and model programs (Durlak & DuPre, 2008; Greenhalgh et al., 2004; Meyers, Durlak, & Wandersman, 2012; Stith et al., 2006). Common themes of successful implementation identified in these reviews are the importance of adequate funding, organizational readiness, a positive work climate, balancing fidelity with local adaptations, shared decision making, coordination with other agencies, effective leadership, program champions, providers' skill proficiency, and training and technical assistance. Over the past few years, a number of other implementation frameworks have been developed (see Meyers, Durlak, & Wandersman, 2012).

While most implementation research is based on local or regional program implementation, less is known about implementation across a statewide system of care. In this chapter, we describe three statewide approaches—in Connecticut, Washington, and Colorado—to disseminating EBPs for victims of child abuse, neglect, and other forms of trauma exposure.

CONNECTICUT

The Connecticut Department of Children and Families (DCF) is an integrated state agency with four mandates: child protective services, behavioral health, juvenile justice, and substance abuse services. For years, administrators at the DCF recognized that many Connecticut chil-

dren, particularly those in the child welfare system, suffered from undiagnosed or untreated traumatic stress symptoms secondary to physical abuse, sexual abuse, violence exposure, and other forms of trauma. Administrators also recognized that Connecticut had very limited availability of EBPs for victims of trauma, particularly in the DCF-contracted outpatient provider network through which most children in the DCF system are served. These factors, along with several previous successful statewide implementations of in-home EBPs, led the DCF to develop plans for disseminating a trauma-focused EBP in Connecticut's outpatient behavioral health agencies to increase the state's capacity to serve victims of child abuse and other forms of trauma.

During the initial planning, DCF staff consulted with the National Child Traumatic Stress Network's (NCTSN) National Center at Duke University and the University of California, Los Angeles. The NCTSN is funded by the Substance Abuse and Mental Health Services Administration (SAMHSA), part of the U.S. Department of Health and Human Services, and comprises a network of more than 60 sites across the country. The NCTSN pioneered adaptation of the Institute for Healthcare Improvement's Breakthrough Series Collaborative model to disseminate EBPs for treating child traumatic stress (Markiewicz et al., 2006) through what were called "learning collaboratives." Confronted with the challenge of bringing health care research to practice, the Institute for Healthcare Improvement (2004) developed the Breakthrough Series Collaborative to implement practice improvements in medical settings. The model involves a 6- to 15-month process that differs from traditional training in several ways and is also compatible with implementation research and Fixsen et al.'s (2005) stages of implementation. For example, the Breakthrough Series includes staff with diverse roles in a team-based learning approach, uses the Model for Improvement (Langley et al., 2009) for spreading practice improvements, emphasizes the use of data for quality improvement, and focuses on organizational change and sustainability of changes in practice.

While initially designed to promote improvements in health care, the Breakthrough Series model is flexible enough to apply to a variety of practices and fields. The NCTSN has adopted the learning collaborative as the primary mechanism for disseminating EBPs across NCTSN sites nationally and has coordinated more than 35 regional or national learning collaboratives. Connecticut was among the first states that adapted the model for a statewide EBP implementation in 2007.

The DCF selected Trauma-Focused Cognitive Behavioral Therapy (TF-CBT) as the initial treatment model for implementation because of its strong empirical support and ability to be used for children with exposure to a broad range of traumatic events, including child abuse (Cary & McMillen, 2012; Cohen, Mannarino, & Deblinger, 2006). In consultation with NCTSN staff, DCF staff designed a proposal outlining the structure of a statewide learning collaborative and released a request for proposals to identify a coordinating center for the initiative. In early 2007, the DCF selected the Connecticut Center for Effective Practice, a division of the Child Health and Development Institute of Connecticut, as the coordinating center. The Center for Effective Practice, functioning as an intermediary organization (Franks, 2011), collaborated with the DCF, TF-CBT treatment developers and trainers, family members, and community providers to develop the structure of the Connecticut TF-CBT Learning Collaborative.

The coordinating center was funded by the DCF at a cost of $244,000 per year (in 2007 dollars) for three years, from 2007 to 2010. Funds were used to establish and support the coordinating center staff and all training, quality assurance, and evaluation activities. The DCF also provided $30,000 for each participating agency implementing TF-CBT to offset lost productivity due to training and to pay for a part-time TF-CBT site coordinator. Agencies were selected for participation in each of three year-long training periods through a competitive procurement process, on the basis of organizational readiness, capacity, and geographic considerations. Sixteen agencies were trained over three years. The primary goals were that the initiative would build capacity for EBP delivery in agencies, that TF-CBT services would be reimbursable through Medicaid and private insurance, and that agencies would be able to sustain TF-CBT programs after training with limited external funding.

The Connecticut TF-CBT Learning Collaborative was largely modeled after a traditional Breakthrough Series Collaborative, with the focus on implementation of TF-CBT in outpatient clinics of community-based agencies (Lang, Franks, & Bory, 2011). A faculty team consisting of coordinating center staff, a DCF program officer, a TF-CBT trainer, an expert in trauma assessment, and a family representative developed training plans and oversaw implementation—similar to the concept of an "implementation team" (Fixsen et al., 2005; Meyers, Durlak, & Wandersman, 2012). Similarly, each provider agency assembled a TF-CBT team of 7–12 staff, including clinicians, supervisors, a senior administrator, a site coordinator, and a family partner, to oversee implementation in the agency. Thus, each training cohort included 40–60 provider staff from four to six agencies.

Prior to the initial training, each agency participated in a site visit with the faculty that focused on enhancing organizational readiness to implement TF-CBT. Team members also completed preparatory work, including the Web-based TF-CBT training (tfcbt.musc.edu), readings on TF-CBT, development of agency plans for trauma screening, and team-building activities. All staff attended three or four learning sessions (seven days of in-person training) during the year. Learning sessions were developed using adult learning principles to favor interactive, skills-based activities and included content on clinical skills, implementation, use of data, and practice improvement, including the Model for Improvement (Langley et al., 2009). Separate training "tracks" and curricula were developed for clinicians, supervisors, senior leaders in the agency, and family partners, who worked with their teams to ensure family-centered, culturally competent practice and to ensure that the consumer perspective was considered throughout implementation and practice change. Between learning sessions, teams received consultation through a series of role-specific telephone calls with faculty, weekly site-based technical assistance from the coordinating center, and a secure intranet site. Monthly "metric" data submitted by all agencies were used by the faculty and each team to monitor implementation and to identify successes and challenges. Additionally, a simple online data system was developed to allow agency staff to have their clinical assessments scored and summarized instantly and to allow the coordinating center to monitor data and provide technical assistance in real time.

Since the end of the learning collaboratives in 2010, the DCF has used $60,000–$160,000 annually in federal mental health block-grant funds for the coordinating center to provide additional support and resources to the 16 agencies. This funding has included a two-day introductory training for new staff, development of a TF-CBT fellowship program for experienced TF-CBT "champions" to gain additional experience, an annual statewide TF-CBT conference, maintenance of a statewide TF-CBT roster and intranet site, monthly metric data collection and reporting, maintenance of online scoring of assessment measures, site-based consultation, consultation calls/webinars, performance incentives, and advanced training opportunities.

More than 400 staff from 16 agencies were trained in TF-CBT between 2007 and 2012. These agencies have cumulatively provided TF-CBT to 2,300 children, and more than 700 have completed the full course of treatment. All 16 agencies continue to maintain a TF-CBT team two to four years after initial implementation, albeit with wide variation in capacity.

The initiative and training were very well received by the participating agencies and staff and are well known among the larger Connecticut provider network as an example of a successful EBP implementation. Staff valued the learning collaborative training approach and the amount of initial and ongoing consultation and support provided. Senior administrators anecdotally reported other benefits from the initiative, including enhanced staff morale and self-efficacy, staff's use of selected TF-CBT components across a broader range of clients, increased family engagement in treatment, shorter length of stay, and reduced no-show rates for clients receiving TF-CBT.

Several consistent challenges have emerged, including staff turnover, the costs of sustaining TF-CBT, and educating other child-serving systems about the availability of EBPs. In an era of significant financial challenges for community providers, the increased costs for providing an EBP without a commensurate enhanced reimbursement rate are a threat to sustainability. Additionally, there continues to be a limited awareness about the availability of TF-CBT, and the benefits of EBPs more broadly, outside the mental health community.

Connecticut continues to pursue expansion of trauma-focused EBPs based on the Breakthrough Series Collaborative model, including training an additional 12 agencies in TF-CBT using this model. In addition, work is underway in other systems to improve awareness about child traumatic stress and the availability of EBPs. Specifically, the DCF is developing plans to implement universal screening for exposure to trauma and child traumatic stress symptoms, along with training all child welfare staff in trauma-informed care and availability of EBPs. The Child Health and Development Institute, in collaboration with the network of TF-CBT agencies, has also begun training pediatricians in trauma-informed care and EBPs through the Educating Practices in the Community program, using academic detailing (Honigfeld, Chandhok, & Spiegelman, 2012).

WASHINGTON

The Washington State TF-CBT and CBT+ Initiative in the public mental health system began in 2007 in response to increasing interest in trauma and posttraumatic stress as significant problems facing children. The public mental health system, primarily supported by Medicaid, serves poor children and those involved in the child welfare system, where the rates of trauma exposure are highest. In Washington, public mental health is managed by regional networks that oversee Medicaid services through contracts with licensed agencies in local communities. The agencies may also accept commercial insurance and provide some subsidized services to children who do not have insurance, but the large majority of clients are poor children receiving Medicaid. The Medicaid benefit is generous; it covers unlimited outpatient care as long as medical necessity criteria are met and also supports intensive services and supports for children with high-acuity needs, including Wraparound teams and access to inpatient care.

The CBT+ Initiative is a collaboration between the Washington State Department of Social and Health Services' Department of Behavioral Health and Recovery, Harborview Center for Sexual Assault and Traumatic Stress, based at a University of Washington teaching hospital, and the University of Washington Evidence-Based Practice Institute. It is fully supported by federal block-grant funds issued year to year at a cost of approximately $100,000 per year. The CBT+ Initiative strategies and elements have evolved over time, strongly informed by developments in the dissemination and implementation literature (e.g., Fixsen et al., 2005). Initially the program was designed as a training support program for TF-CBT (Cohen, Mannarino, & Deblinger, 2006). Over time the intervention model expanded to incorporate CBT for anxiety and depression and parent management training for behavior problems. The rationale was that posttraumatic stress, the clinical target for which TF-CBT is designed, affects only a small percentage of children seeking care in public mental health, whereas a broader CBT and parent management training

approach would encompass the clinical needs of 80% of children seeking service. One lesson learned in the early years was that providers did not generalize the CBT skills contained in TF-CBT to other clinical targets. Thus the initiative is now known as CBT+ (CBT plus TF-CBT). The goal of the initiative is to extend the reach of evidence-based practice within the public mental health system for children with a broad range of clinical needs.

A modified and streamlined learning collaborative model was adopted for training, using elements of the Breakthrough Series Collaborative (Institute for Healthcare Improvement, 2004). The CBT+ implementation model consists of a pre-training organizational consultation, a three-day learning session for 60–100 providers, and biweekly telephone case consultations for six months in groups of 10–15. The organizational consultation proactively establishes the expectation that the goal is a change in practice, which requires organizational commitment and supports. Originally it was handled in a lecture format with supporting documentation from research. Over time it has become a conversation with administrators about expectations, potential challenges, tips and suggestions, and anticipatory problem solving, and the clear communication that practice change is the goal. Minimally, a verbal commitment to the initiative is required before an organization can send staff to the training.

The three-day learning session has increasingly become skills and practice oriented. The CBT+ team has stripped away most of the lecture to concentrate on key clinical skills, all of which are practiced by participants during the class. The teaching approach for the providers is presented as a process parallel to that for delivering CBT+ with clients: brief psychoeducation, then modeling and rehearsal of the skill. The training uses case examples for practicing the key skills and is presented in a highly interactive, fun, fast-paced, and lively fashion. Providers are asked to make a stated intention of new practices they intend to undertake following the learning session, and this list is mailed to them after the first consultation call. Organizations must initially send a team consisting of a clinical supervisor and two clinicians; once the organization has a trained supervisor on site, it can just send clinicians.

The consultation calls are scheduled to begin within three weeks after the training. Consultants send introductory emails containing standardized measures, tip sheets, and other materials to stimulate enthusiasm for changing practice. Initially, the requirement was to attend 9 of 12 calls and to present a case during the six months of biweekly telephone consultations in order receive a certificate of completion. Recently, a requirement was added to enter online data documenting delivery of a course of CBT+ to at least one client. The consultants often send summary emails after calls, and tips are shared among consultants and their groups.

In addition to the trainings and consultations, the initiative has been involved in numerous other activities designed to support and provide reinforcement to providers, supervisors, and organizations in changing practice. The CBT+ team has developed resources for clinicians and for clients, including tip sheets and informational sheets on each clinical target. These resources are available on the CBT+ website maintained by Harborview (http://depts.washington.edu/hcsats/PDF/TF-%20CBT/CBT_Plus_NB.html). There is also a CBT+ listserv through which new resources are disseminated. Special attention has been focused on clinical supervisors, who are seen as crucial to sustainment of EBP; resources include a supervisor listserv maintained by Harborview, a monthly consultation call for supervisors, and an annual supervisors peer meeting. Highly motivated supervisors are selected to serve as co-consultants and are paid a modest fee to co-consult for a subsequent training cohort. An annual "advanced training" opportunity led by a nationally recognized speaker is also provided to staff who have completed the learning collaborative.

An online public roster and provider toolkit have been developed to support ongoing quality assurance and sustainment. The roster is a public website that lists qualified providers (http://ebproster.org) and is designed to promote consumer education and advocacy in selecting providers who offer EBP. It contains information about EBP, the various clinical targets and their treatments, and tips for choosing a provider. The toolkit is a provider-only section where providers enter information on their qualifications, on their cases, including standardized measures that are scored and immediately made available graphically, and on session structure and content. The toolkit is used to establish the criteria for rostering but is also being developed for use as an organizational and supervisory tool for establishing competence and collecting outcomes data and for active use by providers with their clients. For example, a provider can instruct a client to enter data on a measure that will be scored instantly and becomes available for feedback and discussion.

The CBT+ Initiative is widely known throughout the public mental health system in the state. Trainings are always fully enrolled, and there is a strong demand for additional learning collaboratives. The university-community collaboration appears to be highly successful. Harborview and the University of Washington Evidence-Based Practice Institute faculty strive to be helpful resources and are perceived as such by the practice community. Harborview is a working clinic and licensed mental health center, which lends credibility to the team. The University of Washington faculty is exceptionally responsive to the public mental health providers. The mutually respectful and collaborative relationship is reflected by the fact that individual providers as well as supervisors, administrators, and organizations frequently seek out team members for evidenced-based assistance with clinical and organizational problems.

The challenges facing public mental health adoption of EBP are well known (e.g., difficulty securing commitment to EBP, insufficient resources for widespread adoption, and lack of incentives and support for sustainment), and Washington State, like all states, is struggling with the practice and policy considerations. To extend its reach as much as possible, the CBT+ Initiative has focused on being practically useful, with the goal of modest but widespread increases in access to EBPs with corresponding improvements in child and family outcomes.

Although the Washington program is modestly supported compared with other states, the key aspect of the strategy has been to use elements of the Breakthrough Series Collaborative model, including organizational commitment, case consultation, and learning sessions. Other crucial aspects include (1) adopting a modular clinical model to extend the reach of EBP to the majority of children seeking services; (2) providing multiple supports to individual staff, their supervisors, and their organizations, including listservs, access to materials, incentives such as advanced training, the roster, and the toolkit; and (3) most important of all, cultivating EBP supervisors to assume leadership roles within their organizations.

COLORADO

In Colorado, the Division of Mental Health Services emphasizes the importance of access to quality and effective public mental health services and supports. Within child welfare, the Colorado Department of Human Services recently increased the demand and the funding support for core service providers to deliver and support evidence-based services that are proven to be effective. The department identified the expansion of access to evidence-based services to achieve successful child, youth, and family outcomes as a high-priority area (Aultman-Bettridge, Hall, & Selby, 2011). To address the service gap identified by key community leaders and professionals and to increase the state's capacity for delivering trauma-focused EBPs, the Evidence-Based Practice Training Initiative (EBTI) began in Colorado in January 2010. The EBTI is based at the Child Trauma Program of the Kempe Center for the Prevention and Treatment of Child Abuse and Neglect, a section of the Department of Pediatrics of the University of Colorado School of Medicine, located in Aurora.

The EBTI aims to build professionals' knowledge and skills related to delivering EBPs to abused and trauma-exposed youths and their families in mental health service settings. More specifically, the program aims to increase knowledge on (1) child abuse and trauma and their impact on mental health, including posttraumatic stress disorder, depression, and behavior problems; (2) evidence-based assessment and treatment for traumatized youths and their families; and (3) methods for ensuring successful implementation of EBPs in diverse practice settings.

The EBTI began with a six-month information-gathering process (including informational calls, meetings, and conferences) among mental health professionals, administrative leaders, and key stakeholders to assess interests, usual practices, barriers, and needs related to serving abused and traumatized children. Based on this informal needs and readiness assessment, TF-CBT was selected as the initial EBP to introduce to the community. Faculty members who are expert trainers in TF-CBT lead the initiative, provide expert clinical training, and oversee the evaluation plan.

The initiative began by offering TF-CBT training and implementation support to clinicians in the Denver Metropolitan area and outlying areas who were serving children and families, as well as to clinicians at the Kempe Center, University of Colorado Denver, and Children's Hospital Colorado. An inclusive and open process allowed any interested clinician with a master's degree (or currently in a master's degree program) to participate, regardless of whether other agency members or supervisors were participating.

Cohorts of approximately 20–40 clinicians receive a two-day, in-person TF-CBT training and are offered 6–12 months of follow-up clinical consultation to support implementation. Of the 416 clinicians who have attended the training thus far, nearly 50% have attended follow-up consultations, with an average of seven calls. This participation level is notable given that, for the initial EBTI cohorts, telephone consultation was not required. While project staff were well aware of the limited impact of training alone on sustained changes in practice (Beidas & Kendall, 2010; Sholomskas et al., 2005), the aim was to encourage clinicians "in the door" as a first step to learning about EBP. After establishing an in-person connection, the project staff strongly encouraged clinicians and agency leaders to engage in the implementation components that are important for sustained adoption of new practices—involvement of supervisors, expert consultation on cases following the in-person training, monitoring the progress of child/family treatment by collecting clinical outcomes metrics, and tracking fidelity. Involvement of administrative leaders was strongly recommended to support and facilitate the implementation effort, to overcome agency barriers, and to build infrastructure to sustain the practice in the agencies (Beidas et al., 2011). The strategies and elements of the EBTI have evolved as interest and demand for TF-CBT has increased and are directly informed by developments in the burgeoning dissemination and implementation science field (Herschell, McNeil, & McNeil, 2004; Kolko et al., 2012).

From the beginning, the bar was set high for participation requirements, while also maximizing engagement with community clinicians. The EBTI currently offers training and consultation packages with a strong recommendation that at least one supervisor be involved in all training and consultation efforts and a preference that supervisors take a TF-CBT "training case." Organizational consultation and involvement of agency leaders are also strongly encouraged. The EBTI model emphasizes inclusiveness of all practitioners who are committed to learning about EBPs, and thus private practitioners are included; these practitioners deliver services to a large number of children in many communities.

Participation in TF-CBT training currently requires that clinicians (1) attend a two-day, in-person learning session; (2) participate in bimonthly 60-minute telephone or videoconference case-consultation calls for a minimum of six months, in groups of 8–12; (3) take eligible cases as TF-CBT "training cases" to practice the use of the model; and (4) use standardized measures to assess and identify trauma exposure, track mental health symptoms, and monitor treatment response and outcomes. Completion of the free Web-based course (TF-CBTWeb) is required for all participants as preparatory work for the in-person training. EBTI faculty hold discussions with agency leaders about enhancing the organizational climate to adopt a new practice before providers attend the training. A subset of agencies in the EBTI are currently participating in more comprehensive implementation efforts, in which they commit to 12 months of ongoing bimonthly consultation, booster trainings at 4- to 6-month intervals, supervisor-specific training, and fidelity evaluation through audiotape reviews.

The teaching approach incorporates adult-learning principles, with modeling and skills rehearsal integrated into training and with small- and large-group skills practice opportunities. Short videotaped demonstrations of skills in real therapy cases are used, as well as engaging case examples to practice skills in small groups. The trainers offer live coaching of clinicians in implementing the skills. These learning approaches are also used during the bimonthly consultation calls, and videoconferencing helps to enhance participation and engagement. The EBTI supports clinicians in integrating standardized trauma measures to track the outcomes of clients receiving TF-CBT. Consultation is offered to agencies that wish to set up data systems to track progress. All participants also receive engaging materials such as worksheets and tip sheets to stimulate enthusiasm for beginning a new practice and to help them structure their TF-CBT work. The EBTI recently incorporated ongoing tracking during consultation calls, including case progress, number of practice cases, and completion of key TF-CBT components. The consultants often send follow-up emails with new tools, resources, and tips. Clinical innovations by EBTI clinicians are featured in a quarterly newsletter sent to all participants. The initiative is also tracking the frequency and quality of supervisors' involvement in consultation calls.

The initiative was launched at extremely low cost to professionals because the coordinating center was partially funded by SAMHSA as part of the NCTSN initiative and by small pockets of local/state funds. The estimated cost of implementing the EBTI ranged from $123,000 to $166,500 per year. The lower end of the range excludes costs for the built-in evaluation component, which includes construction of the Web-based survey, data management, and support for pre- to post-training follow-up administration and data summary for EBTI participants. Training packages are offered with different levels of implementation support, including introductory training in TF-CBT, clinical consultation calls on TF-CBT, supervisors' consultation calls, advanced booster trainings, audiotape reviews to assess TF-CBT fidelity and competency, and organizational support that includes incorporation of fidelity-monitoring tools, assessment selection, and development of systems to track child and family outcomes. As interest in and demand for TF-CBT increased, a required commitment to follow-up consultation was added. This requirement did not reduce demand for TF-CBT but, rather, increased engagement in and use of the model. The training packages vary in cost, depending on the number of implementation-support components chosen by the individual or agency. Because the EBTI offers "open trainings" in addition to closed trainings for specific agencies, low-cost alternatives are available, and payment installment options are offered to clinicians or students with financial barriers. After three years, the EBTI is now fully sustained by training and consultation income.

The EBTI is gaining positive recognition in the Colorado mental health community as a resource for clinicians, and there has been a strong, consistent demand for additional trainings. From January 2010 to October 2012, 416 mental health professionals from diverse practice settings (e.g., community mental health agencies, juvenile justice, residential treatment, private practice) participated in 16 training cohorts. Clinicians currently participating in the EBTI serve children and their families in 51 of the 64 Colorado counties, in the public and private mental health sectors. An ongoing evaluation offers feedback for improving the training efforts. Preliminary data from pre-training and six months' post-training show significant increases in the reported use of EBPs, such as a 44% increase in the reported use of standardized measures to assess trauma exposure and symptoms and a 58% increase in the reported use of TF-CBT in general practice with youths who are eligible for this therapy. Summarized findings are aggregated and presented for clinicians and agency leaders in quarterly newsletters and are discussed with interested agencies. Sustaining a new practice is always challenging, but successful strategies have been developed to sustain TF-CBT, such as clinicians organizing local peer TF-CBT consultation groups and "open" brown-bag lunches. The EBTI is continually providing implementation support to the trained clinicians. Evaluation data will provide information about the types and dosages of implementation support that correlate with sustained practice change. New SAMHSA/NCTSN funding will support efforts to bolster the supervisor arm of the initiative and the administrative support components and provide implementation support to EBTI clinicians who are interested in but have not yet attended the follow-up consultations or booster training. A Web-based learning portal is also being developed to support a listserv, to facilitate the sharing of clinical materials and use of screening tools, and to support the implementation and sustainment of TF-CBT.

CONCLUSIONS AND RECOMMENDATIONS

The examples from Connecticut, Washington, and Colorado provide three different approaches to statewide implementation of EBPs for children experiencing abuse or other forms of trauma. These approaches differ in many ways, including the focus of implementation (agency, clinician/supervisor team, or individual provider), training approach (ranging from a two-day training plus consultation to a year-long learning collaborative), training focus (a specific EBP or a components-based approach applicable to a range of children), and funding sources (state agencies, grants, and/or participants). These differences are primarily due to local conditions and funding, which has ranged from $100,000 to more than $400,000 annually.

Despite the different approaches and resources available in each of these states, the three implementation efforts share a number of elements informed by implementation science (e.g., Fixsen et al., 2005). First, each has made efforts to develop and maintain stakeholders' buy-in and a commitment to implementation and sustained practice change from the beginning. These efforts include assessing organizational readiness and capacity, requiring a commitment to practice change (either contractually or verbally), and other pre-training and ongoing work to support implementation. A strong demand for the implemented EBPs has allowed a competitive process for selection and/or the setting of a high bar for interested participants and agencies. This may have "filtered out" more casual and less committed agencies or staff, thus directing the limited resources to those providers most likely to successfully implement practice changes.

Second, each initiative has a training plan that goes beyond traditional clinical training. Didactic training is minimized in favor of interactive practice-based skills training, using adult-learning principles. An organizational commitment from senior administrators is required at least initially and sometimes throughout and even following the training period. Ongoing consultation is provided after the training through a variety of methods, including consultation calls, webinars, intranet sites, or additional trainings, and this is seen as integral to practice change and sustainment. The identification and use of "champions" to serve as peer supports or co-trainers is integrated into programs to further build experience and training capacity. Supervisors are seen as essential to implementation and warrant special attention and training, including the requirement that they become experienced in providing the EBP themselves.

Third, each initiative uses data to monitor treatment progress (standardized assessment measures) and implementation (e.g., number of children served), ranging from the use of limited data on one or more cases during training to the ongoing reporting of all cases during and after implementation. There is an emphasis on data systems that are simple and quick to use, provide helpful information to participants (e.g., scoring measures with graphed data), and provide feedback to staff and agencies about their implementation progress.

It is also clear that practice change takes time and that these efforts are just the beginning of statewide EBP implementations for child victims of abuse or other forms of trauma exposure. Common challenges continue to be the limited funding, staff turnover, increased time necessary to utilize EBPs, and limited financial or policy incentives for sustaining EBPs. For example, many staff and agencies report that the implementation and sustainment of an EBP take additional staff and agency time beyond that required for "treatment as usual"—for learning the model, receiving model-specific clinical supervision, preparing for sessions, reporting data, and other related tasks. These additional costs are typically not reimbursable and can be a burden for community mental health agencies. Despite these challenges and the limited research on the most effective approaches to implementation and sustainment, Connecticut, Washington, Colorado, and other states continue to actively pursue the expansion of EBPs. Over the next several years, the burgeoning implementation research field should further inform how to best channel limited resources for implementing and sustaining EBPs. To that end, we make the following recommendations for statewide EBP implementations:

1. Statewide dissemination efforts should be based on current implementation science and should include ongoing consultation, the use of data and quality-improvement approaches, and a focus on organizational change. The use of the Institute for Healthcare Improvement's Breakthrough Series model and learning collaboratives is one promising approach.

2. Before embarking on a statewide implementation initiative, states should devote considerable planning and capacity building to identify and gain buy-in from key stakeholders, identify resources and funding mechanisms, and develop a comprehensive implementation and sustainability plan.

3. Agencies and staff should be carefully selected based on a strong commitment to implementing and sustaining the practice, including completion of readiness assessments, a transparent selection process, clearly defined and high expectations for participation, and securing a commitment to implement and sustain the practice through memoranda of understanding and, if possible, contractual relationships.

4. Implementation should not be focused solely on clinicians and must include clinical supervisors, administrators, intake staff, and any other internal or external staff that intersect with the practice.

5. Ongoing collection of outcome and implementation data should be built into the implementation efforts to monitor successes and challenges and for quality improvement purposes.

6. Plans for sustaining the practice should be developed from the beginning, including ongoing training, data reporting, and promotion of EBP "champions."

7. Policies at the agency, local, and state levels, as well as reimbursement mechanisms that support the practice, must be aligned to support the implementation and sustainment of EBPs.

8. Statewide implementation efforts can use economies of scale to leverage limited resources to support multiple agencies and increase the scope and speed of practice change (e.g., having a central location or intermediary organization that is used for training and quality improvement).

9. Statewide implementation efforts in children's mental health should consider how the practice intersects with, and how to include, other child-serving systems and professionals, including child welfare, juvenile justice, education, early childhood, adult mental health, and pediatric practices.

10. Research is needed to compare different implementation strategies, including benefit-cost analyses. Strong evaluations should also be built into statewide implementation efforts to inform the direction of the field.

References

American Psychological Association. (2005). *Policy statement on evidence-based practice in psychology.* www.apa.org/practice/resources/evidence/evidence-based-statement.pdf

Aultman-Bettridge, T., Hall, E., & Selby, P. (2011). *Core services program evaluation annual report: State fiscal year 2010–2011.* Boulder, CO: Colorado Department of Human Services, Office of Children, Youth and Family Services, Division of Child Welfare Services.

Beidas, R. S., & Kendall, P. C. (2010). Training therapists in evidence-based practice: A critical review of studies from a systems-contextual perspective. *Clinical Psychology: Science and Practice, 17*(1), 1–30.

Beidas, R. S., Koerner, K., Weingardt, K. R., & Kendall, P. C. (2011). Training research: Practical recommendations for maximum impact. *Administration and Policy in Mental Health, 38*(4), 223–237.

Burns, B. J., Phillips, S. D., Wagner, H. R., Barth, R. P., Kolko, D. J., Campbell, Y., & Landsverk, J. (2004). Mental health need and access to mental health services by youth involved with child welfare: A national survey. *Journal of the American Academy of Child and Adolescent Psychiatry, 43*, 960–970.

Cary, C. E., & McMillen, J. C. (2012). The data behind the dissemination: A systematic review of Trauma-Focused Cognitive Behavioral Therapy for use with children and youth. *Children and Youth Services Review, 34*(4), 748–757.

Chadwick Center for Children and Families. (2004). *Closing the quality chasm in child abuse treatment: Identifying and disseminating best practices.* San Diego, CA: Author. www.chadwickcenter.org/Documents/Kaufman Report/ChildHosp-CTA brochure.pdf

Cohen, J. A., Mannarino, A. P., & Deblinger, E. (2006). *Treating trauma and traumatic grief in children and adolescents.* New York, NY: Guilford Press.

DeAngelis, T. (2010). Getting research into the real world. *Monitor on Psychology (American Psychological Association), 41*(10), 60.

Durlak, J. A., & DuPre, E. P. (2008). Implementation matters: A review of research on the influence of implementation on program outcomes and the factors affecting implementation. *American Journal of Community Psychology, 4*(3–4), 327–350.

Fixsen, D., Naoom, S., Blase, K., Friedman, R., & Wallace, F. (2005). *Implementation research: A synthesis of the literature* (FMHI publication No. 231). Tampa, FL: University of South Florida, Louis de la Parte Florida Mental Health Institute, National Implementation Research Network.

Franks, R. (2011). Role of the intermediary organization in promoting and disseminating best practices. *Emotional and Behavioral Disorders in Youth, 10*(4), 87–93.

Ganju, V. (2003). Implementation of evidence-based practices in state mental health systems: Implications for research and effectiveness studies. *Schizophrenia Bulletin, 29*(1), 125–131.

Greenhalgh, T., Robert, G., MacFarlane, F., Bate, P., & Kyriakidou, O. (2004). Diffusion of innovations in service organizations: Systematic review and recommendations. *Milbank Quarterly, 82*(4), 581–629.

Herschell, A. D., McNeil, C. B., & McNeil, D. W. (2004). Clinical child psychology's progress in disseminating empirically supported treatments. *Clinical Psychology: Science and Practice, 11*, 267–288.

Honigfeld, L., Chandhok, L., & Spiegelman, K. (2012). Engaging pediatricians in developmental screening: The effectiveness of academic detailing. *Journal of Autism and Developmental Disorders, 42*(6), 1175–1182.

Institute for Healthcare Improvement. (2004). The Breakthrough Series: IHI's Collaborative Model for Achieving Breakthrough Improvement. *Diabetes Spectrum, 17*(2), 97–101.

Institute of Medicine. (2004). *The chasm in quality: Select indicators from recent reports.* Washington, DC: Author. www.iom.edu /subpage.asp?id=14980

Jensen-Doss, A., Cusack, K. J., & de Arellano, M. A. (2008). Workshop-based training in trauma-focused CBT: An in-depth analysis of impact on provider practices. *Community Mental Health Journal, 44*, 227–244.

Kolko, D. J., Baumann, B. L., Herschell, A. D., Hart, J. A., Holden, E. A., & Wisniewski, S. R. (2012). Implementation of AF-CBT by community practitioners serving child welfare and mental health: A randomized trial. *Child Maltreatment, 17*(1), 32–46.

Landsverk, J. A., Burns, B. J., Stambaugh, L. F., & Rolls-Reutz, J. A. (2006). *Mental health care for children and adolescents in foster care: Review of research literature.* www.casey.org /Resources/Publications/pdf/MentalHealthCareChildren.pdf

Landsverk, J. A., Burns, B. J., Stambaugh, L. F., & Rolls-Reutz, J. A. (2009). Psychosocial interventions for children and adolescents in foster care: Review of research literature. *Child Welfare, 88*(1), 49–69.

Lang, J. M., Franks, R. P., & Bory, C. (2011, July). Statewide implementation of best practices: The Connecticut TF-CBT Learning Collaborative. *Impact.* Farmington, CT: Child Health and Development Institute of Connecticut. www.chdi .org/impact-tf-cbt-learningcollab

Langley, G. J., Moen, R. D., Nolan, K. M., Nolan, T. W., Norman, C. L., & Provost, L. P. (2009). *The improvement guide: A practical approach to enhancing organizational performance.* San Francisco, CA: Jossey-Bass.

Markiewicz, J., Elbert, L., Ling D., Amaya-Jackson, L., & Kisiel, C. (2006). *Learning collaborative toolkit: Raising the standard of care for traumatized children and their families.* Los Angeles, CA, and Durham, NC: National Child Traumatic Stress Network. www.nctsn.org/nctsn_assets/pdfs/lc/Module_all.pdf

McHugh, R. K., & Barlow, D. H. (2010). Dissemination and implementation of evidence-based psychological interventions: A review of current efforts. *American Psychologist, 65*(2), 73–84.

McLennan, J. D., Wathen, C. N., MacMillan, H. L., & Lavis, J. N. (2006). Research-practice gaps in child mental health. *Journal of the American Academy of Child and Adolescent Psychiatry, 45*(6), 658–665.

Meyers, D. C., Durlak, J. A., & Wandersman, A. (2012). The quality implementation framework: A synthesis of critical steps in the implementation process. *American Journal of Community Psychology, 50*(3–4), 462–480.

Sholomskas, D. E., Syracuse-Siewert, G., Rounsaville, B. J., Ball, S. A., Nuro, K. F., & Carroll, K. M. (2005). We don't train in vain: A dissemination trail of three strategies of training clinicians in cognitive-behavioral therapy. *Journal of Consulting and Clinical Psychology 73*(1), 106–115.

Stahmer, A. C., Leslie, L. K., Hurlburt, M., Barth, R. P., Webb, M. B., Landsverk, J., & Zhang, J. (2005). Developmental and behavioral needs and service use for young children in child welfare. *Pediatrics, 116*(4),891–900.

Stith, S., Pruitt, I., Dees, J., Fronce, M., Green, N., Som, A., & Linkh, D. (2006). Implementing community-based prevention programming: A review of the literature. *Journal of Primary Prevention, 27*(6), 599–617.

Weiss, B., Catton, T., & Harris, V. (2000). A 2-year follow-up of the effectiveness of traditional child psychotherapy. *Journal of Consulting and Clinical Psychology, 68*, 1094–1101.

Creating a Culture of Wellness for Providers in Harm's Way

GENERAL CONSIDERATIONS

Providers who work with children, families, and adults who have been exposed to trauma consistently report experiences of work-related distress. Regardless of providers' age, profession, training, or years on the job, exposure to a client's or patient's trauma has a profound, unique impact on each individual. For some, there are lingering traumatic stress reactions such as avoidance, hyperarousal, or intrusive thoughts. For others, trauma triggers related to their own trauma history are most distressing. Some report traumatic stress related to being directly in harm's way in the process of doing their work; others just feel a sense of burnout, stress, and fatigue. In seeking to understand the inherent complexity of trauma experiences in general, we are learning more about the impact of factors such as prior trauma exposure, promotive and protective factors, neurobiology, culture, somatic and emotional responses, safety concerns, breeches in social contracts, and environmental stressors on the effects of and recovery from trauma exposure. These same factors come into play in understanding providers' secondary trauma reactions, creating a particular challenge in defining and addressing their impact on the individual, organization, and larger systems. The goals of this chapter are to highlight these risk factors and the strategies needed to develop a network of wellness-focused support systems for early intervention.

Increased knowledge of the impact of trauma on both mental and physical well-being expands our awareness of the inherent risk of providing services to those who have been in harm's way. By better understanding the potential exposure to multiple risk factors for providers who work with victims of trauma, individuals and organizations can identify and implement intervention strategies to create a network of support and wellness. As we expand implementation of trauma-informed models of practice, this wellness component for providers increasingly becomes a challenging issue for both individuals and organizations. In a truly trauma-informed system, the impact of secondary traumatic stress (STS), vicarious trauma (VT), and compassion fatigue (CF) would be integrated into early-intervention policy and self-care and resiliency-building practice. Organizations and training institutions have been working diligently to keep up with the proliferation of trauma-focused evidence-based treatment models, but few training protocols or implementation guidelines formally address the impact of the work on students, interns, medical providers, legal practitioners, child welfare workers, and mental health providers. This, then, becomes a critical time to begin to establish a network of support to build resilience and sustainability into professional trauma-focused practice.

Both graduate school programs and postgraduate trauma-focused evidence-based treatment training typically fail to include topics related to prevention of and intervention in the occupational hazards for the provider associated with actually doing the work. Professional training for social workers, mental health workers, and other first-responder providers rarely includes any training on the impact of working with victims of trauma, on primary trauma, or on compassion fatigue. Thus our workforce is unprepared for the potential psychological and physiological toll of the work ahead of them. This also becomes a missed opportunity to create networks of support in a training environment so that students can learn and begin to practice self-care and early-intervention skills before they have a critical incident in their professional careers. This oversight contributes to isolation and perpetuation of the unspoken message that to be successful, providers should be able to handle whatever stress or distress is related to this work. To establish a viable network of support, it is critical that, as part of the training process, we change this unspoken culture so that the field begins to acknowledge the inherent risk to providers in caring for traumatized children and families. Students and trainees must get the message that to do good work, we must be able to identify the risks and develop the skills for early intervention, resiliency, and wellness. This shift alone would greatly enhance the development of stronger networks of research, policy change, and a supported and sustainable workforce.

The current inconsistent application of training and organizational policies that promote workforce wellness and resiliency in the implementation of trauma-informed models of practice can often make cross-system collaboration and communication challenging. Often, staff and organizations are overwhelmed with providing services in high-need environments with few resources, leaving little time and organizational support for wellness interventions for secondary traumatic stress, compassion fatigue, and burnout. In an era when trauma-informed practice models are becoming key to system collaboration, it is surprising that inclusion of the impact of trauma exposure for the provider is typically not part of the conversations about implementing best practice. As a trainer and consultant in this area, I am frequently called upon to come up with solutions to help staff, supervisors, and managers cope with this issue; however, change in systems models is slow and resistant. The focus of this chapter is to bring to light the many resources and networks available to individuals and organizations doing this work. Many agencies and institutions recognize the problem but are not able to build into their policy and procedures effective strategies to manage it, and little research is available on effective strategies for individuals or organizations. The increase in training and implementation in trauma-focused practices makes our providers more adept at addressing the impact and recovery for trauma victims but increases the likelihood that they will be given more cases with increased severity, which means higher risk for secondary trauma exposure, compassion fatigue, and burnout. The current focus on trauma-informed practice associated with higher provider exposure makes the need for viable solutions a critical next step in the field of trauma work.

There is a growing movement to address this need by both individuals and organizations across the country. The National Child Traumatic Stress Network (NCTSN) has developed a series of Core Concepts on Child Trauma that include the impact on providers when working with traumatized children and families. Other training materials developed in the NCTSN include training and information on reducing the impact of secondary traumatic stress, vicarious trauma, primary exposure, and compassion fatigue. Some of these professional NCTSN training products are available to download (without charge) from the NCTSN website. Examples include the Child Welfare Trauma Training Toolkit and the Resource Parent Workshop training materials, developed to help child welfare workers and parents increase trauma-informed practice. The Resilience Alliance Handbook developed by Administration of Children's Services–New York University, also available at no cost on the NCTSN website, is a workbook designed to promote resilience and reduce secondary trauma among child welfare staff. Also available are NCTSN factsheets that provide general information on secondary traumatic stress, as well as a series of webinars by STS experts for judges and legal professionals, for providers working with young children, on trauma in schools, terrorism, and disaster, and on the impact of culture on secondary trauma. Many evidence-based trauma intervention developers and trainers are also beginning to include material on risk factors, self-care practices, and reflective supervision models that support resiliency along with best practice in treatment implementation. The cumulative effect of this shift is to create more awareness and change in the way we define best practice to include workforce wellness in trauma-informed model implementation, organizational policy, and systems collaboration. This gives credibility and validity to the idea that organizations and systems should assume a level of accountability, not only for the bottom-line productivity of their workers, but also to create sustainable best practices that include policy, training, and implementation of wellness strategies to address the occupational risks associated with working with victims of trauma and abuse.

Strategies must include individuals and organizations working together to promote protection and resiliency practices to create a sustainable and supportive environment. Establishing a growing network of awareness and support requires both individuals and organizations to change the way they think about their work and work environment. For individual providers or students, valuing wellness and understanding their own personal risk factors increases their ability to do their best work and to be mindful of when they need to reduce the number of trauma cases, prepare for a challenging client, or know when to reach out for help from a supervisor, coach, or clinician trained in this area. Organizations must recognize the value in implementing strategies to promote wellness and resilience and see the results: reduced absenteeism, staff turnover, and low performance and improved system outcomes. This organizational and individual shift toward improved practice, policy, and awareness can nurture a growing network of support, risk reduction, and reversal of the pervasive experience of compassion fatigue and traumatic stress reactions in the workforce.

KEY CONCEPTS AND DEFINITION OF TERMS

Some of the current challenges in developing effective organizational strategies to address traumatic stress reactions among providers are related to the inconsistencies with which the various terms have been used and defined. Although the common terms are complementary, there are some distinctions that are critical in understanding the individual impact and experience of each, and it is important to know that there is still ongoing development and refinement of these definitions.

Primary Trauma

To best understand the impact of working with children and families exposed to trauma in often stressful and challenging work environments, it is important to clarify some of the major risk factors discussed in the literature. Each factor has a different origin, impact, and response needed to sustain work-life balance. Intervention strategies can then be personalized to enhance resiliency, recovery, and protective factors related to each individual's history, exposure, and personal vulnerability. *Primary trauma* is most commonly defined as direct exposure to traumatic events, but this is often broken down further into direct exposure in the past or in early childhood and direct exposure experienced by some workers as part of their job.

TRAUMA HISTORY. Those in the helping professions often come to the work because of their own exposure to negative life experiences from early childhood and beyond. Just as the clients that we serve are vulnerable to trauma triggers, flashbacks, numbing, hypervigilance, and other trauma response symptoms in certain situations, so providers, in the process of doing their professional work, also are vulnerable to experiencing a trauma reaction or trigger related to their own trauma history. Depending on the severity of the reaction and exposure to other risk factors, this response can range from mild to severe. Developing awareness about this vulnerability and being mindful at any given moment of one's own capacity to manage trauma triggers from past experiences are essential elements in practicing self-care. Laura van Dernoot Lipsky, in *Trauma Stewardship* (2009), talks about "trauma mastery" as an ongoing process of managing and processing one's own past traumatic experiences. This is often a primarily unconscious way of coping with trauma triggers, hyperarousal, avoidance, and intrusive experiences such as flashbacks or nightmares. She encourages processing these experiences from a place of self-compassion and empathy, but she highlights the importance of becoming more aware of the specific risk factors associated with working in the field of trauma and being triggered by these past events. This can also create more vulnerability to vicarious trauma and shifts in personal worldviews with prolonged exposure.

DIRECT EXPOSURE. The term *direct exposure* can refer to current personal exposure to traumatic events, such as a natural disaster or assault, and to trauma experienced by work-related exposure. Françoise Mathieu, in *Compassion*

Fatigue Workbook (2012), describes this kind of impact—a "primary" impact because it is happening to the individual. During a dangerous or frightening experience that occurs in the line of duty, the individual can potentially be in harm's way or overwhelmed by the horror or terror of the situation. Many providers, such as workers in crisis response, disaster, and terrorism, as well as first-responders such as fire, police, and emergency medical workers, experience this every day. There can be both a lingering response to an individual event and a cumulative stress response over time.

Secondary Trauma

Secondary trauma refers to indirect exposure to traumatic events. Typically, this means that there is no real danger and that the individual is not actually present at the scene of the event but rather comes to know about the incident or experience by hearing about it, reading or listening to material, or working with victims who are retelling the details of their experiences. Babette Rothschild, in *Help for the Helper* (2006), describes an additional risk factor of "mirror empathy" and the neurophysiology of experiencing another person's experience. *Empathy* is described as an autonomic nervous system state that mirrors the emotional experience of another person. So one not only hears the story but can be affected both mentally and physically by the experience of empathizing with the storyteller.

SECONDARY TRAUMATIC STRESS. According to Charles Figley (2012), *secondary traumatic stress* is a set of observable reactions to working with traumatized people and mirrors the symptoms of posttraumatic stress disorder (PTSD). The source of this trauma does not emanate directly from an event; rather, it comes to us indirectly. Others define STS as the result of bearing witness to a traumatic event (or series of events) that leads to PTSD-like symptoms of avoidance, hyperarousal, and intrusive thoughts or imagery (Mathieu, 2012). Rothschild (2006) gives a detailed description of the literature associated with the idea that empathic engagement with victims or survivors increases vulnerability to traumatic stress reactions through unconscious mirroring. This process induces associated feelings and autonomic nervous system reactions. Empathy is a highly integrative process involving somatic, cognitive, and neurological processes that may lead to PTSD-like reactions. Just as in direct exposure to traumatic events, protective and promotive factors such as resiliency, a supportive network of family, friends, and coworkers, and self-care practices can reduce the impact of STS reactions.

VICARIOUS TRAUMA. The term *vicarious trauma* is defined by Saakvitne and Pearlman (1996) as a transformation of the helper's inner experience resulting from empathic engagement with survivors' trauma material and a sense of responsibility or commitment to help. The authors go on to describe the social cost of VT manifesting in cynicism and despair that results in a loss to society of hope and the positive action it fuels. Many of us enter the helping professions with a commitment to making a difference in the lives of others and creating positive change in the world. We are often unprepared for the toll this work takes. When we lose hope, we lose an important part of what we have to offer our patients and clients; we lose the capacity to share our belief in the possibility of healing and change.

VT responses may manifest as changes in one's belief about the self or the world, one's spiritual beliefs, or one's sense of emotional stability and groundedness. Some experience changes in trust of their own judgment or the judgment of others, changes in their sense of personal or family safety, or a feeling of losing control over their life or the ability to affect others. Other noted changes can involve the ability to be alone or to be with others, as well as changes in intimacy and the relationship with one's own body. There may be a diminished perception of self-capacity or inner sense of balance, and decreased work satisfaction and motivation for doing the work are also common (Greenwald, 2005; Saakvitne & Pearlman, 1996). Unlike STS, VT cannot be measured directly, but it can be evaluated using a number of trait-based tendencies in responding to trauma (Figley, 2012).

BURNOUT. The experience of *burnout* is conceptualized as a psychological and physiological response to prolonged occupational exposure to demanding interpersonal situations that produce psychological strain and provide inadequate support (Meichenbaum, 2003). This can be reflected in the kind of stress and frustration caused by the workplace, such as poor pay, unrealistic work demands, heavy workload, long shifts, poor management, or inadequate supervision. Burnout can be seen in any occupation where these elements are present and is a unique stressor that increases vulnerability to VT and STS (Mathieu, 2012).

COMPASSION FATIGUE. The idea of *compassion fatigue* was redefined in 1995 by Figley in his book of the same name. He suggested that human service providers, both professional and volunteer, absorb the pain that they treat, leading to health consequences. Caregivers' needs can be overlooked, not only by supervisors and fellow caregivers, but by the providers themselves. This kind of stress response can be measured and linked to decreased immune system function (Figley, 2012). CF often can be seen in relief workers and disaster responders when they are immersed in overwhelming need by large numbers of victims. It also can be prevalent in systems where the needs of the community far exceed the resources of the individuals and organizations that serve them, such as child welfare and community mental health organizations. Often, workers in these organizations do not recognize that their compassionate work can lead to a sense of being overwhelmed and exhausted.

SIGNS AND SYMPTOMS: HOW DO YOU KNOW IF IT'S HAPPENED TO YOU?

The risk factors described above have a specific set of signs and symptoms associated with each kind of experience. Individuals are affected by this work in their own way and may experience one or all of these risk factors. Thus, in developing strategies to reduce the impact—ways to generate real solutions and interventions—it is critical to be able to identify what gets to us and why.

As stated above, *secondary traumatic stress* results from a trauma reaction in response to trauma experienced by others, often in the workplace. Its symptoms are often indistinguishable from those of direct exposure and may include:

- Re-experiencing: nightmares, intrusive thoughts, triggers
- Avoidance: efforts to avoid reminders, numbing, detachment, withdrawal
- Arousal: hypervigilance, trouble concentrating, being quick to anger

Signs of *vicarious trauma* can be related more to personal schemas or beliefs about the self and the world (Saakvitne & Pearlman, 1996) than to direct or indirect trauma exposure. VT can include changes in:

- Beliefs about the world
- Spiritual beliefs
- Sense of self, groundedness, and emotional stability
- Sense of personal and family safety
- Trust of oneself and/or others
- Way of judging people
- Sense of control
- Ability to be alone, or to be with others
- Relationship to one's own body

Other signs related to *compassion fatigue* and *burnout* include cognitive effects such as:

- Negative bias, pessimism
- All-or-nothing thinking
- Loss of perspective and critical thinking skills
- Threat focus (i.e., seeing clients, peers, supervisor as the enemy)
- Decreased self-monitoring
- Intrusive thoughts
- Minimizing

The *social impact* can be seen, both in the workplace and at home, as:

- Reduction in collaboration
- Withdrawal and loss of social support
- Factionalism
- Conflicts—easily angered
- Isolation
- Difficulty trusting—worry about getting close
- Avoidance

The *emotional toll* can also include experiences of:

- Helplessness
- Hopelessness
- Feeling overwhelmed
- Depression
- Worry—realistic and unrealistic fears
- Anger/irritability
- Feeling numb

Physical complaints are also commonly reported, such as:

- Headaches
- Tense muscles
- Fatigue / sleep difficulties
- Nightmares
- Stomach problems / nausea
- Feeling jittery
- Frequent illness

Clearly, individual well-being and client care can be compromised if a provider is affected by the signs and symptoms described above. Some may believe they can no longer provide services to their clients and end up leaving their profession altogether.

WHO IS AT RISK?

There are many studies indicating that signs of vicarious trauma, compassion fatigue, secondary trauma, and burnout occur across the various helping professions, including teachers, mental health professionals, advocates, clergy, nurses, physicians, prison staff, judges, lawyers, police officers, and so on. Secondary traumatic stress is becoming recognized in the literature as a common occupational hazard for professionals working with trauma. Studies show that 6%–26% of therapists working with trauma victims and up to 50% of child welfare workers are at high risk (National Child Traumatic Stress Network, 2011). A few of these groups are highlighted here.

Child welfare workers deal with child abuse, neglect, family violence, community violence, and stressful work environments and may be particularly vulnerable to signs and symptoms of cynicism, anger, or irritability, as well as anxiety or new fears about their safety or the safety of their family. They may experience emotional detachment, a sense of numbness, depression, and sadness. They often report intrusive imagery about victims, patients, or clients, as well as nightmares or difficulty sleeping. They may also experience changes in worldview and a sense of futility or pessimism, changes in spiritual beliefs, and diminished self-care. Increased physical ailments and illness or use of alcohol/drugs to forget about work or relax are also reported (Osofsky, Putnam, & Lederman, 2008). Common sources of secondary trauma and stress can also include the death of a child or adult among one's cases, an investigation about a particular client, traumatic grief and loss experienced by a grieving family, concerns about adequate funding and agency resources, and constant concerns about public scrutiny and scapegoating.

Mental health providers and supervisors working with clients who have experienced trauma are vulnerable to many of the same risk factors as child welfare workers. An additional factor that has been characterized as both protective and a risk is important to mention here. Studies have shown that training in the implementation of trauma-focused evidence-based practices can provide the structure and support needed to reduce compassion fatigue and burnout. However, those with specialized training in trauma treatment usually have a higher trauma caseload, which has been associated with increased risk (Sprang, Clark, & Whitt-Woosley, 2007).

Judges and legal professionals are often affected by their large caseloads and increased stress levels at work, by the need to maintain a nonbiased perspective, by isolation related to the confidential nature of their work, by a nonsupportive culture in dealing with the impact of STS, and by compassion fatigue, burnout, anger, frustration, and a sense of helplessness or hopelessness about their cases (Osofsky, Putnam, & Lederman, 2008). Domestic violence lawyers and immigration judges are found to have significantly higher levels of burnout and secondary trauma (Mathieu, 2012).

Medical professionals such as nurses and physicians report high levels of burnout, and working in chronic care or with terminally ill patients is reportedly a significant factor (Osofsky, Putnam, & Lederman, 2008). A study by Sprang and colleagues (2007) showed that psychiatrists were particularly susceptible to secondary trauma when compared with other health care workers who provide direct care. Surgeons report suicidal ideation 1.5–3 times more often than the general population; studies indicate that this is strongly related to symptoms of depression and a surgeon's degree of burnout (Mathieu, 2012).

ASSESSMENT STRATEGIES

Self-assessment is the most common approach for individuals' identification and management of risk factors associated with working with traumatized populations. This is an important part of any intervention strategy. By tracking the onset, duration, and severity of the many signs and symptoms described above, individuals can begin to become mindful of their personal risk factors and devise strategies, both in the workplace and at home, to support a wellness plan. See the Resources section below for some self-assessment suggestions.

Organizations can take a more formal approach and implement various assessment strategies, as simple as including reflective supervision on the risk factors associated with work or periodically requiring staff to complete formal measures such as the Professional Quality of Life Scale (ProQOL), developed by Charles Figley and Beth Stamm (Figley & Stamm, 1996; Stamm, 1995, 1996). The results of formal assessments can be used both to give feedback to staff and to assess the prevalence of STS, vicarious trauma, and burnout agency-wide. An additional benefit to using the ProQOL is a scale on compassion satisfaction, which measures individuals' levels of satisfaction with their work.

INTERVENTION STRATEGIES

Different experiences require different strategies. Primary trauma, secondary traumatic stress, vicarious trauma, compassion fatigue, and burn out—each requires a slightly different response to create an effective self-care plan. Initially, some kind of evaluation strategy is needed to identify the type and severity of distress. Early-intervention strategies— including psychoeducation, clinical supervision, flextime scheduling, self-care "buddy relationships," and workplace self-care groups such as meditation or yoga—can be implemented in the workplace. Organizations can also provide training on intervention and self-care strategies, such as mindfulness training, reflective supervision, and self-care practices, as well as provide time for informal gatherings for peer support, referrals for employee assistance by trained providers, and/or changes in job assignment. Use of evidence-based practices can also reduce risks, as long as caseload management is an integral part of implementation.

A multidimensional approach including direct practitioners, coworkers, supervisors, administrators, board members, and community members should all be included in self-care training and planning. Successful organizational intervention strategies include the triad of psychoeducation, skills training, and supervision. As workers gain knowledge and experience about managing the stress reactions associated with their work, they are empowered to integrate self-care and early-intervention practices into their work, creating a profound cultural shift in the concept of best practice. This, combined with policy change to create a supportive work environment and the resources to implement these strategies, can create a network of support for providers.

There are numerous opportunities and networks to create support for individuals and organizations to address the occupational hazards associated with working with those who have experienced trauma (see the Resources section). By beginning to implement these strategies, we can create a cultural change in the concept of "best practice" that includes a supportive network of individuals who prioritize wellness and supportive work environments as essential components of our professions.

RESOURCES

The following websites can connect you to valuable, comprehensive resources.

- The Compassion Fatigue Awareness Project (http:// compassionfatigue.org) is described on its website as "dedicated to educating caregivers about authentic, sustainable self-care and aiding organizations in their goal of providing healthy, compassionate care to those whom they serve." The website has many resources, including training materials, workbooks, and texts for caregivers working in many professions.
- Compassion Fatigue Solutions (http://compassionfatigue.ca) provides skill-based workshops, consulting services, and training materials focusing on compassion fatigue, self-care, and workplace wellness. The website has a variety of resources, including videos, an extensive bibliography of books and workbooks, assessment tools, and a blog related to compassion fatigue and vicarious trauma.
- The Figley Institute (http://figleyinstitute.com /indexMain.html) offers cutting-edge training and continuing education programs developed by Dr. Charles R. Figley, Dr. Kathleen Regan Figley, and adjunct faculty for those who provide relief to emotionally traumatized individuals and communities. The website has information on a variety of courses and trainings to support professionals in "reducing the impact of working with traumatized populations."
- Fisher and Associates (www.fisherandassociates.org) focuses on organizational health and workplace wellness in sectors with high risk for stress, burnout, and exposure to direct and vicarious trauma. The tools on this website are geared toward managers working in diverse fields, including the comprehensive e-course "When Working Hurts: Effectively Addressing Stress in Trauma-Informed Workplaces."
- The Headington Institute (www.headington-institute .org/Default.aspx?tabid=2648) provides "Care for Caregivers Worldwide" by promoting the physical hardiness, emotional resilience, and spiritual vitality of humanitarian relief and development personnel. Through this website you can access a variety of resources for care providers, including counseling services and trainings.
- The Joyful Heart Foundation's (http://joyfulheart foundation.org) mission is to heal, educate, and empower survivors of sexual assault, domestic violence, and child abuse and to shed light into the darkness that surrounds these issues. Through this website you can find resources to support healers as well as survivors in creating a practice of self-care and developing a sense of balance in life.

Additional resource websites include the following:

- Compassion Fatigue Self-Test (www.ptsdsupport.net /compassion_fatigue-selftest.html)
- Cops Alive (www.copsalive.com), with information strategies and tools to help cops plan happy, healthy, and successful careers, relationships, and lives
- The National Center on Family Homelessness (http:// 508.center4si.com/SelfCareforCareGivers.pdf), includ-

ing "What about You? A Workbook for Those Who Work with Others."

- The National Child Traumatic Stress Network (http://nctsn.org); search for Resiliency Manual; Secondary Traumatic Stress Fact Sheet; Secondary Traumatic Stress Webinar Series
- The National Health Care for the Homeless Council (www.nhchc.org), described as "Breaking the links between poor health and homelessness"; search for Self-Care; Compassion Fatigue
- ProQOL, Professional Quality of Life Elements Theory and Measurement (http://proqol.org)
- Trauma Stewardship Institute (http://traumasteward ship.com)

References

Figley, C. R. (1995). *Compassion fatigue: Coping with secondary traumatic stress disorder in those who treat the traumatized.* New York, NY: Brunner-Mazel.

Figley, C. R. (2012, spring). Helping that hurts: Child welfare secondary traumatic stress reactions. In *CW 360°: Secondary trauma and the child welfare workforce* (pp. 4–5). Saint Paul, MN: Center for Advanced Studies in Child Welfare, School of Social Work, College of Education and Human Development, University of Minnesota.

Figley, C. R., & Stamm, B. H. (1996). Psychometric view of Compassion Fatigue Self Test. In B. H. Stamm (Ed.), *Measurement of stress, trauma, and adaptation.* Lutherville, MD: Sidran Press.

Greenwald, R. (2005). *Child trauma handbook: A guide for helping trauma-exposed children and adolescents.* Binghamton, NY: Haworth Press.

Mathieu, F. (2012). *The compassion fatigue workbook: Creative tools for transforming compassion fatigue and vicarious traumatization.* New York, NY: Routledge / Taylor & Francis Group.

Meichenbaum, D. (2003). Stress inoculation training. In W. O'Donohue, J. E. Fisher, & S. C. Hays (Eds.), *Cognitive behavior therapy: Applying empirically supported techniques in your practice* (pp. 407–410). Hoboken, NJ: John Wiley & Sons.

National Child Traumatic Stress Network, Secondary Traumatic Stress Committee. (2011). *Secondary traumatic stress: A fact sheet for child-serving professionals.* Los Angeles, CA, and Durham, NC: National Center for Child Traumatic Stress.

Osofsky, J. D., Putnam, F. W., & Lederman, C. S. (2008). How to maintain emotional health when working with trauma. *Juvenile and Family Court Journal, 59*(4), 91–102.

Rothschild, B. (2006). *Help for the helper: Self-care strategies for managing burnout and stress.* New York, NY: W. W. Norton and Company.

Saakvitne, K. W., & Pearlman, L. A. (1996). *Transforming the pain. A workbook on vicarious traumatization.* New York, NY: Traumatic Stress Institute and Center for Adult & Adolescent Psychotherapy.

Sprang, G., Clark, J. J., & Whitt-Woosley, A. (2007). Compassion fatigue, compassion satisfaction, and burnout: Factors impacting a professional's quality of life. *Journal of Loss and Trauma: International Perspectives on Stress & Coping, 12*(3), 259–280.

Stamm, B. H. (1995). *Secondary traumatic stress: Self-care issues for clinicians, researchers, and educators.* Baltimore, MD: Sidran Press.

Stamm, B. H. (1996). *Measurement of stress, trauma, and adaptation.* Lutherville, MD: Sidran Press.

van Dernoot Lipsky, L. (2009). *Trauma stewardship: An everyday guide to caring for self while caring for others.* San Francisco, CA: Berrett-Koehler Publishers.

Additional Reading

Anderson, D. G. (2000). Coping strategies and burnout among veteran child protection workers. *Child Abuse & Neglect, 24*(6), 839–848.

Bober, T., & Regehr, C. (2006). Strategies for reducing secondary or vicarious trauma: Do they work? *Brief Treatment and Crisis Intervention, 6*(1), 1–9.

Bober, T., Regehr, C., & Zhou, N. (2006). Development of the Coping Strategies Inventory for trauma counselors. *Journal of Loss and Trauma, 11,* 71–83.

Bride, B. E. (2007). Prevalence of secondary traumatic stress among social workers. *Social Work, 52*(1), 63–70.

Bride, B. E., & Figley, C. R. (2007). The fatigue of compassionate social workers: An introduction to the Special Issue on Compassion Fatigue. *Clinical Social Work Journal, 35,* 151–153.

Bride, B. E., Radey, M., & Figley, C. R. (2007). Measuring compassion fatigue. *Clinical Social Work Journal, 35,* 155–163.

Depanfilis, D. (2006). Compassion fatigue, burnout, and compassion satisfaction: Implications for retention of workers. *Child Abuse & Neglect, 30,* 1067–1069.

Figley, C. R. (Ed.). (2002). *Treating compassion fatigue.* New York, NY: Brunner-Routledge.

Folette, V. M., Polusny, M. M., & Milbeck, K. (1994). Mental health and law enforcement professionals: Trauma history, psychological symptoms, and impact of providing services to child sexual abuse survivors. *Professional Psychology: Research and Practice, 25*(3), 275–282.

Kanter, J. (2007). Compassion fatigue and secondary traumatization: A second look. *Clinical Social Work Journal, 35,* 289–293.

Killian, K. D. (2008). Helping till it hurts? A multimethod study of compassion fatigue, burnout, and self-care in clinicians working with trauma survivors. *Traumatology, 14,* 32.

Kravits, K., McAllister-Black, R., Grant, W., & Kirk, C. (2010). Self-care strategies for nurses: A psycho-educational intervention for stress reduction and the prevention of burnout. *Applied Nursing Research, 23,* 130–138.

O'Halloran, M. S., & O'Halloran, T. (2001). Secondary traumatic stress in the classroom: Ameliorating stress in graduate students. *Teaching of Psychology, 28,* 92.

Radey, M., & Figley, C. R. (2007). The social psychology of compassion. *Clinical Social Work Journal, 35,* 207–214.

Schauben, L. J., & Frazier, P. A. (1995). Vicarious trauma: The effects on female counselors of working with sexual violence survivors. *Psychology of Women Quarterly, 19,* 49.

Weinstein, N., Brown, K. W., & Ryan, R. M. (2009). A multimethod examination of the effects of mindfulness on stress attribution, coping, and emotional well-being. *Journal of Research in Personality, 43,* 374–385.

MARCELA M. TORRES, PH.D.
MONICA M. FITZGERALD, PH.D.
KIMBERLY L. SHIPMAN, PH.D.

25

The Importance of Therapist and Family Engagement in Treatment Implementation

GENERAL CONSIDERATIONS

As noted throughout this book, there are several evidence-supported and innovative approaches for treating children and families who have experienced abuse and other types of traumatic events. Unfortunately, these evidence-supported treatments are still not readily available and accessible to all children and families who need them (Burns et al., 2004). In particular, children affected by maltreatment and trauma exposure may be less likely than other children with mental health needs to be identified and referred for services (Chadwick Center for Children and Families, 2004) and also less likely to be engaged and retained in services once their family makes contact with a treatment provider (Lau & Weisz, 2003). Thanks to burgeoning research, there is a growing understanding of the factors that contribute to the service-need gap for families in community care settings and urban areas, and we have identified specific evidence-based strategies and skills for engaging families in effective services (e.g., McKay et al., 2004; Nock & Kazdin, 2001; Szapocznik et al., 1990).

In this chapter we define what is meant by engagement, review common challenges to engaging families affected by child maltreatment and trauma in treatment, and focus on the role of the therapist in family engagement and the importance of cultural competence. We describe specific examples of effective and theoretically derived therapeutic engagement strategies for connecting children and families with evidence-supported treatments (ESTs).

DEFINITIONS AND DESCRIPTIONS OF ENGAGEMENT IN CHILD MENTAL HEALTH SERVICE DELIVERY

Several definitions of "engagement" in the context of child and family mental health service delivery have been offered in the literature, along with attempts by researchers to develop a common understanding of the term. For the purposes of this chapter, *engagement* is defined as including both (1) active and collaborative *participation* in treatment and (2) a *process* involving all activities from identification of families in need of mental health services to completion of treatment. Both of these components are keys to understanding the effective engagement of families in treatment.

Engagement as Participation in Treatment

Our conceptualization of engagement as participation emphasizes *quality* of participation in treatment, in addition to attendance. Although important, attendance alone does not correspond to genuine engagement, effort, response to treatment, or improved behavioral outcomes as much as does *active and collaborative participation* in treatment (Cunningham & Henggeler, 2004; Nix, Bierman, & McMahon, 2009; Yatchmenoff, 2005). Active and collaborative participation thus implies some level of client intentionality or motivation in completing treatment tasks and requires the therapist and client to participate equally in the treatment process. Engagement, from this perspective, has both behavioral components (e.g., attendance, completion of homework) and attitudinal components (e.g., motivation, commitment, belief in the treatment, confidence in the therapist) (Staudt, 2007; Yatchmenoff, 2005). Attitudinal components can distinguish between those who complete treatment and achieve the treatment goals and those who drop out prematurely or do not achieve behavioral change. For example, research shows that families are more likely to drop out of treatment early if they do not have confidence that the treatment will help and if they have not established a comfortable working relationship with their therapist (Kazdin, Holland, & Crowley, 1997;

McKay et al., 2001; Morrissey-Kane & Prinz, 1999; Spoth & Redmond, 1995).

Engagement as a Process: From Identification of Need through Treatment Completion

Engagement has also been conceptualized more broadly as a process or series of events by which children and families are first identified within the community as in need of mental health treatment, then referred or connected to a mental health provider, and effectively engaged in appropriate services (Coatsworth et al., 2001; Liddle, 1995; McKay et al., 2004; Tryon & Winograd, 2002). This definition of engagement also includes an expectation that some or all treatment goals will be met.

An illustration of successful engagement as a process of shared responsibility may include a scenario in which a teacher is the first to notice or *identify* a child welfare concern and mental health need of a child at school. She may discuss her concerns with the child's parents and school counselor and, as a mandated reporter, disclose the abuse or neglect to the local child welfare agency. In doing so, she *connects* the child to a mental health referral source, and in turn, the caseworker or school counselor may *refer* the family to a mental health treatment center that can meet the child's and family's specific mental health needs. This agency is responsible for *providing treatment*, and the family is responsible for *participating in treatment*. Therapists are responsible for *creating goals* and *reducing barriers to treatment* in a collaborative manner with the family. For children who have experienced abuse or neglect, the referral source may also *communicate* its goals for the family to enhance the safety, permanency, and well-being of the child. Lastly, the process must include follow-up whereby therapists, family, caseworkers, and other professionals are *monitoring progress* and working together to support the family's participation and completion of the treatment goals. Successful engagement and treatment implementation are greatly aided by ongoing collaboration and coordination among the systems of care, including the family.

This level of coordination is, unfortunately, uncommon, even for children brought to the attention of a child welfare agency. Those who refer families to treatment often do not remain involved in monitoring its progress after making the initial referral. The ability to effectively identify mental health problems requiring treatment and to connect families with effective, appropriate, and available mental health treatment requires specialized knowledge and targeted follow-up (Dorsey et al., 2012; Kerns et al., 2010). Professionals who are in the best position to identify and refer abused or neglected children to treatment (e.g., teachers, caseworkers, primary care providers) typically do not have the training or support necessary to do so effectively and may lack the ability or mandate to monitor treatment progress. Thus, although contact with child welfare agencies increases the likelihood that children will have their mental health needs

identified and be referred for treatment, a large disparity remains between need and access to care for this group of children, particularly those who remain in their homes (Leslie et al., 2005; Stiffman et al., 1997).

When conceptualizing engagement as a process, it becomes evident that successful engagement is not reliant on family behavior alone. Successful engagement depends also on the referring professional's awareness of (1) children's mental health treatment needs; (2) types of ESTs that can meet those needs; and (3) the type of communication and collaboration required to link families with appropriate treatment and to monitor treatment progress. Much work remains to be done in this area, although some promising pilot programs have been developed to address this need. For example, Project Focus is a training and consultation program for caseworkers and supervisors in child welfare. It is designed to enhance caseworkers' awareness of mental health needs for children involved with child welfare and to provide training and consultation around linking children and families to ESTs (Dorsey et al., 2012; Kerns et al., 2010). Communication and collaboration with therapists is heavily emphasized to identify treatment components that address specific child mental health problems and effectively monitor a child's progress during treatment. Project Focus has been piloted in Washington State (Dorsey et al., 2012) and adapted for use in Colorado, with promising evidence for improving coordination among systems of care (Kerns & Gorrono, 2012) for children and families involved with child welfare.

RATES OF TREATMENT ENGAGEMENT AMONG MALTREATED CHILDREN AND THEIR FAMILIES

Identification and referral to mental health services for children and families in need are important first steps to engagement, but engagement efforts cannot stop at the door of the therapist's office. Among those who make initial contact with a mental health service provider, many will never attend a first appointment. McKay and colleagues (2001) found that more than one-third of families who were scheduled for an initial intake appointment at an urban mental health clinic (in response to their request for mental health services) failed to attend. Among those who do make it "through the door" to an initial meeting with a mental health provider, relatively few complete treatment (McKay, Lynn, & Bannon, 2005; Saxe et al., 2012).

Further, youths experiencing maltreatment or trauma are more likely to drop out of community-based mental health services early in treatment than youths who do not have maltreatment or trauma histories (Lau & Weisz, 2003). For example, Meezan and O'Keefe (1998) reported that only 30% of low-income child welfare–involved families referred for maltreatment had a planned termination from traditionally delivered family therapy. Saxe and colleagues (2012) found that in an urban community outpatient treatment setting, more than two-thirds of children and adolescents dropped out of treatment for childhood traumatic stress within their first seven sessions. McKay and colleagues (2005) similarly reported that in an urban community setting, only 9% of children with trauma histories were still participating in traditional outpatient mental health services at 12 weeks.

These reports are particularly discouraging because most evidence-based treatments for child mental health problems and for child maltreatment and trauma include a minimum of 8–12 sessions (L. Miller, Southam-Gerow, & Allin, 2008; see also California Evidence-Based Clearinghouse for Child Welfare, www.cebc4cw.org). Further, only a few community-based treatment settings use evidence-based programs (Landsverk et al., 2006), which demonstrate the greatest effects in the shortest amount of time. Settings where ESTs are not available may take even longer to produce the desired outcomes. In summary, then, only a very small percentage of maltreated children and their families in need of mental health services will complete treatment or remain in treatment long enough to achieve meaningful outcomes.

ENGAGING CAREGIVERS OF MALTREATED CHILDREN

Meaningful engagement in child mental health services often requires parents or caregivers to participate actively in the treatment and/or dedicate themselves to supporting their child's mental health needs. This type of commitment may be particularly challenging for caregivers who have abused or neglected their children (Lau & Weisz, 2003). Caregivers' fear or suspicion that discussion of childrearing practices could result in removal of the child from the home or the termination of parental rights can impede the process of engagement (Azar & Wolfe, 1998). Adding to the challenge for clinicians, parents who are experiencing higher levels of child behavior problems and difficulties with discipline are less likely to keep their treatment appointments, despite requesting services (Harrison, McKay, & Bannon, 2004; McKay et al., 2001). Also, physically abusive parents are often referred, and sometimes mandated, to treatment that emphasizes parenting skills and nonphysical discipline for child behavior problems—the principles of which may be incongruent with their long-held beliefs about or models of child rearing (Azar & Wolfe, 1998).

Many evidence-based parenting programs emphasize praise and positive attention as a strategy for preventing behavior problems (e.g., Barkley, 1997; Eyberg & Boggs, 1998; Kazdin, 2005; Webster-Stratton, 2001), which may feel uncomfortable to parents who are unaccustomed to relating to their children in these ways. These programs also tend to incorporate the use of tangible rewards for behavioral compliance with adults' requests. Many parents erroneously equate such practices with "bribery" or simply feel that compliance is an expected child behavior and should not need to be rewarded (Forehand & Kotchick, 2002). In addition, most evidence-based parenting programs pur-

posefully sequence teaching skills related to praise, positive attention, child-directed play, and rewards before teaching skills for effective discipline strategies (e.g., time-out, removal of privileges). While the rationale for this sequencing of skills is theoretically and empirically sound, maltreating parents may feel particularly unsupported around managing behavior problems during the initial few weeks of treatment (e.g., "I'm not allowed to spank him anymore, but you won't tell me what to do, besides praise him, until session five?!"). In these situations, caregivers' engagement may depend on the therapist's ability to explain the rationale for the sequencing of skills in a manner that conveys empathy, instills hope, and is sensitive to maltreating caregivers' parenting beliefs.

Nonmaltreating caregivers are more likely than maltreating parents to engage in mental health treatment for their children (Lau & Weisz, 2003). However, even when brought to treatment by nonabusive caregivers, maltreated children are still more likely than nonmaltreated children to terminate treatment early and against the advice of their therapists. Nonabusive caregivers of maltreated children may be struggling with a host of stressors that can interfere with engagement in treatment. For example, at the time the child maltreatment is discovered and children are referred for treatment, caregivers may be dealing with stressful transitions or role changes (e.g., transition to single parenthood; moving from home; changes in financial stability). In addition, they may be experiencing guilt or denial related to failure to protect their child, which may not be fully or carefully addressed in child-focused treatment.

Some of the difficulties in engaging maltreated children and their caregivers may be inherent in family characteristics that are part of the etiology of maltreatment. Maltreating families are typically characterized by multiple and varied problems, each of which may pose barriers to children's ability to benefit from typical interventions or to complete treatment. Parental psychopathology or substance use, psychiatric comorbidity, parenting skill deficits, intergenerational perpetration of abuse, domestic violence, neighborhood violence, and/or high levels of financial or daily stress—these are just some of the possible family-level barriers to successful treatment engagement for maltreating families (Berger, 2005; Cicchetti & Lynch, 1993; Egeland, Breitenbucher, & Rosenberg, 1980). The chaotic or disorganized patterns of interaction that often characterize maltreating families pose additional challenges to treatment engagement. For example, Howes et al. (2000) found, through observation and coding of family interactions, that maltreating families experience greater levels of chaos, more difficulty with emotional regulation, less flexibility in interactions, poorer adaptive relationship skills, and less clarity of roles within the family than nonmaltreating families. The implications for treatment engagement are critical, as these types of maladaptive patterns of interaction are known to predict poor engagement in family therapy and are associated with poor treatment outcomes (Kazdin, 1995; Perrino et al., 2001). Empathy, openness, and respect for caregivers' experiences and roles are powerful engagement tools when working with struggling families. In addition, engagement with vulnerable families can benefit from treatment approaches that identify and build on strengths.

Children in Out-of-Home Placement

Among maltreated children, those in out-of-home placements are the most likely to engage in mental health treatment (Leslie et al., 2005); however, engagement with foster families poses some unique challenges. Many foster parents express motivation to be involved in service and treatment planning for the children in their care (Denby, Rindfleisch, & Bean, 1999; Hudson & Levasseur, 2002; Rhodes, Orme, & Buehler, 2001). Yet, the extent to which they are invited to participate in the child's treatment, kept informed of the child's progress in therapy, or taught specific skills for managing child behavior problems varies greatly (Dorsey & Deblinger, 2012). Foster parents do not typically receive much specific support or coaching to deal with child mental health difficulties. Opportunities for foster parents to learn how to manage difficult behavior and emotional problems are often limited by therapists' perceptions of the role of foster parents in a child's life. For example, treatment providers—or foster parents themselves—may believe that it is detrimental to the child to get too close or emotionally involved with the foster family because this might set the child up for another loss if or when there is a change in placement. And when reunification is the focus of treatment, foster parents may be excluded in favor of supporting a relationship with the biological parents.

Engagement of foster parents, however, is critical. Research shows that the likelihood of multiple foster placements increases when foster parents do not receive needed assistance in managing children's mental health needs (Dorsey & Deblinger, 2012). A greater awareness of the positive impact of even one temporary yet supportive caregiver on a child's mental health and development is essential, as are greater efforts to engage foster parents in treatment. For example, Trauma-Focused Cognitive Behavioral Therapy (TF-CBT), an EST for child trauma that uses nonoffending caregiver support, is effective even when the supportive caregiver is a teacher, residential facility staff member, foster parent, or someone in the child's extended family (Cohen, Mannarino, & Deblinger, 2012).

Additional Barriers to Treatment Engagement

LOGISTICAL BARRIERS. Additional external or logistical barriers may also impede engagement, particularly for low-income or single-parent families. For example, lack of transportation, scheduling conflicts, coordination of child care for siblings, and financial cost or lack of insurance are common and real barriers for many families. These types of barriers have been linked to difficulty with engagement and early, unplanned termination from treatment (Kazdin, Holland, & Crowley, 1997; Spoth & Redmond, 2000). Many maltreating families find themselves mandated to participate in several, often uncoordinated services as part of the requirement for case closure and autonomy from the child welfare system. For these families, having to attend multiple weekly appointments as part of child welfare involvement often poses greater than usual logistical barriers to treatment participation, as well as increased stress among caregivers (Staudt, 2007). Furthermore, missed appointments are too often interpreted as "resistance," "noncompliance," or simply "failure" on the part of the family, with little attention to helping families overcome these barriers to participation. The effort required on the part of families to overcome logistical barriers to attending treatment may far outweigh the perceived benefits, particularly if attending treatment adds to their level of stress (e.g., Kazdin, Holland, & Crowley, 1997; Kazdin & Wassell, 2000; Kruzich et al., 2003; MacNaughton & Rodrigue, 2001).

It is important to note, too, that although logistical barriers represent very real obstacles to engagement, perceptual barriers (e.g., attitudes and beliefs about therapy) may carry even more weight with families when determining whether treatment is worthwhile (Kazdin, Holland, & Crowley, 1997; McKay et al., 2001). This highlights the importance of addressing both types of barriers as part of treatment.

AGENCY POLICIES. Agencies play an important role in posing or reducing both logistical and perceptual barriers for families, through policies related to attendance, child care, scheduling, insurance, waitlists, arrangement of transportation services, hours of operation, and mobility of services. In addition, the number of families served by a particular agency and the number of providers available influence the frequency and duration of sessions, the amount of supervision and support for providers, and the level of provider turnover—all of which can impact family engagement (Azar, 2000). Although agency-level factors have an important influence on family engagement, many agencies are challenged with balancing the needs of the clients they serve and maintaining financial sustainability. Financial sustainability and compliance with state and federal mandates often take precedence, leading to enactment of policies that may not always be consistent with providing the most effective services to all families (Yoo, 2002). For example, agencies may respond to a family's difficulties with attendance by terminating treatment rather than by exploring barriers and discussing with the family the rationale for why treatment may be worth the effort required to attend regularly. Similarly, agencies may not have the funds to cover costs associated with attending therapy (e.g., parking or transportation), which may make treatment participation prohibitively expensive for some families. Staff turnover and burnout due to high caseloads or low pay may limit therapists' ability to project confidence about the treatment to skeptical families. Increased local, state, and federal support aimed at helping agencies and staff provide the most effective services, particularly to low-income families, is greatly needed.

CAREGIVER AND FAMILY STRESS. Caregivers with high levels of personal stress are likely to experience barriers to treatment participation as more difficult to overcome than those with lower levels of stress (Kazdin & Wassell, 2000; Owens et al., 2002). Caregiver and family stress can stem from numerous circumstances, as noted earlier, including financial hardship, mental health challenges (e.g., depression, posttraumatic stress), marital or partner conflict, daily hassles related to juggling the demands of working and parenting, and challenges in parenting children with behavior problems. Caregivers may not readily bring many of these challenges to a therapist's attention, especially if they do not perceive a link between their own personal stress and their child's mental health difficulties. Therapists should spend time assessing the sources and levels of caregivers' stress in the early stages of treatment and should emphasize caregiver self-care as an important treatment goal.

The impact of caregivers' stress on treatment engagement can be mitigated by the presence of a second, supportive adult partner in the home (McKay et al., 2001). In addition, social support from friends, extended family, the community, and even other families in treatment is positively related to treatment engagement and attendance (Harrison, McKay, & Bannon, 2004) and can buffer families against the negative effects of stress. Beyond the ability to provide support for keeping appointments, friends and community members can influence a family's "buy-in" to treatment or can challenge a family's reluctance to engage in treatment. Dadds and McHugh (1992) found better outcomes from a parent management training intervention for families who received social support from friends. Meezan and O'Keefe (1998) found that families participating in treatment for child abuse and neglect in a group with other families had fewer unplanned terminations and better outcomes than families who participated in treatment individually. Although rarely a focus of treatment, interventions to increase social support or to include supportive extended-family members, friends, or community members in treatment may improve engagement and outcomes for at-risk families. This may be particularly important for families at risk for child abuse or neglect, as stress and lack of social support have also been associated with child maltreatment (Bishop & Leadbeater, 2010; Whipple & Webster-Stratton, 1991).

THE THERAPEUTIC RELATIONSHIP—KEY TO ENGAGEMENT

The therapeutic relationship is central to the process of engagement for many families. Although families are often perceived as the entity engaged in therapy, therapists carry great responsibility in promoting and maintaining engagement (Cunningham & Henggeler, 2004; Elvins & Green, 2008; Liddle, 1995; McGinty et al., 2003; McKay et al., 1995; Santisteban & Szapocznik, 1994). For example, therapists who seek family input about the course and targets of treatment are more likely to successfully engage the family in treatment. Part of seeking family input involves learning about the family's belief system regarding children's mental health, discipline, roles within the family, and therapy itself, as well as learning about the family's cultural or spiritual background and the extent to which this influences engagement with a particular treatment approach. Seeking and incorporating family input is particularly important when working with maltreating families, because it may reduce perceptions of coercion (Platt, 2006).

Therapists can also be effective in promoting engagement by openly discussing therapeutic relationship problems. One study found that a problem in the therapeutic relationship was the strongest predictor of completion versus drop-out among families receiving treatment in community clinics (Garcia & Weisz, 2002). Relationship problems identified by families included feeling that the therapist was ignoring relevant problems and targeting less relevant ones, that the treatment approach was not adequately explained, that the therapist was not competent to provide effective services, or that the therapist did not spend enough time with the child or the caregiver, or the family simply did not like the therapist. By their nature and social construction, helping relationships—particularly those involving a professional as helper—often imply an imbalance in strength, knowledge, or power (Azar & Wolfe, 1998). This dynamic may make it difficult for families to voice their concerns about the therapist, the therapeutic relationship, or the treatment provided without being invited to do so.

Discussing such concerns may be even more daunting for families mandated to treatment because of child abuse or neglect or those who feel shame or embarrassment related to their reasons for seeking treatment. It is often easier for families to leave treatment than to tell their therapists they are not comfortable with an aspect of treatment or with the relationship. The therapist is responsible for inviting discussion about the therapeutic relationship. Doing so requires confidence and experience. It is not always easy to ask a family to share their impressions of the therapeutic relationship and concerns about treatment, particularly if the therapist is feeling overwhelmed about the nature of the family's problems. In fact, many therapists enter the field of child mental health without adequate training in working with and engaging families around issues of child maltreatment (Azar, 2000; McGinty et al., 2003), highlighting the importance of supervisory support for less experienced providers. When therapists are able to experience problems with collaboration as opportunities for communication rather than as signs that a family is not ready or not able to benefit from treatment, they are likely to achieve greater success in implementing treatment (Liddle, 1995; Santisteban & Szapocznik, 1994).

CULTURAL COMPETENCE

Cultural competence is increasingly recognized as a therapist- and agency-level characteristic that is important to providing effective mental health services to diverse populations (Hernandez & Isaacs, 1998; Kumpfer et al., 2002). It can be defined as a dynamic process that involves obtaining cultural knowledge, developing an ability to see when and how cultural differences between therapist and client affect the therapeutic discourse, and learning how to adjust practices accordingly (Betancourt et al., 2003; López, 1997). Central to cultural competence is an understanding of culture itself. Whaley and Davis (2007) note that most definitions of culture include traditions, values, norms, beliefs, and coping behaviors that are passed from generation to generation. It is important to recognize the overlap between this description of culture and factors central to family engagement in treatment. Many families have long-held beliefs about parenting, coping, trauma, and help-seeking behavior, extending back for several generations, that influence the circumstances in which they arrive at therapy and the set of expectations they bring to the process (Cardemil, 2010; Morrissey-Kane & Prinz, 1999; Prinz & Miller, 1994). An awareness of the importance of cultural influence to successful engagement is essential to success in implementing treatment for all families.

Cultural competence may be particularly important in working with families from minority backgrounds. Racial/ethnic minority children and families are less likely than nonminority children and families to make use of mental health services when they are needed (Kataoka, Zhang, & Wells, 2002; Yeh et al., 2003) and are more likely to drop out prematurely when they do access services (McKay et al., 2004; L. Miller, Southam-Gerow, & Allin, 2008). At their core, strategies for engaging racial/ethnic minority families do not differ greatly from strategies developed with all families in mind, in that they directly address beliefs and attitudes about mental health treatment and families' views of the world more generally (role of family, parenting, help-seeking behavior, coping with trauma, etc.). There are, however, several additional strategies that are important to enhancing treatment engagement for racial/ethnic minority families. For example, agencies should have on hand therapists or interpreters that speak a family's native language and offer the family a choice about the language they feel most comfortable using in therapy. Because the nuances of different languages may be particularly important to the expression of emotion and description of relationships, there is tremendous benefit to engagement and the therapeutic process when families have the option of using their native language.

Agency administrators should also be aware of how treatment setting can affect different racial/ethnic minority groups and be ready to modify these factors when needed. For example, families may experience discomfort in therapy settings where the racial/ethnic backgrounds of staff members are homogeneous and different from their own. It is important to strive to create clinic environments that are diverse and representative of the families served. Similarly, therapists can enhance engagement by openly acknowledging and discussing cultural and racial/ethnic differences when they exist, as well as by understanding their own culturally based worldview and biases. Therapists should learn about specific minority groups' collective history of trauma, oppression, or discrimination within the larger majority culture. This knowledge base serves as a helpful foundation for learning about and understanding each family's unique experience and the set of beliefs they bring to treatment.

Infusion of culturally relevant content in the treatment program may also enhance engagement and treatment implementation for racial/ethnic minority families. Most child mental health treatments were developed and tested with majority families and may not be as relevant for some minority families. Of these, cognitive behavioral approaches have the strongest evidence for effectiveness with racial/ethnic minority children and families (Huey & Polo, 2008). However, there may still be a need for adaptations that account for a family's cultural beliefs but do not compromise the integrity or effectiveness of the treatment (Cardemil, 2010; Liddle, Jackson-Gilfort, & Marvel, 2006). For example, narrative approaches may best suit members of cultural groups that value collective storytelling, whereas solution-focused approaches may be best for members of cultural groups that do not believe in dwelling on past issues. Essential to being able to adapt interventions to the cultural beliefs of different families is a thorough assessment of a family's specific beliefs.

INTERVENTION APPROACHES SPECIFICALLY ADDRESSING ENGAGEMENT

Thus far we have described several important considerations relevant to improving engagement in mental health treatment, particularly for families experiencing child maltreatment. This section focuses on some specific intervention strategies that have been developed to address this need (these are summarized in table 25.1).

Pre-treatment Strategies

Phone calls prior to the first appointment, specifically structured to identify and begin problem solving for logistical and perceptual barriers to treatment, have proved successful in increasing family buy-in to treatment and improving the likelihood of initial engagement. For example, McKay, McCadam, and Gonzales (1996) developed and evaluated an effective pre-intake telephone interview designed to clarify with the caregiver the goals and need for the child's

Table 25.1. Summary of Specific Engagement Strategies

Pre-treatment strategies	Pre-intake telephone interview	• Join with the family • Instill hope • Assess goals • Determine level of motivation • Explore beliefs about treatment • Problem-solve barriers
First-session strategies	Initial appointment(s)	• Describe intake process, policies, and provider roles • Clarify fit between family goals and treatment options • Describe therapy as collaboration • Learn about family expectations • Problem-solve immediate logistical concerns • Make a plan to address ongoing barriers
Ongoing strategies	Throughout treatment	*Appointment reminders:* • Call client prior to sessions *Motivational Interviewing techniques:* • Express empathy • Avoid disagreements • Highlight discrepancies between client's goals and behavior • Elicit motivational self-talk • Collaborate to achieve desired goals

mental health treatment, to validate and support the caregiver's effort and motivation for seeking and engaging in treatment, and to identify and begin to problem-solve barriers to engagement. This telephone interview significantly increased attendance at the first appointment when compared with a traditional telephone intake process.

Similarly, Strategic Structural-Systems Engagement (SSSE; Coatsworth et al., 2001; Santisteban et al., 1996; Szapocznik et al., 1988) is another effective pre-treatment intervention for family engagement in therapy that is implemented by phone prior to the first therapy appointment. SSSE strategies include direct questioning about family concerns and values, empathic "joining" around perceived barriers, instillation of hope, and the therapist's projection of confidence that he or she can successfully address family-identified problems and goals during treatment. In some cases, the family member on the phone is taught to negotiate with difficult-to-engage family members and to reframe those family members' negative beliefs about therapy before the first session. Sometimes, as part of this intervention, the therapist may make contact with family members other than the original caller, or even nonfamily significant others, who can support the whole family's buy-in. Rigorous testing of this approach revealed that significantly more families receiving the SSSE intervention completed early treatment sessions and remained in treatment longer when compared with those not receiving the intervention (Coatsworth et al., 2001; Santisteban et al., 1996; Szapocznik et al., 1988).

First-Session Strategies

The first session is an important opportunity to strengthen a family's engagement and, indeed, can "make or break"

successful engagement for many families. McKay, Nudelman, and McCadam (1996) developed engagement strategies specifically for initial treatment appointments, focused solely on family expectations about treatment and problem solving with the family around logistical concerns. During the first session, therapists also help families understand the intake process and the provider's roles, clarify how the family's needs fit with treatment options, describe therapy as a collaboration between family and therapist, problem-solve immediate practical concerns, and create a plan to address barriers that might affect treatment in an ongoing manner. When combined with the pre-intake telephone interview described above, these strategies are effective at enhancing initial engagement (McKay et al., 1998).

Ongoing Engagement Strategies

With regard to retention and ongoing engagement, a simple intervention that has been found to reduce missed appointments involves reminder phone calls to parents before each therapy session (Kourany, Garber, & Tornusciolo, 1990; Shivack & Sullivan, 1989; Watts et al., 2007). This strategy may be most helpful for families juggling a busy schedule and is relatively easy to implement.

Motivational Interviewing (MI) approaches (W. Miller & Rollnick, 2002) focused on reducing perceptual barriers can also be used to enhance families' retention and engagement in treatment. These techniques were originally developed for improving engagement in adult mental health and substance abuse services and have recently been adapted for use with children and families (Chaffin et al., 2009; Nock & Kazdin, 2001). MI was designed to target clients' ambivalence about making therapeutically meaningful changes by expressing empathy, avoiding disagreements, highlighting discrepancies between clients' goals and their current functioning or behavior, eliciting motivational self-talk, and collaborating to achieve desired goals. A benefit of MI is that it can be incorporated into any number of existing treatment models to promote engagement and motivation throughout the treatment process and can be delivered in brief doses. For example, Nock and Kazdin (2001) found that MI techniques, infused into a parent training intervention in just three 5- to 10-minute conversations during the course of treatment, were effective in enhancing caregivers' motivations to participate in the treatment and increased the number of sessions they attended. At higher doses, MI was found to be effective in improving engagement and retention for child welfare–involved families reporting low levels of motivation for treatment. Specifically, Chaffin and colleagues (2009) found that families receiving six sessions of MI, which included testimonials from parents who had successfully completed treatment, were more likely to complete an evidence-based parenting program successfully.

CONCLUSIONS

Engagement in child mental health treatment can be defined as a process that begins with the identification of mental health needs and ends with the successful achievement of treatment goals, and includes the active and collaborative participation of both families and therapists. Many unique challenges to engagement exist for children and families referred for child maltreatment or trauma. Successful engagement with this group of children and families typically requires that (1) therapists directly address engagement issues with the family in the early stages of treatment, and in some cases before treatment begins; (2) therapists directly ask about expectations, goals, concerns, and barriers and create plans, in collaboration with families, to overcome these barriers; and (3) strategies are easily integrated into an existing treatment structure or setting.

References

Azar, S. T. (2000). Preventing burnout in professionals and paraprofessionals who work with child abuse and neglect cases: A cognitive behavioral approach to supervision. *Journal of Clinical Psychology, 56*(5), 643–663.

Azar, S. T., & Wolfe, D. A. (1998). Child physical abuse and neglect. In E. J. Mash & R. A. Barkley (Eds.), *Treatment of childhood disorders* (2nd ed., pp. 501–544). New York, NY: Guilford Press.

Barkley, R. A. (1997). *Defiant children: A clinician's manual for assessment and parent training.* (2nd ed.). New York, NY: Guilford Press.

Berger, L. M. (2005). Income, family characteristics, and physical violence toward children. *Child Abuse & Neglect, 29*(2), 107–133.

Betancourt, J. R., Green, A. R., Carrillo, J. E., & Ananeh-Firempong, O. (2003). Defining cultural competence: A practical framework for addressing racial/ethnic disparities in health and health care. *Public Health Reports, 118*(4), 293–302.

Bishop, S. J., & Leadbeater, B. J. (2010). Maternal social support patterns and child maltreatment: Comparison of maltreating and nonmaltreating mothers. *American Journal of Orthopsychiatry, 69*(2), 172–181.

Burns, B. J., Phillips, S. D., Wagner, H. R., Barth, R. P., Kolko, D. J., Campbell, Y., & Landsverk, J. (2004). Mental health need and access to mental health services by youths involved with child welfare: A national survey. *Journal of the American Academy of Child and Adolescent Psychiatry, 43*(8), 960–970.

Cardemil, E. V. (2010). Cultural adaptations to empirically supported treatments: A research agenda. *Scientific Review of Mental Health Practice, 7*(2), 8–21.

Chadwick Center for Children and Families. (2004). *Closing the quality chasm in child abuse treatment: Identifying and disseminating best practices.* San Diego, CA: Author.

Chaffin, M., Valle, L. A., Funderburk, B., Gurwitch, R., Silovsky, J., Bard, D., et al. (2009). A motivational intervention can improve retention in PCIT for low-motivation child welfare clients. *Child Maltreatment, 14*(4), 356–368.

Cicchetti, D., & Lynch, M. (1993). Toward an ecological/transactional model of community violence and child maltreatment: Consequences for children's development. *Psychiatry, 56*(1), 96–118.

Coatsworth, J. D., Santisteban, D. A., McBride, C. K., & Szapocznik, J. (2001). Brief strategic family therapy versus community control: Engagement, retention, and an exploration of the moderating role of adolescent symptom severity. *Family Process, 40*(3), 313–332.

Cohen, J. A., Mannarino, A. P., & Deblinger, E. (Eds.). (2012). *Trauma-focused CBT for children and adolescents: Treatment applications.* New York, NY: Guilford Press.

Cunningham, P. B., & Henggeler, S. W. (2004). Engaging multiproblem families in treatment: Lessons learned throughout the development of multisystemic therapy. *Family Process, 38*(3), 265–281.

Dadds, M. R., & McHugh, T. A. (1992). Social support and treatment outcome in behavioral family therapy for child conduct problems. *Journal of Consulting and Clinical Psychology, 60*(2), 252.

Denby, R., Rindfleisch, N., & Bean, G. (1999). Predictors of foster parents' satisfaction and intent to continue to foster. *Child Abuse & Neglect, 23*(3), 287–303.

Dorsey, S., & Deblinger, E. (2012). Children in foster care. In J. A. Cohen, A. P. Mannarino, & E. Deblinger (Eds.), *Trauma-focused CBT for children and adolescents: Treatment applications* (pp. 49–72). New York, NY: Guilford Press.

Dorsey, S., Kerns, S. E., Trupin, E. W., Conover, K. L., & Berliner, L. (2012). Child welfare caseworkers as service brokers for youth in foster care: Findings from Project Focus. *Child Maltreatment, 17*(1), 22–31.

Egeland, B. R., Breitenbucher, M., & Rosenberg, D. (1980). Prospective study of the significance of life stress in the etiology of child abuse. *Journal of Consulting and Clinical Psychology, 48*(2), 195.

Elvins, R., & Green, J. (2008). The conceptualization and measurement of therapeutic alliance: An empirical review. *Clinical Psychology Review, 28*(7), 1167–1187.

Eyberg, S. M., & Boggs, S. R. (1998). Parent-child interaction therapy: A psychosocial intervention for the treatment of young conduct-disordered children. In J. Briesmeister & C. Schaefer (Eds.), *Handbook of parent training: Parents as co-therapists for children's behavior problems* (2nd ed., pp. 61–97). Hoboken, NJ: John Wiley & Sons.

Forehand, R., & Kotchick, B. A. (2002). Behavioral parent training: Current challenges and potential solutions. *Journal of Child and Family Studies, 11*(4), 377–384.

Garcia, J. A., & Weisz, J. R. (2002). When youth mental health care stops: Therapeutic relationship problems and other reasons for ending youth outpatient treatment. *Journal of Consulting and Clinical Psychology, 70*(2), 439.

Harrison, M. E., McKay, M. M., & Bannon, W. M. (2004). Inner-city child mental health service use: The real question is why youth and families do not use services. *Community Mental Health Journal, 40*(2), 119–131.

Hernandez, M. E., & Isaacs, M. R. (Eds.). (1998). *Promoting cultural competence in children's mental health services.* Baltimore, MD: Paul H. Brookes Publishing.

Howes, P. W., Cicchetti, D., Toth, S. L., & Rogosch, F. A. (2000). Affective, organizational, and relational characteristics of maltreating families: A system's perspective. *Journal of Family Psychology, 14*(1), 95.

Hudson, P., & Levasseur, K. (2002). Supporting foster parents: Caring voices. *Child Welfare: Journal of Policy, Practice, and Program, 81*(6), 853–866.

Huey, S. J., Jr., & Polo, A. J. (2008). Evidence-based psychosocial treatments for ethnic minority youth. *Journal of Clinical Child and Adolescent Psychology, 37*(1), 262–301.

Kataoka, S. H., Zhang, L., & Wells, K. B. (2002). Unmet need for mental health care among US children: Variation by ethnicity and insurance status. *American Journal of Psychiatry, 159*(9), 1548–1555.

Kazdin, A. E. (1995). Child, parent and family dysfunction as predictors of outcome in cognitive-behavioral treatment of antisocial children. *Behaviour Research and Therapy, 33*(3), 271–281.

Kazdin, A. E. (2005). *Parent management training: Treatment for oppositional, aggressive, and antisocial behavior in children and adolescents.* New York, NY: Oxford University Press.

Kazdin, A. E., Holland, L., & Crowley, M. (1997). Family experience of barriers to treatment and premature termination from child therapy. *Journal of Consulting and Clinical Psychology, 65*(3), 453.

Kazdin, A. E., & Wassell, G. (2000). Predictors of barriers to treatment and therapeutic change in outpatient therapy for antisocial children and their families. *Mental Health Services Research, 2*(1), 27–40.

Kerns, S. E. U., Dorsey, S., Trupin, E.W., & Berliner, L. (2010). Project Focus: Promoting emotional health and wellbeing for youth in foster care through connections to evidence-based practices. *Emotional and Behavioral Disorders of Youth, 10*, 30–38.

Kerns, S. E. U., & Gorrono, J. (2012, October). *New approaches to supporting caseworkers as "brokers" in addressing child and family wellbeing.* Paper presented at the meeting of the National Staff Training and Development Association, Portland, OR.

Kourany, R. F., Garber, J., & Tornusciolo, G. (1990). Improving first appointment attendance rates in child psychiatry outpatient clinics. *Journal of the American Academy of Child and Adolescent Psychiatry, 29*, 657–660.

Kruzich, J. M., Jivanjee, P., Robinson, A., & Friesen, B. J. (2003). Family caregivers' perceptions of barriers to and supports of participation in their children's out-of-home treatment. *Psychiatric Services, 54*(11), 1513–1518.

Kumpfer, K. L., Alvarado, R., Smith, P., & Bellamy, N. (2002). Cultural sensitivity and adaptation in family-based prevention interventions. *Prevention Science, 3*(3), 241–246.

Landsverk, J. A., Burns, B. J., Stambaugh, L. F., & Rolls Reutz, J. A. (2006). *Mental health care for children and adolescents in foster care: Review of research literature.* Casey Family Programs. www.casey.org/Resources/Publications/pdf/MentalHealthCareChildren.pdf

Lau, A. S., & Weisz, J. R. (2003). Reported maltreatment among clinic-referred children: Implications for presenting problems, treatment attrition, and long-term outcomes. *Journal of the American Academy of Child and Adolescent Psychiatry, 42*(11), 1327–1334.

Leslie, L. K., Hurlburt, M. S., James, S., Landsverk, J., Slymen, D. J., & Zhang, J. (2005). Relationship between entry into child welfare and mental health service use. *Psychiatric Services, 56*(8), 981.

Liddle, H. A. (1995). Conceptual and clinical dimensions of a multidimensional, multisystems engagement strategy in family-based adolescent treatment. *Psychotherapy: Theory, Research, Practice, Training, 32*(1), 39.

Liddle, H. A., Jackson-Gilfort, A., & Marvel, F. A. (2006). An empirically supported and culturally specific engagement and intervention strategy for African American adolescent males. *American Journal of Orthopsychiatry, 76*(2), 215–225.

López, S. R. (1997) Cultural competence in psychotherapy: A guide for clinicians and their supervisors. In C. E. Watkins, Jr. (Ed.), *Handbook of psychotherapy supervision* (pp. 570–588). Hoboken, NJ: John Wiley & Sons.

MacNaughton, K. L., & Rodrigue, J. R. (2001). Predicting adherence to recommendations by parents of clinic-referred children. *Journal of Consulting and Clinical Psychology, 69*(2), 262.

McGinty, K. L., Diamond, J. M., Brown, M. B., & McCammon, S. L. (2003). Training child and adolescent psychiatrists and child mental health professionals for systems of care. In A. J. Pumariega & N. Winters (Eds.), *Handbook of community-based systems of care: The new child & adolescent community psychiatry* (pp. 487–507) San Francisco, CA: Jossey-Bass.

McKay, M. M., Bennett, E., Stone, S., & Gonzales, J. (1995). A comprehensive training model for inner city social workers. *Arete, 20*, 56–65.

McKay, M. M., Hibbert, R., Hoagwood, K., Rodriguez, J., Murray, L., Legerski, J., & Fernandez, D. (2004). Integrating evidence-based engagement interventions into "real world" child mental health settings. *Brief Treatment and Crisis Intervention, 4*(2), 177.

McKay, M. M., Lynn, C. J., & Bannon, W. M. (2005). Understanding inner city child mental health need and trauma exposure: Implications for preparing urban service providers. *American Journal of Orthopsychiatry, 75*(2), 201–210.

McKay, M. M., McCadam, K., & Gonzales, J. J. (1996). Addressing the barriers to mental health services for inner city children and their caretakers. *Community Mental Health Journal, 32*(4), 353–361.

McKay, M. M., Nudelman, R., & McCadam, K. (1996). Involving inner-city families in mental health services: First interview engagement skills. *Research in Social Work Practice, 6*, 462–472.

McKay, M. M., Pennington, J., Lynn, C. J., & McCadam, K. (2001). Understanding urban child mental health service use: Two studies of child, family, and environmental correlates. *Journal of Behavioral Health Services & Research, 28*(4), 475–483.

McKay, M. M., Stoewe, J., McCadam, K., & Gonzales, J. J. (1998). Increasing access to child mental health services for urban children and their care givers. *Health & Social Work, 23*, 9–15.

Meezan, W., & O'Keefe, M. (1998). Evaluating the effectiveness of multifamily group therapy in child abuse and neglect. *Research on Social Work Practice, 8*(3), 330–353.

Miller, L. M., Southam-Gerow, M. A., & Allin, R. B. (2008). Who stays in treatment? Child and family predictors of youth client retention in a public mental health agency. *Child and Youth Care Forum, 37*(4), 153–170.

Miller, W. R., & Rollnick, S. P. (2002). *Motivational interviewing: Preparing people for change.* New York, NY: Guilford Press.

Morrissey-Kane, E., & Prinz, R. J. (1999). Engagement in child and adolescent treatment: The role of parental cognitions and attributions. *Clinical Child and Family Psychology Review, 2*(3), 183–198.

Nix, R. L., Bierman, K. L., & McMahon, R. J. (2009). How attendance and quality of participation affect treatment response to parent management training. *Journal of Consulting and Clinical Psychology, 77*(3), 429.

Nock, M. K., & Kazdin, A. E. (2001). Parent expectancies for child therapy: Assessment and relation to participation in treatment. *Journal of Child and Family Studies, 10*(2), 155–180.

Owens, P. L., Hoagwood, K., Horwitz, S. M., Leaf, P. J., Poduska, J. M., Kellam, S. G., & Ialongo, N. S. (2002). Barriers to children's mental health services. *Journal of the American Academy of Child and Adolescent Psychiatry, 41*(6), 731–738.

Perrino, T., Coatsworth, J. D., Briones, E., Pantin, H., & Szapocznik, J. (2001). Initial engagement in parent-centered preventive interventions: A family systems perspective. *Journal of Primary Prevention, 22*(1), 21–44.

Platt, D. (2006). Threshold decisions: How social workers prioritize referrals of child concern. *Child Abuse Review, 15*, 4–18.

Prinz, R. J., & Miller, G. E. (1994). Family-based treatment for childhood antisocial behavior: Experimental influences on dropout and engagement. *Journal of Consulting and Clinical Psychology, 62*(3), 645.

Rhodes, K. W., Orme, J. G., & Buehler, C. (2001). A comparison of family foster parents who quit, consider quitting, and plan to continue fostering. *Social Service Review, 75*(1), 84–114.

Santisteban, D. A., & Szapocznik, J. (1994). Bridging theory, research and practice to more successfully engage substance abusing youth and their families into therapy. *Journal of Child & Adolescent Substance Abuse, 3*(2), 9–24.

Santisteban, D. A., Szapocznik, J., Perez-Vidal, A., Kurtines, W. M., Murray, E. J., & LaPerriere, A. (1996). Efficacy of intervention for engaging youth and families into treatment and some variables that may contribute to differential effectiveness. *Journal of Family Psychology, 10*(1), 35.

Saxe, G. N., Ellis, B. H., Fogler, J., & Navalta, C. P. (2012). Innovations in practice: Preliminary evidence for effective family engagement in treatment for child traumatic stress–trauma systems therapy approach to preventing dropout. *Child and Adolescent Mental Health, 17*(1), 58–61.

Shivack, I. M., & Sullivan, C. W. (1989). Use of telephone prompts at an inner-city outpatient clinic. *Hospital & Community Psychiatry, 40*(8), 851–853.

Spoth, R., & Redmond, C. (1995). Parent motivation to enroll in parenting skills programs: A model of family context and health belief predictors. *Journal of Family Psychology, 9*(3), 294.

Spoth, R., & Redmond, C. (2000). Research on family engagement in preventive interventions: Toward improved use of scientific findings in primary prevention practice. *Journal of Primary Prevention, 21*(2), 267–284.

Staudt, M. (2007). Treatment engagement with caregivers of at-risk children: Gaps in research and conceptualization. *Journal of Child and Family Studies, 16*(2), 183–196.

Stiffman, A. R., Chen, Y. W., Elze, D., Dore, P., & Cheng, L. C. (1997). Adolescents' and providers' perspectives on the need for and use of mental health services. *Journal of Adolescent Health, 21*(5), 335–342.

Szapocznik, J., Perez-Vidal, A., Brickman, A. L., Foote, F. H., Santisteban, D., Hervis, O., & Kurtines, W. M. (1988). Engaging adolescent drug abusers and their families in treatment: A strategic structural systems approach. *Journal of Consulting and Clinical Psychology, 56*(4), 552.

Szapocznik, J., Perez-Vidal, A., Hervis, O. E., Brickman, A. L., & Kurtines, W. M. (1990). Innovations in family therapy: Overcoming resistance to treatment. In R. Wells & V. Gianetti (Eds.), *Handbook of brief psychotherapy* (pp. 93–114). New York, NY: Plenum Press.

Tryon, G. S., & Winograd, G. (2002). Goal consensus and collaboration. In J. C. Norcross (Ed.), *Psychotherapy relationships that work: Therapist contributions and responsiveness to patients* (pp. 109–125). Oxford, UK: Oxford University Press.

Watts, B. V., Shiner, B., Pomerantz, A., Stender, P., & Weeks, W. B. (2007). Outcomes of a quality improvement project integrating mental health into primary care. *Quality and Safety in Health Care, 16*(5), 378–381.

Webster-Stratton, C. (2001). The Incredible Years: Parents, teachers, and children training series. *Residential Treatment for Children and Youth, 18*(3), 31–46.

Whaley, A. L., & Davis, K. E. (2007). Cultural competence and evidence-based practice in mental health services: A complementary perspective. *American Psychologist, 62*(6), 563.

Whipple, E. E., & Webster-Stratton, C. (1991). The role of parental stress in physically abusive families. *Child Abuse & Neglect, 15*(3), 279–291.

Yatchmenoff, D. K. (2005). Measuring client engagement from the client's perspective in nonvoluntary child protective services. *Research on Social Work Practice, 15*(2), 84–96.

Yeh, M., McCabe, K., Hough, R. L., Dupuis, D., & Hazen, A. (2003). Racial/ethnic differences in parental endorsement of barriers to mental health services for youth. *Mental Health Services Research, 5*(2), 65–77.

Yoo, J. (2002). The relationship between organizational variables and client outcomes. *Administration in Social Work, 26*(2), 39–61.

26

NICHOLAS C. HECK, PH.D.
DANIEL W. SMITH, PH.D.

The Roles of Web-Based Technology in the Dissemination and Implementation of Evidence-Based Treatments for Child Abuse

GENERAL CONSIDERATIONS

When the Internet was launched in 1989, an estimated 28% of American adults used a computer at home, work, or school (U.S. Census Bureau, 1991). Between the years 2000 and 2010, the percentage of American adults using computers increased from 65% to 77%, and the percentage of adults using the Internet increased from 53% to 79% (U.S. Census Bureau, 2012). The launches of the Internet and the World Wide Web (in 1992) have led to a global shift in how knowledge is stored, disseminated, and consumed in modern society (Harasim, 2000; Hilbert & Lopez, 2012). Knowledge about mental health treatment is no exception. Innovations in the development, dissemination, and implementation of psychosocial interventions accompanied the technological revolution of the late twentieth century. Web-based technology, in particular, is being used in a variety of mental health applications, including the delivery of treatments for smoking cessation (Shahab & McEwen, 2009), depression and anxiety (Andersson & Cuijpers, 2009; Andrews et al., 2010), and post-disaster emotional psychopathology (Ruggiero et al., 2006), as well as child in maltreatment prevention efforts (cf. Self-Brown & Whitaker, 2008).

Over the past 10–15 years there has been a simultaneous trend within mental health treatments to increasingly emphasize "evidence-supported treatments" (ESTs), those treatments that research has demonstrated to be either efficacious or promising in relieving psychological symptoms. These first efforts at systematically identifying and promoting ESTs (e.g., Chambless & Hollon, 1998) were motivated in large part by an American Psychological Association Task Force (1995) and initially focused on major psychological disorders or populations (e.g., adults, children). Similar efforts followed shortly thereafter within some specialty areas, including child maltreatment (e.g., Saunders, Berliner, & Hanson, 2004).

The timing of these two trends, while probably coincidental, has provided novel opportunities for mental health professionals to learn about ESTs. In the broader context of clinical training models, we are seeing a clear trend toward the incorporation of Web-based technology in the spread and utilization of evidence-based mental health interventions. The purpose of this chapter is to summarize the current impact that such technology is having on the dissemination and implementation of ESTs for child maltreatment and to foreshadow ways in which such technology might be applied to solve existing training-related problems in the field.

IDENTIFYING, DISSEMINATING, AND IMPLEMENTING TREATMENTS

Before beginning an analysis of technology's impact on the process, it is useful to summarize briefly how treatments are determined to be ESTs and how they are disseminated and implemented. The classification system developed by Chambless and Hollon (1998), and subsequently adapted by Saunders and colleagues (2004) for child maltreatment, emphasizes treatment efficacy data produced by randomized controlled clinical trials (ideally) or other methods as the main determinant of "empirical support." Although this decision was not without controversy, it has led to useful and widely promulgated systems of ranking treatments according to their level of support within specified criteria. Saunders and colleagues, for example, identified six ranks ranging from "well-supported, efficacious" to "concerning," based on the type and quality of outcome studies available, as well as other factors. Saunders and colleagues reviewed 24 treatment protocols, each associated with a specific intervention, and assigned an empirical support rating. Excluding the 2 interventions targeting offenders, 14 interventions were classified as having some degree of empirical support. One intervention, Trauma-Focused Cognitive Behavioral Therapy (TF-CBT; Cohen, Mannarino, & Deblinger, 2006), was classified as "well-supported and efficacious."

After an intervention (such as TF-CBT) is developed and evaluated, it must be transferred to and adopted by clinicians who treat maltreated children. This is referred to as dissemination and implementation. According to Gotham (2004, p. 164), "Dissemination is the process of informing others or spreading the word about a new technology. Dissemination ends with the decision to adopt. Implementation picks up after the adoption decision has been made and refers to how the technology is realized in practice." For the purposes of mental health interventions, it is useful to think of dissemination as providing therapists with information about the underlying theory, methods, and procedures associated with a treatment. Implementation involves translating that knowledge into performance in a practical context or environment. As an intervention is transferred and adopted, clinicians make changes or modifications to the intervention to fit their therapeutic style, the idiosyncrasies of clients, and/or the organizational characteristics of their practice site. Training clinicians to adopt an EST fully, therefore, involves both dissemination and implementation activities.

In an ideal world, clinicians would be highly adept in delivering an array of ESTs, selecting an appropriate intervention for each maltreated child they serve. Yet numerous obstacles hinder the successful dissemination and implementation of ESTs. The Institute of Medicine (2000) estimated that an average of 17 years passes before knowledge of best practices, as generated in empirical settings, is routinely incorporated into everyday clinical practices. Web-based technologies may prove to be particularly useful methods for hastening this process.

HOW ARE THERAPISTS CURRENTLY TRAINED?

Generally speaking, therapists learn how to provide clinical treatments through two traditional training models. These models are not mutually exclusive; indeed, virtually all clinicians have experienced training through both models at different points in their careers. The first model, the university-based supervision model, predominates during graduate training in all clinical training programs in the United States. The second model, the intensive workshop, characterizes postgraduate training. We briefly review each model here, highlighting the strengths and weaknesses of each with respect to producing clinicians who can deliver ESTs with fidelity and competence, and focusing on ESTs relevant to child maltreatment victims.

In university settings, where basic interviewing and therapy skills (reflection, validation, paraphrasing, etc.) are often first developed, trainees acquire knowledge by reading course materials, attending lectures, observing instructors, practicing skills in controlled settings, and receiving feedback or supervision (Sommers-Flanagan & Heck, 2012). Because training in a university setting is often sequential, trainees may not be exposed to specific interventions, such as ESTs, until they have mastered foundational skills. Subsequent coursework is often organized according to broad theoretical orientations (e.g., "Behavior Therapy," "Psychodynamic Psychotherapy") in which specific ESTs are provided as examples of a larger treatment model. In such cases, in our experience, supervised practice in delivering an EST in a clinic ("implementation") is a hit-or-miss proposition. Training is not uniform across (or even within) disciplines, either. Although the American Psychological Association's accreditation standards require instruction in ESTs, they do not provide a rigid structure for how such training is to be delivered. In one less than encouraging study, for example, Weissman and colleagues (2006) reported that the percentage of professional clinical psychology (Psy.D.) and social work programs not requiring didactic training and clinical supervision in at least one EST exceeded 60%.

The emphasis on training in ESTs across the mental health professions is a relatively new phenomenon, and many training program faculty and affiliates may themselves lack adequate training in specific ESTs. With respect to interventions for maltreated children, many psychology graduate and internship training programs offer opportunities to learn at least one EST for child abuse (Sigel & Silovsky, 2012a, 2012b). However, training programs have limited numbers of faculty, and it is unreasonable to assume that they can be expert trainers in all conceivable ESTs.

The reality is that with our current methods of providing clinical training, professionals finish their education without being exposed to a considerable amount of information about specific ESTs. Both personal and professional incentives (e.g., continuing education requirements) require clinicians to continue learning after their formal, university-based education is finished. By far the most common model for such learning is the intensive training workshop. The workshop model involves the dissemination, often at workshops and professional conferences, of didactic training (e.g., reviewing theory associated with an intervention, demonstrating intervention techniques, practicing specific skills through role plays). Research has consistently demonstrated, however, that such training is insufficient to produce changes in clinical practice and meaningful implementation of ESTs (e.g., King et al., 2002; Sholomskas et al., 2005). Clinicians are more likely to implement a newly learned EST with fidelity if they receive competency training comprising feedback and coaching (Beidas & Kendall, 2010; Sholomskas et al., 2005). Borrowing McHugh and Barlow's (2012) analogy, didactic training in the absence of competency training is akin to purchasing a computer that does not have an operating system and other important software.

Time and money serve as two, often interrelated barriers to disseminating information about ESTs via the workshop model. Attending multiday workshops may be cost-prohibitive for mental health professionals and agencies. Time and money are also barriers to competency training. The limited availability and the cost of professional supervision/consultation may deter mental health professionals and agencies from pursuing training in ESTs, especially when considered in the context of a system where reimbursement for services is often decreasing while administrative requirements to receive reimbursement are increasing. Research to identify best practices in the training of clinicians is limited. Questions remain about the intensity, duration, and mechanisms of training necessary to ensure treatment fidelity, competence, and sustainability, as well as the measurement strategies used to operationalize clinician competence, client outcomes, and cost-effectiveness (McHugh & Barlow, 2012).

With these two models of training and their associated barriers in mind, we turn our attention to how technology is changing the way two ESTs for child abuse and maltreatment are disseminated, highlighting how technology can be used to eliminate or reduce identified barriers to dissemination and implementation.

WEB-BASED TECHNOLOGY AND DISSEMINATION: TF-CBTWEB

As noted above, Trauma-Focused Cognitive Behavioral Therapy was identified in 2004 as the only "well-supported and efficacious" treatment for child maltreatment victims. This coincided with the proliferation of the National Child Traumatic Stress Network, a national effort funded by the Substance Abuse and Mental Health Services Administration to produce more trauma-informed service systems for families and children. Many centers and agencies around the country were funded to identify and implement promising services for child trauma victims. Given its empirical support, many agencies were naturally interested in TF-CBT, resulting in a high demand for workshop training. In response, the co-developers of the treatment, Drs. Judith Cohen, Esther Deblinger, and Anthony Mannarino, collaborated with the National Crime Victims Research & Treatment Center at the Medical University of South Carolina to create an online training system that would supplement the workshop-based training they were providing. The resulting product, known as TF-CBTWeb (www.musc.edu/tfcbt; see also Smith & Saunders, 2006), is a 10-hour, Web-based, asynchronous, distance learning course that teaches mental health professionals and students the basic skills associated with TF-CBT and serves as a foundation for the in-person workshop training.

While developing TF-CBTWeb, we conducted extensive reviews of the distance education, Web-based learning, and

adult learning literatures. Provision of asynchronous, Web-based learning for adult professionals is quite different from teaching a graduate course or even providing a traditional training workshop. Therefore, the design of TF-CBTWeb was based on specific principles of learning related to its target audience and modality. In particular, making the website attractive and using engaging technology were a high priority because most learners would be taking TF-CBTWeb voluntarily for the learning experience, rather than as part of a degree-granting program (although several training programs now require students to complete the course).

TF-CBTWeb contains learning modules that present information about each component of TF-CBT. Each module includes:

- Pre- and post-tests assessing knowledge of the treatment component
- Learning objectives
- A text description of the intervention techniques associated with the specific component
- Sample scripts of therapist-client interactions
- Multiple streaming video demonstrations of techniques being implemented by trained therapists with simulated clients
- Homework or follow-up exercises that can be used with clients
- Relevant cultural considerations for applying the techniques
- A discussion of common clinical challenges
- Directions for engaging parents or guardians in the intervention

The course was designed to be used by busy, frontline practitioners who often have little time and few resources for traditional approaches to professional education. The asynchronous, modular, self-study approach allows practitioners to learn at their own pace at a time that is convenient. They can access the training at any time, from virtually any computer with Internet access. The modular approach means they can space their learning over time and return to the course whenever they like. TF-CBTWeb is offered at no charge, and mental health professionals who complete the course (i.e., finish all post-test modules and the course evaluation) are eligible for 10 contact hours of continuing education from the Medical University of South Carolina.

TF-CBTWeb was launched on October 1, 2005, and learner evaluation data reveal that it has been successful in achieving several of its purposes. A more thorough evaluation is currently underway (Heck, Saunders, & Smith, 2013), but data from 9,149 learners who registered for the course during its first full year of operation (October 1, 2005, to September 30, 2006) are very encouraging. The full report is available online (National Crime Victims Research & Treatment Center, 2007). Course evaluation data from the 3,558 (39%) course completers indicate statistically significant knowledge gains in every module, as measured by changes in pre-post test scores. Learner satisfaction scores were also quite high, with over 90% of learners either "agreeing" or "strongly agreeing" that each element of the course we assessed (including ease of navigation, "look and feel," clarity of content, streaming video content) was helpful or satisfactory. The learner profile for the first year also suggests that the course reached our target audience: mental health professionals from a variety of disciplines who are relatively early in their careers (or students). The large majority of learners lived in the United States, but a significant minority (8%) were international learners (in 60 different countries).

Registration for the course continues to grow; as of September 30, 2012, more than a hundred thousand learners had registered for the course, and a preliminary analysis indicated that the overall completion rate was approximately 50% (Heck, Saunders, & Smith, 2013). Therefore, from a dissemination point of view, TF-CBTWeb has clearly been a success. Literally tens of thousands of people have received basic instruction in the foundational principles and methods of the treatment via the Web in a format approved by (and developed in collaboration with) the treatment developers. Indeed, all participants in authorized TF-CBT workshop trainings are now required to complete TF-CBTWeb prior to workshop attendance.

Of course, the course does have its limitations. For example, since the launch in 2005, the treatment developers have slightly modified the way that TF-CBT training is organized, and the content of the modules has evolved somewhat. Due to a lack of resources, TF-CBTWeb has not yet been updated to reflect these modifications. However, funding for "TF-CBTWeb 2.0" was recently obtained. In addition, our outcome evaluation data thus far are limited to user satisfaction and knowledge gain—both appear to be excellent—but we have no information on utilization of the treatment, therapists' skill acquisition, or fidelity to the treatment for course completers. Information about these crucial aspects of implementation are needed before TF-CBTWeb can be viewed as fully successful.

WEB-BASED TECHNOLOGY AND IMPLEMENTATION: PARENT-CHILD INTERACTION THERAPY

Originally developed to treat disruptive behavior problems in children and, more broadly, in families with unhealthy styles of interaction, Parent-Child Interaction Therapy (PCIT; Hembree-Kigin & McNeil, 1995) has been successfully adapted to treat physically abusive families (Saunders, Berliner, & Hanson, 2004). Traditionally, PCIT has been disseminated in university-based settings where the trainee receives didactic training, followed by approximately six months of co-therapy in which a trainer observes, coaches, and provides feedback to the trainee (Funderbunk et al., 2008). In community settings, PCIT training typically requires as many as 40 hours of didactic training, followed by

regular consultation and coaching. Historically, such consultation and coaching involved the trainer and trainee speaking over the telephone. With the trainer unable to directly observe or review the trainee's work, however, the value of such consultation was limited because it relied on trainees' self-reports of their performance, which might not accurately reflect their fidelity to the PCIT model (Funderbunk et al., 2008). An additional barrier to implementing PCIT in community settings was the cost associated with hiring a full-time trainer, and the limited availability of such trainers, to provide on-site coaching for three to six months. Simply put, the co-therapy model of PCIT training, which involved direct observation of trainees' performance, was highly impractical outside university-based settings.

Advances in Web-based communication technologies may help address this barrier. Funderbunk and colleagues (2008) developed and are evaluating a method of videoconferencing that can approximate the traditional co-therapy model of training. The following vignette illustrates this advance.

> Dr. Brennan has recently completed a week of didactic training in PCIT and has returned to his community-based counseling center in a small town in West Virginia. Dr. Brennan has been working with a father-child dyad and is planning to observe and coach the father in a child-directed dyadic play session. The father and child are in the playroom, and Dr. Brennan is in the observation room. In addition, Dr. Stewart, a PCIT trainer working at a medical center in North Carolina, is providing live coaching remotely to Dr. Brennan as Dr. Brennan coaches the father.
>
> In the corner of the playroom, a small camera is affixed above two videoconferencing screens (both similar in size to a computer monitor). The camera is equipped with a microphone and speaker system so that Dr. Brennan and Dr. Stewart can hear what is happening in the room and provide coaching to the father. On the screens, the father can see Dr. Brennan and Dr. Stewart. In the observation room sits another camera and two screens that allow Dr. Brennan to communicate with the father and with Dr. Stewart. Finally, in Dr. Stewart's office sit two small screens and a camera allowing her to communicate with both the father and Dr. Brennan. Using videoconferencing technology, Dr. Stewart is able to see, hear, and speak both with the father as he interacts with the child and with Dr. Brennan as he coaches the father from the observation room.

Videoconferencing technology allows the PCIT trainer to remain in the co-therapist role that is typical of university-based training settings. This technology is feasible, and surveys indicate that clinicians are satisfied with the consultation delivered by videoconferencing (Funderbunk et al., 2008). One drawback, noted by Funderbunk and colleagues, is the cost of such technology, which may be prohibitive for many community-based organizations and providers. However, the authors note that videoconferencing supervision takes place during a billable client-contact hour, which may offset some costs associated with forgoing a billable hour for weekly telephone supervision.

In the absence of co-therapy, a Video Analysis Tool (VAT; www.videoanalysistool.com) may serve as a viable, cost-effective method to provide ongoing coaching in PCIT to other trainees. According to Wilsie and Brestan-Knight (2012), a VAT allows a trainee to receive feedback from a trainer, who reviews videos of therapy sessions online using a Web interface compliant with HIPAA (Health Insurance Portability and Accountability Act of 1996). Trainers can review the video and insert comments that are linked to specific time points in the session, and once the trainer has finished his or her review, the trainee can review the feedback associated with the most important points of the therapy session (Wilsie & Brestan-Knight, 2012).

In summary, technological advances, including videoconferencing and VATs, increase access to off-site experts who can provide the ongoing coaching and feedback needed for successful implementation of PCIT. Additionally, the use of technology can be used in "train-the-trainer" approaches as a way to increase the number of community clinicians who can receive supervision in a specific EST. Such approaches are ideal—and probably cost-effective—because they increase the availability of on-site supervision, which, given the high turnover rates in community settings, can help to ensure newly hired clinicians' access to feedback and coaching (Cahill et al., 2006). Although the current cost of acquiring videoconferencing technology may be prohibitive, as time progresses the costs of technology tend to decrease, and alternative methods such as VATs may be used more frequently. Clearly, research is needed into how new technologies can best facilitate the dissemination of ESTs.

FUTURE DIRECTIONS

We have highlighted the ways in which technology is currently being used to improve dissemination and implementation of ESTs related to child maltreatment. However, technology is not standing still. As advances in technology occur, we hope that corresponding advancements in training will follow. Although it is extremely difficult to predict what will and will not "take" as a technological advance (for every Blu-ray there is a Betamax), we are aware of several exciting new directions in existing or emerging technology that we plan to follow closely.

First, although extensive empirical evidence demonstrates the efficacy of TF-CBT (for a review, see Cary & McMillen, 2012), emerging evidence also suggests that fidelity to TF-CBT may be suboptimal in some community settings (Allen & Johnson, 2012). In an effort to increase fidelity and child and family engagement in TF-CBT, researchers at the Medical University of South Carolina, the University of Medicine and Dentistry of New Jersey, and Allegheny General Hospital, with funding from the National Institute of Mental Health, are developing and evaluating an "eTF-CBT" toolkit. Comprising technology-based applications (videos, interactive content, drawing tools, etc.) that mental health professionals can download to mobile devices such as tablets and smartphones for use in or out of session, the eTF-CBT toolkit will include applications that correspond to each component of TF-CBT. The selection of applications for the toolkit is ongoing but will be grounded in qualitative data obtained from TF-CBT training experts regarding their impressions of aspects of TF-CBT that present challenges to implementation with fidelity. With the proliferation of tablets and smartphones, it is exciting to consider how their capabilities can be leveraged in mental health interventions, whether for TF-CBT or any other EST.

A second potentially exciting development addresses one of the main shortcomings in the training impact of TF-CBTWeb. In its current form, the learning course cannot measure skill acquisition in a feasible way that is not resource intensive. We have considered a variety of methods for obtaining learners' performance data, but each has had significant shortcomings. However, recent applications of virtual reality (VR) simulation technology to clinical interactions have led to the development and feasibility analysis of "virtual clients" (Rizzo et al., 2010). Clinical researchers and computer programmers are collaborating to create low-cost, desktop computer–based avatars that can be programmed to mimic clinical patients in a believable fashion. VR technology has been used for some time in exposure-based treatments for phobia and posttraumatic stress disorder (e.g., Rothbaum et al., 2001). Unlike those systems, however, the technology being proposed does not involve wearing VR glasses or goggles or the subjective sense of immersion into a "virtual setting." Rather, a "virtual client" is created on the computer screen who interacts aurally and orally with the therapist. A feasibility study of this technology for augmenting suicide assessment training is currently underway (Carpenter, Osterberg, & Sutcliffe, 2012). If the technology proves feasible, similar functionality could be applied to online training courses, such as TF-CBTWeb, that would permit remote data collection via computer of a feasible and reasonably standardized interaction with a client or patient, which could in turn be evaluated for competence and treatment model fidelity. Refinement of this technology may be years away, but if it can be readily adapted to different treatment models, its potential for training could indeed be revolutionary.

Although these future possibilities are exciting, it would be imprudent not to mention the caveats and concerns that must accompany technological advances. Although many videoconferencing programs have been deemed HIPAA-compliant, we may still have a lot to learn about how to protect the confidentiality of learners and clients/patients when using technology. This is especially true if applications or programs that contain therapeutic elements are downloaded to smartphones, tablets, or other portable devices. The storage of information on such devices, or on "cloud" servers associated with many computer platforms, requires careful consideration.

CONCLUSIONS

As Hensler, Wilson, and Sadler (2004) noted, the human tendency to resist change and maintain homeostatic systems is an omnipresent force that we must overcome if we are to disseminate and implement ESTs more broadly. History is filled with examples of technological advances precipitating enormous cultural changes. In the early eighteenth century, Jethro Tull's horse-drawn seed drill and horse-drawn hoe revolutionized the agricultural industry. James Hargreaves's spinning jenny and James Watt's steam engine gave rise to the industrial revolution of the late eighteenth and early nineteenth centuries. And recently, personal computers, the Internet, and the World Wide Web gave rise to a technological revolution that changed the way knowledge is stored, disseminated, and consumed in our society. In the mental health professions, technology is changing how we train and deliver mental health services. The potential for creating better providers, for improving the efficiency of clinical training and the client/patient care system, and for increasing clients' access to excellent care is enticing and exciting. We have already seen remarkable progress in dissemination and implementation spurred by Web-based technology within, but not limited to, the child maltreatment field. We must continue to capitalize on advances in technology, but we must do so responsibly, never forgetting our obligations to our profession and to the safeguarding of our clients' well-being.

References

Allen, B., & Johnson, J. C. (2012). Utilization and implementation of trauma-focused cognitive-behavioral therapy for the treatment of maltreated children. *Child Maltreatment, 17,* 80–85. doi:10.1177/1077559511418220

American Psychological Association Task Force on Promotion and Dissemination of Psychological Procedures. (1995). Training in and dissemination of empirically-validated psychological treatments: Report and recommendations. *Clinical Psychologist, 48,* 3–23.

Andersson, G., & Cuijpers, P. (2009). Internet-based and other computerized psychological treatments for adult depression: A meta-analysis. *Cognitive Behaviour Therapy, 38,* 196–205. doi:10.1080/16506070903318960

Andrews, G., Cuijpers, P., Craske, M. G., McEvoy, P., & Titov, N. (2010). Computer therapy for the anxiety and depressive disorders is effective, acceptable and practical health care: A meta-analysis. *PLoS ONE, 5,* e13196. doi:10.1371/journal.pone.0013196

Beidas, R. S., & Kendall, P. C. (2010). Training therapists in evidence-based practice: A critical review of studies from a systems-contextual perspective. *Clinical Psychology: Science and Practice, 17*(1), 1–30.

Cahill, S. P., Foa, E. B., Hembree, E. A., Marshall, R. D., & Nacash, N. (2006). Dissemination of exposure therapy in the treatment of posttraumatic stress disorder. *Journal of Traumatic Stress, 19,* 597–610. doi:10.1002/jts.20173

Carpenter, C., Osterberg, L. D., & Sutcliffe, G. (2012, May). *SAMHT—Suicidal avatars for mental health training.* Paper presented at the International FLAIRS Conference, Buena Vista, FL.

Cary, C. E., & McMillen, J. C. (2012). The data behind the dissemination: A systematic review of Trauma-Focused Cognitive Behavioral Therapy for use with children and youth. *Children and Youth Services Review, 34,* 748–757. doi:10.1016/j.childyouth.2012.01.003

Chadwick Center for Children and Families. (2004). *Closing the quality chasm in child abuse treatment: Identifying and disseminating best practices.* San Diego, CA: Author. www.chadwickcenter.org/Kauffman/kauffman.htm

Chambless, D. L., & Hollon, S. D. (1998). Defining empirically supported therapies. *Journal of Consulting and Clinical Psychology, 66,* 7–18. doi:10.1037/0022-006X.66.1.7

Cohen, J. A., Mannarino, A. P., & Deblinger, E. (2006). *Treating trauma and traumatic grief in children and adolescents.* New York, NY: Guilford Press.

Funderbunk, B. W., Ware, L. M., Altshuler, E., & Chaffin, M. (2008). Use and feasibility of telemedicine technology in the dissemination of Parent-Child Interaction Therapy. *Child Maltreatment, 13,* 377–382. doi:10.1177/1077559508321483

Gotham, H. J. (2004). Diffusion of mental health and substance abuse treatments: Development, dissemination, and implementation. *Clinical Psychology: Science and Practice, 11,* 160–176. doi:10.1093/clipsy/bph067

Harasim, L. (2000). Shift happens: Online education as a new paradigm in learning. *Internet and Higher Education, 3,* 41–61. doi:10.1016/S1096-7516(00)00032-4

Heck, N. C., Saunders, B. E., & Smith, D. W. (2013). *Web-based training in evidence supported treatment: Training completion and knowledge acquisition in a global sample of learners.* Manuscript submitted for publication.

Hembree-Kigin, T. L., & McNeil, C. B. (1995). *Parent-Child Interaction Therapy.* New York, NY: Springer.

Hilbert, M., & Lopez, P. (2012). How to measure the world's technological capacity to communicate, store, and compute information: Part I. Results and scope. *International Journal of Communication, 6,* 956–979.

Institute of Medicine. (2000). *Crossing the quality chasm: A new health system for the 21st century.* Washington, DC: Author.

King, M., Davidson, O., Taylor, F., Haines, A., Sharp, D., & Turner, R. (2002). Effectiveness of teaching general practitioners skills in brief cognitive behaviour therapy to treat patients with depression: Randomized controlled trial. *BMJ, 324,* 947–950. doi:10.1136/bmj.324.7343.947

McHugh, R. K., & Barlow, D. H. (2012). Training in evidence-based psychological interventions. In R. K. McHugh & D. H. Barlow (Eds.), *Dissemination and implementation of evidence-based psychological interventions* (pp. 43–58). New York, NY: Oxford University Press.

National Crime Victims Research & Treatment Center. (2007). *TF-CBTWeb: First year report.* Charleston, SC: Author. http://academicdepartments.musc.edu/ncvc/resources_pro/TFCBTWebFirstYearReport%20final%202-1-07.pdf

Rizzo, A., Parsons, T., Buckwalter, G., & Kenny, P. (2010, March). *A new generation of intelligent virtual patients for clinical training.* Proceedings of the IEEE Virtual Reality Conference, Waltham, MA.

Rothbaum, B. O., Hodges, L. F., Ready, D., Graap, K., & Alarcon, R. D. (2001). Virtual reality exposure therapy for Vietnam veterans with posttraumatic stress disorder. *Journal of Clinical Psychiatry, 62,* 617–622.

Ruggiero, K. J., Resnick, H. S., Acierno, R., Coffey, S. F., Carpenter, M. J., Ruscio, A. M., et al. (2006). Internet-based intervention for mental health and substance use problems in disaster-affected populations: A pilot feasibility study. *Behavior Therapy, 37,* 190–205.

Saunders, B. E., Berliner, L., & Hanson, R. F. (Eds.). (2004, April 26). *Child physical and sexual abuse: Guidelines for treatment* (Revised report). Charleston, SC: National Crime Victims Research & Treatment Center.

Self-Brown, S., & Whitaker, D. J. (2008). Parent-focused child maltreatment prevention: Improving assessment, intervention and dissemination with technology. *Child Maltreatment, 13,* 400–416. doi:10.1177/1077559508320059

Shahab, L., & McEwen A. (2009). Online support for smoking cessation: A systematic review of the literature. *Addiction, 104,* 1792–1804. doi:10.1111/j.1360-0443.2009.02710.x

Sholomskas, D. E., Syracuse-Siewert, G., Rounsaville, B. J., Ball, S. A., Nuro, K. F., & Carroll, K. M. (2005). We don't train in vain: A dissemination trial of three strategies of training in cognitive-behavioral therapy. *Journal of Consulting and Clinical Psychology, 73,* 106–115. doi:10.1037/0022-006X.73.1.106

Sigel, B. A., & Silovsky, J. F. (2011a). Psychology graduate school training on interventions for child maltreatment. *Training and Education in Professional Psychology, 3,* 229–234. doi:10.1037/a0024467

Sigel, B. A., & Silovsky, J. F. (2011b). Psychology internship training on interventions for children with maltreatment

histories. *Training and Education in Professional Psychology, 5,* 237–243. doi:10.1037/a0025867

Smith, D. W., & Saunders, B. E. (2006). Dissemination of empirically supported, trauma-focused treatment via the internet: TF-CBTWeb. *Traumatic StressPoints, 20*(2), 1, 10.

Sommers-Flanagan, J., & Heck, N. C. (2012). Counseling skills: Building the pillars of professional counseling. In D. Perera-Diltz & K. MacCluskie (Eds.), *The counselor educator's survival guide: Designing and teaching outstanding courses in community mental health counseling and school programs* (pp. 153–170). New York, NY: Routledge.

U.S. Census Bureau. (1991). *Statistical brief: The growing use of computers.* Washington, DC: Author. www.census.gov/hhes /computer/publications

U.S. Census Bureau. (2012). *Adult computer and adult Internet users by selected characteristics: 2000 to 2011.* Washington, DC: Author. www.census.gov/hhes/computer/publications

Weissman, M. M., Verdeli, H., Gameroff, M. J., Bledsoe, S. E., Betts, K., Mufson, L., et al. (2006). National survey of psychotherapy training in psychiatry, psychology and social work. *Archives of General Psychiatry, 63,* 925–934. doi:10.1001/ archpsyc.63.8.925

Wilsie, C. C., & Brestan-Knight, B. (2012). Using and online viewing system for Parent-Child Interaction Therapy consulting with professionals. *Psychological Services, 9,* 224–226. doi:10.1037/a002618

27

ROBERT D. SEGE, M.D., PH.D.
GENEVIEVE PREER, M.D.
KIMBERLY A. SCHWARTZ, M.D., FAAP

Education of Emergency Department Physicians

Emergency medicine physicians are at the frontline of caring for children with abusive injuries. This chapter focuses on the essential educational content that emergency medicine physicians require to identify, manage, and report child maltreatment in the emergency department.

THE PROBLEM

Injured children may be seen in emergency departments in children's hospitals, in specialized pediatric emergency departments in general hospitals, or in emergency departments of hospitals without on-site pediatric expertise. In general, less than half of American children entering emergency departments are seen in pediatric specialty emergency settings. At the same time, many American children are evaluated in the emergency department for physical injuries that result from abuse or for concerns about sexual abuse. According to the Centers for Disease Control and Prevention's (2012) National Epidemiologic Injury Surveillance System, in 2010 more than twenty-six thousand children under the age of 5 years (132 per 100,000) were seen in emergency departments for violence-related injuries.

The overall statistics most likely represent an underestimate of the overall number of children treated for abuse-related injuries, as recent research has shown that abusive injuries are frequently missed in emergency departments that do not have pediatric-specific services. For example, children with abdominal injuries resulting from abuse are less likely to be diagnosed if they are treated in a general emergency department than if treated at a pediatric emergency facility (Trokel, Discala, et al., 2006). Similarly, abuse-related fractures are more likely to be missed in a general emergency department than in a pediatric emergency facility setting (Ravichandiran et al., 2010). Even af-

ter a significant educational intervention, emergency departments often fail to document key aspects of childhood abuse–related injuries (Guenther et al., 2009).

Emergency medicine training requirements include general knowledge of interpersonal violence, including child maltreatment, elder abuse, and intimate partner violence, but do not include any specific requirements for the recognition and management of specific syndromes associated with child abuse (Perina et al., 2012). In fact, emergency medicine residents receive relatively little training in child abuse pediatrics. In 2009, Starling et al. reported that less than 20% of emergency medicine physicians received eight hours or more of didactic instruction in child abuse and only 11% received eight hours or more of clinical teaching in child abuse, even though one-third of respondents had seen seven or more cases of child sexual abuse during their residencies.

Given the high likelihood that physicians working in emergency department settings will encounter child maltreatment, it is critically important that emergency physicians receive specialized training on the recognition, evaluation, and management of common forms of child maltreatment. This training is even more important because of strong evidence for the presence of bias in the medical assessment of suspected child maltreatment. In a landmark study, Lane and colleagues (2002) showed that African American children were more likely to have a skeletal survey than white children in the same emergency department. Furthermore, Laskey and colleagues (2012) found that given a child with the same history and injury, pediatricians were more likely to consider child abuse in families of lower socioeconomic status, confirming earlier results obtained in a national prospective primary care study (Flaherty et al., 2008). Hence, objective evaluation at the time of a patient's initial presentation is necessary to formulate a clinical rationale guided by specific facts while minimizing bias. In addition, access to consultation with qualified pediatric personnel experienced in child maltreatment is essential to navigating the possible pitfalls that these complex cases often present (Hansen & Hill, 2011).

DIAGNOSIS OF SUSPECTED MALTREATMENT

Proper diagnosis of child maltreatment hinges on early recognition of patterns that are concerning for abuse or neglect. This includes objective identification of sentinel injuries and injuries suggestive of physical abuse. In addition, emergency physicians should be familiar with the medical response to other types of maltreatment, including sexual abuse and medical neglect.

Table 27.1 lists common presentations of child maltreatment that may be detected in the emergency medicine setting. Because an exhaustive list of each concerning injury would be neither practical nor useful, this table includes the most prevalent and dangerous conditions. In every case of suspected child maltreatment, the clinician must remember that there is no substitute for a thoughtful workup coupled with sound clinical judgment.

Physicians evaluating children for suspected maltreatment should conduct a complete history and physical examination. Consultation with a pediatrician trained in child abuse pediatrics can yield invaluable guidance on how to proceed with the history and medical evaluation.

Infants and preverbal children are particularly vulnerable to injury, including maltreatment-related fatalities. Bruises are very rare in children who are not yet independently mobile and should always prompt consideration of maltreatment. In toddlers and children, bruises behind the ears, bruises on the buttocks, and patterned bruises are particularly worrisome. In contrast, bruises on the shins and other bony prominences are common in toddlers and children and generally do not elicit concern for maltreatment.

Head trauma raises specific concerns in young children. Children who are found obtunded or with injuries around the head and neck should be evaluated promptly and thoroughly. Abusive head trauma often includes subdural hematoma or other intracranial bleeding, evidence of diffuse axonal injury, retinal hemorrhages, and changes in neurological status. These may occur even in the absence of skull fractures or other external signs of injury. Child abuse must be considered in the evaluation of any infant who appears obtunded or presents with altered mental status in the absence of clear trauma history (such as a motor vehicle accident) or acute medical problem. Indeed, even when another medical etiology may explain the child's presentation, it is critically important to recall that children with chronic medical problems can also be the victims of child maltreatment and, in fact, are at higher risk than their healthy peers (Jones et al., 2012).

Child neglect is a common reason for presentation to the emergency department. Typical presentations include ingestions, children found wandering alone, and children who have sustained injuries from burns, falls, and other avoidable mechanisms resulting from lack of supervision. When the antecedent history reveals a failure to supervise, particularly when family violence, mental illness, or parental substance abuse may have contributed to the child's presentation, child neglect must be diagnosed and reported. For example, when any motor vehicle accident results from a parent driving under the influence with a child passenger, a mandatory report should be filed for neglect, regardless of whether the child was injured.

Table 27.1. Selected Emergency Department Presentations of Child Maltreatment

Age (Developmental Stage)	Presentation/Injury	Initial Evaluation
Under 6 months (not yet cruising or walking)	Any bruise, any fracture, any burn, any injury without a history	Full history and physical, CBC with platelets, PT/PTT, ALT, AST, PTH, vitamin D 25-OH, Ca, Mg, Phos, photodocumentation of bruises; consider head imaging and skeletal survey
Under 1 year	Obtunded or other evidence of head injury without clear explanation	Full history and physical, head imaging, skeletal survey; if head injury, lab tests as above and retinal exam recommended
Over 1 year (independently mobile)	Bruises behind ears, on neck, abdomen, or buttocks, or in the pattern of a hand or object	Full history and physical, CBC with platelets, PT/PTT, ALT, AST, Ca, Mg, Phos, photodocumentation of bruises
Any age	Child found alone without adult supervision, other signs of neglect	Full history and physical, assessment of social situation
Any age	Disclosure of sexual abuse	Forensic evidence collection if contact within 72 hours, external exam for bruising or injuries, urine tests for chlamydia and gonorrhea, referral to child advocacy center for forensic interview and full exam
Any age	Motor vehicle crash	Specific history of driver drug or alcohol use and whether child passenger was restrained
Any age	Serious unintentional injury	Complete history, with specific evaluation of circumstances of injury and adult supervision; see table 27.2
Any age	Unexplained death	Refer to medical examiner; *if* protective concerns (i.e., other children in the home), refer to child protective services and law enforcement for evaluation

Burns, while not highly specific for child maltreatment, should be evaluated with care. These may be symptoms of child physical abuse or supervisory neglect. Patterns of burns that are highly suspicious for child maltreatment include pattern burns from cigarettes, irons, or other hot objects and hot water immersion burns. Burns that do not match the history given or that otherwise raise concerns for abuse or neglect should be discussed with a child abuse pediatrician. Additionally, photographing cutaneous injuries to provide a visual record should be standard practice in cases where maltreatment is suspected.

New disclosures of child sexual abuse often prompt parents or other adults to bring the child to the emergency department for evaluation. In general, definitive evaluation of these children should occur at child advocacy centers, which are located in every state and can conduct both forensic interviews and examinations. In the emergency department, evaluation centers on the collection of forensic evidence, if there has been contact with the alleged perpetrator within the past 72 hours, and a physical examination as outlined above for any other signs of injury. Detailed guidelines for when to initiate evidence collection in the acute setting are outlined in policy from the American Academy of Pediatrics (Kellogg & Committee on Child Abuse and Neglect, 2005).

Due to the risk for over-interpretation and misinterpretation, specialized examinations for sexual abuse should not be conducted by emergency department personnel. Makoroff and colleagues (2002) showed that when pediatric emergency room physicians identified abnormal findings in cases of prepubertal nonacute sexual abuse, a child abuse physician frequently found the exam results to be normal or nonspecific in follow-up. Adams and colleagues (2012)

demonstrated the importance for nonspecialists who see fewer than five cases of child sexual abuse per month to keep their knowledge current by reviewing the sexual abuse literature and engaging in regular case review with an expert in child sexual abuse in order to avoid diagnostic errors.

In addition to the specific presentations described above, it is not uncommon for emergency medicine providers to encounter protective concerns when a parent or adult caregiver presents to the emergency department with a medical condition related to domestic violence, drug abuse, alcohol intoxication, or psychiatric decompensation. In each of these cases, consultation with a child abuse specialist is critically important in order not to miss reportable instances of abuse or neglect of the children in these parents' care.

EVALUATION OF SUSPECTED CHILD MALTREATMENT

Tables 27.1 and 27.2 provide an overview of the initial evaluation and history required when child maltreatment is suspected. In all cases, a thorough nondirected history and physical is required. The key elements of distinguishing unintentional injury from injury resulting from child maltreatment come from the history. Table 27.2 contains a detailed description of an injury history that will assist the clinician in differentiating the two types of causes. Inconsistent histories, histories that do not match the child's developmental status, or injuries without any history offered at all are also highly suspicious for child maltreatment (Hettler & Greenes, 2003). When possible, a review of the patient's medical history for prior concerning injuries, medical neglect, or

Table 27.2. Childhood Injury History

Information to Be Documented	Questions	Considerations
Who?	Who are you speaking with? Did the person witness the injury? Is there someone who witnessed the injury?	Obtain history from verbal child without parent or guardian present. Obtain history from adults separately and not in presence of verbal child.
When?	When was the last time the child appeared well? When did the injury occur? When did the child first display symptoms and what were they?	For infants, review events of the past 24 hours chronologically, with particular attention to who has cared for the infant during this period.
What?	Find out and document as many details as possible. Was there a fall? How far? From where to where? Onto what surface? What happened as the child fell? What was the infant/child doing before? What part of the child's body hit what? What was the infant/child doing after? What position was the infant/child in?	Try to visualize the injury event. If you cannot picture the exact episode, you need more details. Inquire specifically about the child's immediate reaction after the injury.
Where?	Where did the injury occur? Where was the infant/child? Was an adult carrying the infant/child?	Was this a place that the infant/child normally visits?
Development?	What is the infant/child able to do? Roll over, crawl, pull to a stand, walk, run, climb?	If the patient is able, a demonstration of the described motor skill is of value.

other circumstances that raise protective concerns is essential. A history of concerning injuries or medical neglect in a sibling can be crucially important and is commonly missed.

The physical examination should always include a complete skin inspection of all children, with specific attention to bruises, scars, and burns, as discussed above. A thorough head, ears, eyes, nose, and throat exam should include inspection of the pinnae and posterior auricular areas for bruising and an otoscopic exam for hemotympanum. Inspection of the oropharynx for signs of trauma, including lesions of the buccal mucosa, trauma to the upper or lower frenula, and damage to the teeth, can identify injuries that may be clinically silent. An external genital examination should be performed for all children. Clinicians should provide a developmentally appropriate explanation for this portion of the examination for children over the age of 3 years. Normal findings on genital examination do not preclude the possibility of sexual abuse, but the exam is essential in order not to miss the presence of injuries or lesions that might not be reported in the history.

Screening for a bleeding disorder should be considered for children with bruising or bleeding as a significant feature of the clinical presentation. While these disorders are quite uncommon in children without a previous history of bleeding, evaluation may be important to avoid misdiagnosing physical abuse. Similarly, children with signs of trauma should have liver transaminases measured (Lindberg et al., 2009), as internal injuries are not uncommonly associated with child physical abuse (Trokel, Discala, et al., 2006) and may not be otherwise evident in the history or on physical examination.

Skeletal surveys (American Academy of Pediatrics, Section on Radiology, 2009), which include a specified set of plain radiographs of the skull, ribs, and axial skeleton, should be performed for children who are premobile and preverbal and whose presentation raises concerns about abusive injury. Although a large number of images (22) are required, the overall radiation dose is much lower than that from a single CT. "Baby grams" and other survey radiographs are insufficiently detailed and nondiagnostic. For example, specific views of the axial skeleton are required to demonstrate classic metaphyseal lesions, which involve growth plates of the long bones in children under the age of 1 year. These injuries are virtually diagnostic of child maltreatment (Kleinman et al., 2011). If at all possible, in cases where abusive injury is suspected, skeletal surveys and other radiographs should be reviewed by a pediatric radiologist, as findings may be subtle. In addition, consideration should be given to repeating the skeletal survey within 10–14 days as some fractures that may not be evident in the acute setting are more easily detected in the healing phase.

REPORTING SUSPECTED CHILD MALTREATMENT

All cases of suspected child abuse and neglect should be reported to the state child protective services (CPS), as is required by law in every state in the United States. There is potential civil and criminal liability for failing to report suspected maltreatment, while there is legal protection for mandated reporters who file in good faith. Child abuse reports allow the reporter to share information with state CPS even in the absence of parental consent. In many states, CPS may also choose to involve law enforcement. The clinician should keep in mind that child abuse is typically a chronic condition, and when suspected abuse is not reported, children may be exposed to further danger. The state CPS response occurs in phases. When a call or report is received by CPS, the first determination is a screening decision. CPS may decide to screen in the report and provide an immediate emergency response when the patient or another child in the home may be at imminent risk of further maltreatment. CPS may also decide to screen in for investigation or assessment, which typically takes place over a 1- to 3-week time frame. During this investigation, CPS will have access to previous reports to the agency and law enforcement history and will typically visit the home and interview other relevant collaterals in making its decision. The child is often in the home or with a relative during this phase of the investigation.

Most states have a variable response mechanism in place. This allows CPS to provide services to families even when the protective concerns are lower. In the bulk of substantiated claims. CPS will provide services for the family. These may range from mental health services for adult caregivers, daycare vouchers, assistance with housing or other concrete needs, or simply counseling and monitoring.

A small number of cases result in children being removed from parents' or guardians' custody to temporary foster care. National statistics from 2010 show that 4% of CPS referrals result in temporary foster placement (U.S. Department of Health and Human Services, 2012). This is more likely to occur in the setting of the type of severe injury typically seen in the emergency department. Most agencies are granted a brief period during which children at risk may be placed in foster care pending a judicial decision regarding custody. Typical judicially mandated foster care arrangements are temporary, allowing stabilization of the child's family situation. When child maltreatment is chronic, however, CPS may take legal measures to retain custody of a child or children at risk, including a longer-term removal from the parents' custody or eventual termination of parental rights.

CONCLUSIONS

Child maltreatment is a medically and legally complex area that frequently plays a role in acute presentations to the emergency department. All emergency medicine physicians deserve adequate training in this critically important area. Improved education that focuses on typical presentations, key elements of the diagnostic evaluation, and the importance of consultation can equip emergency department physicians with the tools they need to care for maltreated children. Training in the proper reporting of suspected child maltreatment to child protective services is a crucial and often overlooked area. Finally, medical professionals who care for children in general hospital emergency departments should have ready access to child abuse pediatricians for consultation and guidance on both the initial assessment and subsequent workup when child maltreatment is suspected.

References

Adams, J. A., Starling, S. P., Frasier, L. D., Palusci, V. J., Shapiro, R. A., Finkel, M. A., & Botash, A. S. (2012). Diagnostic accuracy in child sexual abuse medical evaluation: Role of experience, training, and expert case review. *Child Abuse & Neglect, 36*(5), 383–392.

American Academy of Pediatrics, Section on Radiology. (2009). Diagnostic imaging of child abuse. *Pediatrics, 123*(5), 1430–1435.

Centers for Disease Control and Prevention, National Center for Injury Prevention and Control. (2012). WISQARS (Web-based Injury Statistics Query and Reporting System). www.cdc.gov/ncipc/wisqars

Flaherty, E. G., Sege, R. D., Griffith, J., Price, L. L., Wasserman, R., Slora, E., et al. (2008). From suspicion of physical child abuse to reporting: Primary care clinician decision-making. *Pediatrics, 122*(3), 611–619.

Guenther, E., Olsen, C., Keenan, H., Newberry, C., Dean, J. M., & Olson, L. M. (2009). Randomized prospective study to evaluate child abuse documentation in the emergency department. *Academic Emergency Medicine, 16*(3), 249–257.

Hansen, N., & Hill, K. S. (2011, October). *Defining the children's hospital role in child maltreatment* (2nd ed.). Alexandria, VA: National Association of Children's Hospitals and Related Institutions. www.childrenshospitals.net/AM/Template.cfm?Section=Child_Abuse_and_Neglect&Template=/CM/ContentDisplay.cfm&ContentID=59013

Hettler, J., & Greenes, D. (2003). Can the initial history predict whether a child with a head injury has been abused? *Pediatrics, 111*(3), 602–607.

Jones, L., Bellis, M. A., Wood, S., Hughes, K., McCoy, E., Eckley, L., et al. (2012). Prevalence and risk of violence against children with disabilities: A systematic review and meta-analysis of observational studies. *Lancet, 380*(9845), 899–907.

Kellogg, N., & Committee on Child Abuse and Neglect, American Academy of Pediatrics. (2005). The evaluation of sexual abuse in children. *Pediatrics, 116*(2), 506–512.

Kleinman, P. K., Perez-Rossello, J. M., Newton, A. W., Feldman, H. A., & Kleinman, P. L. (2011). Prevalence of the classic metaphyseal lesion in infants at low versus high risk for abuse. *AJR, American Journal of Roentgenology, 197*(4), 1005–1008.

Lane, W. G., Rubin, D. M., Monteith, R., & Christian, C. W. (2002). Racial differences in the evaluation of pediatric fractures for physical abuse. *JAMA, 288*(13), 1603–1609.

Laskey, A. L., Stump, T. E., Perkins, S. M., Zimet, G. D., Sherman, S. J., & Downs, S. M. (2012). Influence of race and socioeconomic status on the diagnosis of child abuse: A randomized study. *Journal of Pediatrics, 160*(6), 1003–1008.

Lindberg, D., Makoroff, K., Harper, N., Laskey, A., Bechtel, K., Deye, K., & Shapiro, R., ULTRA Investigators. (2009). Utility of hepatic transaminases to recognize abuse in children. *Pediatrics, 124*(2), 509–516.

Makoroff, K. L., Brauley, J. L., Brandner, A. M., Myers, P. A., & Shapiro, R. A. (2002). Genital examinations for alleged sexual abuse of prepubertal girls: Findings by pediatric emergency medicine physicians compared with child abuse trained physicians. *Child Abuse & Neglect, 26*(12), 1235–1242.

Perina. D. G., Brunett, P., Caro, D. A., Char, D. M., Chisholm, C. D., Counselman, F. L., et al. (2012, May 31). The 2011 model of the clinical practice of emergency medicine. *Academic Emergency Medicine.* Advance online publication. doi:10.1111/j.1553-2712.2012.01385

Ravichandiran, N., Schuh, S., Bejuk, M., Al-Harthy, N., Shouldice, M., Au, H., & Boutis, K. (2010). Delayed identification of pediatric abuse-related fractures. *Pediatrics, 125*(1), 60–66.

Starling, S. P., Heisler, K. W., Paulson, J. F., & Youmans, E. (2009). Child abuse training and knowledge: A national survey of emergency medicine, family medicine, and pediatric residents and program directors. *Pediatrics, 123*(4), e595–602.

Trokel, M., Discala, C., Terrin, N. C., & Sege, R. D. (2006). Patient and injury characteristics in abusive abdominal injuries. *Pediatric Emergency Care, 22*(10), 700–704.

Trokel, M., Waddimba, A., Griffith, J., & Sege, R. (2006). Variation in the diagnosis of child abuse in severely injured infants. *Pediatrics, 117*(3), 722–728.

U.S. Department of Health and Human Services, Administration for Children and Families, Administration on Children, Youth and Families, Children's Bureau. (2012). *Child maltreatment, 2010: Summary of key findings.* www.childwelfare.gov/pubs/factsheets/canstats.pdf

28

KATHI MAKOROFF, M.D., M.ED.

Education of Physicians in Residency Training

GENERAL CONSIDERATIONS

Child abuse (maltreatment) is an enormous public health issue, with significant morbidity and mortality. Residents in training frequently see children with suspected child abuse and neglect, and no matter what field of practice the graduates of residency programs enter, they will continue to evaluate children with suspected maltreatment. It is important that the resident learns to recognize the signs and symptoms of child abuse, knows what to do once it is recognized, has the skills to talk with a caregiver about concerns of suspected abuse, and knows how to take care of herself or himself during difficult cases. Residents should also be knowledgeable about preventing maltreatment and have the skills to do so. Finally, residents should be armed with the knowledge of how child abuse and neglect influence behaviors and affect physical and mental health outcomes in later years, into adulthood, and how clinicians can influence parents, community professionals, and the public in preventing or decreasing sources of adversity in childhood.

The long-term effects of child abuse have been recognized and studied in recent years. Certain types and degrees of childhood adversity can have lasting effects on behavior and health, well into adulthood. By studying a large number of adults who were being seen for preventive health care, the ACE (Adverse Childhood Experiences) studies looked at the connection between childhood exposure to adversities and health-related outcomes (Felitti et al., 1998). The ACE studies have demonstrated that exposure to certain types of childhood adversity (each one is considered an individual ACE)—including physical, emotional, or sexual abuse; exposure to violence; household substance abuse; and mental illness—is more likely to affect risk factors for behaviors and diseases in adulthood (Brown et al., 2010; Dong et al., 2004; Felitti et al., 1998; Williamson et al., 2002).

Some of these risk factors involve behaviors, such as smoking, illicit drug use, and alcoholism, and some involve prevalent adult diseases, such as cardiovascular diseases and cancer; other studies have analyzed general health and functioning and mental health problems, such as depression, anxiety, and poor anger control. The studies have shown that as the number of ACEs experienced in childhood increases, the risk of early death increases (Felitti et al., 1998).

It is now better understood that long-term and adult diseases, as well as behavior, learning, and cognition problems in childhood, are linked to toxic stress in childhood and that toxic stress may alter early brain architecture and functioning. Toxic stress is defined as excessive stress that leads to activation of the physiological stress response systems (including stress hormone levels, immune system functioning) in the absence of an external buffering protection from the stress (such as the presence of nurturing parents or other caregivers, stable responsive relationships). An eco-bio-developmental framework is used to better understand health and disease prevention; this framework combines genetic predispositions, environmental influences, and personal experiences (Shankoff & Garner, 2012).

This growing body of literature, community experiences, and science that demonstrate how early adverse experiences and toxic stress are connected to impairments in physical and mental health should be part of resident education.

The importance of discovering and preventing child maltreatment to prevent problems in childhood and adulthood is increasingly recognized. The immediate importance of accurately detecting child abuse has also been documented. In a landmark article, Jenny and colleagues (1999) found that 31.2% of shaken baby cases (now more commonly referred to as abusive head trauma) were not initially recognized by physicians. Twenty-eight percent of the patients were reinjured after the missed diagnosis; 9.3% died. All of these patients had at least one prior visit to an emergency department or to a primary care provider and received diagnoses including gastroenteritis, otitis media, and colic. The diagnosis was more likely to be missed in children who presented with milder symptoms, children whose parents were living together, and children who were not minorities. Education of all physicians, beginning in residency training, helps them to accurately diagnose cases of child abuse.

CURRENT STATE OF RESIDENT EDUCATION IN CHILD ABUSE PEDIATRICS

Child abuse pediatrics was first recognized as a board-certified pediatric subspecialty by the American Board of Pediatrics in 2009. Child abuse pediatrics fellowship training programs have been accredited by the Accreditation Council for Graduate Medical Education since 2010.

Child abuse pediatrics is not currently an additional required subspecialty experience, according to the Residency Review Committee requirements. Where possible, it is included as an elective experience. The Common Program Requirements maintain that pediatric residents must demonstrate medical knowledge (and application to patient care) in the evolving biomedical, clinical, epidemiological, and social behavioral sciences; this includes knowledge of physical and sexual abuse (Accreditation Council for Graduate Medical Education, 2012). Thus, there is great variation among residency programs in how much child abuse training residents receive. Some programs have a two- to four-week mandatory rotation, some offer an elective, and some do not have the capability for any resident experience in this area.

Many studies indicate that physicians lack knowledge, training, and confidence in cases of child abuse, including identification, reporting, and treatment of child abuse and identification of child abuse mimics. A survey study showed that a quarter of all accredited pediatric residency programs did not offer any rotation in child abuse pediatrics (Narayan, Socolar, & St. Clair, 2006). Didactic education ranged from 0 to 10 hours annually, and less than half of the residents reported that they attended more than 75% of these didactic talks. Not surprisingly, most of the programs surveyed reported that more time and more patient experience with abused children were needed. This survey result has been echoed in research. Studies of pediatric chief residents (Dubow et al., 2005) and primary care physicians (Ladson, Johnson, & Doty, 1987) found that these physicians were unable to correctly identify genital structures in a prepubertal child. In the Dubow et al. study (2005), only half of the pediatric chief residents thought that their training in sexual abuse evaluation was "adequate."

A few studies have examined residents' knowledge and comfort in the identification and management of cases of child abuse. One large national study evaluated pediatric, family medicine, and emergency medicine residents, comparing the amount of child abuse–related training received and number of child abuse cases seen during residency and residents' knowledge and comfort about child abuse cases (Starling, Heisler, & Paulson, 2009). Residents who had more training and saw a greater number of patients with child abuse scored higher on the knowledge portion of the survey. Residents' knowledge also correlated positively with institutions that had a child abuse pediatrician, a multidisciplinary child abuse team, or a child abuse assessment center. Knowledge was also greater when training programs had a required child abuse rotation or a written curriculum.

In another study of residents' knowledge that used a 30-question test, the pediatric residents (n = 61) had a mean score of 60.4%. There was no significant difference in score based on year of training (Menoch et al., 2011).

PRIMARY CARE TRAINING IN CHILD ABUSE EVALUATION AND PREVENTION

Primary care physicians are often the first to evaluate children with suspected child abuse, and therefore it is imperative that they are able to recognize injuries and differentiate child abuse from other medical conditions or accidents.

Physicians should be involved in the diagnosis and treatment of suspected child abuse and should also serve as resources for patients and families, as well as for community agencies, law enforcement, and the court system. Physicians should also be actively involved in administering prevention programs, including prevention as part of anticipatory guidance during patient visits.

Appropriate evaluations for child abuse and neglect, which include a history, physical examination, and interpretation of laboratory and radiographic findings, benefit the interests of the child, the family, and society. Yet, cases of child abuse can be difficult to correctly diagnose. The symptoms and signs of child abuse, particularly in young children, can be similar to symptoms and signs resulting from accidental injury or medical illness. A complete evaluation also will ensure the child's health and safety, will detect conditions and diseases, and may discover occult injuries that can then be treated and documented for forensic purposes. An inadequate or improper evaluation can harm the child and family.

Prevention of child maltreatment is needed to reduce the burden of child abuse and neglect and to protect children and families. Many current prevention strategies focus on home visitation programs. More recently, screening for psychosocial risk factors has been shown to be an important facet of prevention of maltreatment. This screening is an essential aspect of the well-child care visit and therefore should be part of residency training. The American Academy of Pediatrics suggests the use of programs such as Practicing Safety and Bright Futures at well-child visits. These programs include asking caregivers about and monitoring risk factors, such as intimate partner violence, maternal depression, and effective disciplinary strategies. Although these programs are well-established and screening for family risk factors is encouraged, practicing physicians voice barriers to implementing such screenings. These barriers include lack of time, but also lack of training and discomfort in addressing potentially sensitive topics. However, there are examples of programs, and evidence supporting them, that train pediatric residents to address psychosocial risk factors.

One such program was piloted in Maryland: the Safe Environment for Every Kid (SEEK) model (Dubowitz et al., 2009). This pilot program was based in an urban resident continuity clinic. The model included training (initial training plus six-month booster trainings) for the pediatric residents, added a social worker to work with the residents and within the model, and used a 20-item parent screening questionnaire to screen for the targeted risk factors. The training aspect of this program included a multidisciplinary teaching faculty and focused on psychosocial risk factors, including violence, depression, and substance abuse, as well as on discipline and food insecurity. The teaching included instruction on assessment of the screening and was also interactive, using cases and role play to practice how to address positive findings. The outcome of the pilot program showed that in the group of patients who received the SEEK program (as opposed to traditional continuity care), there were 31% fewer reports to child protective services. From a review of the medical records, children in the SEEK group also had fewer instances of medical neglect and less inappropriate discipline, as reported by their parents (Dubowitz et al., 2009).

This model is important because it moves ahead of simply teaching residents about identification of child abuse and reporting laws and focuses on prevention of child maltreatment. The residents who used this model also demonstrated improvements in knowledge, perceived competence, and level of comfort in many of the psychosocial issues shown to be risk factors for child abuse (Feigelman et al., 2011).

Additional educational programs have been piloted to teach pediatric residents about domestic violence, or intimate partner violence (IPV). The negative effects of IPV on the health and functioning of children have been studied and are becoming better recognized. After an educational intervention with pediatric residents in a large urban continuity care setting, the residents improved the frequency of screening for IPV during well-child visits (Berger et al., 2002). The educational intervention consisted of a didactic session, articles, and a reference guide. This was followed a few months later with an interactive role-play session.

Primary care interactions offer an opportunity to pay attention to social and behavioral issues. It is important to be aware that certain types of abuse are more common at certain ages. Signs and symptoms of child abuse manifest differently at different ages. Knowing both the child and parental characteristics that can increase the risk for child abuse is necessary for early detection. The "child variables" differ at different ages, such as crying in infancy, separation anxiety in older infants, and toilet training in toddlers. The types of evaluation, physical examination, and laboratory/radiographic studies will also differ for children at different ages. Parental mental health issues, isolation, substance abuse, IPV, family stressors, frequently missed appointments, or excessive care seeking—all are other issues to be considered. The resident should ask appropriate screening questions that might uncover family issues or risk factors for abuse. By observing how the parent bonds with the infant and responds to the child's needs and activity level and observing to what degree the parent uses positive rather than negative terms when talking about the child, the resident can gain a sense of the risk of maltreatment. An unreasonable developmental expectation of a child, such as expecting an 18-month-old to toilet train, is a major risk factor for physical abuse.

Anticipatory guidance related to physical or sexual abuse should be provided at each visit. These messages should start at the prenatal and newborn visits with the information that it is normal for an infant to cry, then move into developmental expectations for toddlers, and continue through strategies for protecting children from sexual abuse, including Internet safety for school-age and adolescent children. Some anticipatory guidance tools include (1) the Period of PURPLE Crying, which gives parents and caregivers a framework to understand that crying in infancy (even long-lasting crying that resists soothing) can be normal (Barr, 1998; National Center on Shaken Baby Syndrome,www.dontshake.org), and (2) Stewards of Children, a child sexual abuse prevention program that was designed for adults but can also be used by youth organizations, which increases awareness of child sexual abuse and teaches strategies for protecting children (Darkness to Light, www.d2l.org).

RESIDENTS AND CHILD ABUSE REPORTING

The mandatory reporting laws in all 50 states maintain that when a practitioner has reasonable suspicion that a child has been abused or neglected, that practitioner must make a report to child protective services (CPS). Failure to make a report can result in a criminal penalty and can also cause action against a practitioner's professional license. The practitioner need not be certain about the diagnosis to make a report.

Although physicians are mandated reporters, one study found that only 4% of total reports of suspected child abuse to CPS came from primary care physicians (Flaherty et al., 2000). These authors surveyed primary care providers and found that barriers to reporting included not believing that their patient would benefit from CPS involvement. The study did show that education on the topic of child abuse (recognition, need to report) increased the probability that the provider would report a case of suspected child abuse.

Residents, as physicians, are mandated reporters. If the report is reasonable and is made in good faith, the resident should not fear legal retaliation even if a report of suspected child abuse is based on a medical diagnosis that is, eventually, not the final diagnosis. This can happen, for example, for a child with multiple bruises who is found to have a bleeding disorder or for a child with fractures who is discovered to have a genetic bony dysplasia. Knowledge of common mimics of child abuse can help decrease the incidence of incorrect diagnoses, again highlighting the importance of education in this area.

When residents and their supervising physicians differ in their decisions to report a case as suspected child abuse, the resident should be offered an alternative, such as consultation with the child abuse pediatrics or child protection consult service (if available) or discussion with the residency program director.

INNOVATIVE TEACHING METHODS

Most physicians feel uncomfortable with the recognition and management of cases of child abuse because they have not received adequate education and training in the area of child maltreatment (Christian, 2008). Child abuse can be seen in all of the subspecialties of medicine. Orthopedic surgeons, general surgeons, radiologists, ophthalmologists, and dentists may be the first health care professionals to come into professional contact with a child who has been abused. The consequences of missing a case of child abuse are great; the consequences of misdiagnosing a case of child abuse are also significant, as a child can be inappropriately removed from a home environment.

Although the subspecialty of child abuse pediatrics was recognized by the American Board of Pediatrics in 2009, the regional distribution of physician specialists in child abuse pediatrics is uneven. Many but not all hospitals and pediatric training programs include specialists in this area. Therefore, not every medical student or pediatric resident is exposed to this subspecialty or receives instruction in recognizing and managing cases of child abuse from experts in the field of child abuse pediatrics.

One way to bridge the divide between the needs of learners and the availability of instructors and resources is through the use of distance education (distance learning). Distance education is an emerging area of education that delivers instruction and materials to learners who are not studying in the same location or at the same time as the instructor is teaching or materials are presented. It encompasses teaching techniques such as Web-based discussion boards, videoconferencing, email assignments, and presentations. Using distance learning, learners from different institutions can have access to the same information and instruction.

A handful of studies have examined the advantages and disadvantages of Web-based instruction in the field of child maltreatment (Blanchet, 2008; Kenny, 2007; Saunders, 2008). Some of the reported advantages are being able to disseminate the instruction easily and fostering social networking. Disadvantages include the loss of face-to-face interactions and the costs of implementation (Saunders, 2008). However, given that child abuse pediatrics education is necessary but is not available to every resident, distance education is one way to bridge this need.

RESIDENTS AND INTERACTIONS WITH THE CHILD PROTECTION SYSTEM AND THE LEGAL SYSTEM

Many cases of child abuse and neglect proceed to agencies for child protection and the legal system, and the physicians who evaluate these children are required to interact with these systems and may be required to testify in court. The child protection system (child protective services, CPS) investigates any case of suspected abuse or neglect; its duty is to protect children from further harm. The legal system (criminal justice) is involved when it is suspected that someone has broken the law. Not every case warrants that both systems be involved, but many cases of child abuse include both.

All states have CPS. Residents should know about the process of making a report of suspected child abuse or neglect in the area where they practice. Some states have a statewide system, and some states have individual county agencies. Once a report is made, CPS determines whether it will accept the report of suspected abuse/neglect or not. If it does accept the report, an investigation begins, and CPS has a set number of days to carry out the investigation and make a determination of abuse/neglect or not. During this investigation, CPS decides whether to keep the child in the home or remove him or her to an alternative home (this can be an out-of-home kinship care home or foster placement). Although CPS will listen to the medical team and the report of the medical evaluation and findings, it is up to CPS to determine the placement and outcome of the child. It would be inappropriate for the physician to make this determination. During the investigation, a physician may be called to juvenile or family court to testify about the child's medical findings.

The criminal justice system becomes involved in cases of child abuse/neglect in which laws have been broken. Not all cases rise to the level of criminal prosecution. Sometimes a serious crime has occurred (severe or life-threatening injuries to a child) but it is impossible to determine the perpetrator. In a criminal justice case, the prosecutor ("State") must prove the case "beyond a reasonable doubt" (Palusci, Hicks, & Vandevort, 2001).

An essential part of residents' training in the area of child abuse and neglect is education about these other systems that become involved after the medical treatment—the child protection system and the legal system. A 1985 study found that 3% of physicians did not report a case of suspected abuse because they were wary of becoming involved with the legal system (Saulsbury & Campbell, 1985).

A pilot study performed at Arkansas Children's Hospital demonstrated that residents wanted to receive court-related information—including the types of questions asked in court, especially on cross-examination, and the court proceeding process—and wanted feedback on their performance (Jones et al., 1990). The participants in the pilot survey also noted that training in the law (such as when to seek legal advise) would be helpful. The residents in this small survey did not perceive the stress of having to testify as very great. However, other interactions with residents and fellows suggest that the idea of having to testify in court, together with their lack of knowledge about legal proceedings, is very stressful and that they do not feel prepared or comfortable with legal proceedings.

The "nonmedical" aspects of child abuse cases, then, should be part of residents' education. Mock trials can be helpful before a resident needs to appear in court. In addition, residents can feel frustrated and angry when the outcome of a case is not what was expected, such as when CPS does not remove a child from the home. A better understanding of the child protection system and its constraints can help lessen the frustration and anger. Direct communication with CPS workers should be encouraged for additional education and experience.

COMMUNICATING WITH FAMILIES ABOUT SUSPECTED CHILD ABUSE

Conversations surrounding suspected child abuse can be difficult and emotionally charged. These conversations are difficult for families to hear but equally difficult for the provider to deliver. Residents should be given the tools to develop and practice communication skills. Many residency programs offer sessions for residents on "death and dying" or "delivering bad news," and many of the tools and skills learned in such programs can be applied when approaching families about suspected child abuse.

One of the best ways to learn skills and to practice skills in a safe environment is through role plays. Many learners do not initially embrace the idea of role-playing. It does have its limitations: many feel that it is artificial and that it is impossible to capture the true physician-patient (or family) relationship. However, role-playing does afford the opportunity to practice new skills, take risks, and make mistakes. Once learners have had some practice with the skills, they will be able to try them in real patient care contexts.

When approaching families about the diagnosis of suspected child abuse, there are some important points to remember. The decision to report a case as suspicious for child abuse should be communicated to the family either before or immediately after contacting CPS and/or law enforcement. Every provider will feel some stress when hav-

ing such a conversation. It is natural to have these feelings and they should be acknowledged. All caregivers or members of a family should be treated with respect. It is not the provider's role to arrest someone or to make a determination of guilt.

When having a discussion with the family, the resident should create an environment that is conducive to effective communication by ensuring privacy, adequate seating, and time for discussion. Residents should ask who else the parent (or guardian) would like to have present for the discussion, and then document that the parent gave permission to have other family or friends present. The use of simple, easily understood language is key, along with frequent checking with the family to ensure they understand what is being said. It is imperative that all information is delivered in a sensitive but straightforward manner. If the family does not understand that the diagnosis is child abuse, then, when CPS and law enforcement become involved, they will feel that the medical team was hiding information from them. The resident needs to know that no resident, or indeed any physician, will know all the answers. Learning to be comfortable with the response of "I don't know" is one of the lessons of residency training.

Outbursts of strong emotion from the family make many physicians uncomfortable. The resident needs to give the family time to react, but at the same time the resident must have a plan for safety before entering the room. It is always best to have another member of the team present. If there is reasonable concern that the safety of the resident cannot be ensured, arrangement for hospital security to be present during the informing session is advisable. If it would be safer to first report concerns to CPS or law enforcement and wait to talk to the family, then this is the appropriate approach.

SECONDARY TRAUMATIC STRESS

Residents need to be educated about secondary traumatic stress (STS), sometimes referred to as vicarious trauma. This can result when a professional caretaker becomes traumatized after hearing victims' accounts of traumatic events. This can happen to anyone who is in a "helping" profession, including counselors, emergency department and other trauma and medical personnel, hospice workers, police, firefighters, and caseworkers (Gates & Gillespie, 2007). Researchers and practitioners now recognize that those who work with or help traumatized persons are indirectly or secondarily at risk of developing the same symptoms as the persons directly affected by the trauma. Symptoms of STS can include physical symptoms (nausea, fatigue, poor sleep, headaches) and emotional symptoms (feeling powerless, inadequate, frustrated, sad). Cognitive effects such as difficulty concentrating, poor decision making, and forgetfulness can result, and behaviors such as withdrawal, avoidance, and absenteeism. Feelings of emotional distance will involve both one's professional and personal life. People with STS have symptoms that are nearly identical to those of posttraumatic stress disorder, including physiological arousal, intrusive imagery, and even avoidance responses (Gates & Gillespie, 2007).

Not all professionals who care for patients who have suffered trauma develop STS. There are individual risk factors that can influence who will develop STS. A history of poor coping mechanisms or a history of prior trauma can increase the risk of developing STS. Women are at higher risk. There is a positive correlation between increasing amounts of victim contact and the likelihood of STS symptoms. Finally, the more a professional can "relate" to a patient—that is, if the patient reminds the professional of a family member or close friend—the greater the risk of developing STS symptoms (Gates & Gillespie, 2007).

Prevention and treatment of STS and of any emotional response must involve a supportive supervisor. With residents, this supportive supervisor can be a program director, an attending mentor, or even a senior resident or chief resident. Residency programs should openly recognize potential risk situations (emergency department rotations, trauma electives, neonatal or pediatric intensive care rotations, child abuse electives/rotations, local disasters) and also establish program-specific or hospital-specific practices and policies. These should include providing education about STS and its signs and risk factors and being open to peer and mentor monitoring. Physicians should never feel that they are immune to any of these feelings because they are physicians. Debriefing and reflecting sessions can be useful around certain traumatic cases and events. Self-care includes maintaining clear professional boundaries and good home-work balance.

Other considerations for the physician in residency training are emotional responses to the situations of child abuse. It should be expected that one would feel outrage and anger toward the alleged perpetrator and even toward a nonoffending caregiver who did not protect a child from harm. There can also be an overall sadness to seeing a badly injured child and knowing that an adult caused the injuries. Fear of immediate or delayed reprisal from the alleged perpetrator and anxiety about court proceedings would also be appropriate feelings. Anticipating and discussing these feelings and reactions should be part of any residency curriculum. Having a supportive and knowledgeable mentor to help work through the emotions and to offer guidance through any court proceedings will also be helpful.

CONCLUSIONS

Residents in every field will be touched by child maltreatment, whether it is the acute care of an abused child or the care of an adult who suffered adverse childhood experiences. Residents who treat children and adolescents will evaluate children with suspected child abuse and will need to communicate their concerns with the child's family,

with CPS, and with law enforcement. Residents are also in a position to prevent child abuse and therefore should have the knowledge and skills to do so. Residents should know how to be advocates for their patients and for all children. Finally, residents and their residency programs should ensure that the residents are well cared for and acknowledge that secondary traumatic stress can occur.

References

Accreditation Council for Graduate Medical Education. (2012, September). *Program director guide to the common program requirements.* www.acgme.org/acgmeweb/tabid/237/GraduateMedicalEducation/InstitutionalReview/ProgramDirectorGuidetotheCommonProgramRequi.aspx

Barr, R. G. (1998). Colic and crying syndromes in infants. *Pediatrics, 102*(5, Suppl. E), 1282–1286.

Berger, R. P., Bogen, D., Dulani, T., & Broussard, E. (2002). Implementation of a program to teach pediatric residents and faculty about domestic violence. *Archives of Pediatrics & Adolescent Medicine, 156,* 804–810.

Blanchet, K. D. (2008). Innovative programs in telemedicine. *Telemedicine and e-Health, 14,* 637–641.

Brown, D. W., Anda, R. F., Felitti, V. J., Edwards, V. J., Malarcher, A. M., Croft, J. B., & Giles, W. H. (2010). Adverse childhood experiences and the risk of lung cancer. *BMC Public Health, 10,* 20.

Christian, C. (2008). Professional education in child abuse and neglect. *Pediatrics, 122,* S13–17.

Dong, M., Giles, W. H., Felitti, V. J., Dube, S. R., Williams, J. E., Chapman, D. P., & Anda, R. F. (2004). Insights into causal pathways for ischemic heart disease: Adverse Childhood Experiences Study. *Circulation, 110,* 1761–1766.

Dubow, S. R., Giardino, A. P., Christian, C. W., & Johnson, C. F. (2005). Do pediatric chief residents recognize details of prepubertal female genital anatomy? A national survey. *Child Abuse & Neglect, 29*(2), 195–205.

Dubowitz, H., Feigelman, S., Lane, W., & Kim, J. (2009). Pediatric primary care to help prevent child maltreatment: The Safe Environment for Every Kid (SEEK) model. *Pediatrics, 123,* 858–864.

Feigelman, S., Dubowitz, H., Lane, W., Grube, L., & Kim, J. (2011). Training pediatric residents in a primary care clinic to help address psychosocial problems and prevent child maltreatment. *Academic Pediatrics, 11,* 474–480.

Felitti, V. J., Anda, R. F., Nordenberg, D., Williamson, D. F., Spitz, A. M., Edwards, V., et al. (1998). The relationship of adult health status to childhood abuse and household dysfunction. *American Journal of Preventive Medicine, 14,* 245–258.

Flaherty, E. G., Sege, R., Binns, H. J., Mattson, C. L., & Christoffel, K. K. (2000). Healthcare providers' experience reporting child abuse in the primary care setting. *Archives of Pediatrics & Adolescent Medicine, 154,* 489–493.

Gates, D. M., & Gillespie, G. L. (2007). Secondary traumatic stress in nurses who care for traumatized women. *JOGNN, 37,* 243–249.

Jenny, C., Hymel, K. P., Ritzen, A., Reinert S. E., & Hay, T. C. (1999). Analysis of missed cases of abusive head trauma. *JAMA, 282,* 621–626.

Jones, J. G., Rickert, C. P., Balentine, J., Lawson, L., Rickert, V. I., & Holder, J. (1990). Residents' attitudes toward the legal system and court testimony. *Child Abuse & Neglect, 14,* 79–85.

Kenny, M. C. (2007). Web-based training in child maltreatment for future mandated reporters. *Child Abuse & Neglect, 31,* 671–678.

Ladson, S., Johnson, C. F., & Doty, R. E. (1987). Do physicians recognize sexual abuse? *American Journal of Diseases in Children, 141*, 411–415.

Menoch, M., Zimmerman, S., Garcia-Filion, P., & Bulloch, B. (2011). Child abuse education: An objective evaluation of resident and attending physician knowledge. *Pediatric Emergency Care, 27*(10), 937–940.

Narayan, A. P., Socolar, R. S., & St. Claire, K. (2006). Pediatric residency training in child abuse and neglect in the United States. *Pediatrics, 117*(6), 2215–2221.

Palusci, V. J., Hicks, R. A., & Vandevort, F. E. (2001). You are hereby commanded to appear: Pediatrician subpoena and court appearance in child maltreatment. *Pediatrics, 107*, 1427–1430.

Saulsbury, F. T., & Campbell, R. E. (1985). Evaluation of child abuse reporting by physicians. *American Journal of Diseases in Childhood, 139*(4), 393–395.

Saunders, B. E. (2008). Commentary on using new technologies in the child maltreatment field. *Child Maltreatment, 13*, 417–423.

Shankoff, J. P., & Garner, A. S. (2012). The lifelong effects of early childhood adversity and toxic stress. *Pediatrics, 129*, e232–246.

Starling, S. P., Heisler, K. W., & Paulson, J. F. (2009) Child abuse training and knowledge: A national survey of emergency medicine, family medicine and pediatric residents and program directors. *Pediatrics, 123*, e595–602.

Williamson, D. F., Thompson, T. J., Anda, R. F., Dietz, W. H, & Felitti V. J. (2002). Body weight, obesity, and self-reported abuse in childhood. *International Journal of Obesity, 26*, 1075–1082.

AMANDA K. FINGARSON, D.O.
EMALEE G. FLAHERTY, M.D.
ROBERT D. SEGE, M.D., PH.D.

29

Education of Community Physicians

GENERAL CONSIDERATIONS

Virtually all American children receive primary care medical services. Community physicians, through their trusted ongoing relationships with children and their caregivers, can detect changes in children's health and well-being and develop important insights into family dynamics. Nevertheless, community physicians often face challenges in properly diagnosing and managing suspected maltreatment. Leading the list of challenges is a lack of physician training and confidence in diagnosing and managing suspected child maltreatment.

THE SCOPE OF THE PROBLEM

Child abuse is a common problem worldwide, which ultimately affects all community practices providing pediatric care. In the United States, approximately three million reports of suspected maltreatment are made to child protective services (CPS) annually (Gaudiosi, 2010). On average, CPS substantiates fewer than one-third of these reports. Numerous studies suggest that the actual incidence of child maltreatment is substantially higher, with many cases going unsuspected or unreported (Centers for Disease Control and Prevention, 2010; Flaherty, Sege, Griffith, et al., 2008; Jenny et al., 1999; MacMillan et al., 1997; Theodore et al., 2005). Through education and awareness, community physicians can help to identify these potentially missed cases.

IDENTIFICATION AND MANAGEMENT OF MALTREATMENT

Despite the relatively high prevalence of child maltreatment, physicians often fail to suspect and report abuse, par-

ticularly in certain patient populations. Family characteristics can play a role. Studies have found that physicians are less likely to suspect and report child abuse in white, intact families (Flaherty, Sege, Griffith, et al., 2008; Jenny et al., 1999; Jones et al., 2008; Lane et al., 2002; Laskey et al., 2012; Ravichandiran et al., 2010). Privately insured patients are also less likely to be evaluated and reported for maltreatment (Flaherty et al., 2002). In addition to the contribution of family traits, child characteristics can influence the likelihood of a physician correctly diagnosing child abuse. In cases of abusive head trauma, children who are younger or have less severe or less specific symptoms are more likely to be missed (Jenny et al., 1999). Among children with abuse-related fractures, male children are less likely to have the abuse recognized (Ravichandiran et al., 2010). By familiarizing themselves with these trends, community physicians can develop an awareness of personal biases that may influence their decisions, decreasing the possibility that these cases will be missed in their own practices.

In addition to the influence of child and family factors, physicians' response to maltreatment also varies by type of abuse or neglect. Physicians indicate that they report most diagnosed cases of sexual abuse and physical abuse (92% and 91%, respectively) but report physical neglect (58%) and medical neglect (43%) significantly less often (Saulsbury & Campbell, 1985).

REPORTING CHILD MALTREATMENT

Failure to properly diagnose and report child abuse leads to a high likelihood of recurring or escalating child maltreatment (Jenny et al., 1999; Oral et al., 2008). With this in mind, it is important to assess barriers to physicians' reporting of child maltreatment in order to focus educational efforts. Physicians fail to report suspected abuse for a number of reasons. Although state laws require reporting of *suspected* maltreatment (Levi & Brown, 2005; Myers, 1992), many physicians are reluctant to report unless absolutely certain that maltreatment has occurred.

Prior negative experiences or lack of trust in CPS may also result in a decision not to report. Physicians who have had negative prior experiences in court may be less likely to report suspected abuse (Flaherty et al., 2000; Gunn, Hickson, & Cooper, 2005). Familiarity with a family can also prevent physicians from properly addressing suspected maltreatment, as they may be falsely reassured by their belief that they know a particular family well and that the family would be incapable of abuse (Jones et al., 2008). Physicians may also believe that they can intervene and protect a child from future harm without involving state CPS (Flaherty et al., 2000; Saulsbury & Campbell, 1985). Physicians sometimes fear that if they report families to CPS, the families will leave their practices, though often this is not the case (Jones et al., 2008; Vulliamy & Sullivan, 2000).

PHYSICIAN CHARACTERISTICS

Many physicians lack both confidence and a sense of competence to identify and manage child maltreatment. Even though many physicians are expected to evaluate children in their community for suspected physical or sexual abuse, most physicians have had little training to prepare them to do so. A study by Alpert et al. (1998) found that most U.S. medical schools reported curricula in child abuse and neglect, but the amount varied, ranging from 0 to 16 hours, with a median of 2 hours. Twenty-one percent of medical students reported that they had received no instruction on child abuse. Resident education is also limited, even among pediatric residency training programs. In a recent survey of chief residents, many did not think that graduating residents were well prepared to address child abuse and neglect; the study reported that fewer than half (41%) of pediatric residency programs had mandatory rotations, 57% had elective rotations, and 25% offered no rotations at all (Narayan, Socolar, & St Claire, 2006). Overall, one-third of the study participants reported that graduating residents were either not well prepared or were only somewhat well prepared to address child maltreatment.

Reflecting the same education gap, a recent survey of practicing pediatricians found that only 47% reported that they had received sufficient training in child maltreatment during their residency. Many practicing physicians reported that they did not feel competent to conduct sexual abuse examinations (52%) or physical abuse examinations (16%). Even more concerning is that many of the physicians who reported not feeling confident were conducting examinations for sexual abuse and physical abuse in their practices (27% and 19%, respectively). Despite feeling unprepared to assess child maltreatment, some of the physicians (14%–57%) reported an interest in gaining education and serving in a child protection role (Arnold et al., 2005; Christian, 2008; Lane & Dubowitz, 2009).

Within the field of child abuse pediatrics, physicians' knowledge and practice in the area of child sexual abuse is the area most studied. Studies over the past several decades have found that many physicians lack the understanding of anatomy necessary to evaluate child abuse. Several studies showed that both physician trainees and practicing physicians struggle to identify basic prepubertal female genital anatomy such as the hymen and urethra. They also often fail to correctly interpret genital findings that may represent either abnormalities or normal variants. Perhaps related to this, physicians also reported that they do not consistently examine children's genitalia in practice (this was true for prepubertal girls in particular) (Lentsch & Johnson, 2000). Physicians also struggle with interpreting the significance of sexually transmitted infections and sexualized behaviors (Dubow et al., 2005; Ladson, Johnson, & Doty, 1987; Lentsch & Johnson, 2000; Starling et al., 2009).

EDUCATIONAL APPROACHES

Despite the recognition that community physicians would benefit from education on child maltreatment, a systematic review of the literature assessing child protection training and procedural interventions found little rigorous evaluation of the impact and effectiveness of educational efforts directed to physicians in practice (Carter et al., 2006).

Some states have mandated that professionals receive training in child abuse and neglect as a requirement for licensing. One study surveyed professionals, including physicians, psychologists, nurses, teachers, and others, who underwent a mandatory two-hour training in New York (Reiniger, Robison, & McHugh, 1995). A substantial portion of the participants reported that they had not been aware of indicators of abuse prior to the training. The majority reported learning new information about identifying and reporting child maltreatment and legal liabilities. Interestingly, overall, the participants' level of experience in their fields did not affect their need for the information they had received.

Pennsylvania has developed a statewide community-based continuing medical education (CME) program called EPIC-SCAN (Educating Physicians in their Community on Suspected Child Abuse and Neglect) to train primary care providers and their entire office staff to identify and report child maltreatment. This program, initially developed in 1999, paired a local physician with a county child protection worker to deliver an educational presentation (Christian, 2008). Community physicians sometimes report feeling left out of the child abuse investigation process. Programs such as EPIC-SCAN can help physicians establish relationships with local child protection investigators and can inform them of how cases are investigated and how services may be provided to families.

A study by Hibbard, Serwint, & Connolly (1987) assessed the effectiveness of a sexual abuse symposium provided to Indiana medical and social work professionals who were interested in training on this topic. The majority of the participants reported no previous training in the medical evaluation of sexual abuse. As demonstrated by their scores on pre-tests versus post-tests, their knowledge improved significantly at both two weeks and six months after the symposium. Of further benefit, some of these participants later contributed to the education of others by organizing training for medical, social work, and legal professionals in their local communities.

While these studies suggest that short conferences or sessions may be useful, a systematic review of multiple areas of medicine did not find that short, formal CME events such as conferences effect change in physicians' practice unless combined with practice-reinforcing strategies (Davis et al., 1995). The study found that other techniques have proved more effective, such as systematic practice-based interventions and outreach visits, though these formats are infrequently used.

While child abuse education can increase professionals' awareness and knowledge, knowledge gaps can remain. A study by Botash et al. (2005) assessed the effectiveness of an educational intervention on medical providers' knowledge and competence regarding child sexual abuse. Practicing physicians and pediatric residents completed a self-study, case-based curriculum on child sexual abuse, including a workbook and videotaped genital examination. On average, participants showed significant improvement on their pre-test to post-test scores. But despite these encouraging cognitive gains, over half of the physicians did not correctly interpret the exam findings, did not correctly reassure the family, and did not indicate an appropriate understanding of the legal implications. This suggests that significant practice gaps may remain after this type of educational intervention. In addition to conferences and self-directed learning, practice-based, individually tailored feedback is another educational option.

In a randomized, controlled trial by Socolar et al. (1998), tailored written feedback based on chart reviews along with relevant articles were sent to physicians who performed sexual abuse evaluations. Knowledge was tested with a pre-test and post-test at the end of the three-month intervention. There was no significant change in documentation or knowledge for physicians who had received the feedback and articles, suggesting that this may not be a useful way to improve physicians' knowledge and performance in this area. Studies in other areas of medicine have found similar results (Davis et al., 1995).

Regardless of the format, studies have shown that physicians' level of concern for abuse can be influenced by recent child abuse education. Flaherty et al. (2002) found that physicians were more likely to classify injuries in their practices as being suspicious for abuse if they had received some sort of education about child abuse in the preceding five years (Flaherty et al., 2002). Studies have also found that physicians' confidence in identifying child abuse increases with recent child maltreatment training (Flaherty et al., 2006). While child abuse training during residency is important, another study by Flaherty et al. (2000) highlighted the importance of post-residency education on child abuse. The authors found that providers who had received some sort of training after residency were 10 times more likely to report all abuse than those who had not received post-residency education.

CONCLUSIONS AND RECOMMENDATIONS

Physicians' education should be tailored to their practice setting and include an awareness of sentinel injuries, including typical history and physical and radiological signs of maltreatment. Educational efforts should address the attitudinal barriers that inhibit reporting, including bias in assessment and a poor understanding of the entire child protective system.

Ideally, physicians would receive exposure to child abuse pediatrics through didactic sessions and clinical rotations before completing medical school and residency training and entering into a primary care practice. The content of training should be specified for all medical trainees. A report published as a result of a national multidisciplinary conference suggested that standards be specified for the "quantity or quality of education that medical students, pediatric residents, or other physicians should receive about child maltreatment" as part of a "comprehensive educational strategy that builds knowledge and experience from medical school and residency through continuing education once a clinician is in practice, including segments that describe prevention, identification, and interaction with the state CPS system" (Flaherty, Sege, Hurley, & Baker, 2008, p. S19).

Once in practice, busy physicians will find CME-based training opportunities a viable option, despite their limitations. Both regional and national conferences focus on child maltreatment. Some conferences are primarily medically oriented, while others provide a broader scope. Many of these conferences are also attended by professionals in related fields, including social workers, law enforcement, and child protection workers. Their perspectives can enhance physicians' experience and learning. Exposure to the investigation process that occurs after child maltreatment is reported can help facilitate community physicians' participation in the interdisciplinary process of child protection.

There are a number of published resources that physicians may find helpful. The American Academy of Pediatrics (AAP) publishes useful practice guidelines addressing various forms of maltreatment and has published visual atlases that may be of assistance in evaluating possible physical and sexual abuse. Resources discussing the role of the physician in court proceedings on child maltreatment are also available (Hanes & McAuliff, 1997). Being called to testify in either family or criminal court can be an anxiety-provoking experience for community physicians, yet their participation can be vital in protecting children. There are articles, books, and conference presentations that can prepare physicians on what to expect in court and how to testify effectively (Horsley & Carlova, 1983; Myers, 1992).

While recognizing and reporting child abuse are important in ensuring children's safety, community physicians also play an important role in the prevention of child abuse. Barton Schmitt (1987) described the "seven deadly sins of childhood," suggesting that these normal phases of a child's development place them at risk of maltreatment. An awareness of how particular stages of development may pose a parenting challenge can help physicians direct their anticipatory guidance during routine pediatric care.

Infant crying is one of the normal developmental phases that can trigger child maltreatment. Studies have shown that infant crying is a main trigger for child abuse (Lee et al., 2007; Reijneveld et al., 2004). A number of brochures, videos, and websites are available to help parents understand and cope with their child's crying.

With older children, abuse sometimes results from caregivers having unrealistic expectations about their children's behaviors. Physicians can empower parents by teaching them about normal child development and behavior (Flaherty & Stirling, 2010). The AAP Bright Futures program is a valuable resource, with materials incorporating child maltreatment prevention counseling into regular health supervision visits. The AAP also publishes parent handouts that address many of the challenges of parenting, including infant crying, toddler discipline, and adolescent behaviors (Sege et al., 2005).

In addition to conferences and written resources, local child abuse experts can be important resources for community physicians. Child abuse pediatrics is now a board-certifiable subspecialty through the American Board of Pediatrics, and child abuse pediatricians can be found in many metropolitan areas. Community physicians should familiarize themselves with their local child abuse pediatricians, who can serve as important resources for education and referrals.

In conclusion, community physicians may feel overwhelmed by the responsibility of preventing, identifying, and addressing child maltreatment in their practices and may feel unqualified to serve in this capacity. Physicians should take advantage of training opportunities at all points during their medical training and practice and should reach out to child abuse pediatricians and other professionals in their region for help when needed. They should remain aware of their mandate to report any suspected child maltreatment. Though the responsibility is great, community physicians serve a vital role in protecting children in their communities.

References

Alpert, E. J., Tonkin, A. E., Seeherman, A. M., & Holtz, H. A. (1998). Family violence curricula in U.S. medical schools. *American Journal of Preventive Medicine, 14*(4), 273–282.

Arnold, D. H., Spiro, D. M., Nichols, M. H., & King, W. D. (2005). Availability and perceived competence of pediatricians to serve as child protection team medical consultants: A survey of practicing pediatricians. *Southern Medical Journal, 98*(4), 423–428.

Botash, A. S., Galloway, A. E., Booth, T., Ploutz-Snyder, R., Hoffman-Rosenfeld, J., & Cahill, L. (2005). Continuing medical education in child sexual abuse: Cognitive gains but not expertise. *Archives of Pediatrics & Adolescent Medicine, 159*(6), 561–566. doi:10.1001/archpedi.159.6.561

Carter, Y. H., Bannon, M. J., Limbert, C., Docherty, A., & Barlow, J. (2006). Improving child protection: A systematic review of training and procedural interventions. *Archives of Disease of Childhood, 91*(9), 740–743. doi:10.1136/adc.2005.092007

Centers for Disease Control and Prevention. (2010). Adverse childhood experiences reported by adults—Five states, 2009. *MMWR Morbidity and Mortality Weekly Report, 59*(49), 1609–1613.

Christian, C. W. (2008). Professional education in child abuse and neglect. *Pediatrics, 122*(Suppl. 1), S13–17. doi:10.1542/peds.2008-0715f

Davis, D. A., Thomson, M. A., Oxman, A. D., & Haynes, R. B. (1995). Changing physician performance: A systematic review of the effect of continuing medical education strategies. *JAMA, 274*(9), 700–705.

Dubow, S. R., Giardino, A. P., Christian, C. W., & Johnson, C. F. (2005). Do pediatric chief residents recognize details of prepubertal female genital anatomy: A national survey. *Child Abuse & Neglect, 29*(2), 195–205. doi:10.1016/j.chiabu.2004.03.017

Flaherty, E. G., Sege, R., Binns, H. J., Mattson, C. L., & Christoffel, K. K., Pediatric Practice Research Group. (2000). Health care providers' experience reporting child abuse in the primary care setting. *Archives of Pediatric & Adolescent Medicine, 154*(5), 489–493.

Flaherty, E. G., Sege, R. D., Griffith, J., Price, L. L., Wasserman, R., Slora, E., et al. (2008). From suspicion of physical child abuse to reporting: Primary care clinician decision-making. *Pediatrics, 122*(3), 611–619. doi:10.1542/peds.2007-2311

Flaherty, E. G., Sege, R. D., Hurley, T. P., & Baker, A. (2008). Strategies for saving and improving children's lives. *Pediatrics, 122*(Suppl. 1), S18–20. doi:10.1542/peds.2008-0715g

Flaherty, E. G., Sege, R., Mattson, C. L., & Binns, H. J. (2002). Assessment of suspicion of abuse in the primary care setting. *Ambulatory Pediatrics, 2*(2), 120–126.

Flaherty, E. G., Sege, R., Price, L. L., Christoffel, K. K., Norton, D. P., & O'Connor, K. G. (2006). Pediatrician characteristics associated with child abuse identification and reporting: Results from a national survey of pediatricians. *Child Maltreatment, 11*(4), 361–369. doi:10.1177/1077559506292287

Flaherty, E. G., & Stirling, J., Jr. (2010). Clinical report: The pediatrician's role in child maltreatment prevention. *Pediatrics, 126*(4), 833–841.

Gaudiosi, J. A. (2010). *Child maltreatment*. Washington, DC: U.S. Government Printing Office.

Gunn, V. L., Hickson, G. B., & Cooper, W. O. (2005). Factors affecting pediatricians' reporting of suspected child maltreatment. *Ambulatory Pediatrics, 5*(2), 96–101. doi:10.1367/A04-094R.1

Hanes, M., & McAuliff, T. (1997). Preparation for child abuse litigation: Perspectives of the prosecutor and the pediatrician. *Pediatric Annals, 26*(5), 288–295.

Hibbard, R. A., Serwint, J., & Connolly, M. (1987). Educational program on evaluation of alleged sexual abuse victims. *Child Abuse & Neglect, 11*(4), 513–519.

Horsley, J. E., & Carlova, J. (1983). *Testifying in court: A guide for physicians* (2nd ed.). Oradell, NJ: Medical Economics Books.

Jenny, C., Hymel, K. P., Ritzen, A., Reinert, S. E., & Hay, T. C. (1999). Analysis of missed cases of abusive head trauma. *JAMA, 281*(7), 621–626.

Jones, R., Flaherty, E. G., Binns, H. J., Price, L. L., Slora, E., Abney, D., et al. (2008). Clinicians' description of factors influencing their reporting of suspected child abuse: Report of the Child Abuse Reporting Experience Study Research Group. *Pediatrics, 122*(2), 259–266. doi:10.1542/peds.2007-2312

Ladson, S., Johnson, C. F., & Doty, R. E. (1987). Do physicians recognize sexual abuse? *American Journal of Diseases of Children, 141*(4), 411–415.

Lane, W. G., & Dubowitz, H. (2009). Primary care pediatricians' experience, comfort and competence in the evaluation and management of child maltreatment: Do we need child abuse experts? *Child Abuse & Neglect, 33*(2), 76–83. doi:10.1016/j.chiabu.2008.09.003

Lane, W. G., Rubin, D. M., Monteith, R., & Christian, C. W. (2002). Racial differences in the evaluation of pediatric fractures for physical abuse. *JAMA, 288*(13), 1603–1609.

Laskey, A. L., Stump, T. E., Perkins, S. M., Zimet, G. D., Sherman, S. J., & Downs, S. M. (2012). Influence of race and socioeconomic status on the diagnosis of child abuse: A randomized study. *Journal of Pediatrics, 160*(6), 1003–1008. doi:10.1016/j.jpeds.2011.11.042

Lee, C., Barr, R. G., Catherine, N., & Wicks, A. (2007). Age-related incidence of publicly reported shaken baby syndrome cases: Is crying a trigger for shaking? *Journal of Developmental and Behavioral Pediatrics, 28*(4), 288–293.

Lentsch, K. A., & Johnson, C. F. (2000). Do physicians have adequate knowledge of child sexual abuse? The results of two surveys of practicing physicians, 1986 and 1996. *Child Maltreatment, 5*(1), 72–78.

Levi, B. H., & Brown, G. (2005). Reasonable suspicion: A study of Pennsylvania pediatricians regarding child abuse. *Pediatrics, 116*(1), e5–12. doi:10.1542/peds.2004-2649

MacMillan, H. L., Fleming, J. E., Trocme, N., Boyle, M. H., Wong, M., Racine, Y. A., et al. (1997). Prevalence of child physical and sexual abuse in the community: Results from the Ontario Health Supplement. *JAMA, 278*(2), 131–135.

Myers, J. E. B. (1992). *Legal issues in child abuse and neglect.* Newbury Park, CA: Sage Publications.

Narayan, A. P., Socolar, R. R., & St Claire, K. (2006). Pediatric residency training in child abuse and neglect in the United States. *Pediatrics, 117*(6), 2215–2221. doi:10.1542/peds.2006-0160

Oral, R., Yagmur, F., Nashelsky, M., Turkmen, M., & Kirby, P. (2008). Fatal abusive head trauma cases: Consequence of medical staff missing milder forms of physical abuse. *Pediatric Emergency Care, 24*(12), 816–821. doi:10.1097/PEC.0b013e31818e9f5d

Ravichandiran, N., Schuh, S., Bejuk, M., Al-Harthy, N., Shouldice, M., Au, H., & Boutis, K. (2010). Delayed identification of pediatric abuse-related fractures. *Pediatrics, 125*(1), 60–66. doi:10.1542/peds.2008-3794

Reijneveld, S. A., van der Wal, M. F., Brugman, E., Sing, R. A., & Verloove-Vanhorick, S. P. (2004). Infant crying and abuse. *Lancet, 364*(9442), 1340–1342. doi:10.1016/S0140-6736(04)17191-2

Reiniger, A., Robison, E., & McHugh, M. (1995). Mandated training of professionals: A means for improving reporting of suspected child abuse. *Child Abuse & Neglect, 19*(1), 63–69.

Saulsbury, F. T., & Campbell, R. E. (1985). Evaluation of child abuse reporting by physicians. *American Journal of Diseases of Children, 139*(4), 393–395.

Schmitt, B. D. (1987). Seven deadly sins of childhood: Advising parents about difficult developmental phases. *Child Abuse & Neglect, 11*(3), 421–432.

Sege, R. D., Flanigan, E., Levin-Goodman, R., Licenziato, V. G., De Vos, E., & Spivak, H. (2005). American Academy of Pediatrics' Connected Kids program: Case study. *American Journal of Preventive Medicine, 29*(5, Suppl. 2), 215–219. doi:10.1016/j.amepre.2005.08.026

Socolar, R. R., Raines, B., Chen-Mok, M., Runyan, D. K., Green, C., & Paterno, S. (1998). Intervention to improve physician documentation and knowledge of child sexual abuse: A randomized, controlled trial. *Pediatrics, 101*(5), 817–824.

Starling, S. P., Heisler, K. W., Paulson, J. F., & Youmans, E. (2009). Child abuse training and knowledge: A national survey of emergency medicine, family medicine, and pediatric residents and program directors. *Pediatrics, 123*(4), e595–602. doi:10.1542/peds.2008-2938

Theodore, A. D., Chang, J. J., Runyan, D. K., Hunter, W. M., Bangdiwala, S. I., & Agans, R. (2005). Epidemiologic features of the physical and sexual maltreatment of children in the Carolinas. *Pediatrics, 115*(3), e331–337. doi:10.1542/peds.2004-1033

Vulliamy, A. P., & Sullivan, R. (2000). Reporting child abuse: Pediatricians' experiences with the child protection system. *Child Abuse & Neglect, 24*(11), 1461–1470.

BRETT SLINGSBY, M.D.
CHRISTINE BARRON, M.D.

30

Child Abuse Pediatricians

Treating Child Victims of Maltreatment

GENERAL CONSIDERATIONS

Whenever there is concern about any form of child maltreatment, the child would benefit from an appropriate medical evaluation. Over the past few years, a new subspecialty has emerged of physicians who are experienced and knowledgeable about the complex aspects within the field of child abuse pediatrics. Their expertise allows them to provide appropriate medical evaluations for child victims of sexual abuse, physical abuse, emotional abuse, and neglect. The subspecialty of child abuse pediatrics and its recognition by the medical, legal, and child protective services communities has led to improved evaluations and care for child victims of abuse. A familiarity with this new group of pediatricians will provide other professionals with a unique resource in the evaluation, diagnosis, and treatment of child abuse and neglect.

CHILD ABUSE PEDIATRICS AS A SUBSPECIALTY

Over the past six decades, child abuse has been recognized as a medical issue. Medical interest in child abuse began in 1946, when John Caffey described six infants who presented to medical care with subdural hemorrhages and long bone fractures. While the causal relationship between these injuries was not clearly stated in his article, Caffey did indicate that the two were somehow related and most likely due to trauma. Then in the early 1960s, C. Henry Kempe described "the battered child syndrome," which acknowledged that children developed injuries from physical abuse and that it is important for the physician to be aware of the possibility of battered child syndrome and to look for inconsistencies between the physical examination and the history provided (Kempe et al., 1965). This article gave rise to increased medical interest in and research into child abuse.

Since the 1960s, the amount of research and clinical knowledge in the field of child abuse has grown considerably. As a result, a need arose for physicians to both continue the advancement of research in the field and provide quality clinical care to suspected victims of abuse. Eventually it became clear that as the medical knowledge grew and clinical skill demands increased, new physicians entering the field would require more training and experience than that obtained during pediatric residency. In 2006, the American Board of Pediatrics established child abuse pediatrics as a subspecialty of pediatrics. This was an acknowledgment of the skills, education, and training required to provide appropriate care to child victims of abuse. Subsequently, the Accreditation Council for Graduate Medical Education (ACGME) standardized the fellowship training requirements for physicians entering this field. As justification for the need of consistent fellowship training in child abuse pediatrics, the organization stated that "the purpose of establishing and recognizing additional training and separate certification in child abuse pediatrics is to ensure that abused and neglected children will receive expert and appropriate care" (Accreditation Council for Graduate Medical Education [ACGME], 2012).

Most pediatricians, immediately after residency training, have very limited experience working with victims of abuse. In addition, they are usually not exposed to the multiple areas of medicine with which a familiarity is required to be a competent child abuse pediatrician (ACGME, 2012). As a result, many practicing physicians are uncomfortable with evaluating children when abuse is suspected. Part of this problem is the lack of uniform education among pediatric residents in the field of child maltreatment. When pediatric chief residents were surveyed about how well the graduating pediatric residents were prepared to address child abuse, 34% thought that their graduates were less than well trained in child abuse (Narayan, Scoloar, & St

Claire, 2006). A study by Starling et al. (2009) found that third-year residents in pediatrics, family medicine, and emergency medicine had minimal training in child abuse, were unable to identify normal female genital anatomy, and were very uncomfortable evaluating children for sexual abuse. These articles support the theory that being skilled at working with pediatric victims of abuse requires more training than can be provided during pediatric residency. In their paper about the need for the subspecialty of child abuse pediatrics, Block and Palusci (2006) wrote that hundreds of hours of training and experience are required before one can competently treat potential victims of abuse. That degree of training is not and cannot be offered during a three-year residency program, and adequate experience cannot be obtained without working as a subspecialist.

Like graduating residents, many primary care physicians are uncomfortable dealing with concerns about abuse or neglect, due to their of lack of knowledge and experience in this specific area (Botash et al., 2005; Flaherty & Sege, 2005; Flaherty, Sege, Griffith, et al., 2008; Flaherty, Sege, Price, et al., 2006; Lane & Dubowitz, 2009). In addition, primary care physicians face other practical problems when concerns of abuse are identified. It can be difficult, after spending years knowing and treating a family, to confront them with concerns about child maltreatment. There can be an unintentional bias from years of positive or negative interactions that would not be influencing factors for a consulted expert who has never met the family. Providers are also concerned about losing patients, angering families, or being sued when they report a suspicion of maltreatment (Flaherty & Sege, 2005; Jones et al., 2008). Establishing a subspecialty in the field of child abuse pediatrics allows primary care physicians to have a resource and expert opinion when confronted with concerns about abuse. The primary care provider is still responsible for identifying concerns about maltreatment, communicating with the child abuse pediatrician (CAP) before and after the consultation, and following up with the family after the evaluation, but the CAP is there as an expert consultant to deal with the acute concerns and questions.

Another practical problem for the primary care provider confronted with a case of suspected child maltreatment is time. An appropriate evaluation of suspected child maltreatment is time-consuming, often requiring two hours for a formal evaluation. When a provider has patients scheduled into 15-minute appointments (Gottschalk & Flocke, 2005), it is difficult to obtain an adequate history, complete and photodocument an examination, make medical recommendations, contact appropriate authorities, and counsel the family about the next steps in the investigation. In addition, many primary care physicians are uncomfortable or unfamiliar with contacting law enforcement and child protective services (CPS) agencies, even when they have adequate time to do so (Flaherty & Sege, 2005; Flaherty, Sege, Griffith, et al., 2008; Flaherty, Sege, Price, et al., 2006; Lane & Dubowitz, 2009). As a result, they do not always know when to call, whom to call, or how to communicate and document their concerns. When state agencies are contacted, families typically have many questions and concerns that many physicians do not have the experience to answer. As a mandated reporter, the provider still has a medical, ethical, and legal obligation to contact these agencies when abuse or neglect is suspected, but calling the CAP first can augment the primary care physician's plan.

In addition, pediatricians are often uncomfortable dealing with child maltreatment due to their fear of involvement in court procedures (Flaherty & Sege, 2005; Flaherty, Sege, Griffith, et al., 2008; Flaherty, Sege, Price, et al., 2006; Jones et al., 2008; Lane & Dubowitz, 2009). After the initial evaluation of suspected child maltreatment, occasionally the treating physician is asked to provide court testimony. Testifying is very inconvenient for the physician, who may need to alter a full schedule of patients with frequently changing court dates. Training programs for general practitioners usually do not provide much, if any, education about how to testify in court. As a result, providers are usually inadequately prepared and less effective when they do testify (Lane & Dubowitz, 2009). CAPs are expected to testify in court as part of their responsibilities and usually have a working plan established to prevent disruption of patient flow when they testify. CAPs also receive a significant amount of training and experience in providing court testimony during their fellowship. As a result, they are able to provide more accurate and clearer courtroom testimony. Despite the establishment of CAPs, other providers and clinicians do still have to testify in court. When subpoenaed, the provider should contact the attorney immediately to discuss the case well in advance of arriving at court.

TRAINING OF CHILD ABUSE PEDIATRICIANS

Since child abuse pediatrics became an official subspecialty of pediatrics in 2006, uniform standards have been put into place for physicians training to become child abuse pediatricians. These requirements now include a child abuse pediatrics board examination, the first of which was given in 2009. Pediatricians eligible to take this board exam (and become a board-certified CAP), must meet the following criteria: graduate from an accredited medical school, complete a three-year ACGME-accredited pediatric residency program, be board-certified in general pediatrics, have a valid medical license, and complete a three-year ACGME-accredited child abuse pediatrics fellowship (American Board of Pediatrics, 2011).

According to the ACGME (2010), the purpose of a fellowship in child abuse pediatrics is to "prepare a physician to diagnose and manage acute and chronic manifestations of child abuse, demonstrate competence in teaching, design and conduct research in child abuse, act as a competent physician in a multidisciplinary field, and become familiar with administrative, legislative and policy issues in child abuse."

Since child abuse pediatrics became a subspecialty, the ACGME (2012) has set forth specific standards for fellowship education to ensure that "training of the next generation of child abuse pediatricians will be done in recognized educational programs by recognized and Board certified experts." The ACGME (2010) currently requires that all fellowship programs be three years in duration and that fellows have ongoing education from at least two board-certified CAPs and access to multiple subspecialists, including those in child and adolescent psychiatry, forensic pathology, child neurology, pediatric radiology, neuroradiology, ophthalmology, orthopedic surgery, pediatric surgery, trauma surgery, and neurological surgery.

The ACGME requires several competencies to be achieved during the three-year fellowship, including patient care, medical knowledge, interpersonal and communication skills, professionalism, and systems-based practice. CAPs must provide appropriate medical care to victims of abuse and neglect. They are expected to recognize and manage all forms of child maltreatment, including sexual abuse, physical abuse, neglect, medical child abuse (Munchausen syndrome by proxy), and emotional abuse. The physician must be able to utilize appropriate examination techniques, photodocument examination findings, and interpret laboratory and radiographic studies. Finally, CAPs must be able to provide appropriate treatment recommendations for both the physical and mental health of their patients (ACGME, 2010).

The CAP is expected to have proficiency in medical knowledge related to the field of child maltreatment. This includes epidemiology of accidental and nonaccidental pediatric injuries, risk factors for child abuse and neglect, biomechanics of pediatric injuries, child development, and typical and atypical sexualized behaviors. The CAP should also be familiar with forensic pathology, toxicology, and relevant social and community services. Finally, the CAP should know the relevant laws and legal processes for reporting, investigating, and prosecuting suspected child abuse (ACGME, 2010).

During fellowship training, the fellow in child abuse pediatrics must demonstrate professionalism and interpersonal and communication skills. CAPs should be able to conduct medical interviews of suspected victims, suspected perpetrators, and nonoffending caregivers. They should be able to provide appropriate ethical medical testimony that is clear and understandable to nonmedical listeners. The CAP must be comfortable communicating and working with other professional organizations, including police departments, the district attorney's office, the child advocacy center, mental health professionals, other physicians, and CPS. During fellowship training, the fellow is expected to have sufficient experience working within a multidisciplinary team with other professionals to discuss cases and improve the care provided to victims of abuse. It is by working as a member of a team that the CAP will be able to provide improved care for child victims (ACGME, 2010).

One of the reasons that the American Board of Pediatrics acknowledged child abuse as a subspecialty was the ever increasing amount of scientific literature in the field and the need for continued research. To encourage such scholarly activity and the pursuit of research, 12 months of the fellowship in child abuse is dedicated to producing a scholarly project. This allows fellows to learn how to conduct research in the field of maltreatment, encourages them to continue the pursuit of research throughout their career, and teaches them essential skills to critically evaluate research published by others.

CONSULTATION OF THE CHILD ABUSE PEDIATRICIAN

One of the principal roles of a CAP is that of a consultant to hospitals, other physicians, and the community. When community providers—counselors, psychiatrists, primary care physicians, and others—have concerns about child maltreatment, they can call and discuss the case with a CAP. The experience of CAPs allows them to provide clear recommendations to other providers, based on their training, experience, medical knowledge, and familiarity with local resources and laws. This resource allows providers to improve the care they provide to child victims and their families.

The purpose of the CAP's consult is to provide expert opinions and recommendations about a case. Most CAPs are associated with a hospital and are able to provide both inpatient and outpatient consultations. Even if the child is not currently in the hospital or being referred to the child abuse outpatient clinic, the CAP is still available by telephone to speak with providers and give advice. A common phone call from physicians occurs when parents arrive at the office concerned about sexual abuse. The concern may have arisen from the child's behaviors, a disclosure, or a physical examination finding. A phone call to the local CAP can be extremely helpful in facilitating an appropriate evaluation for the child or avoiding unnecessary trips to the emergency department.

The CAP is also an excellent resource for when a provider is faced with unusual or concerning examination findings. By calling the CAP immediately, the provider can receive expert interpretation of examination findings to avoid misinterpretation. Depending on the history and examination findings, CAPs can occasionally arrange to see the child immediately, either in the clinic or in the emergency department. This allows improved visualization of findings, photodocumentation, and immediate answers for the family and investigators.

Another common type of consultation involves concerns about physical abuse. When the child is in the emergency department or the hospital, the CAP can easily evaluate the injuries, speak with the family and patient, and provide an evidence-based and experience-based opinion about the cause of the injuries. When the child is not easily available for the CAP to evaluate, the CAP can still be reached by telephone to discuss with local professionals any examination findings or disclosures made by the child. As in sexual abuse, the CAP can then refer the provider to the appropriate agencies or can have the child sent directly to his or her office for an evaluation and photodocumentation. This immediate availability of a CAP at most large children's hospitals gives professionals in the community direct access to an expert source of information that should prevent misdiagnosis, prevent delayed diagnosis, and support mandatory reporting.

ACUTE TREATMENT BEGINS AT THE CHILD ABUSE PEDIATRICIAN'S OFFICE

The child's evaluation at the child abuse clinic begins long before the child arrives for the appointment at the CAP's office. Most children presenting to the clinic are referred by law enforcement, the emergency department, CPS, mental health professionals, or their primary care providers. In these cases, it is important for the medical provider to obtain as much information as possible from each source involved in the case prior to the child's presentation at the clinic. Having this information initially not only allows a more efficient and effective evaluation of the child but also influences when the child will be scheduled in the clinic. For example, if a physician calls concerned about an acute examination finding, that child would be evaluated by the CAP immediately to photodocument the injuries and develop a safety plan. If a child has had some nonspecific behaviors that have concerned the parents but the pediatrician is unconcerned, the child may be scheduled for the next available appointment, usually in one to two weeks.

Information that the child may have provided to other professionals also influences the medical evaluation and how much information is obtained from the child. For example, if a child has made a clear disclosure of penile-oral penetration to the police or the forensic interviewer and has denied any other type of sexual contact, knowing that information allows the medical provider to more appropriately determine what tests to order, how to diagnose the child, and what recommendations to make. In addition, having that information ahead of time can prevent unnecessary repetitive history taking and allow the physician to focus on questions or concerns that the child may have about his body. Another common issue addressed is when parents do not support or protect their child because they question the validity of his disclosure. If CPS has spoken to the caregivers and they do not believe or are not supportive of the child, that information guides the focus of the medical evaluation and discussions with the caregivers (Elliot & Carnes, 2001).

When a child is referred to the child abuse clinic, it is comforting to the caregivers and child to know what is going to happen prior to the evaluation. A referring professional who is knowledgeable about the evaluation process can inform the family, answer some of their questions, and most importantly, ease some of their anxieties about the medical evaluation. The initial part of the evaluation, as in most pediatric visits, is obtaining a medical history from the caregivers. These evaluations require individual interviews of all caregivers, away from the child. During these interviews, the child may be in the waiting room with an appropriate adult or may be providing her own medical history to providers. When there is concern about sexual abuse, the history provided by the child is critical in the diagnosis and treatment. Depending on the child's age, previous disclosure(s), and concerns, the history provided by the child may be very brief or take up to 20 minutes. After all the relevant information is gathered, the child has a full medical examination, including an anogenital examination. Depending on the medical history provided, the child may have laboratory studies. After all this has been accomplished, the medical evaluation is reviewed with the caregivers, and they receive appropriate medical recommendations and referrals.

Obtaining a medical and social history from all the caregivers available is important to the medical evaluation. Each individual may have a different perspective on the child's disclosure, changes in the child's behavior, and changes in the family since the child's disclosure. These histories are usually obtained separately so that each individual can provide information without being influenced by other caregivers. The clinician asks about when the child first disclosed, to whom he disclosed, the context surrounding the disclosure, and the exact wording used by the child at the time of disclosure. Questions also focus on the child's behavior, physical symptoms, and mental health before, immediately after, and since the disclosure. Finally, information on other social concerns is elicited: Has the child ever been abused before? Is the family supportive of the child since the disclosure? Are caregivers protective? Are there any other social stressors in the home (domestic violence, poverty, drug use, unstable housing, etc.)?

After speaking with the caregivers, the clinician interviews the child separately to obtain additional medical history. It is important for children, especially as they get older, to have an active role in their medical evaluation. The child is asked whether she has any questions or concerns about the evaluation or her body. This medical interview gives the child a chance to voice her thoughts, concerns, and questions about her body, the changes at home since the disclosure, her feelings, or why she is getting an examination. The child is given a chance to disclose concerns that she may not have been able to tell other individuals (Finkel, 2008; Finkel & Alexander, 2011). Occasionally, child victims have concerns about their bodies such as objects remaining in their genitals, HIV, and pregnancy. These concerns can remain for months to years following a sexual assault, and the child may not voice these thoughts to family members or other providers. These concerns are extremely valid to the child, and a discussion with a medical provider, and sometimes simple medical imaging or noninvasive tests, can address the child's concerns and offer a great deal of comfort.

In most cases, the child has already made a disclosure to another professional, usually a forensic interviewer, the police, or CPS. If the child has not disclosed to another person, the physician should obtain a detailed medical history for the purposes of medical diagnosis and treatment. This information provided by the child not only allows the physician to make a medical diagnosis but also guides the physician in determining any additional testing and follow-up care that may be necessary.

Following the interview with caregivers and the child, the physical examination is performed. The examination is done for multiple reasons, not just to look for evidence of sexual abuse. The vast majority of children who have been sexually abused have normal findings on the genital exam (Adams et al., 1994; Anderst, Kellogg, & Jung, 2009; Kellogg, Menard, & Santos, 2004). The purposes of the examination are to identify any abnormal findings and, if there is such a finding, to explain its significance; to identify signs of infection; and to document the examination, in case of a repeat examination or any potential future legal issues. No child is forced to have an examination, and the exam is usually tolerated extremely well. On the very rare occasion when a genital examination must be performed and the child refuses or is uncomfortable with it, a sedated examination can be done; sedated examinations are infrequently required. In the even more unusual event of a prepubescent girl with acute vaginal bleeding, a genital examination can be performed with the child under anesthesia.

Before starting the examination, the clinician explains to the child the purpose of the exam and each step of the procedure. Older children and adolescents are provided with a choice of which caregiver, if any, they would like in the examination room with them. Some medical providers have the benefit of a child life specialist as part of their treatment team. This individual is an additional person who can support the child during the examination if no caregiver is present or if the caregiver is unsupportive or too emotional to be present. The examination is always performed with at least two staff members in the room—usually a nurse and a physician. Most of the time a caregiver is also present.

The examination is similar to a well-child examination completed by primary care physicians, including examination of the head, eyes, ears, nose, and mouth, auscultation of the heart and lungs, an abdominal examination, and a thorough skin evaluation, making sure that as much as possible of the body remains draped to keep the child comfortable. Finally, the child's anogenital region is examined using photocolposcopy. Girls are placed in either the lithotomy position (using stirrups) or the supine frog-leg position, with feet together and knees apart. Each genital structure is examined using labial traction. The examination is usually tolerated well by children and adolescents (Steward et al.,

1995; Wailbel-Duncan, 2001, 2004). A speculum is rarely used during the evaluation. Boys are examined in the supine position, with visual inspection of the penis, scrotum, and testicles. Finally, the anus is examined in boys and girls, using photocolposcopy. The patient lies supine and brings the knees to the chest, and separation is then provided of the buttocks allowing visual inspection of the anus.

The final part of the medical evaluation is reviewing the medical recommendations with the child and family. Any examination findings, including normal findings, are discussed with the family, and the significance of those findings is explained. The clinician frequently explains to parents that the genital examination is normal but that this does not mean the child was not sexually abused and does not exclude the possibility of penetration. This is often difficult for families to understand, but there are multiple reasons that, despite sexual abuse, the genitals appear normal. Some episodes of sexual abuse involve touching that would not be expected to cause injury. There can be labial penetration, where a finger, penis, or object passes the labia majora but does not cause injury, or it may cause an injury to the mucosal surface that will have healed normally by time the examination is completed, if not done soon after the sexual abuse incident. There can be vaginal penetration that does not cause injury, even in a prepubescent girl (Anderst, Kellogg, & Jung, 2009). Finally, there can be injury to the genital area that heals prior to the medical evaluation so that no evidence remains of the injury.

After discussing the child's examination, the clinician explains the need for laboratory studies; laboratory testing, when indicated, frequently includes not only studies required on leaving the clinic but repeat testing in several months. Caregivers are evaluated to determine their capacity to support and protect their children (Elliot & Carnes, 2001). Finally, the clinician makes recommendations for counseling of both the child and the caregiver.

Caregivers frequently have multiple questions for the CAP regarding the next steps with CPS, law enforcement, and custody. The CAP's experience in working with these agencies allows him or her to inform the family about the usual process and provide them with appropriate recommendations and contact information for the involved agencies (Leventhal, Murphy, & Asnes, 2010).

As a mandated reporter, the CAP reports abuse or neglect to all appropriate agencies. Frequently, multidisciplinary team meetings are held that improve communication between the various agencies involved. The team members are professionals, including forensic interviewers, social workers, medical providers, law enforcement, CPS workers, and representatives from the district attorney's office and the children's advocacy center.

Medical providers also serve as educators to caregivers throughout the evaluation. The physician can review with parents the normal and abnormal sexualized behaviors of children of different age groups (Leventhal, Murphy, & Asnes, 2010). The physician can also provide the family with strategies to intervene and redirect, rather than punishing, abnormal sexual behavior. Basic safety advice is also reviewed, including choosing appropriate caregivers, teaching children about appropriate and inappropriate touches, teaching children not to keep secrets from their parents, reviewing safety measures with cellphones, Internet, and television, and prevention information. This information can be reiterated to families by other professionals, including the primary care physician and mental health provider. Such information is helpful to all caregivers, even when there is no concern about sexual abuse.

LONG-TERM TREATMENT

Either prior to or following the medical evaluation, many children and young adolescents may be scheduled for a forensic interview at the children's advocacy center, which provides a neutral, child-friendly environment devoted to advocacy for child victims of abuse. The National Children's Alliance accredits child advocacy centers, which bring together professionals from multiple disciplines, including medicine, law enforcement, the district attorney's office, and CPS, to investigate child abuse and to intervene appropriately.

The forensic interview of a child, according to the National Children's Alliance, should be a coordinated, neutral, fact-finding mission that is legally sound. It should be coordinated with a multidisciplinary team to avoid re-interviewing of the child. The goal of the forensic interview is to "obtain a statement from a child, in a developmentally and culturally sensitive, unbiased and fact-finding manner that will support accurate and fair decision making by the involved multidisciplinary team in the criminal justice and child protection systems" (National Children's Alliance, www.nationalchildrensalliance.org).

In addition to obtaining information from the child during the forensic interview, the children's advocacy center also provides an advocate for the child or adolescent. The advocate provides support to the family and child throughout the investigation and trial. The prosecutor's office can also provide the child with an advocate, who orients the child to the courtroom, educates the child about the court proceedings, and accompanies the child during the trial. These advocates can also help to maintain counseling for the child and family and help them deal with additional social stressors (housing, transportation, etc.) (National Children's Alliance, www.nationalchildrensalliance.org).

Following their initial evaluation with the child abuse clinic, many children return to the clinic for various reasons. One of the most common reasons for follow-up at the clinic is to document the healing of an acute, questionable, or undetermined finding. When acute trauma is found in the anogenital examination, having the child return to the clinic in a few weeks allows the provider to document that the injury has completely healed, then to reassure the child that their body is now normal or to document a healed in-

jury. A change in examination findings over the course of two weeks can demonstrate that there was an acute finding as opposed to a normal variant, which would not change in two weeks (Gavril, Kellogg, & Nair, 2012). This is also true in cases of physical abuse. Occasionally, birth marks such as dermal melanoses can be confused with bruising. A repeat examination two weeks later will differentiate the two, as bruises change and heal whereas dermal melanoses do not change over the course of a few weeks.

Patients are also asked to return to the child abuse clinic for documentation of the long-term effects of the physical abuse or neglect. In some jurisdictions, an inflicted injury that results in a scar is prosecuted differently from an injury that completely resolves. In cases of abusive head trauma, reevaluation of the child's development several months following the injury is helpful from an educational and prosecutorial perspective.

Finally, children are often asked to return to the child abuse clinic for a reevaluation of their emotional/psychiatric state and their safety and support in the home. One significant concern following children's disclosures of sexual abuse is the reaction of the family, especially when the alleged perpetrator is a member of the family (Elliot & Carnes, 2001). In these situations, it is helpful to provide children with an opportunity to discuss with the medical provider any concerns they are having, any issues they have had with nonsupportive family members, or any reexposure to the alleged perpetrator. It also gives the medical provider a chance to make sure that parents have complied with the medical recommendations, such as laboratory testing, counseling, and appropriate supervision.

The most important aspect of treatment following the medical evaluation of child abuse, especially child sexual abuse, is long-term counseling. Child sexual abuse has short- and long-term negative mental health effects. Adult victims of child sexual abuse are more likely to have major depression, substance abuse, posttraumatic stress disorder, dissociative disorders, suicidality, and bulimia nervosa (Dinwiddie et al., 2000; Putnam, 2003). In addition, children who have been sexually abused have more sexualized behaviors, have higher-risk sexual behaviors, and are more likely to become pregnant at a younger age. Because the majority of children who have been sexually abused will develop mental health sequelae, long-term mental health treatment is necessary for this population. The treatment should be with a professional who is skilled and experienced in working with children who have been sexually abused. Currently, Trauma-Focused Cognitive Behavioral Therapy with the child, in addition to counseling for the nonoffending parent, has produced the best outcomes for children (Cohen & Mannarino, 1998; Cohen et al., 2000; King et al., 2000; Putnam, 2003).

Even after the medical evaluation and any follow-up appointments, the CAP remains involved in the case and is available as a resource for future providers. If the counselor has questions about the medical evaluation, the lawyer needs expert testimony in court, or the primary care physician has questions about future sexualized behaviors, the CAP is always available to discuss both new patients and new or continuing concerns about previous patients.

References

Accreditation Council for Graduate Medical Education (ACGME). (2010). *ACGME program requirements for graduate medical education in child abuse pediatrics.* www.acgme.org /acWebsite/downloads/RRC_progReq/339_child_abuse _peds_02062010.pdf

Accreditation Council for Graduate Medical Education (ACGME). (2012). *ACGME impact/justification statement: Proposed program requirements for fellowship education in child abuse pediatrics.* www.acgme.org/acWebsite/reviewComment /ChildAbuseImpact.pdf

Adams, J. A., Harper, K., Knudson, S., & Revilla, J. (1994). Exam findings in legally confirmed child sex abuse: It's normal to be normal. *Pediatrics, 94,* 310–317.

American Board of Pediatrics. (2011). *Eligibility criteria for certification in child abuse pediatrics.* Chapel Hill, NC: Author. www.abp.org

Anderst, J., Kellogg, N., & Jung, I. (2009). Reports of repetitive penile-genital penetration often have no definitive evidence of penetration. *Pediatrics, 124,* e403–409.

Block, R. W., & Palusci, V. J. (2006). Child abuse pediatrics: A new pediatric subspecialty. *Journal of Pediatrics, 148(6),* 711–712.

Botash, A. S., Galloway, A. E., Booth, T., Ploutz-Snyder, R., Hoffman-Rosenfeld, J., & Cahill, L. (2005). Continuing medical education in child sexual abuse: Cognitive gains but no experience. *Archives of Pediatric & Adolescent Medicine, 159,* 561–566.

Caffey, J. (1946). Multiple fractures in the long bones of infants suffering from chronic subdural hematoma. *American Journal of Roentgenology, 56,* 163–173.

Cohen, J., & Mannarino, A. (1998). Interventions for sexually abused children: Initial treatment outcome findings. *Child Maltreatment, 3,* 17–26.

Cohen, J., Mannarino, A., Berliner, L., & Deblinger, E. (2000). Trauma-Focused Cognitive Behavioral Therapy for children and adolescents: An empirical update. *Journal of Interpersonal Violence, 15,* 1202–1223.

Dinwiddie, S., Heath, A. C., Dunne, K. K., Bucholz, P. A., Madden, W. S., Slutske, L. J., et al. (2000). Early sexual abuse and lifetime psychopathology: A co-twin–control study. *Psychological Medicine, 30,* 41–52.

Elliot, A. N., & Carnes, C. N. (2001). Reactions of nonoffending parents to the sexual abuse of their child: A review of the literature. *Child Maltreatment, 6(4),* 314–331.

Finkel, M. A. (2008). "I can tell you because you're a doctor." *Pediatrics, 122(2),* 442.

Finkel, M. A., & Alexander, R. A. (2011). Conducting the medical history. *Journal of Child Sexual Abuse, 20(5),* 486–504.

Flaherty, E. G., & Sege, R. (2005). Barriers to physician identification and reporting of child abuse. *Pediatric Annals, 34(5),* 349–356.

Flaherty, E. G., Sege, R. D., Griffith, J., Price, L. L., Wasserman, R., Slora, E., et al. (2008). From suspicion to report: Primary care clinician decision-making. *Pediatrics, 122(3),* 611–619.

Flaherty, E. G., Sege, R., Price, L. L., Christoffel, K. K., Norton, D. P., & O'Connor, K. G. (2006). Pediatric characteristics associated with child abuse identification and reporting: Results from a national survey of pediatricians. *Child Maltreatment, 11(4),* 361–369.

Gavril, A. R., Kellogg, N. D., & Nair, P. (2012). Value of follow-up examinations of children and adolescents evaluated for sexual abuse and assault. *Pediatrics, 129(2),* 282–289.

Gottschalk, A., & Flocke, S. A. (2005). Time spent in face-to-face patient care and work outside the examination room. *Annals of Family Medicine, 3(6),* 488–493.

Jones, R., Flaherty, E. G., Binns, H. J., Price, L. L., Slora, E., Abney, D., et al. (2008). Clinicians' description of factors influencing their reporting of suspected child abuse: Report of the Child Abuse Reporting Experience Study Research Group. *Pediatrics, 122,* 259–266.

Kellogg, N., Menard, S. W., & Santos, A. (2004). Genital anatomy in pregnant adolescents: "Normal" does not mean "nothing happened." *Pediatrics, 113,* e67–69.

Kempe, C. H., Silverman, F. N., Steele, B. F., Droegmueller, W., & Silver, H. K. (1965). The battered-child syndrome. *Child Abuse & Neglect, 9,* 143–154.

King, N. J., Tonge, B. J., Mullen, P., Meyerson, N., Heyne, D., Rollings, S., et al. (2000). Treating sexually abused children with posttraumatic stress symptoms: A randomized clinical trial. *Journal of the American Academy of Child and Adolescent Psychiatry, 39,* 1347–1355.

Lane, W. G., & Dubowitz, H. (2009). Primary care physician's experience, comfort, and competence in the evaluation and management of child maltreatment: Do we need child abuse experts? *Child Abuse & Neglect, 33,* 76–83.

Leventhal, J. M., Murphy, J. L., & Asnes, A. G. (2010). Evaluations of child sexual abuse: Recognition of overt and latent family concerns. *Child Abuse & Neglect, 34(5),* 289–295.

Narayan, A. P., Scoloar, R. R. S., & St Claire, K. (2006). Pediatric residency training in child abuse and neglect in the United States. *Pediatrics, 117,* 2215–2221.

Putnam, F. W. (2003). Ten year research review update: Child sexual abuse. *Journal of the American Academy of Child and Adolescent Psychiatry, 42(3),* 269–278.

Starling, S. P., Heisler, K. W., Paulson, J. F., & Youmans, E. (2009). Child abuse training and knowledge: A national survey of emergency medicine, family medicine, and pediatric residents and program directors. *Pediatrics, 123,* e595–602.

Steward, M. S., Schmitz, M., Steward, D. S., Joye, N. R., & Reinhart, M. (1995). Children's anticipation of and response to colposcopic examination. *Child Abuse & Neglect, 19(8),* 997–1005.

Wailbel-Duncan, M. K. (2001). Medical fears following alleged child abuse. *Journal of Child and Adolescent Psychiatric Nursing, 14(4),* 179–185.

Wailbel-Duncan, M. K. (2004). Identifying competence in the context of the pediatric anogenital exam. *Journal of Child and Adolescent Psychiatric Nursing, 17(1)* 21–28.

31

SIGALIT HOFFMAN, M.D.
JOHN SARGENT, M.D.

Training Child Psychiatry Fellows to Provide Trauma-Informed Care

GENERAL CONSIDERATIONS

The goals of training child psychiatrists include familiarizing them with the manifestations of trauma, developing their understanding of the impact of trauma on children at various developmental stages, and making them aware of treatment approaches, as outlined in other chapters of this book. This task can be divided into three components: building a foundation of knowledge, developing skills, and fostering appropriate attitudes toward providing trauma-informed care.

KNOWLEDGE

The first requirement for building a trauma-informed knowledge base is to understand the impact of abuse on child development and to appreciate the range of trauma-related symptoms at various ages. Child psychiatry training should offer the trainee ample settings in which to identify trauma and in which trauma symptoms are likely to present. The trainee may encounter trauma in infants during well-child visits or when in the emergency room. In infants, trauma may manifest overtly when the child is brought to medical attention after being shaken or with broken limbs. In less overt cases, the child might present with emotional withdrawal or failure to thrive—though the child psychiatry trainee must be aware that abuse is the etiology for failure to thrive in a minority of cases (Egan, Chantoor, & Rosen, 1980).

Trauma in very young children manifests differently from trauma in older children or teenagers. Young children who have been victims of abuse or neglect might present with disorders of attachment (Iwaniec, 1997), commonly referred to as reactive attachment disorder of infancy or early childhood. These children are unable to initiate or respond to social interactions in a developmentally appropriate way (Sadock & Sadock 2003). Their interactions can vary between being excessively inhibited or diffuse. Those who are inhibited in their interactions are hypervigilant or ambivalent or demonstrate contradictory responses—which are often very frustrating to the parents, who rightly feel as though their efforts to establish a reciprocally affectionate relationship are continuously thwarted or actively sabotaged. Children whose attachments are diffuse fail to establish appropriately selective attachments, thus behaving in an excessively familiar way with strangers. Child and adolescent psychiatry trainees must be able to appreciate both the disturbance in attachment in children who have experienced abuse or neglect throughout infancy or early childhood and the impact of these attachment difficulties on caregivers. They must be cognizant of the feelings of inadequacy that attachment disorders engender in caregivers with respect to their parenting skills, as well as the resulting sense of anger, frustration, and helplessness they feel toward their children (George & Solomon, 2011).

In older children, trauma may manifest as dysregulated mood or behavior, attention difficulties, cognitive delays, and disturbances in interactions with peers and caregivers (Ford et al., 2012). These interactions might include defiance toward authority figures or severe disturbances in conduct. Taken in a developmental context, when trauma is the etiology of these symptoms, a child will begin to fail at school and not meet academic, social, or emotional milestones. A child psychiatry trainee must be aware of the various ways in which trauma can present and the reciprocal relationship with development. On the one hand, trauma influences development by distorting, slowing, or inhibiting it. On the other hand, how the child is affected by trauma depends on the developmental stage at which it occurs. Trainees must be aware of the growing body of evidence on the interaction between trauma and development that has delineated the neurobiological, epigenetic, and endocrine effects of trauma on physical as well as cognitive and emotional development (McCrory, De Brito, & Viding, 2012).

Trauma in adolescents manifests differently from that in children. Trauma in teens more commonly presents as a disturbance in mood, disturbance in affect regulation, self-injurious behavior, suicide attempts, substance abuse, promiscuity, or antisocial behaviors such as bullying or intimidation. Trainees must be aware of these various presentations so that they know to screen for these risk factors and understand the possible motivation behind these behaviors. Taking a developmental approach, the child psychiatrist must remain cognizant that while teens who are not trauma survivors are navigating the normal developmental stage of identity versus identity diffusion, teens who have suffered abuse might still be negotiating earlier developmental stages and struggling with questions related to basic trust, autonomy, guilt, and inferiority (McCann & Pearlmann, 1990). Their behaviors can be understood in the context of trying to gain a sense of agency over a situation in which they have had no control and in testing limits to see whether the world is a place where their needs will be met.

In addition to understanding how trauma manifests throughout development, child psychiatrists must be aware of the various approaches to trauma assessment. Specifically, they must be knowledgeable about the scales commonly used to assess trauma-related symptoms and comorbidities. They must also be aware of the evidence-based treatment approaches to trauma and its comorbid illnesses.

SKILLS

The skill set needed by a child psychiatrist depends on the context in which the child is examined. In any setting, psychiatrists are expected to be sensitive in examining the patient. While they are expected to be thorough in their evaluation, they must not force the patient to reveal more than he or she is comfortable doing or can do safely and must avoid asking leading questions or asking questions using an emotionally laden tone (Giardino, Lyn, & Giardino, 2010), especially when very young children are involved. At the same time, however, the psychiatrist must not give the impression that a particular subject is out of bounds for discussion. In other words, the child psychiatrist must work to create an environment that is open, supportive, validating, and most importantly, nonjudgmental to minimize any guilt, shame, or self-blame the patient might be carrying as a result of trauma.

Providing training experiences in a variety of environments will expose the child psychiatrist to the broad field of psychiatric work. It will also build the skill sets needed in these different areas.

Emergency Room

The emergency room (ER) is a setting in which child psychiatrists commonly find themselves. In the ER, it is the child psychiatrist's primary responsibility to ensure the physical safety of the child. The goal of training in this setting is to be able to provide a timely and relatively comprehensive evaluation of the child in a condensed timeframe. Despite the eagerness of many trainees to glean every piece of information possible due to the acuity with which the patient often presents, and because of their relative inexperience in the emergency setting, they should be encouraged to perform a focused assessment that centers on safety and to provide a placement recommendation that offers the least restrictive environment needed to ensure the child's safety (Tasman et al., 2011).

In terms of trauma, the child psychiatrist must be aware that any self-destructive behavior or suicidal statements might be related to a traumatic experience that is either discrete or ongoing (Briere, 1992). The child psychiatrist must also be conversant with the legal resources available to ensure the child's safety. As a mandated reporter, a child psychiatrist cannot hospitalize a child against a parent's will but can report the parent to child protective services if the parent is found to be neglectful of the child's physical or mental health (Giardino, Lyn, & Giardino, 2010). A child psychiatry trainee must feel empowered to use the risk management services available should medico-legal questions arise. While trainees must not be encouraged to take an adversarial stance toward parents, it can often be therapeutic for children who feel dismissed or invalidated to find that someone who is a caregiver is concerned enough about them to resort to extreme measures to ensure their health and safety. Child psychiatry trainees should be encouraged to ally themselves with parents by reminding them that, like the parent, the psychiatrist has the child's best interest at heart and that recommendations are based on a disinterested clinical evaluation. This can often be helpful in diffusing tense situations that arise in acute settings such as the ER.

Another skill important to the training of child psychiatrists in the ER is information gathering. Especially for adolescent patients, it is not uncommon for them to minimize the situation that brought them to the ER. (One study found that adolescents were far more likely to report suicidal ideation or a history of prior attempts when allowed to do so in a context of anonymity; see Safer, 1997.) An example is an adolescent who is sent to the ER by his or her school after making suicidal statements. Gathering collateral information from the school and other people who know the child is crucial to being able to make a decision about an appropriate level of care. Although a teen might deny current suicidal ideation while in the ER, he or she may have made some gestures or statements that would indicate the contrary, such as writing a suicide note, giving away possessions, or making prior attempts that went unreported. The child psychiatrist must be able to weigh the information gathered and present it in a manner that is both clear and convincing so that there is little doubt in the minds of the accepting facility or the insurer of the need to place the child in an inpatient level of care. If what the teen has said contradicts his or her actions, the child psychiatry trainee should err on the side of caution. While the law has made it clear that health care providers must be mindful of the human rights of minors, child psychiatrists must also be mindful of the limitations inherent to children's developmental stage. Prior research has identified impulsivity as a major risk factor in suicide attempts (Brent et al., 1993), and recent research finds impaired decision making as a further risk factor associated with suicide attempts (Bridge et al., 2012). In cases of younger children and suicidality, it is possible that a lack of understanding of the permanence of death might also affect their judgment as it relates to risk-taking behavior and acting out (Webb, 2011). It is for this reason that the child psychiatrist has been granted some latitude within the law to make decisions in a child's best interest (Webb, 2011), especially when, for emotional or developmental reasons, the child is not able to do so for himself or herself.

A skill that is not much discussed but is crucial to providing competent care is the ability of the child psychiatrist to work in a team and tolerate the angry feelings that often surface in treating children who have had trauma. Members of the treating medical team can often have a sense of anger and powerlessness. Medical caregivers might be horrified at the level of abuse or neglect a child has suffered, but, given the expectations of professionalism, they cannot confront perpetrators directly. Sometimes the perpetrator is not present to be confronted and the child has been sent to the ER from a foster home or residential treatment facility. This too can be challenging for medical providers in that they feel as though they don't understand the mental health system from which the child came or how to navigate it. They might feel very angry about the often long wait time between making a placement recommendation and finding a bed. They may feel anger toward the patient because traumatized patients can sometimes act in ways that reject help (Muller, 2009), which can color the treatment team's view of the patient as being ungrateful. Though it is not expressly a part of their core competencies, child psychiatrists are also charged with managing the emotions of the medical staff (Lipowski, 1974). It is important for a trainee to know that frustrations stemming from all of the above might manifest as anger toward the psychiatrist. The trainee must learn to manage the frustration, confusion, and hopelessness that trauma patients engender in the medical team by providing psychoeducation on why a patient might be acting in a way that elicits such negative emotion. The psychiatrist can also help clarify the process and possible timeframe of psychiatric placement. Trainees should strive to empathize with, normalize, and validate the conflicting feelings of the medical team, helping team members balance their desire to help the patient and their anger at the child.

Finally, an exploration of the role of the child psychiatrist in the ER would not be complete without mentioning one last skill: the ability to maintain clear boundaries within this setting. In a highly stressful environment in which a patient engenders numerous and complex feelings in the staff, it is common for child psychiatrists to be asked to step outside their role as consultant, either to take on complete responsibility for the patient or to complete tasks outside the scope of the psychiatrist's role of making a clinical assessment and treatment recommendation (Roberts & Steele, 2009). In the ER, it is essential that trainees keep in mind that as a consultant, their legal responsibility toward the patient includes a reasonable evaluation and disposition recommendation (Applebaum & Gutheil, 2007). In some cases, the medical team might have an opinion that conflicts with that of the consultant and might request that the consultant change his or her opinion so that it is consonant with that of the medical team. Just as a training program would expect a trainee to be able to stay within clinical boundaries in an outpatient setting, the same holds true for the emergency setting. Trainees must be empowered by supervisors to maintain that they are charged with making a recommendation based on their best clinical judgment. When the medical team disagrees with this assessment, it is always free to disregard the consultant's recommendations, as long as the team is aware that by doing so, it takes on any liability it may incur as a result of such a decision. In the era of managed care, it does remain the child psychiatrist's responsibility to "engage in vigorous advocacy" with the managed care company so that the patient can receive the treatment he or she needs while an appeal on coverage is made (Applebaum & Gutheil, 2007).

In a high-stress setting and resource-restricted environment, a trainee might be asked to do administrative work such as performing a bed search for a child in need of inpatient hospitalization. With the support of the training program, trainees should be empowered to focus on the work for which they have undergone years of medical training. Although the field of psychiatry has always been surrounded with a certain aura of separateness from the medical field, we might draw a parallel between expecting a psychiatry trainee to place a patient in a psychiatric hospital and the absurdity of asking an orthopedic surgeon to place a postoperative patient in a rehabilitation facility.

Court

The role of a child psychiatry trainee is different in a forensic setting. Doing court evaluations is often part of the forensic experience of child and adolescent psychiatry training. Once again, trainees must be aware of their role and must understand the lack of doctor-patient confidentiality that this type of patient interaction entails. While the court's mandate is to act in the best interests of the child (Applebaum & Gutheil, 2007), the trainee must be cognizant of the court's dual role in acting as surrogate parent to the child when caregivers are unable to do so (in parens patriae) and protecting society from harm. Some of the skills required in a forensic evaluation are common to those required in any setting for the child psychiatrist, such as gathering collateral information. A trainee must be aware of the impact the evaluation might have on the child's future and thus must make every effort to provide as comprehensive and objective an evaluation as possible. The trainee must also make the child aware of the limits of confidentiality in a forensic setting (Applebaum & Gutheil, 2007).

Although child psychiatrists must never misrepresent the facts they have gathered, they can play a role in mitigating a sentence by educating the court. Providing a cogent and concise explanation as to why a child who has suffered trauma or who has a history of early childhood abuse or neglect might have difficulty maintaining himself or herself in a therapeutic setting could encourage the judge to consider alternatives to incarceration. The psychiatrist may also be helpful in elucidating possible explanations for self-destructive behaviors such as drug use or gang involvement. Highlighting the role of trauma and its comorbidities—such as untreated depression, posttraumatic stress disorder, and anxiety, as well as academic failure and peer rejection—as triggers for such behaviors may help steer a court in the direction of rehabilitation and treatment. In the case of status offenses such as truancy or running away from home, it is imperative that the psychiatrist be aware of whether the trauma is ongoing and the child's reaction is not necessarily a maladaptive behavior, given the context of the situation.

Schools

In the school setting, the child psychiatrist can provide direct or indirect case consultation for a child. In direct consultation, the psychiatrist evaluates the child directly and suggests treatments that can be provided by other professionals. In indirect consultation, the psychiatrist assesses an issue (e.g., a behavior problem) articulated by the school staff rather than assessing the child directly (Dulcan, 2010). The role of the trainee is to learn how to be a consultant and to provide information to help the child benefit maximally from the school setting. This is generally achieved by a review of the child's academic performance, listening to reports of the child's social and emotional functioning, and observing the child in class. In cases of suspected child abuse, the child psychiatrist must help teachers be attuned to signs that might be indicative of trauma. Overt examples might include bruises or injuries that have no plausible explanation; other examples include multiple unexplained absences, withdrawal from other children, changes of affect,

irritability, acting out, or acting in. The child psychiatrist can help guide teachers in accessing youth protective services if they have a serious concern and in engaging the child and the parents in a nonthreatening way. The psychiatrist can also help a school decide on the kinds of intervention it would like to offer and identify the children who would be most appropriate to receive the intervention. For example, schools can choose to provide universal interventions that are general or specific. Specific intervention programs may focus on suicide or violence prevention in school. Prevention programs can be selective for children who are at high risk or for students who exhibit symptoms of emotional, behavior, or social problems but do not meet the full criteria for a specific diagnosis.

For the child psychiatrist, the need for appropriate boundaries is also important in the school setting (Dulcan, 2010). When engaging in a consultative relationship with a school, it is important that the consultation model is agreed upon beforehand and the limits of the consultant's role are clarified up front.

Pediatric Inpatient Unit

As in the ER, a child psychiatry trainee must be able to work in a collaborative way with the consulting medical team in the pediatric inpatient unit. Estimates of the prevalence of somatization disorder vary, but two major studies found a lifetime prevalence of between 12% and 13% and a 12-month prevalence of 7% (Essau, Conradt, & Petermann, 2000; Lieb et al., 2000; Schulte & Petermann, 2011). When completing a psychiatric evaluation of a child with a somatoform disorder, the child psychiatrist must keep in mind the increased prevalence of sexual or physical abuse history in children with conversion disorders (Shapiro et al., 1987). Theories regarding the etiology of factitious disorders also include a history of physical or sexual abuse (Plassmann, 1994).

In working up these cases, the child psychiatry trainee should be cognizant of the feelings of the medical team toward the patient and family. Team members may feel that their efforts are being "wasted" on an illness that is not medical in nature (Smith, 1985). They might also be frustrated with a patient or parents who they feel are creating symptoms as a cry for attention or an act of selfishness. In the case of a conversion disorder, it is the role of the child psychiatrist to support the medical team in understanding the unconscious nature of the symptoms and the possibility that the child is trying to use his or her body to communicate something that, for whatever reason, he or she is unable to communicate through words. The role of the child psychiatrist is to help sensitize the medical treatment team to the possible cultural taboos related to mental illness and the much greater validity and palatability that a medical illness offers to children. The trainee must also be aware, in the case of a somatoform disorder, that the hospital might be the only safe place a child can be if abuse is occurring in the home or another setting from which the child cannot escape. In performing a psychiatric assessment of the child, the trainee must be able to create a safe space in which any current or past abuse can be revealed without fear of blame, retribution, or judgment. This is best achieved by being a consistent, predictable member of the treatment team. By establishing themselves as trusted caregivers, psychiatry trainees might be able to help patients make the leap of faith to trust them and reveal the source of the emotional pain that has led to the current presentation.

Once again, the issue of boundaries is an important one. The medical treatment team might feel uncomfortable delivering the news to a family that there is no medical etiology to the child's presentation and ask the psychiatry team to do so in its place, but the trainee's role as a consultant is to work with the medical team to help reduce its discomfort in informing the family of the findings. In the workup of an illness for which there is a high index of suspicion for conversion disorder, the child psychiatrist must encourage the medical team to incorporate a psychiatric assessment as part of the general workup. This gives parents and child the opportunity to create a working alliance with the psychiatry consultant and places in their minds the possibility that there might be a psychiatric finding. This way, once the news is delivered, the parents and child are not left with the idea that the psychiatric assessment was an afterthought and a result of the failure of the team to provide an adequate medical explanation for the child's symptoms. The psychiatrist can support the team in explaining to the patient and family that sometimes the body unconsciously expresses through physical symptoms what it is unable to express in words (Shapiro et al., 1987). This kind of explanation helps provide a nonblaming rationale for the disorder while also validating the physical symptoms, which can be very real for the child.

When abuse is uncovered through a factitious disorder by proxy or a conversion disorder, the child psychiatrist must be proactive in taking appropriate steps to ensure the child's safety. It is important to clarify that even though Munchausen by proxy is an uncommon presentation of child abuse, it is still considered abuse, and the child is still entitled to care and protection provided by the legal system and child protective services (Muscari & Brown, 2010). The child psychiatrist might encourage the medical team to get in contact with the various entities in place to ensure the child's safety. These might include a child protection team, risk management, the social work department, state youth protective services, and when necessary, the hospital's security personnel. While the child remains in the inpatient unit, the child psychiatrist can offer support and psychoeducation to the medical team to provide trauma-informed care and avoid unintentionally replicating some aspects of a child's abuse history—for example, avoiding unnecessary diagnostic procedures. The team might try to avoid a situation in which the child feels coerced. In addition, if the offending parent is also the parent in the room with the child,

the psychiatrist should recommend a sitter so that the child is not alone with the parent. For cases in which youth protective services has been called, the psychiatrist should encourage the medical team to inform the parent of the decision to do so. Once the diagnosis is confirmed, the offending parent must be confronted and told that the physicians are aware of the behavior (Martin & Volkmar, 2007). It is through open and honest communication that the medical team might help maintain an alliance with the family and start a dialogue that can refocus everyone's energies on the child rather than who is to blame for the current situation. The trainee has the opportunity to help the medical team keep its countertransference in check so that it can provide medical care to the best of its ability.

Psychiatric Inpatient Unit

In contrast to the settings discussed thus far, the inpatient psychiatric unit is where the child psychiatrist is the primary care provider rather than a consultant. With this difference in roles come different responsibilities. While most models of inpatient units include a team approach that values the contribution of each member, the child psychiatrist has traditionally acted as the team leader who is ultimately responsible for making decisions on patient care and is ultimately liable for the outcome of treatment.

In her book *Creating Sanctuary*, Dr. Sandra Bloom (1997) describes how she and her team came to better understand their patients by becoming aware of the impact of trauma on their lives. This new trauma awareness began to inform every aspect of their approach with trauma survivors, such as setting gentle and firm limits around self-injurious behaviors. It also helped enhance the team's understanding of patients and thus helped lower the sense of frustration and helplessness in moving patients along a trajectory of recovery.

Child psychiatry trainees should strive to create a similar environment in their own inpatient units. This is done by completing an assessment that is trauma-informed, by educating staff in the various ways trauma can manifest in children, by avoiding a setting that uses coercive methods to change behavior, and not tolerating self-harm behavior in hospitalized patients. Unit staff must be encouraged to be judicious in their use of physical restraint or avoid it altogether if possible. In addition, to avoid retraumatizing a child, staff must be mindful of the patient mix in the units, being careful not to place a trauma survivor in the path of a perpetrator. As in the medical unit, the child psychiatrist and the team must work to create a therapeutic alliance with the children so that they feel they have a safe space to reveal their trauma history. The team must also be ready to use the tools in its power to ensure a child's safety once a disclosure is made. The trainee and the team must be able to work with state agencies such as youth protective services, juvenile justice, the department of mental health or developmental disabilities, and schools to coordinate care and ensure a smooth transition after discharge.

Outpatient Clinic

The outpatient clinic is a unique setting in which the focus is less on diagnosis, stabilization, and safety and more on establishing trust and rapport and working through trauma experiences. It is common for a child to present with a set of symptoms that may not initially appear to be trauma-related; however, child psychiatry trainees must use their knowledge base to construct a thoughtful differential diagnosis, keeping in mind the manifold forms that trauma may take. In the office, trainees must be able to create a space in which children feel at ease and able to unburden themselves of whatever emotional baggage they have been carrying. Trainees must establish themselves as a trusted adult who can provide a warm, consistent, and predictable environment in which the behavioral expectations are also clear. Before approaching the trauma work per se, the child psychiatrist must first ensure that the child is stable and safe. Safety and stability can be achieved by first making sure that the child is no longer in harm's way and is not engaging in overly self-destructive behavior This can be done by addressing common comorbidities of trauma such as substance abuse, suicidality, and self-injury. Only once the child is stable can he or she begin the process of healing.

Child psychiatry trainees must be familiar with and comfortable using the many evidence-based modalities such as Trauma-Focused Cognitive Behavioral Therapy, narrative storytelling, prolonged exposure, and other therapies outlined in this book that have proved safe and effective in treating child and adolescent trauma survivors. Trainees must be cognizant of the main difficulties from which a child is suffering and tailor the treatment modality to the symptoms that cause the most distress and interfere the most with function. For example, they might choose to use Dialectical Behavioral Therapy for teens who are impulsive and self-injuring (American Academy of Child and Adolescent Psychiatry, 2011). Alternatively, they may prefer mentalization therapy for individuals who have difficulties with affect regulation (Bateman & Fonagy, 2010). They may also want to bolster the child's natural sources of resilience, such as engaging support from trusted family members or community leaders with whom the child already has a good rapport. In sum, the child psychiatrist has a multitude of approaches to choose from in treating child abuse survivors. If all roads lead to Rome, each trainee is free to choose the one that she or he finds the most intuitive and the best suited for a particular child's journey.

ATTITUDES

Balancing Validation with Expectations of Progress

While the instinct of most providers might be to treat a trauma victim as one would a wounded bird, it is important to balance a child's need for validation with the expectation that whatever the trauma history, all individuals are still accountable for their decisions and their behavior. This can sometimes prove difficult, as many trauma survivors view themselves as helpless onlookers in their own lives. This perception is probably based on their abuse experience, during which they were powerless and helpless. Among the many tasks of trauma work is the need to change individuals' perception of themselves from someone who once was helpless to someone who no longer is. Trauma survivors might view their lives as a long chain of victimization, much like the child who is abused at home and then bullied at school. Although child psychiatry trainees must respect children's experiences of victimhood, they must work to not enable them to adopt these experiences as their identity. This can be achieved by challenging children and adolescents to take steps that negate their view of themselves as victims. A trainee can encourage a child to do something that he or she generally avoids as a result of the trauma, such as going to a location or participating in an activity that reminds him or her of the trauma. Of course, any exposure activity should not put the child in danger. Narrative-based treatments are also a form of exposure, as many children don't like to talk or think about their trauma. By addressing thoughts and situations that are trauma triggers, children foster a sense of mastery over these tasks, which, in turn, will challenge their perception of themselves as a powerless or fearful person (Deblinger et al., 2011).

Self-Care

A passage about self-care is crucial in any text directed at those who work with trauma survivors. While the work is very rewarding, the journey to trauma recovery is fraught with challenges. For those who specialize in treating trauma survivors, especially when those survivors are children, it can be extremely emotionally taxing to listen to stories in which people are treated in a way that challenges one's beliefs about the goodness of humanity. When treating trauma survivors, providers must take care not to be vicariously traumatized by patients' stories. This is initially done by using some of the same techniques that patients are encouraged to use—remaining grounded and mindful of the emotions being stirred up. Just as psychiatrists encourage patients to use self-care skills such as taking space, reserving time to spend in activities they enjoy, and leaning on support systems if they have them, so too can trainees use these approaches to keep themselves healthy and present for their patients. Trainees can use exercise to let off emotional steam, stay grounded in their families and their community, and use colleagues as sounding boards or safe places to vent about the complexities and injustice of people and systems (North American Drama Therapy Association, 2013). Faith can be very comforting for some, as can appreciating the incremental changes that, over time, result in major shifts toward improvement of patients' lives. Given the emotional intensity of the work, it is important that the child psychiatry trainee who chooses to work with this patient population is aware of the challenges in doing so (International Society for Traumatic Stress Studies, 2013). Most people who work in trauma see it as a calling rather than just a job and, as a result, bring much drive and energy to their work. It is crucial that this energy is channeled and gauged appropriately so that these committed treaters do not fall victim to their own enthusiasm.

A Culture of Communication

There are many instances in which a child psychiatrist interacts with caregivers and with other professionals concerning a child trauma survivor. Psychiatrists are also likely to find themselves as ambassadors of sorts, helping mitigate the negative reactions a child's behavior might trigger in caregivers by placing it in the context of common trauma reactions. And they have to balance this with the expectation that the child will continue to be involved in everyday activities such as attending school, extracurricular activities, and family or social events.

Professionalism

Working with children who have suffered trauma or with families who have perpetrated abuse is a trying task even for an experienced provider. Helping trainees to maintain a neutral and nonjudgmental stance in treating these children and families (assuming the caregiver is no longer engaged in abusive behavior toward the child) is among the most important parts of training. There are many reasons for the need to maintain neutrality and a nonjudgmental stance. First, it is unlikely that the family will engage in treatment if they feel the psychiatrist perceives them in a negative light. Second, however abusive the relationship between caregiver and child might have been, the child has a very practical need to maintain an emotional bond with the parents as he or she continues to depend on them materially and emotionally (Shapiro et al., 1987).

People who choose to work in mental health are a self-selecting group. Most choose the field out of a desire to help others. Especially when working with young children, it is difficult not to have a fantasy of rescuing a child from adverse circumstances. Trainees must be aware not only of their rescue fantasies but also of how they might present themselves to the child and the parents. While the trainee might in fact be a better parent than the child's caregiver, the reality is that the child must learn to live with the caregiver, however flawed his or her parenting skills may be. It is important for trainees to keep in mind that their job is to help caregivers be accountable for their behavior toward the child and interact with the child in a healthy, loving, and constructive way. The child psychiatrist's job is to help children forgive parents for their behavior and to feel a greater sense of agency in their relationship with the parent and with the world. The psychiatrist's responsibilities also include helping staff manage their feelings toward the parents and the child. The trainee can set an example for the medical staff by treating the family with the same respect and courtesy as the family of any other hospitalized child. By so doing, one can avoid creating an antagonistic relationship between health care providers and the family. This will help ensure that the child does not get lost in the fray, and it might help the parents be more open to owning their behavior and accepting whatever interventions might be indicated to address the abuse.

Lastly, it is sometimes the traumatized child or adolescent who acts in a hateful way toward the trainee and the medical staff. The push and pull of a patient with borderline personality disorder can make even the most patient mental health providers want to tear their hair out. It may be very difficult for a provider to tolerate a child who engages in self-harm and undermines the treater's efforts to promote his or her safety and well-being. Trainees must be aware of the countertransference such a patient elicits. They must curb their own desire to act in an angry and punitive way toward the child, while continuing to provide firm and consistent limits (Gabard & Wilkinson, 2000).

The Importance of Practice and Humility

In his book *Outliers: The Story of Success*, Malcolm Gladwell (2008) makes the case that to be an expert, one must put in more than 10,000 hours of practice. Similarly, the only way to gain mastery in providing trauma-informed care is by seeking out as many experiences as possible where one can do so. Psychiatry training can provide an opportunity to work in a multitude of settings and with a variety of patients. Trainees must be encouraged to seek out diverse training experiences so they can practice working with individuals or families, with single-event or chronic trauma. Most importantly, trainees must be made aware that although there are similarities in the way most trauma survivors present and in the numerous treatment approaches available, each child or adolescent must be seen as a unique challenge or mystery to be unraveled. Trainees must be open to the meaning that each individual has made of the trauma and the imprint it has made on his or her life. Although much of any medical training centers around demonstrating one's knowledge and skills, it is only by taking a stance of not knowing, of openness and curiosity, that a child psychiatry trainee can help a child or adolescent take the necessary steps to begin the journey to recovery.

References

American Academy of Child and Adolescent Psychiatry. (2011, March). Psychotherapies for children and adolescents. *Facts for families,* No. 86. Washington, DC: Author.

Applebaum, P. A., & Gutheil, T. G. (2007). *Clinical handbook of psychiatry and the law.* Philadelphia, PA: Lippincott Williams & Wilkins.

Bateman, A., & Fonagy, P. (2010). Mentalization based treatment for borderline personality disorder. *World Psychiatry, 9*(1), 11–15.

Bloom, S. (1997). *Creating sanctuary: Towards the evolution of sane societies.* New York, NY: Routledge / Taylor & Francis Group.

Brent, D. A., Johnson, B., Bartle, S., Bridge, J., Rather, C., Matta, J., et al. (1993). Personality disorder, tendency to impulsive violence, and suicidal behavior in adolescents. *Journal of the American Academy of Child and Adolescent Psychiatry, 32,* 69–75.

Bridge, J. A., McBee-Strayer, S. M., Cannon, E. A., Sheftall, A. H., Reynolds, B., Campo, J. V., et al. (2012). Impaired decision making in adolescent suicide attempters. *Journal of the American Academy of Child and Adolescent Psychiatry, 51*(4), 394–403.

Briere, J. (1992). *Child abuse trauma: Theory and treatment of the lasting effects.* New York, NY: Sage Publications.

Deblinger, E., Mannarino, A. P., Cohen, J., Runyon, M. K., & Steer, R. A. (2011). Trauma-Focused Cognitive Behavioral Therapy for children: Impact of the trauma narrative and treatment length. *Depression and Anxiety, 28,* 67–75.

Dulcan, M. K. (2010). *Dulcan's textbook of child and adolescent psychiatry.* Arlington, VA: American Psychiatric Publishing.

Egan, J., Chantoor, I., & Rosen, G. (1980). Nonorganic failure to thrive: Pathogenesis and classification. *Clinical Proceedings: Children's Hospital National Medical Center, 34,* 173–182.

Essau, C. A., Conradt, J., & Petermann, F. (2000). Haeufigkeit und Komorbiditaet somatoformer Stoerungen bei Jugendlichen. Ergebnisse der Bremer Jugendstudie [Prevalence and comorbidity of somatoform disorders in adolescents: Results of the Bremen Youth Study]. *Zeitschrift fur klinische Psychologie und Psychotherapie, 29,* 97–108.

Ford, J., Chapman, J., Connor, D., & Cruise, K. (2012). Complex trauma and aggression in secure juvenile justice settings. *Criminal Justice and Behavior, 39*(6), 694–724.

Gabard, G. O., & Wilkinson, S. A. (2000). *Management of countertransference in borderline patients.* Lanham, MD: Rowman & Littlefield Publishers.

George, C., & Solomon, J. (2011). *Caregiving helplessness: The development of a screening measure for disorganized maternal caregiving.* New York, NY: Guilford Press.

Giardino, A. P., Lyn, M. A., Giardino, E. R. (Eds.). (2010). *A practical guide to the evaluation of child physical abuse and neglect.* New York, NY: Springer Publishing.

Gladwell, M. (2008). *Outliers: The story of success.* Boston, MA: Little, Brown and Company.

International Society for Traumatic Stress Studies. (2013). *Treating trauma: Self-care for providers.* www.istss.org/Self CareForProviders.htm

Iwaniec, D. (1997). An overview of emotional maltreatment and failure to thrive. *Child Abuse Review, 6,* 370–388.

Lieb, R., Pfister, H., Mastaler, M., & Witcchen, H.-U. (2000). Somatoform syndromes and disorders in a representative sample of adolescents and young adults: Prevalence, comorbidity and impairment *Acta Psychiatrica Scandinavica, 101,* 194–208.

Lipowski, Z. J. (1974). Consultation-liaison psychiatry: An overview. *American Journal of Psychiatry, 13,* 623–630.

Martin, A., & Volkmar, F. R. (2007). *Lewis's child and adolescent psychiatry: A comprehensive textbook* (4th ed.). Philadelphia, PA: Lippincott Williams & Wilkins.

McCann, L. I., & Pearlmann, L. A. (1990). *Psychological trauma and the adult survivor: Theory, therapy, and transformation.* Hove, UK: Brunner-Routledge.

McCrory, E., De Brito, S. A., & Viding, E. (2012). The link between child abuse and psychopathology: A review of neurobiological and genetic research. *Journal of the Royal Society of Medicine, 105,* 151–156.

Muller, R. T. (2009). Trauma and dismissing (avoidant) attachment: Intervention strategies in individual psychotherapy. *Psychotherapy: Theory, Research, Practice, Training, 46*(1), 68–81.

Muscari, M. E., & Brown, K. M. (2010). *Quick reference to child and adolescent forensics: A guide for nurses and other health care professionals.* New York, NY: Springer Publishing.

North American Drama Therapy Association. (2013). *Self-care for therapists.* www.nadt.org/membership/selfcare-for-therapists .html

Plassmann, R. (1994). The biography of the factitious-disorder patient. *Psychotherapy and Psychosomatics, 62*(1–2), 123–128.

Roberts, M. C., & Steele, R. G. (2009). *Handbook of pediatric psychology* (4th ed.). New York, NY: Guilford Press.

Sadock, B. J., & Sadock, V. A. (2003). *Kaplan and Sadock's synopsis of psychiatry: Behavioral sciences / clinical psychiatry* (9th ed.). Philadelphia, PA: Lippincott Williams & Wilkins.

Safer, D. J. (1997). Self reported suicide attempts by adolescents. *Annals of Clinical Psychiatry, 9*(4), 263–269.

Schulte, I. E., & Petermann, F. (2011). Somatoform disorders: 30 years of debate about criteria. What about children and adolescents? *Journal of Psychosomatic Research, 70*(3), 218–228.

Shapiro, E. G., Rosenfeld, A. A., Cohen, N., Levine, D. A., & Renken, B. (1987). *The somatizing child: Diagnosis and treatment of conversion and somatization disorders.* New York, NY: Springer Publishing.

Smith, R. C. (1985). A clinical approach to the somatizing patient. *Journal of Family Practice, 21*(4), 294–301.

Tasman, A., Jerald, K., Lieberman, J. A., First, M. B., & Maj, M. (2011). *Psychiatry* (3rd ed.). New York, NY: John Wiley & Sons.

Webb, N. B. (2011). *Grief after suicide: Understanding the consequences and caring for the survivors.* New York, NY: Routledge / Taylor & Francis Group.

PART VI New Directions

32

SHANNON W. SIMMONS, M.D., M.P.H.
MICHAEL W. NAYLOR, M.D.

Psychopharmacology

GENERAL CONSIDERATIONS

Childhood abuse and neglect are associated with a range of emotional and behavioral disturbances. In some cases, pharmacotherapy to treat posttraumatic psychiatric symptoms is a significant element of the treatment plan. This chapter describes the link between child maltreatment and mental illness, the underlying neurobiological and neuroendocrine changes that may occur following abuse (and which may increasingly serve as targets for medicines as our knowledge base expands), and indications for medications. The scientific data on various classes of medications used to treat childhood posttraumatic stress disorder (PTSD) are summarized, followed by a brief discussion of the treatment of acute stress disorder and medications used for prevention of PTSD. Special considerations related to the use of medications for foster children are also presented. The chapter concludes with a summary of outstanding questions in the understudied area of pharmacotherapy of childhood PTSD.

Child abuse and neglect are associated with a variety of psychiatric and behavioral disturbances. PTSD can be a direct outcome of abuse. Studies have also shown a link between childhood abuse and anxiety and mood disorders (such as major depressive disorder and bipolar disorder) and psychosis—including schizophrenia (Alvarez et al., 2011; Bebbington et al., 2011; Schafer & Fisher, 2011; Sugava et al., 2012). Abused children have a greater risk of developing an eating disorder or abusing drugs and alcohol, with earlier and more severe drug use, compared with nonmaltreated youths (Cisler et al., 2011; Douglas et al., 2010; Nomura, Hurd, & Pilowsky, 2012; Rayworth, Wise, & Harlow, 2004).

Children who develop PTSD are at risk of developing other comorbid conditions. A study of female juvenile offenders showed that girls with PTSD had more psychiatric diagnoses than those without. The comorbid conditions often arose concurrently with or after the PTSD, suggesting a link between the trauma and various psychopathologies. Common comorbid disorders in this population included substance abuse, conduct disorder, depression, psychosis, and generalized anxiety disorder. Suicide attempts were more likely in girls with PTSD (Dixon, Howie, & Starling, 2005). Though this study was of a specialized population, it highlights the variety and extent of comorbid psychopathology that can accompany PTSD.

NEUROBIOLOGY OF CHILD ABUSE

Child abuse causes changes in the brain. Technological advances have led to an improved but still evolving understanding of these changes on a structural and neurochemical level. Children who are traumatized have higher levels of peripheral sympathetic nervous system activity, such as circulating norepinephrine (Pervanidou, 2008). Cortisol, a hormone that is released in response to stress, has a variety of physiological effects, such as mobilizing glucose stores and suppressing immune function. In children, the cortisol response to trauma is perhaps even more complicated than in adults, and study findings have not been completely consistent. Child maltreatment is known to have long-term effects on the developing hypothalamic-pituitary-adrenal axis that are mediated by a variety of individual biological and environmental risk and protective factors (Tarullo & Gunnar, 2006).

A functional MRI study of adults who experienced childhood trauma showed increased amygdala responsiveness when exposed to threatening facial expressions. Reduced gray matter in the hippocampus and other brain regions was also seen (Dannlowski et al., 2012). Notably, these adults were studied decades after the traumatic events, suggesting long-lasting structural and functional brain changes.

THE ROLE OF GENES

Certain genetic polymorphisms may predispose individuals to or protect them from psychiatric sequelae when also exposed to environmental stressors. An example is the serotonin transporter gene, *5-HTTLPR* (serotonin-transporter-linked polymorphic region). Several studies have shown that the short allele confers a greater risk for depression in the presence of stressful life conditions (Aguilera et al., 2009; Brown et al., 2013). The long allele may be associated with a heightened response to selective serotonin reuptake inhibitor (SSRI) medications (Mushtag et al., 2012; Rundell et al., 2011). Testing for this allele is not used clinically at this time.

There are other examples of this gene-environment interaction. A corticotropin-releasing hormone receptor gene (*CRHR1*) haplotype is associated with adult depression if there is exposure to childhood adverse events such as abuse (Bradley et al., 2008; Grabe et al., 2010). A lower level of monoamine oxidase-A (MAOA) expression in the setting of mild to moderate trauma has been linked with higher levels of aggressive behavior and conduct disorder (Ferguson et al., 2011; Foley et al., 2004). There may also be a gene-environment link between certain catechol-O-methyltransferase gene (*COMT*) polymorphisms and childhood trauma. Studies have shown a predisposition for impulsive aggression in women with borderline personality disorder, dissociation, and/or schizotypal personality traits in those with certain polymorphisms of this gene (Savitz, van der Merwe, Newman, Solms, et al., 2008; Savitz, van der Merwe, Newman, Stein, & Ramesar, 2010; Wagner et al, 2010). As our knowledge base increases, these genes may represent specific targets for therapy.

DIAGNOSTIC ISSUES

Lenore Terr introduced the idea of type I and type II trauma in 1991. Type I trauma is a "single blow," an isolated event, more likely to result in classic PTSD symptoms. Type II traumas are recurrent and longstanding; they result in chronic mood dysregulation, dissociation, character identity problems, and rage (often self-directed). Some studies have suggested that physical abuse is more strongly associated with disruptive behavior and aggression in its victims, whereas neglected children may be more likely to display internalizing disorders (Petrenko et al., 2012). Clinicians should perform a thorough diagnostic assessment on each child, as these patterns are certainly not universal.

An increasing body of literature in developmental psychology has explored the effects of chronic, early-life relational trauma on a child's emotional regulation abilities. These effects include difficulty managing negative emotional states such as anger and a greater risk for problematic impulsivity and self-destructive behavior (Ehring & Quack, 2010).

Traumatized children may present with "extreme dysregulation of physical, affective, behavioral, cognition, and/or interpersonal functioning that is not adequately captured in current descriptions of PTSD diagnostic criteria" (American Academy of Child and Adolescent Psychiatry, 2010, p. 416). Children with these symptoms might be misdiagnosed as having bipolar disorder or other psychiatric illnesses if the examiner does not consider the role of trauma. Conversely, all emotional or behavior problems in a child with trauma may erroneously be attributed to PTSD when, in fact, the youngster has another mental illness (Griffin et al., 2011). The timing of the symptoms—in particular, if their onset coincides with a traumatic event—may aid with diagnosis; however, in cases of chronic trauma, a discrete timeline might not be possible.

A child's developmental stage may affect PTSD symptom presentation. The *Diagnostic and Statistical Manual of Mental Disorders* (4th edition, text revision; *DSM-IV-TR*) provides some modifications of criteria for children. For example, instead of intrusive traumatic recollections (which may be difficult for a child to describe), repetitive trauma-themed play is acceptable evidence of re-experiencing the traumatic event (American Psychiatric Association, 2000). Other PTSD criteria, however, do not provide specific guidance or allowances for young children. For example, studies have shown that traumatized youths may demonstrate a wide range of emotional states in response to trauma, not just "fear, helplessness, or horror . . . disorganized or agitated behavior" (*DSM-IV-TR*). Children, particularly preschool-age, may not be able to express feelings of detachment from others. It is not realistic to expect a young child to experience a sense of a foreshortened future or to be able to report avoiding trauma-related stimuli (Scheeringa, Zeanah, & Cohen, 2011).

A white paper by the National Child Traumatic Stress Network (2003) explores complex trauma in depth, asserting that our current diagnostic system does not account for its range of impacts on a developing child. Complex trauma is defined in this paper as multiple simultaneous or sequential traumas within the caretaking environment, beginning in childhood, as well as the multi-domain impairment and symptomatology that often result. The domains of impairment include attachment, biology, affect regulation, dissociation, behavioral control, cognition, and self-concept. The white paper includes recommendations for clinicians, researchers, and policymakers regarding complex trauma.

INDICATIONS FOR PSYCHOPHARMACOLOGY IN TRAUMA

Medications can be helpful in certain cases of trauma-related symptomatology but are not indicated in every case. First, the patient must have a psychiatric disorder or symptoms that are amenable to pharmacotherapy. Years of data show that medications can treat PTSD, major depressive disorder, bipolar disorder, psychosis, and generalized and other anxiety disorders. In cases of mild symptoms, starting with psychotherapy is typically prudent (American Academy of Child and Adolescent Psychiatry, 2010). Though medications should be reserved for more severe cases, unfortunately there is often an inverse relationship between symptom severity and response to treatment. A suboptimal response to psychotherapy is one indication to consider the addition of medication. The presence of comorbidities that are also responsive to medications might more strongly suggest a role for pharmacotherapy; a discussion of the treatment of potential comorbid conditions is beyond the scope of this chapter. When medications are used, the ideal approach is to combine pharmacotherapy with psychotherapy.

GENERAL APPROACH TO TREATMENT

When initiating treatment of a child who has been the victim of abuse, the first step should be a thorough diagnostic assessment. As discussed above, childhood trauma is associated with many psychiatric conditions and can present with a range of emotional and behavioral disturbances not fully described by our current diagnostic criteria. Thus, the child should be assessed for symptoms of PTSD, mood disorders, psychosis, anxiety disorders, and substance abuse. The evaluator should explore how the symptoms affect the child's functioning. A thorough medical history is essential. The evaluator should closely assess for ongoing abuse, neglect, or trauma, as treatment will be less effective if the child continues to be victimized. Prenatal, birth, and developmental history should be obtained when possible. Family psychiatric history can be useful when formulating a differential diagnosis. The clinician should consider further workup with laboratory or other diagnostic tests if there are symptoms that could be explained by medical illness. The Practice Parameters for the Assessment and Treatment of Children and Adolescents with Post-Traumatic Stress Disorder, available through the American Academy of Child and Adolescent Psychiatry (2010), provides further discussion of assessment and treatment planning.

Once a preliminary diagnosis has been established, a treatment plan can be developed. The selection of a medication should be tailored to the diagnosis and symptoms. The high rate of psychiatric comorbidity in this population requires a thoughtful approach, to avoid unnecessary polypharmacy while still addressing the symptoms at hand.

MEDICATIONS

Data on the safety and effectiveness of psychotropic medications in treating PTSD in youths are limited. Clinical practice is outpacing current research in this area. Given the paucity of research, clinical decision making often relies on interpolating data from the adult literature. Developmental considerations must be taken into account, such as the neurobiological differences between children and adults and the poorly understood long-term effects of psychotropic medications on the developing brain. Thus, a cautious and judicious approach to pharmacotherapy should be undertaken. Table 32.1 summarizes the evidence.

Selective Serotonin Reuptake Inhibitors

Selective serotonin reuptake inhibitors are used for treating a variety of psychiatric illnesses, including major depressive disorder and various anxiety disorders. They are generally considered first-line agents for PTSD in adults, given their effectiveness against all three symptom clusters (re-experiencing, hyperarousal, and avoidance). However, data for children are less robust. One double-blind, placebo-controlled trial of sertraline showed a comparable response to placebo in 131 study participants (Robb et al., 2010). In another study, in which sertraline or placebo was added to Trauma-Focused Cognitive Behavioral Therapy (TF-CBT), both groups improved in a similar fashion, suggesting no additional benefit to adding an SSRI (Cohen et al., 2007). A study comparing response to citalopram of 24 children and 14 adults showed no difference between the response rates of the two age groups (Seedat et al., 2002). An open-label trial of citalopram for 8 patients showed significant improvements in PTSD symptoms (Seedat et al., 1999). In most of these studies, the children had suffered chronic, multiple traumas.

In a child with PTSD and a comorbid depressive or anxiety disorder, an SSRI might be a reasonable choice. However, some traumatized children experience severe mood dysregulation or have comorbid bipolar disorder, which might be worsened by an antidepressant. SSRIs are generally well tolerated, but patients should be monitored for side effects. Gastrointestinal upset and headaches may occur but are likely to resolve as treatment continues. Some children report sedation, which can often be addressed by moving the medication to bedtime. A transient increase in anxiety might occur at the start of therapy. In some cases, more concerning symptoms of behavioral activation can arise, including restlessness, insomnia, and agitation.

In 2003, the U.S. Food and Drug Administration issued a public health advisory about an increased risk of suicidal ideation or behaviors in children or adolescents prescribed antidepressants. Patients being treated with an SSRI, particularly in the early stages, should be monitored closely for the emergence of any suicidal thoughts or behaviors.

Though these studies do not demonstrate a robust response to SSRIs, it should be noted that, combined, they included fewer than 200 participants. Thus, it is difficult to derive strong conclusions about SSRIs' effectiveness or lack thereof for traumatized children. In many cases an SSRI may be a reasonable first choice, particularly if there is comorbid anxiety or depression.

Antiadrenergic Agents

As mentioned earlier, children with PTSD have higher circulating levels of sympathetic nervous system hormones such as norepinephrine. Medications that decrease sympathetic tone can be used to address the hyperarousal sometimes seen in PTSD. Centrally acting alpha-2 agonists such

Table 32.1. Summary of PTSD Medication Studies

Authors	Medication	Study Design	N	Trauma Type*	Target Symptoms	Results
Cohen et al., 2007	Sertraline added to TF-CBT	Randomized, placebo-controlled	24	II	Three core symptom clusters	Sertraline offered no benefit over psychotherapy alone
Robb et al., 2010	Sertraline	Double-blind, placebo-controlled	131	V	Three core symptom clusters	Sertraline offered no benefit vs. placebo
Seedat et al., 2002	Citalopram	Open-label, comparing children and adults	24	V	Three core symptom clusters	Teens and adults had symptom reduction
Seedat et al., 1999	Citalopram	Open-label	7	V	Three core symptom clusters	Reduction in all three symptom clusters
Harmon & Riggs, 1996	Clonidine	Open-label	7	II	Multiple (see text discussion)	Most or all had reductions in target symptoms
Horrigan, 1996	Guanfacine	Case report	1	II	Nightmares	Nightmares resolved
Fraleigh et al., 2009	Prazosin	Case report	1	II	Nightmares	Nightmares resolved
Strawn et al., 2009	Prazosin	Case report	1	I	Nightmares, hyperarousal, avoidance	Nightmares resolved; hyperarousal improved; avoidance persisted
Famularo et al., 1988	Propranolol	Case series, on-off-on design	11	V	Three core symptom clusters	Improvement in all symptom clusters; return of symptoms when drug stopped
Yeh et al., 2010	Aripiprazole to augment SSRI	Case report	1	I	Nightmares	Nightmares improved
Wheatley et al., 2004	Clozapine	Retrospective case series	6	V	Self-injury, aggression, hallucinations	4/6 had reduced aggression; 5/6 had fewer hallucinations
Keeshin & Strawn, 2009	Risperidone added to valproex (valproic acid) and clonidine	Case report	1	II	Three core symptom clusters	Decreased re-experiencing; improved sleep; fewer hospitalizations
Stathis et al., 2005	Quetiapine	Case series	6	II (3/6), U (3/6)	Three core symptom clusters	Less dissociation, anxiety, depression, anger in all 6
Looff et al., 1995	Carbamazepine	Case series	28	II	Three core symptom clusters	22/28 became asymptomatic; 6/28 had significant improvements
Steiner et al., 2007	Valproex (valproic acid)	Randomized controlled trial, high vs. low dose	12	U	Three core symptom clusters	High-dose led to greater reduction in PTSD symptoms

*I = single-episode trauma; II = chronic trauma; V = varied; U = unknown.

as clonidine and guanfacine work by decreasing the release of norepinephrine. The one identified open study of clonidine use for severely, chronically abused preschool children involved youngsters, ages 3–6 years, in a day treatment program who had had at least one month of family therapy without resolution of symptoms. A trial of clonidine reduced aggression in all children and reduced emotional outbursts, hyperarousal and hypervigilance, generalized anxiety, and oppositionality in the majority of children (Harmon & Riggs, 1996). Guanfacine reduced PTSD-related nightmares in a case report of a chronically abused 7-year-old (Horrigan, 1996).

Prazosin is an alpha-1 receptor antagonist that decreases adrenergic tone. Randomized, placebo-controlled studies of adults with PTSD have suggested the efficacy of this drug in reducing trauma-related nightmares. In children, a few case reports suggest that this medication may be beneficial. In one report, a 16-year-old girl with PTSD following a violent robbery at work was prescribed prazosin. She reported a robust decrease in nightmares and hyperarousal symptoms but no change in avoidance (Strawn, DelBello, & Geracioti, 2009). In another case report, a 16-year-old boy with PTSD resulting from several traumatic experiences also reported elimination of nightmares with prazosin (Fraleigh et al., 2009).

Propranolol is a beta-blocker with a variety of medical uses, such as treatment of hypertension and migraines; it is also used for some anxiety disorders, such as performance-related social phobias. It decreases the heart rate and blood pressure by reducing noradrenergic activity. An open-label pilot study investigated propranolol's effectiveness in treating PTSD symptoms in a group of 11 school-age children who had been physically and/or sexually abused. There was a statistically significant reduction in PTSD symptoms (Famularo, Kinscherff, & Fenton, 1988).

These medicines are sometimes used in combination with other agents (such as an SSRI) to address hyperarousal symptoms that are suboptimally treated by the other medication. Alpha-2 agonists are also used, often adjunctively with psychostimulants, in treating attention-deficit/hyperactivity disorder (ADHD) to target motor hyperactivity and impulsivity. In a child with PTSD and ADHD, this class of medications could be strongly considered.

Given their cardiovascular effects, these medications should not be prescribed for children with cardiac problems without clearance by a cardiologist or pediatrician. Vital signs should be monitored, as low blood pressure and tachycardia (or bradycardia with propranolol) may develop; patients should be warned of possible orthostatic hypotension. These drugs can be mildly sedating but are otherwise fairly well tolerated.

Atypical Antipsychotics

A child or teen with PTSD may experience psychotic symptoms such as hallucinations, mood lability, or aggression. Also, as mentioned above, bipolar or psychotic disorders may be comorbid with PTSD. In these cases, SSRIs may only partially address the full array of symptoms. Some case series and case reports suggest that atypical antipsychotics, either alone or as augmentation, may be helpful.

A case report described the use of risperidone for a 13-year-old boy with a history of chronic sexual abuse and neglect and multiple hospitalizations for aggression and self-harm. He had prominent symptoms of hypervigilance, auditory hallucinations, and flashbacks and was diagnosed with PTSD. Risperidone was added to his regimen of divalproex (valproic acid) and clonidine, which resulted in resolution of his symptoms (Keeshin & Strawn, 2009).

In another case report, a 14-year-old girl developed PTSD following a physical assault. Symptoms of re-experiencing, avoidance, and hyperarousal were treated successfully with escitalopram, but she continued to suffer nightmares related to the trauma. The addition of aripiprazole at bedtime resulted in resolution of her nightmares (Yeh, Hsieh, & Chou, 2010).

Quetiapine was studied in a case series of six teens in a youth detention center, ages 15–17 years. These teens, who met the criteria for PTSD, were given low doses of quetiapine, which resulted in an overall reduction in PTSD symptoms, particularly dissociation, anxiety, depressed mood, and anger. Many of the youths reported sedation, though this was felt to be beneficial given the high rates of insomnia. Weight gain was significant during this six-week study (Stathis, Martin, & McKenna, 2005).

Clozapine, when used for schizophrenia or bipolar disorder, is reserved for treatment-resistant cases due to the low but serious risk of agranulocytosis. A case series suggested a possible benefit in teens with treatment-resistant symptoms of PTSD. In one series, six patients, ages 17–19 years, with PTSD from both acute and chronic traumas were treated with clozapine. They experienced symptoms of psychosis, had a history of aggression or self-injury, and had had at least two failed trials of other antipsychotic drugs. Patients reported improvements in psychosis and sleep (Wheatley et al., 2004). When clozapine is being considered, the ability of the patient to obtain weekly blood draws to monitor granulocyte counts should be a factor in determining the appropriateness of this medicine. Clozapine also carries the highest risk of weight gain and metabolic syndrome, but the lowest risk of tardive dyskinesia. In adults with schizophrenia, clozapine is indicated only after failed trials of at least two antipsychotics, including one atypical antipsychotic (American Psychiatric Association, 2004). In the understudied population of youths with PTSD, equally if not more stringent criteria should be applied.

This class of medication carries a significant side-effect profile, including metabolic syndrome, extrapyramidal symptoms, and other medication-specific effects. Monitoring of metabolic parameters and for abnormal involuntary movements should be performed at baseline and at regular intervals. No pediatric studies were found for olanzapine, ziprasidone, or some of the newer antipsychotics such as paliperidone, asenapine, lurasidone, and iloperidone.

Mood Stabilizers

Mood stabilizers are traditionally used for the manic or maintenance phase of bipolar disorder. They also have been used in the treatment of other conditions, including PTSD in adults. As with other classes of medications, data supporting their use in children or adolescents are limited. No studies were found on the use of lithium for this population.

A small study of 12 incarcerated adolescent males diagnosed with PTSD and conduct disorder randomized the subjects to either high- or low-dose divalproex sodium for seven weeks; the type of trauma was not specified. The 6 teens in the high-dose group showed greater reductions in overall symptom severity, as well as a greater decrease in the three PTSD core symptom areas (Steiner et al., 2007). Divalproex sodium can cause weight gain, sedation, hepatic injury, alopecia, tremor, elevated ammonia, teratogenicity if taken during pregnancy, and pancreatitis. Regular blood work is required for monitoring blood levels, complete blood counts, and liver function tests.

Carbamazepine has not been evaluated in randomized trials. In a case series of 28 children, ages 8–17 years, with PTSD resulting from repeated sexual abuse, 22 were asymptomatic by the end of the study and the other 6 were markedly improved. Concurrent treatment with an SSRI, a stimulant for ADHD, or clonidine was seen in a minority of cases (Looff et al., 1995). Regular blood work is required for monitoring drug levels, complete blood counts (due to the risk of thrombocytopenia or, rarely, pancytopenia), and liver function tests (due to the risk of hepatic injury). Drug interactions are an important consideration with carbamazepine, which is a strong inducer of multiple hepatic cytochrome P450 subsystems.

Benzodiazepines

Benzodiazepines are used to treat PTSD in adults, though the data suggest a cautious approach. The U.S. Department of Veterans Affairs and Department of Defense's (2010) Clinical Practice Guidelines for the Management of Post-Traumatic Stress recommends against the use of benzodiazepines due to their unclear efficacy and the risk of dependence. Some evidence has suggested an increased risk of developing PTSD when benzodiazepines are administered in the acute posttrauma period (Gelpin et al., 1996). Other concerns include the potential for worsening anxiety symptoms when these medications are discontinued and the risk of cognitive side effects. In children, benzodiazepines may have a paradoxically disinhibiting effect rather than an anxiolytic effect. No studies on the use of benzodiazepines in children or adolescents with PTSD were found; however, benzodiazepines may have some utility in some childhood anxiety disorders.

EARLY INTERVENTION

Treatment of Acute Stress Disorder

Some studies have investigated potential treatments for acute stress disorder (ASD); table 32.2 summarizes the evidence. Many studies in this area involve burn patients because they present quickly following the trauma and often require lengthy hospitalizations and close medical follow-up. However, these studies often do not specify the prevalence of abuse or suspected abuse.

Robert et al. (1999) found that treatment with low-dose imipramine, a tricyclic antidepressant, resulted in more symptom reduction than chloral hydrate. A comparative, non-placebo-controlled study of imipramine and fluoxetine found that 89% of patients responded to either medicine (Tcheung et al., 2005), while another comparison of imipramine, fluoxetine, and placebo showed no statistically significant difference between the three groups (Robert et al., 2008). A case series in which risperidone was used for three preschoolers who suffered burns due to child abuse showed improvements in all children (Meighen, Hines, & Lagges, 2007). A study of propranolol did not show a significant reduction in development of ASD symptoms compared with placebo (Sharp et al., 2010). Tricyclic antidepressants have a more significant side-effect burden than SSRIs and are more dangerous in overdose due to cardiac toxicity. It is difficult to know what clinical practices to derive from these limited data.

Table 32.2. Summary of Acute Stress Disorder and Prevention of PTSD Medication Studies

Authors	Medication	Study Design	N	Duration of Treatment	Results
Acute stress disorder					
Meighen et al., 2007	Risperidone	Case series	3	Followed for 8 weeks	Rapid reduction in all symptom clusters
Robert et al., 1999	Imipramine or chloral hydrate	Randomized, double-blind	25	7 days	83% responded to imipramine; 38% responded to chloral hydrate (statistically significant)
Robert et al., 2008	Imipramine, fluoxetine, or placebo	Randomized, placebo-controlled, double-blind	60	7 days	55% responded to placebo; 60% to imipramine; 72% to fluoxetine (not statistically significant)
Sharp et al., 2010	Propranolol	Retrospective chart review of prior placebo-controlled, randomized controlled trial	363	—	No difference in rates of ASD between treatment and placebo groups
Tcheung et al., 2005	Imipramine or fluoxetine	Retrospective chart review; switch medicines if no response after 7 days	128	7 days on each medication	Initially, 81% responded to imipramine and 75% to fluoxetine; 89% eventually responded to either medication
PTSD prevention					
Nugent et al., 2010	Propranolol	Double-blind placebo-controlled	29	10 days (monitored 6 weeks)	No difference between groups; boys had a nonsignificant decrease in symptoms with propranolol
Saxe et al., 2001	Morphine	Open-label	24	2–26 days (monitored 6 months)	Higher dose of morphine correlated with fewer PTSD symptoms at 6 months
Stoddard et al., 2011	Sertraline	Double-blind placebo-controlled	26	12 weeks (monitored 24 weeks)	Children reported no difference; parents reported decrease in observed PTSD symptoms with sertraline
Stoddard et al., 2009	Morphine	Open-label	70	Varied (monitored 6 months)	Correlation between total daily morphine dose and reduction in PTSD symptoms

—= Not applicable

Prevention of PTSD

An important emerging area of research is the prevention of PTSD following exposure to a trauma. As for ASD, many studies of PTSD prevention involve patients who have suffered burn injuries. Two studies of children and adolescents with severe burn injuries showed that the dosage of morphine administered in the immediate posttrauma period is inversely related to the risk of later developing PTSD. This may be due to morphine's inhibition of noradrenergically medicated overconsolidation of traumatic memories that is postulated to occur in PTSD (Saxe et al., 2001; Stoddard et al., 2009). Adult studies have yielded similar results. Whether these findings can be applied to abused children is unclear. More research may shed light on the utility of this intervention.

Sertraline has also been investigated for its possible efficacy in preventing PTSD. A placebo-controlled, double-blind, randomized controlled trial of 26 children and young adults, ages 6–20 years, showed mixed results. Participants reported no difference between the active medication and placebo after 24 weeks, whereas parents of those in the sertraline group reported a decrease in observed child PTSD symptoms compared with parents of those in the placebo group (Stoddard et al., 2011). A study of propranolol administered to traumatized children did not show a significant difference in ultimate development of PTSD symptomatology compared with placebo (Nugent et al., 2010). Again, in these studies, the traumas suffered were not abuse or neglect.

OVERSIGHT OF THE USE OF PSYCHOTROPIC MEDICATIONS FOR FOSTER CHILDREN

Children and adolescents in the child welfare system represent a special subset of youths who have experienced trauma. The use of psychotropic medications for this vulnerable population has recently received a great deal of attention in the press and in government oversight programs (U.S. Administration for Children and Families, 2012).

Foster children—who are, by definition, Medicaid-eligible—are at higher risk for developing emotional and behavioral disturbances and mental illness (Burns et al., 2004; dos Reis et al., 2001; Harman, Childs, & Kelleher, 2000; Landsverk et al., 2006; White et al., 2007), use mental health services at higher rates (Burns et al., 2004; dos Reis et al., 2001; Halfon, Berkowitz, & Klee, 1992; Harman, Childs, &Kelleher, 2000), and are more likely to receive psychotropic medications than other Medicaid-eligible youths (Breland-Noble et al., 2004; dos Reis et al., 2001; Raghavan, 2005).

The use of psychotropic medications for the treatment of youths in the general population who have severe emotional and behavioral disturbances has increased dramatically over recent years (Olfson et al., 2002; Zito et al., 2003). This increase is paralleled by an increase in the rate of poly-

pharmacy, the concurrent administration of two or more psychotropic medications (Bhatara et al., 2004; Olfson et al., 2002; Safer, Zito, & dos Reis, 2003). Similar findings have been reported for foster children (Anderson et al., 2002).

In 2011, the U.S. Government Accountability Office published a report comparing the use of psychotropic medications for foster children and nonfoster children receiving Medicaid benefits in five states. It found that foster children were up to 4.5 times more likely than nonfoster children to be prescribed a psychotropic medication, up to 52.5 times more likely to be prescribed five or more psychotropic medications concurrently, and nearly 9 times more likely to be prescribed medications at doses exceeding published guidelines. States varied widely in the implementation of published guidelines on the oversight of psychotropic medications for children in state custody (American Academy of Child and Adolescent Psychiatry, 2005). The authors of the U.S. Government Accountability Office (2011) study recommended that the Department of Health and Human Services should consider endorsing guidelines for the states on best practices for monitoring psychotropic medication use in foster children.

In response to concerns raised about the high rate of use of psychotropic medications for foster children, Congress passed the Child and Family Services Improvement and Innovation Act of 2011. This piece of legislation required states to submit a description of their protocol (planned or in place) to oversee and monitor psychotropic medication use among children and youths in foster care. States were specifically asked to address the following:

- Strategies for screening and assessment to identify children with emotional, behavioral, or psychiatric disturbances that may require psychotropic medications
- Mechanisms for enhancing shared decision making on mental health treatment, including means of obtaining informed consent and assent and methods to facilitate effective communication between the prescriber, the child, and his or her caregivers
- Monitoring of the use of psychotropic medications at the individual and statewide level
- Availability of psychiatric consultation for clinical decision making (specifically as related to the consent process)
- Means for accessing and sharing accurate and up-to-date information and educational materials related to mental health and trauma-related interventions for clinicians, child welfare staff, youths, and caregivers

There are several models of psychotropic medication consent and oversight. Consent for children and adolescents who are wards of the state can be provided by a person or office within the child welfare agency, by someone appointed by the court to provide consent, by the court, by foster parents, or by child welfare caseworkers. Oversight can be prospective or retrospective. In prospective models, medications are reviewed, typically in conjunction with a centralized consent process, prior to their prescription. In retrospective models, the responsibility for consent usually resides with foster parents or caseworkers. The use of psychotropic medication is monitored through review of Medicaid payment data. (For a review, see Leslie et al., 2010.)

OUTSTANDING QUESTIONS

Numerous outstanding questions emerge on the use of medications to treat posttraumatic symptoms in children and adolescents. Randomized controlled trials are needed to help clinicians better understand which medications are effective in this heterogeneous population. The impact of trauma type on symptomatology has been studied to some extent, but there has been no examination of how this might predict responses to specific treatments. How treatment affects long-term outcomes for patients is another understudied but important area. Whether monitoring of the use of psychotropic medications for foster children improves quality or cost-effectiveness of care is currently unknown. Additional research is also needed to clarify the distinctions between symptoms of trauma and psychiatric illness and how this affects clinical decision making.

References

Aguilera, M., Arias, B., Wichers, M., Barrantes-Vidal, N., Moya, J., Villa, H., et al. (2009). Early adversity and *5-HTT/BDNF* genes: New evidence of gene-environment interactions on depressive symptoms in a general population. *Psychological Medicine 39*(9), 1425–1432. doi:10.1017/S0033291709005248

Alvarez, M. J., Roura, P., Oses, A., Foguet, Q., Sola, J., & Arrufat, F. X. (2011). Prevalence and clinical impact of childhood trauma in patients with severe mental disorders. *Journal of Nervous and Mental Disease, 199*(3), 156–161. doi:10.1097/NMD.0b013e31820c751c

American Academy of Child and Adolescent Psychiatry. (2005). *Oversight of psychotropic medication use for children in state custody: A best principles guideline.* www.aacap.org/galleries/PracticeInformation/FosterCare_BestPrinciples_FINAL.pdf

American Academy of Child and Adolescent Psychiatry. (2010). Practice parameters for the assessment and treatment of children and adolescents with post-traumatic stress disorder. *Journal of the American Academy of Child and Adolescent Psychiatry, 49*(4), 414–430. doi:10.1016/j.jaac.2009.12.020

American Psychiatric Association. (2000). *Diagnostic and statistical manual of mental disorders* (4th ed., text rev.). Washington, DC: Author.

American Psychiatric Association. (2004). Practice guidelines for the treatment of patients with schizophrenia, second edition. *American Journal of Psychiatry, 161*, 1–54. doi:10.1176/appi.books.9780890423363.45859

Anderson, T. R., Naylor, M. W., Kruesi, M., & Stoewe, J. (2002, October). *Co-pharmacy and poly-pharmacy in children and adolescents in substitute care.* Paper presented at 49th annual meeting of the American Academy of Child and Adolescent Psychiatry, San Francisco, CA. Abstract No. C-31.

Bebbington, P., Jonas, S., Kuipers, E., King, M., Cooper, C., Brugha, T., et al. (2011). Childhood sexual abuse and psychosis: Data from a cross-sectional national psychiatric survey in England. *British Journal of Psychiatry, 199*, 29–37. doi:10.1192/bjp.bp.110.083642

Bhatara, V., Feil, M., Hoagwood, K., Vitiello, B., & Zima, B. (2004). National trends in concomitant psychotropic medication with stimulants in pediatric visits: Practice versus knowledge. *Journal of Attention Disorders, 7*, 217–226.

Bradley, R., Binder, E., Epstein, M., Tang, Y., Nair, H., Liu, W., et al. (2008). Influence of child abuse on adult depression: Moderation by the corticotropin-releasing hormone receptor gene. *Archives of General Psychiatry, 65*(2), 190–200.

Breland-Noble, A. M., Elbogen, E. B., Farmer, E. M., Dubs, M. S., Wagner, H. R., & Burns, B. J. (2004). Use of psychotropic medications by youths in therapeutic foster care and group homes. *Psychiatric Services, 55*, 706–708.

Brown, G., Ban, M., Craig, T., Harris, T., Herbert, J., & Uher, R. (2013). Serotonin transporter length polymorphism, childhood maltreatment, and chronic depression: A specific gene-environment interaction. *Depression and Anxiety, 30*(1), 5–13. doi:10.1002/da.21982

Burns, B. J., Phillips, S. D., Wagner, H. R., Barth, R. P., Kolko, D. J., Campbell, Y., & Landsverk, J. (2004). Mental health need and access to mental health services by youths involved with child welfare: A national survey. *Journal of the American Academy of Child and Adolescent Psychiatry, 43*, 960–970.

Cisler, J., Amstadter, A., Begle, A., Resnick, H., Danielson, C., Saunders, B., & Kilpatrick, D. (2011). PTSD symptoms, potentially traumatic event exposure, and binge drinking: A prospective study with a national sample of adolescents. *Journal of Anxiety Disorders, 25*, 978–987. doi:10.1016/j.janxdis.2011.06.006

Cohen, J., Mannarino, A., Perel, J., & Staron, V. (2007). A pilot randomized controlled trial of combined trauma-focused CBT and sertraline for childhood PTSD symptoms. *Journal of the American Academy of Child and Adolescent Psychiatry, 46*(7), 811–819. doi:10.1097/chi.0b013e3180547105

Dannlowski, U., Stuhrmann, A., Beutelmann, V., Zwanzger, P., Lenzen, T., Grotegerd, D., et al. (2012). Limbic scars: Long-term consequences of childhood maltreatment revealed by functional and structural magnetic resonance imagining. *Biological Psychiatry, 71*, 286–293. doi:10.1016/j.biopsych.2011.10.021

Dixon, A., Howie, P., & Starling, J. (2005). Trauma exposure, posttraumatic stress, and psychiatric comorbidity in female juvenile offenders. *Journal of the American Academy of Child and Adolescent Psychiatry, 44*(8), 798–806. doi:10.1097/01.chi.0000164590.48318.9c

dos Reis, S., Zito, J. M., Safer, D. J., & Soeken, K. L. (2001). Mental health services for youths in foster care and disabled youths. *American Journal of Public Health, 91*, 1094–1099.

Douglas, K., Chan, G., Gelernter, J., Arias, A., Anton, R., Weiss, R., et al. (2010). Adverse childhood events as risk factors for substance dependence: Partial mediation by mood and anxiety disorders. *Addictive Behaviors, 35*, 7–13. doi:10.1016/j.addbeh.2009.07.004

Ehring, T., & Quack, D. (2010). Emotion regulation difficulties in trauma survivors: The role of trauma type and PTSD symptom severity. *Behavior Therapy, 41*(4), 587–598. doi:10.1016/j.beth.2010.04.004

Famularo, R., Kinscherff, R., & Fenton, T. (1988). Propranolol treatment for childhood posttraumatic stress disorder, acute type. *American Journal of Diseases of Children, 142*(11), 1244–1247.

Ferguson, D., Boden, J., Horwood, L., Miller, A., & Kennedy, M. (2011). MAOA, abuse exposure and antisocial behavior: 30-year longitudinal study. *British Journal of Psychiatry, 198*(6), 457–463. doi:10.1192/bjp.bp.110.086991

Foley, D., Eaves, L., Wormley, B., Silberg, J., Maes, H., Kuhn, J., & Riley, B. (2004). Childhood adversity, monoamine oxidase A genotype, and risk for conduct disorder. *Archives of General Psychiatry, 61*(7), 738–744. doi:10.1001/archgenpsychiatry .2011.2116

Fraleigh, L., Hendratta, V., Ford, J., & Connor, D. (2009). Prazosin for the treatment of posttraumatic stress disorder–related nightmares in an adolescent male. *Journal of Child and Adolescent Psychopharmacology, 19*(4), 475–476. doi:10.1089/ cap.2009.0002

Gelpin, E., Bonne, O., Peri, T., Brandes, D., & Shalev, A. (1996). Treatment of recent trauma survivors with benzodiazepines: A prospective study. *Journal of Clinical Psychiatry, 57*(9), 390–394.

Grabe, H., Schwahn, C., Appel, K., Mahler, J., Schulz, A., Spitzer, C., et al. (2010). Childhood maltreatment, the corticotropin-releasing hormone receptor gene and adult depression in the general population. *American Journal of Medical Genetics, 153B*(8), 1483–1493. doi:10.1002/ajmg.b.31131

Griffin, G., McClelland, G., Holzberg, M., Stolbach, B., Maj, N., & Kisiel, C. (2011). Addressing the impact of trauma before diagnosing. *Child Welfare, 90*(6), 69–89.

Halfon, N., Berkowitz, G., & Klee, L. (1992). Mental health service utilization by children in foster care in California. *Pediatrics, 89*, 1238–1244.

Harman, J. S., Childs, G. E., & Kelleher, K. J. (2000). Mental health utilization and expenditures by children in foster care. *Archives of Pediatrics & Adolescent Medicine, 154*, 1114–1117.

Harmon, R., & Riggs, P. (1996). Clonidine for posttraumatic stress disorder in preschool children. *Journal of the American Academy of Child and Adolescent Psychiatry, 35*(9), 1247–1249.

Horrigan, J. (1996) Guanfacine for PTSD nightmares [Letter to the editor]. *Journal of the American Academy of Child and Adolescent Psychiatry, 35*(8), 975.

Keeshin, B., & Strawn, J. (2009, July/August). Risperidone treatment of an adolescent with severe posttraumatic stress disorder [Letter to the editor]. *Annals of Pharmacotherapy, 43*, 1374. doi:10.1345/aph.1M219

Landsverk J., Burns B., Stambaugh L. F., & Rolls-Reutz J. A. (2006). *Mental health care for children and adolescents in foster care: Review of research literature.* Seattle, WA: Casey Family Programs.

Leslie, L. K., Mackie, T., Dawson, E. H., Bellonci, C., Schoonover, D. R., Rodday, A. M., et al. (2010). *Multi-state study on psychotropic medication oversight in foster care.* Boston, MA: Tufts Clinical and Translational Science Institute. http:// 160.109.101.132/icrhps/prodserv/docs/Executive_Report_09 -07-10_348.pdf

Looff, D., Grimley, P., Kuller, F., Martin, A., & Shonfield, L. (1995). Carbamazepine for PTSD [Letter to the editor]. *Journal of the American Academy of Child and Adolescent Psychiatry, 34*(6), 703.

Meighen, K. G., Hines, L. A., & Lagges, A. M. (2007). Risperidone treatment of preschool children with thermal burns and acute stress disorder. *Journal of Child and Adolescent Psychopharmacology, 17*(2), 223–232. doi:10.1089/cap.2007.0121

Mushtag, D., Ali, A., Margoob, M., Murtaza, I., & Andrade, C. (2012). Association between serotonin transporter gene promoter-region polymorphism and 4- and 12-week treatment response to sertraline in posttraumatic stress disorder. *Journal of Affective Disorders, 136*(3), 955–962. doi:10.1016/j.jad .2011.08.033

National Child Traumatic Stress Network Complex Trauma Task Force. (2003). *Complex trauma in children and adolescents* (White paper). http://nctsn.org/sites/default/files/assets/pdfs/Complex Trauma_All.pdf

Nomura, Y., Hurd, Y., & Pilowsky, D. (2012). Lifetime risk for substance abuse among offspring of abusive family environment from the community. *Substance Use and Misuse, 47*(12), 1281–1292. doi:10.3109/10826084.2012.695420

Nugent, N., Christopher, N., Crow, J., Browne, L., Ostrowski, S., & Delahanty, D. (2010). The efficacy of early propranolol administration at reducing PTSD in pediatric injury patients: A pilot study. *Journal of Traumatic Stress, 23*(2), 282–287. doi:10.1002/jts.20517

Olfson, M., Marcus, S. C., Weissman, M. M., & Jensen, P. S. (2002). National trends in the use of psychotropic medications by children. *Journal of the American Academy of Child and Adolescent Psychiatry, 41*, 514–521.

Pervanidou, P. (2008). Biology of post-traumatic stress disorder in childhood and adolescence. *Journal of Neuroendocrinology, 20*, 632–638. doi:10.1111/j.1365-2826.2008.01701.x

Petrenko, C., Friend, A., Garrido, E., Taussig, H., & Culhane, S. (2012). Does subtype matter? Assessing the effects of maltreatment on functioning in preadolescent youth in out-of-home care. *Child Abuse & Neglect, 36*(9), 633–644. doi:10.1016/j.chiabu.2012.07.001

Raghavan, R., Zima, B. T., Anderson, R. M., Leibowitz, A. A., Schuster, M. A., & Landsverk, J. (2005). Psychotropic medication use in a national probability sample of children in the child welfare system. *Journal of Child and Adolescent Psychopharmacology, 15*, 97–106.

Rayworth, B., Wise, L., & Harlow, B. (2004). Child abuse and risk of eating disorders in women. *Epidemiology, 15*(3), 271–278. doi:10.1097/01.ede.0000120047.07140.9d

Robb, A., Cueva, J., Sporn, J., Yang, R., & Vanderburg, D. (2010). Sertraline treatment of children and adolescents with posttraumatic stress disorder: A double-blind, placebo-controlled trial. *Journal of Child and Adolescent Psychopharmacology, 20*(6), 463–471. doi:10.1089/cap.2009.0115

Robert, R., Blakeney, P., Rosenberg, L., & Meyer, W. J. (1999). Imipramine treatment in pediatric burn patients with symptoms of acute stress disorder—A pilot study. *Journal of the American Academy of Child and Adolescent Psychiatry, 38*(7), 873–882.

Robert, R., Tcheung, W. J., Rosenberg, L., Rosenberg, M., Mitchell, C., Villareal, C., et al. (2008). Treating thermally injured children suffering symptoms of acute stress disorder with imipramine and fluoxetine: A randomized, double-blind study. *Burns, 34*(7), 919–928. doi:10.1016/j.burns.2008.04.009

Rundell, J., Staab, J., Shinozaki, G., & McAlpine, D. (2011). Serotonin transporter gene promoter polymorphism (5-HTTLPR) associations with number of psychotropic medication trials in a tertiary care outpatient psychiatric consultation practice. *Psychosomatics, 52*(2), 147–153. doi:10.1016/ j.psym.2010.12.013

Safer, D. J., Zito, J. M., & dos Reis, S. (2003). Concomitant psychotropic medication for youth. *American Journal of Psychiatry, 160*, 438–449.

Savitz, J., van der Merwe, L., Newman, T., Solms, M., Stein, D., & Ramesar, R. (2008). The relationship between childhood abuse and dissociation. Is it influenced by catechol-O-methyltransferase (COMT) activity? *International Journal of Neuropsychopharmacology, 11*(2), 149–161. doi:10.1017/ S1461145707007900

Savitz, J., van der Merwe, L., Newman, T., Stein, D., & Ramesar, R. (2010). Catechol-O-methyltransferase genotype and childhood trauma may interact to impact schizotypal personality traits. *Behavior Genetics, 40*(3), 415–423. doi:10.1007/s10519-009-9323-7

Saxe, G., Stoddard, F., Courtney, D., Cunningham, K., Chawla, N., Sheridan, R., et al. (2001). Relationship between acute morphine and the course of PTSD in children with burns.

Journal of the American Academy of Child and Adolescent Psychiatry, 40(8), 915–921.

Schafer, I., & Fisher, H. (2011). Childhood trauma and psychosis—What is the evidence? *Dialogues in Clinical Neuroscience, 13*(3), 360–365.

Scheeringa, M., Zeanah, C., & Cohen, J. (2011). PTSD in children and adolescents: Towards a more empirically based algorithm. *Depression and Anxiety, 28,* 770–782. doi:10.1002/da.20736

Seedat, S., Lockhat, R., Kaminer, D., Zungu-Dirwayi, N., & Stein, D. (1999). An open trial of citalopram in adolescents with post-traumatic stress disorder. *International Clinical Psychopharmacology, 16,* 21–25.

Seedat, S., Stein, D., Ziervogel, C., Middleton, T., Kaminer, D., Emsley, R., & Rossouw, W. (2002). Comparison of response to a selective serotonin reuptake inhibitor in children, adolescents, and adults with posttraumatic stress disorder. *Journal of Child and Adolescent Psychopharmacology, 12*(1), 37–46.

Sharp, S., Thomas, C., Rosenberg, L., Rosenberg, M., & Meyer, W. (2010). Propranolol does not reduce risk for acute stress disorder in pediatric burn trauma. *Journal of Trauma, Injury, Infection, and Critical Care, 68*(1), 193–197. doi:10.1097/TA.0b013e3181a8b326

Stathis, S., Martin, G., & McKenna, J. (2005). A preliminary case series on the use of quetiapine for posttraumatic stress disorder in juveniles within a youth detention series. *Journal of Clinical Psychopharmacology, 25*(6), 539–544. doi:10.1097/01.jcp.0000186901.79861.e2

Steiner, H., Saxena, K., Carrion, V., Khanzone, L., Silverman, M., & Chang, K. (2007). Divalproex sodium for the treatment of PTSD and conduct disordered youth: A pilot randomized controlled clinical trial. *Clinical Psychiatry and Human Development, 38,* 183–193. doi:10.1007/s10578-007-0055-8

Stoddard, F., Luthra, R., Sorrentino, E., Saxe, G., Drake J., Chang, Y., et al. (2011). A randomized controlled trial of sertraline to prevent posttraumatic stress disorder in burned children. *Journal of Child and Adolescent Psychopharmacology, 21*(5), 469–477. doi:10.1089/cap.2010.0133

Stoddard, F., Sorrentino, E., Ceranoglu, A., Saxe, G., Murphy, M., Drake, J., et al. (2009). Preliminary evidence for the effects of morphine on posttraumatic stress disorder symptoms in one- to four-year-olds with burns. *Journal of Burn Care and Research, 30*(5), 836–843. doi:10.1097/BCR.0b013e3181b48102

Strawn, J., DelBello, M., & Geracioti, T. (2009). Prazosin treatment of an adolescent with posttraumatic stress disorder. *Journal of Child and Adolescent Psychopharmacology, 19*(5), 599–600. doi:10.1089/cap.2009.0043

Sugava, L., Hasin, D., Olfson, M., Lin, K. H., Grant, B., & Blanco, C. (2012). Child abuse and adult mental health: A national study. *Journal of Traumatic Stress, 25*(4), 384–392. doi:10.1002/jts.21719

Tarullo, A., & Gunnar, M. (2006). Child maltreatment and the developing HPA axis. *Hormones and Behavior, 50,* 632–639. doi:10.1016/j.yhbeh.2006.06.010

Tcheung, W., Robert, R., Rosenberg, L., Rosenberg, M., Villareal, C., Thomas, C., et al. (2005). Early treatment of acute stress disorder in children with major burn injury. *Pediatric Critical Care Medicine, 6*(6), 676–681.

Terr, L. (1991). Childhood traumas: An outline and overview. *American Journal of Psychiatry, 148*(1), 10–20.

U.S. Administration for Children and Families. (2012). *Information memorandum: Promoting the safe, appropriate, and effective use of psychotropic medication for children in foster care.* www.acf.hhs.gov/programs/cb/laws_policies/policy/im/2012/im1203.pdf

U.S. Department of Veterans Affairs & Department of Defense. (2010, October). *VA/DoD clinical practice guidelines for the management of post-traumatic stress* (Version 2.0). www.healthquality.va.gov/PTSD-FULL-2010c.pdf

U.S. Food and Drug Administration. (2003, October 27). *FDA public health advisory: Reports of suicidality in pediatric patients being treated with antidepressant medications for major depressive disorder.* www.fda.gov/cder/drug/advisory/mdd.htm

U.S. Government Accountability Office. (2011). *HHS guidance could help states improve oversight of psychotropic prescriptions.* www.gao.gov/products/GAO-12-201

Wagner, S., Baskaya, O., Anicker, N., Dahmen, N., Lieb, K., & Tadic, A. (2010). The catechol-O-methyltransferase (COMT) val(158)met polymorphism modulates the association of serious life events (SLE) and impulsive aggression in female patients with borderline personality disorder (BPD). *Acta Psychiatrica Scandinavica, 122*(2), 110–117. doi:10.1111/j.1600-0447.2009.01501.x

Wheatley, M., Plant, J., Reader, H., Brown, G., & Cahill, C. (2004). Clozapine treatment of adolescents with posttraumatic stress disorder and psychotic symptoms. *Journal of Clinical Psychopharmacology, 24*(2), 167–173. doi:10.1097/01.jcp.0000116650.91923.1d

White, C. R., Havalchak, A., Jackson, L. J., O'Brien, K., & Pecora, P. J. (2007). *Mental health, ethnicity, sexuality, and spirituality among youth in foster care: Findings from the Casey Field Office Mental Health Study.* Seattle, WA: Casey Family Programs.

Yeh, C., Hsieh, M. H., & Chou, J. (2010). Aripiprazole augmentation for the treatment of an adolescent with posttraumatic stress disorder [Letter to the editor]. *Progress in Neuro-Psychopharmacology & Biological Psychiatry, 34,* 722–723. doi:10.1016/j.pnpbp.2010.03.018

Zito, J. M., Safer, D. J., dos Reis, S., Gardner, J. F., Magder, L., Soeken, K., et al. (2003). Psychotropic practice patterns for youth: A 10-year perspective. *Archives of Pediatrics & Adolescent Medicine, 157,* 17–25.

ANANDA B. AMSTADTER, PH.D.
ERIN C. DUNN, SC.D., M.P.H.
RUTH C. BROWN, PH.D.
ERIN C. BERENZ, PH.D.
NICOLE R. NUGENT, PH.D.

33

Treatment Implications of Gene-Environment Interplay in Childhood Trauma

GENERAL CONSIDERATIONS

Many fields have had a longstanding interest in questions regarding "nurture" and "nature" as they relate to the development and maintenance of psychopathology. Ample evidence suggests that exposure to traumatic events during specific developmental periods such as childhood substantially elevates the risk for two key internalizing disorders—depression and posttraumatic stress disorder (PTSD), the disorders of focus in this chapter (Dunn et al., 2012; Kendler et al., 2000; Molnar, Buka, & Ronald, 2001)—among many other conditions. As we discuss in detail, it is well documented that liability to developing these psychological disorders, referred to as *phenotypes* in genetically informed research (see table 33.1 for definitions of commonly used genetic terminology), is influenced by genetic factors (Nelson et al., 2012). It is now well accepted that these phenotypes are probably a result of the complex interplay between a multitude of biological and environmental factors. One area of research that has seen significant growth and widespread interest, as well as controversy, in recent years is gene-environment interaction (G×E).

The purpose of this chapter is to put in context the G×E literature on depression and PTSD, two of the most common phenotypes associated with childhood trauma exposure, and to provide commentary on how these findings may impact intervention science. We begin by describing the key findings from behavioral genetic studies of traumatic events, depression, and PTSD, then turn our attention to molecular G×E studies of depression and PTSD and the limited literature on genetically informed treatment studies relevant to these phenotypes. Following this summary of the literature, we highlight the critical methodological considerations and potential confounds of this line

of research and propose some new directions for this budding area of study.

BEHAVIORAL/QUANTITATIVE GENETIC STUDIES

Heritability of Depression and PTSD

Twin studies underscore the importance of genetic factors in the etiology of depression and PTSD, as they have shown that a substantial proportion of the variance in depression and PTSD is related to genetic factors, termed *heritability*. A meta-analysis of genetic epidemiology studies on major depression in twins suggests that approximately 37% of the liability to depression is heritable (Sullivan, Neale, & Kendler, 2000). Twin studies of PTSD also suggest a moderate genetic contribution to this phenotype. The heritability of PTSD is estimated to range from 30% in an all-male sample (Stein et al., 2002; True et al., 1993) to 70% in an all-female sample (Sartor et al., 2011), even after controlling for trauma exposure. Unfortunately, the two twin studies that included both sexes were not adequately powered to determine whether there was a sex difference in the contributing role of genetics (Nelson et al., 2012; Stein et al., 2002); however, these studies found more modest heritability estimates for PTSD (~38% by Stein et al., 2002; 47% by Nelson et al., 2012). Genetic epidemiological studies of PTSD and depression also suggest that the genetic liability to these phenotypes highly overlaps (Fu et al., 2007; Nelson et al., 2012).

Gene-Environment Correlation

Twin studies have also contributed to our understanding of factors related to exposure to different environmental

Table 33.1. Commonly Used Genetic Terminology

Allele A variation of a gene at a specific location along a chromosome. An individual inherits one allele from each parent. If both alleles are the same, that person is said to be *homozygous* for that gene. If the two alleles are different, that person is said to be *heterozygous* for that gene.

Ancestry Race/ethnicity. It can be determined by self-report or by using ancestral informative markers across the genome.

Candidate gene A gene selected based on extant research—such as information about the putative function of a particular gene and/or theory or knowledge about the pathophysiology of a condition—to be tested for potential associations with the disorder.

Gene The fundamental, physical, and functional unit of heredity.

Genotype The specific combination of alleles at a specific location on the chromosome that makes up a gene.

G×E Gene-environment interaction. It can be thought of in terms of genetic variation modifying the relationship between environmental exposure and the phenotype *or* the environment modifying the effect of genetic variation on an outcome

Hardy-Weinberg equilibrium The algebraically determinable genotype ratios expected in a randomly breeding population.

Heritability The proportion of variance in a phenotype that is attributed to genetic factors.

Phenotype The observable characteristics of an organism, thought to result from genetic and environmental influences.

Polymorphism The existence of two or more variants (alleles) in a specific gene.

Population stratification A situation occurring when a sample includes subpopulations characterized by little mating between them such that the subsamples show different allelic frequencies that are unrelated to the phenotype under investigation.

rGE Gene-environment correlation, the extent to which individuals create and influence their own environment.

SNP Pronounced "snip"; single nucleotide polymorphism, occurring when a single nucleotide in the DNA sequence is altered, forming different alleles (i.e., various forms of a genetic locus).

VNTR Variable tandem repeat polymorphism, consisting of segments of repeated base pairs forming various alleles of different lengths (e.g., *5-HTTLPR*).

events. The term *gene-environment correlation*, or rGE, refers to the extent to which individuals create and influence their own environments (e.g., Rutter, 2010). In other words, rGE reflects the passive and active ways in which an individual's genetic constitution influences his or her exposure to various environments. A review of genetic influences on environmental measures, including stressful life events, parenting, and social support, found that heritability estimates fell between 7% and 39%, with a weighted heritability estimate for all environmental measures of 27% (Kendler & Baker, 2007). As related to exposure to traumatic events, twin studies of adults have demonstrated a modest heritable component to various forms of such events (Lyons et al., 1993; Nelson et al., 2012; Stein et al., 2002). In a recent investigation, Amstadter and colleagues (2012) found that approximately one-third of the liability to exposure to a traumatic event was shared with the contingent liability to PTSD. These gene-environment correlations are probably due in part to individual differences in personality. Personality characteristics are moderately heritable and influence the tendency for individuals to select themselves into potentially harmful environments. For example, longitudinal investigations have found that childhood adjustment and neuroticism predicted subsequent stressful life events in adulthood (Van Os & Jones, 1999).

MOLECULAR G×E STUDIES

Whereas the behavioral genetic studies aim to demonstrate the degree to which latent genetic factors account for variability in phenotype expression, molecular genetic studies seek to identify the specific variants in the human genome that differ among individuals and contribute to this heritability. These gene-finding efforts are aimed at the identification of sites across the genome where one form of an allele is present in a higher percentage of cases versus controls. Beyond the main effect of genes, G×E studies examine the way genes interact to influence a phenotype. The environment may interact with genes by (1) *triggering* the expression of a genetic vulnerability, (2) *compensating* for a genetic predisposition, (3) *determining expression* of a genetic predisposition, and/or (4) *potentiating* a genetic predisposition (Shanahan & Hofer, 2005).

Molecular G×E and Depression

Research on G×E interactions in depression has become widespread in psychiatry, psychology, and public health, spanning studies of children, adolescents, and adults, as well as a variety of genetic and environmental exposures. As of late 2012, more than a hundred empirical articles had been published examining the statistical interaction between a specific genetic variant, some aspect of the environment, and depression. In these molecular G×E studies, researchers identify the extent to which individuals with specific alleles (alternative forms of DNA sequence at a specific locus) or genotypes (the combination of alleles that an individual carries at a specific locus) are more or less sensitive to the effects of their environment.

Interest in molecular G×E studies for depression and other mental health outcomes can be traced to an article published in the journal *Science* in 2003. In this article, Caspi and colleagues used data from a 26-year longitudinal study in New Zealand to test whether a functional polymorphism in the promoter region (*5-HTTLPR*) of the serotonin transporter gene (*SLC6A4*) interacted with stressful life events to increase risk for depression. The serotonin transporter gene, which encodes the transporter for the neurotransmitter serotonin, was considered a good "candidate gene," as serotonin is the main target of action for antidepressant medications (e.g., selective serotonin reuptake inhibitors, SSRIs) and serotonin has been implicated in the neurobiology of depression (Owens & Nemeroff, 1994; Thase, 2009). Results of the Caspi et al. study suggested that individuals with at least one *s* allele (i.e., with the *s/s* or *s/l* genotype of the biallelic coded version)* had more depression, whether measured in terms of level of depressive symptoms, a depression diagnosis, or incident depression, as well as more suicidality, in response to stressful life events when compared with people with other genotypes. The researchers also found that *s* allele carriers had a greater probability than those without an *s* allele of experiencing depression as a result of exposure to probable or severe childhood maltreatment. The Caspi et al. article had a tremendous impact on the field. According to Google Scholar, as of fall 2012, it had been cited more than four thousand times. This figure is impressive relative to that for other seminal papers in the field. For example, to date, David Finkelhor's reviews on child sexual abuse have been cited about two thousand times each (Browne & Finkelhor, 1986).

In the years following the Caspi et al. publication, numerous attempts were made to replicate its findings. Many of these studies focused on child maltreatment and other early adversities; table 33.2 lists these 42 studies. As shown in the table, most replication efforts focused on *SLC6A4*, though other genetic variants were also studied, including *BDNF* (brain derived neurotropic factor, a member of the nerve growth factor family that supports neuronal survival, growth, and differentiation), *MAOA* (monoamine oxidase A, an enzyme that degrades neurotransmitters thought to be associated with depression, including dopamine, norepinephrine, and serotonin), *CRHR1* (corticotropin-releasing hormone receptor 1, an important component of the biological stress response), *COMT* (catechol-*O*-methyltransferase, an enzyme that degrades catecholamines, including dopamine, epinephrine, and norepinephrine), and *CREB1* (also known as CAMP responsive element binding protein 1, which stimulates transcription). Indicators of child maltreatment most often came from self-report questionnaires, and some studies also looked at the effects of recent stressful life events in addition to early childhood adversities. Although some studies examined the effects of child sexual abuse or physical abuse, most looked at maltreatment generally. The joint effect of genetic variants and childhood maltreatment was also studied across the lifespan, with studies focusing on depression among children and adolescents as well as adults. In addition to studying depression, some researchers also looked at other processes related to depression (e.g., rumination) or factors considered to be involved in the causal pathway between childhood maltreatment and depression, particularly brain structures (e.g., amygdala and hippocampus).

Among these 42 studies, 32 (76.2%) found at least one significant gene-environment interaction between child

abuse and a genetic variant—a finding that of course could be influenced by publication biases against null effects. Additionally, some of these effects were detected only in specific subgroups (e.g., females) and only in the context of another genetic variant (a three-way or G×G×E interaction). Interestingly, many studies did not find a main effect of the gene—that is, the effect of the gene was present only in the context of exposure to child maltreatment. Moreover, the most direct replication of the Caspi et al. findings, which came from the Fergusson et al. (2011) study, did not find evidence in support of the original findings.

The large number of empirical studies on G×E in depression has given way to several review papers and meta-analyses. In fact, more than a dozen reviews have been published on candidate G×E in depression (e.g., Brown & Harris, 2008; Dunn et al., 2011; Karg et al., 2011; Monroe & Reid, 2008; Munafo et al., 2009; Nugent et al., 2011; Risch et al., 2009; Thapar et al., 2007; Uher & McGuffin, 2008, 2010; Vergne & Nemeroff, 2006; Wankerl, Wust, & Otte, 2010; Zammit & Owen, 2006). These reviews unearthed many important findings about the state of G×E science and, when combined with the original report, ultimately fueled a debate on the plausibility of the Caspi et al. findings. Including largely identical investigations, reviews drew opposing conclusions about the support for G×E effects, with some studies finding consistent G×E effects and others failing to detect them (Munafo et al., 2009; Uher & McGuffin, 2008, 2010). Meta-analyses were conducted to provide a more definitive conclusion about the evidence for G×E. However, the results of two meta-analyses (Munafo et al., 2009; Risch et al., 2009), which found evidence against a consistent G×E effect, differed from a third meta-analysis (Karg et al., 2011), which concluded there was strong evidence to support the serotonin G×E effect.

The heterogeneity in G×E findings, both in the individual replication papers and in the meta-analyses, has been attributed to the heterogeneity in methods used to detect G×E for depression. Indeed, as a recent article highlights, there were considerable methodological differences across individual studies, making it difficult to evaluate the strength of the evidence for G×E (Dunn et al., 2011). Meta-analyses also were affected by these methodological differences, in that each applied different criteria for the studies included in the review. As a result, the validity and reliability of these G×E findings have been questioned, particularly for the serotonin transporter variant. Many are skeptical, noting that the "remarkable finding had a beguiling and seductive plausibility" (Hardy & Low, 2011, p. 455), but "the beautiful story that was too good to be true may, in fact, not be true" (Nierenberg, 2009, p. 463). However, several reviews indicate that the findings for G×E are more robust and consistent for childhood maltreatment than for other adversities, including recent stressful life events (Karg et al., 2011; Uher & McGuffin, 2008, 2010). Despite such findings, the debate and controversy continue.

---

*In addition to the biallelic coding based on size variation, short (*s*) and long (*l*), of the alleles of the *5-HTTLPR* polymorphism, a functional SNP (L_G) that results in functioning comparable to that of the *s* allele has been identified. Accordingly, the polymorphism is typically categorized triallelically, with the L_G and *s* alleles grouped together as *s'* and the remaining *l* alleles labeled *l'*. In this chapter, *s* and *l* refer to the biallelically coded length of the allele, and *s'* and *l'* refer to the triallelically coded alleles.

Table 33.2. Gene-Environment Studies of PTSD and Depression

Study	Trauma Types Assessed	Sample Selection	Outcome: Assessments	N (% male)	Age (yr)	Country/ Nationality: Race/Ethnicity	GENE dbSNP	Findings
				Depression				
Aguilera et al., 2009	Child adversity: CTQ, self-report	Healthy subjects recruited from university and community	Depression symptoms: self-report, SCL-90-R (depressive scale)	N = 532 (45%)	Range: 18–50 M = 23.9 (SD = 5.4)	Spain: HW	*s-HTTLPR BDNF Val66Met*	Main effect of child sexual abuse, emotional abuse, emotional neglect on depressive symptoms, *p* <0.001. Physical abuse, physical neglect ns. No main effect for either gene. G×E interaction significant for *s-HTTLPR* and child sexual abuse on depression symptoms. Interaction significant for high levels of child sexual abuse and *s* carriers. G×E interaction significant for *Val66Met* and child sexual abuse on depression symptoms. Interaction significant for high levels of child sexual abuse. G×E interaction not significant for other types of adversity.
Antypa &Van der Does, 2010	Childhood emotional abuse: CTQ, self-report	University students	Cognitive reactivity: LEIDS-R, self-report Neuroticism: NEO-PI-R, self-report Depression (current and lifetime): Major Depression Questionnaire, self-report Anxiety and depression (current): HADS, self-report	N = 250 (24%)	M = 22.5 (SD = 4.7)	NL: NHW	*s-HTTLPR rs25531*	No main effect of genotype on current anxiety, depression, childhood emotional abuse scores. Main effect of emotional abuse on cognitive reactivity and neuroticism. No E or G main effect or G×E interaction on probable depression diagnosis. G×E interaction significant for *s-HTTLPR* and childhood emotional abuse on cognitive reactivity: *s/s* carriers had lowest cognitive reactivity when abuse was low. No difference when abuse was high. G×E interaction significant for *s-HTTLPR* and childhood emotional abuse on rumination: *s/s* had lowest rumination when abuse was low. No difference when abuse was high.
Aslund et al., 2009	Child maltreatment, study-made questionnaire, self-report	Survey of all high school students in Swedish county	Depression: DSRS, self-report	N = 1,482	Range: 17–18	Sweden: Scandinavian	*s-HTTLPR*	Main effect of maltreatment and depression. No main effect of gene on depression for whole population. G×E interaction significant for *s-HTTLPR* and maltreatment for girls with *s/s*

Study	Sample	Measures	N (%)	Age	Location	Gene	Findings
							genotype. Girls with *s/s* had lower levels of depression, controlling for maltreatment. Girls with maltreatment and *s/s* had higher risk for depression. No significant gene main effect or *5-HTTLPR* and maltreatment interaction for boys.
Beach et al., 2010	Adult adoptees from Iowa adoption studies	Child maltreatment: Child Maltreatment Index, self-report; MDD and antisocial personality disorder: SSAGA-II, clinical interview	N=536 (45%)	Men: M=46.48, Women: M=44.95	US: 94% NHW	MAOA	G×E interaction significant for MAOA and maltreatment MDD. For those with child maltreatment, high-activity alleles predict MDD symptoms; low-activity alleles predispose to ASPD.
Bet et al., 2009	Random, stratified sample of men and women aged 55–85 for Longitudinal Aging Study Amsterdam	Childhood adversity: self-report; Depression symptoms: CES-D, self-report	N=906	Range: 55–85	NL	GR, 22/23EK, N363S, 9beta, Bc1I	G×E interaction significant for 22/23EK and 9beta, with child adversity on depression symptoms. No risk for depression present in absence of childhood adversity. G×E interaction significant for 22/23EK and childhood adversity on free cortisol index. G×E interaction significant for Bc1I variants and childhood adversity on recurrent depression symptoms. Carriers of heterozygous Bc1I variant had lower serum levels of cortisol-binding globulin and no increased risk for recurrent depression compared with wild-type and Bc1I homozygotes.
Carver et al., 2011	University students	Childhood adversity: RF, self-report; MDD: SCID, clinical interview	N=133 (26%)	M=18.71	US: 57.1% NHW, 24.1% HW, 7.5% As, 4.5% AA	5-HTTLPR, BDNF	G×E interaction significant for 5-HTTLPR and childhood adversity for MDD. Adversity predicted lower risk for MDD among *l/l* genotype, higher risk for MDD among *s* allele carriers. G×E interaction significant for BDNF and childhood adversity. Adversity predicted higher risk for MDD among Met allele carriers, no association among Val/Val allele carriers.
Chipman et al., 2007	2 population-based samples: PATH20 (see Chipman et al., 2010), 20- to 24-yr-olds; Australian Temperament Project (ATP)	Childhood adversity: self-report of 17 adversities (e.g., parental emotional problems, sexual abuse); Recent stressors: self-report of 12 "threatening experiences"; Depression and anxiety symptoms: GDAS, self-report	PATH20: N=2,095 (47.9%), ATP: N=2,443 (49.4%–51.5%)	PATH20: Range: 20–24, ATP: 2 cohorts ranges: 15–16, 17–18	Australia: NHW	5-HTTLPR	PATH20: No main effect for gene. Significant main effect for sex, recent stressors, childhood adversity on depression and anxiety. ATP: No main effect of gene. Significant main effect for sex.

(continued)

Table 33.2. (continued)

Study	Trauma Types Assessed	Sample Selection	Outcome: Assessments	N (% male)	Age (yr)	Country/ Nationality: Race/Ethnicity	GENE dbSNP	Findings
								No GxE interaction for recent stressors. 17- to 18-yr-olds with l/l genotype and persistently high levels of family adversity at higher risk for depression compared with no or low levels of adversity.
Chipman et al., 2010	Childhood adversity: self-report of 17 adversities (e.g., parental emotional problems, sexual abuse) Recent adult stressors: self-report of 12 "threatening experiences"	Population-based survey: Personality and Total Health Through Life project (PATH)	Depression and anxiety symptoms: GDAS, self-report	N = 6,445 (47.3%–52%)	3 cohorts Ranges: 20–24, 40–44, 60–64	Australia: NHW	HTR1A rs6295C/G	No main effect of gene. GxE interaction not significant for childhood or adult stressors when corrected for multiple testing.
Chorbov et al., 2007	Traumatic life events occurring at or before 18 yr: 10-item self-report	MDD affected (case) and nonaffected (control) female-female twin pairs, Missouri birth records	Depression: C-SSAGA, phone interview	N = 247	MDD cases: M = 22.1 (SD = 3.2) Control: M = 21.9 (SD = 3.3)	US: NHW	5-HTTLPR rs25531	For s/l classification: No main effect for gene. No GxE interaction with trauma. For low (s/s), medium (s/l'), or high (l'l') activity classification: Main effect for l' allele and MDD. Significant GxE interaction. Number of l' alleles elevated risk for MDD in presence of single adverse event.
Cicchetti et al., 2007	Child maltreatment: emotional, physical, sexual abuse, neglect, MCS: DHS records	Youths in research summer camp for maltreated and nonmaltreated youths identified through DHS records	Depression: DISC, clinical interview Internalizing: YSR, self-report	N = 339 (54.3%) Maltreated: 207 Nonmaltreated: 132	M = 16.70 (SD = 1.31)	US: 61.7% AA 23.3% NHW 12.7% HW 2.4% Other	MAOA 5-HTTLPR	GxE interaction significant for MAOA and maltreatment. Elevated depression symptoms in severely maltreated youths with low MAOA activity. Severely maltreated youths with high MAOA activity had better self-coping. GxGxE interaction significant for 5-HTTLPR, MAOA, and sexual abuse. Sexually abused youths with s/s genotype predicted higher depression, anxiety, somatic symptoms in the presence of low-activity MAOA.
Cicchetti et al., 2010	Child maltreatment: emotional, physical, sexual abuse, neglect, MCS: DHS records	Youths in research summer camp for maltreated and nonmaltreated youths identified through DHS records	Depression and suicidal ideation: CDI, self-report	N = 850 (54.2%) Maltreated: 478 Nonmaltreated: 372	Range: 6–13 M = 9.19 (SD = 1.70)	US: 60.6% AA 21.4% NHW 15.5% HW 2.5% Other	5-HTTLPR	Main effect for maltreatment on suicidal ideation. No main effect for gene. No GxE interaction for depression. GxE interaction significant for suicidal ideation. Youths with lower levels of maltreatment and s/s or s/l genotype at higher risk for suicidal ideation than

(continued)

Study	Abuse/stress measure	Sample	Outcome	N	Age	Country	Genes	Findings
								youths with l/l genotype. No difference at high levels of maltreatment.
Cicchetti et al., 2011	Early abuse: physical/ sexual abuse age <5 yr; Child maltreatment: emotional, physical, sexual abuse, neglect, MCS: DHS records	Youths in research summer camp for maltreated and nonmaltreated youths identified through DHS records	Diurnal cortisol regulation: saliva; Internalizing and depressive symptoms: CDI, self-report; TRF, counselor report	N = 493: Early abuse: 51; Maltreated: 187; Nonmaltreated: 255	M = 10.08 (SD = 1.87)	US: 64% AA 15% HW 19% NHW 2% Other	CRHR1 rs7209436 rs1104202 rs242924 5-HTTLPR	Interaction between maltreatment and internalizing symptoms predicts cortisol dysregulation. G×E interaction significant for CRHR1. CRHRI related to cortisol dysregulation for maltreated children. G×G×E interaction significant between CRHR1, 5-HTTLPR, and child maltreatment significant for internalizing symptoms. Maltreated youths with two-copy CRHR1 and l/l genotype had higher internalizing symptoms than nonmaltreated youths.
Conway et al., 2010	Chronic family stress: composite score of youth, maternal self-report and interview data	Community sample from longitudinal birth cohort; assessed age 15, 20 yr; blood samples collected 22–25 yr	Depression symptoms age 20 yr: BDI-II; Depression diagnosis between 15 and 20 yr: SCID	N = 384	Range: 22–25	Australia: NR	5-HTTLPR COMT Val158Met	No main effect for 5-HTTLPR. G×G×E interaction for 5-HTTLPR significant only for COMT homozygosity. Lower risk for depression among Val158Met homozygotes with l' allele.
Drury et al., 2010	Early social deprivation in institutional care	Abandoned preschool children randomized to standard institutional care (CAU) or enriched foster care (FCG)	Depression symptoms: PAPA, caregiver interview	N = 136	54 months	Romania	COMT Val158Met	Main effect of COMT significant. Lower risk for depression symptoms among Met/Met or Met/Val carriers. G×E interaction significant for COMT and caregiver group. Protective effect of Met allele significant only for CAU (institutional care). Effect of Met allele not significant for FCG (enriched foster care).
Eley et al., 2004	Family environmental risk: social adversity, SPQ, parental education	Children of parents in genetics of depression and anxiety study; mailed questionnaires; top and bottom 15% of depression scores selected for follow-up	Depression symptoms: short MFQ, self-report	N = 377 (43%)	Range: 12–19	NR	5-HTTLPR HTR2A HTR2C MAOA TPH	No main effect for environmental risk on depression. Main effect for HTR2A and TPH significant. G×E interaction for 5-HTTLPR and environmental risk for depression significant only for females. Number of s alleles associated with risk for depression in high environmental risk.
Elzinga et al., 2011	Child abuse: physical, emotional, sexual abuse, neglect, structured interview; Recent stress: LTE-Q, self-report	Participants with lifetime MDD drawn from larger prospective cohort study	Lifetime MDD: CIDI, clinical interview	N = 1,435 (30.7%)	M = 42.2 (SD = 12.4)	NL: North European	BDNF Val66Met	Among lifetime MDD. Main effect for recent life events on BDNF serum levels. G×E interaction significant on BDNF serum levels among individuals with MDD without comorbid anxiety. BDNF Met carriers with child abuse histories had reduced BDNF serum levels. BDNF Met carriers without child abuse had higher BDNF serum levels than Val/Val carriers.

Table 33.2. (continued)

Study	Trauma Types Assessed	Sample Selection	Outcome: Assessments	N (% male)	Age (yr)	Country/ Nationality: Race/Ethnicity	GENE dbSNP	Findings
Fergusson et al., 2011	Child adversity: composite of retrospective reports and parent/child observation Adolescent/adult stressful life events: life-event checklist, self-report; composite index	Participants from 30-yr prospective birth cohort study	MDD diagnosis: CIDI, clinical interview	N = 893	Assessed at: 18, 21, 25, 30	New Zealand: 85% White 15% Maori / Pacific Islander	*s-HTTLPR*	No main effect or G×E interaction.
Gatt et al., 2009	Early life stress: ELSQ, self-report	Healthy, nonclinical participants without Axis I history	Amygdala-hippocampal-prefrontal gray matter volume: structural MRI Heart rate: average and variability Neuroticism: NEO-PI Cognition: IntegNeuro Depression: DASS, self-report	N = 374	M = 36.2 (SD = 12.7)	NHW	*BDNF Val66Met*	Main effects significant for early life stress on resting heart rate, anxiety, and depression. No significant main effects for *BDNF*. G×E interaction significant for *BDNF* and early life stress on brain volume, heart rate, and working memory. *BDNF Met* carriers exposed to elevated early life stress have smaller hippocampal and amygdala volume, higher heart rate, and decline in working memory. Reduced gray matter predicted depression, and depression predicted poor working memory. Elevated heart rate in *BDNF Met* carriers with early life stress also predicted neuroticism, depression, and anxiety. *BDNF Val/Val* carriers with early life stress predicted increase in gray matter, which predicted heart rate variability and higher anxiety. Elevated anxiety associated with verbal memory and impulsivity.
Gatt et al., 2010	Early life stress: ELSQ, self-report	Healthy, nonclinical participants without Axis I history	Fronto-limbic gray matter loss: MRI Depression symptoms: DASS, self-report	N = 397 (52.1%)	M = 36.3 (SD = 12.8)	European	*HTR3A*	Main effect for gene on gray matter loss in right hippocampus (*CC* greater loss than *CT*). No main effect for gene on depression symptoms. Main effect for early life stress on gray matter loss in right hippocampus and lateral prefrontal cortex. G×E interaction significant for *HTR3A* and early life stress on gray matter. *CC* carriers, compared with *T* carriers, had greater loss of gray matter in hippocam

Study	Stress measure	Sample	Outcome measure	N (%)	Age	Gene	Findings
Goodyer et al., 2010	Childhood recent life events, interview	Medically well school children at risk for depression in 1-yr prospective study	Morning salivary cortisol; MDD: K-SADS-PL, clinical interview; Depression symptoms: MFQ, self-report	N = 401 (53%)	Range: 12–16 M = 14	5-HTTLPR BDNF Val66Met rs6265	pal structures. Gray matter loss extended to frontal cortices for CC carriers exposed to early life stress. G×E interaction significant for HTR3A and early life stress on depression symptoms. CC carriers exposed to 3+ early life stressors had greater depression symptoms than CT carriers. Main effects for higher initial depression symptoms, higher morning cortisol, and undesirable life events on new-onset depression. G×G×E interaction for Val66Val variant of BDNF, and s variant 5-HTTLPR moderating risk of morning salivary cortisol on depression onset.
Grabe et al., 2010	Child maltreatment: CTQ, self-report	Community-based sample	Depression symptoms: BDI, self-report	N = 1,638 (47.5%)	M = 53.6 (SD = 13.6)	CRHR1 28 total SNPs	No significant main effect of gene on depression. G×E interaction not significant for TAT haplotype and child abuse or emotional neglect. G×E interaction significant for TAT haplotype and physical neglect on depression. G×E interaction significant for 23 of 28 SNPs and physical neglect on depression; rs17698882 reached gene-wide significance.
Grabe et al., 2012	Child abuse: emotional, physical, sexual abuse, CTQ, self-report	Stratified population-based sample	Depression symptoms: BDI-II, self-report	N = 2,035 (47.5%)	M = 55.6 (SD = 13.8)	5-HTTLPR rs25531 BDNF Val66Met rs6265	G×E interaction significant for 5-HTTLPR and child abuse on depression. G×G×E interaction significant for 5-HTTLPR, BDNF, and child abuse on depression. Carriers of s'/s' and Val/Val allele had higher depression symptoms. Largest effect for emotional abuse.
Haeffel et al., 2008	Perceived maternal rejection, self-report	Male adolescents from Northern Russian juvenile detention	MDD: BDI, self-report; K-SADS-PL, clinical interview	N = 176 (100%)	M = 16.2 (SD = 0.8)	DAT1 rs40184	G×E interaction for rs40184 and maternal rejection on depression and suicidality. Not significant for anxiety.
Hammen et al., 2010	Chronic family stress (<15 yr): composite parent and youth interviews and self-reports; Acute life events (15–19 yr): UCLA Life Stress Interview	Community sample from longitudinal birth cohort; assessed age 15, 20 yr; blood samples collected 22–25 yr	Depression symptoms at age 20 yr: BDI-II	N = 346	M = 23.7 (SD = 0.89)	5-HTTLPR rs25531	G×E interaction significant for 5-HTTLPR and chronic stress at age 15 yr on depression at age 20 yr. Females with chronic stress and 1 or 2 s' alleles at higher risk for depression. G×E interaction for acute stress not significant.

(continued)

Table 33.2. (continued)

Study	Trauma Types Assessed	Sample Selection	Outcome: Assessments	N (% male)	Age (yr)	Country/ Nationality: Race/Ethnicity	GENE dbSNP	Findings
Juhasz et al., 2009	Adult negative life events—previous year: self-report Childhood adversity: CTQ, self-report	Community sample recruited from general practice patient lists and a study website; 48% history of depression	Personality: BFI-44, self-report Depression symptoms: BSI, self-report	N = 1,269 (32%)	Range: 18–60 M = 34.04 (SD = 0.028)	UK: 92% NHW	CNR1 haploblock1 rs806379 rs1535255 rs2023239 haploblock2 rs806369 rs1049353 rs470436 rs12720071 rs806368 rs806366 rs3766029	Main effect for gene on depression, neuroticism, and agreeableness. G×E interaction significant for CNR1 (rs3766029) and recent negative life events on depression (e.g., main effect of gene dropped from significance when life events included in model). G×E interaction not significant for CNR1 and child adversity on depression.
Juhasz et al., 2011	Adult life events—previous year: LTE, self-report Childhood adversity: CTQ, self-report	3-level community cohorts: Level-1 sent questionnaires and genetic sampling by mail (see Juhasz et al., 2009) Level-2 invited for clinical interview Level-3 invited for fMRI of emotional face processing	Level-1: depression symptoms: BSI, self-report Level-2: MDD: SCID, interview; depression symptoms: MADRS, self-report	Level-1: n = 1,269 (30%) Level-2: n = 264 (30%) Level-3: n = 33 (33%)	Range: 18–60	UK: NHW	BDNF Val66Met rs6265 rs12273363 rs962369 rs988748 rs7127507 CREB1 rs2253206 NTRK2 rs1187323 rs1187326	G×E interaction significant for BDNF-rs6265 and CREB1-rs2253206 and childhood adversity on depression symptoms in level-1 cohort. Minor-allele carriers with history of childhood adversity exhibited higher risk for depression. Results validated on MDD level-2 cohort. Healthy controls with minor alleles of BDNF-rs6265 and CREB1-rs2253206 exhibited greater depressive reactivity during fMRI when viewing sad faces.
Kaufman et al., 2004	Childhood maltreatment, from multiple informants and case records	Maltreated children in state custody and nonmaltreated controls	MDD: K-SADS-PL, interview Depression severity: MFQ, self-report Social support: ASSIS, interview	N = 101 Maltreated: 57 Control: 44	Range: 5–15 M = 10.0 (SD = 2.3)	US: 21% NHW 32% AA 25% HW	5-HTTLPR	Main effects significant for 5-HTTLPR, maltreatment, and social support. G×E interaction significant for 5-HTTLPR and maltreatment on depression symptoms. Highest depression risk in maltreated children with s/s genotype. G×E×E interaction significant for 5-HTTLPR, maltreatment, and social support on depression. Maltreated children with no positive social support and with s/s genotype had highest risk for depression (scores twice as high as nonmaltreated with s/s genotype).

Study	Adversity measure	Sample	N	Age	Location/Ethnicity	Outcome measure	Genes	Findings
Kaufman et al., 2006	Childhood maltreatment, from multiple informants and case records	Extension of sample in Kaufman et al., 2004. Maltreated children in state custody and nonmaltreated controls	N = 196 Maltreated: 109 Control: 87	Range: 5–15 M = 9.3 (SD = 2.4)	US: 28% NHW 28% AA 24% HW	MDD: K-SADS-PL, interview Depression severity: MFQ, self-report Social support: ASSIS, interview	5-HTTLPR BDNF Val66Met	GxGxE interaction significant for 5-HTTLPR, BDNF, and child maltreatment on depression. Maltreated children with Met allele of BDNF and two s alleles of 5-HTTLPR at highest risk of depression. GxGxExE interaction significant for 5-HTTLPR, BDNF, child maltreatment, and social support on depression.
Kranzler et al., 2011	Adverse childhood experiences: SSADDA, clinical interview	Participants from family-based linkage study of substance dependence; most had lifetime substance use disorder	N = 3,080 (57%)	AA: M = 42 NHW: M = 38	US: 61% AA 39% NHW	MDE and alcohol dependence: SSADDA, clinical interview	CRHR1 rs7209436 rs110402 rs242924	No main effect of haplotype on alcohol dependence. No GxE interaction. GxE interaction significant for haplotype and childhood adversity on depression only in AA women. Each copy of the TAT haplotype reduced risk for depression by 40%. AA women without childhood adversity and two copies of TAT increased risk of MDE.
Nederhof et al., 2010	Childhood adversity, prenatal and delivery adversity, long-term difficulties: parent report	Prospective cohort study of Dutch adolescents: Tracking Adolescents' Individual Lives Survey; assessments at 11, 13.5., and 16 yr of age	N = 1,096	Wave 3: M = 16.13 (SD = 0.59)	NL	Depression symptoms: YSR, self-report	5-HTTLPR rs25531 BDNF Val66Met rs6265	Main effects significant for gender, childhood adversity, and long-term difficulty (e.g., disability, chronic illness). No main effect of genes. No GxE interaction.
Nikulina et al., 2012	Child abuse and neglect	Prospective cohort of cases of court-substantiated child abuse and neglect and matched controls	N = 575 (51.3%)	M = 41 (SD = 3.85)	US: 60.8% NHW 35.1% AA 4.1% HW	MDD, dysthymia, alcohol abuse: DIS-III-R, interview	MAOA	GxESex interaction significant for MAOA, child abuse, and sex on dysthymia. Low-activity MAOA protective for multiply maltreated women. GxERace interaction significant for MAOA, sexual abuse, and race for all outcomes. Low-activity MAOA protective for sexually abused NHW participants. High-activity MAOA protective for nonwhite sexually abused participants.
Nilsson et al., 2009	Childhood psychosocial adversity: single- vs. multifamily housing; nuclear family vs. separated parents, interview	Stratified sample of secondary and third-year college students	N = 200	16, 19	Sweden	Depression symptoms: DSRS, self-report	AP-2β	GxE interaction significant for AP-2β and housing quality on depression symptoms. GxE interaction significant for AP-2β and parental separation on depression symptoms. Adolescents with s/s genotype, from multifamily housing, and with separated parents had highest risk for depression.

(continued)

333

Table 33.2. (continued)

Study	Trauma Types Assessed	Sample Selection	Outcome: Assessments	N (% male)	Age (yr)	Country/ Nationality: Race/Ethnicity	GENE dbSNP	Findings
Polanczyk et al., 2009	Childhood maltreatment: E-Risk study: CTQ, self-report Dunedin study: composite score of mother-child interactions at age 3 yr, parent report of harsh discipline, multiple changes in primary caregiver, retrospective report of physical and sexual abuse	Participants from 2 studies: E-Risk study (UK, N = 1,116) and Dunedin study (New Zealand, N = 1,037)	MDD: DIS, clinical interview	N = 2,153 E-Risk: n = 1,116 (0%) Dunedin: n = 1,037 (52%)	E-Risk: M = 40 Dunedin: M = 32	E-Risk: UK: 90% NHW Dunedin: New Zealand: 90%+ NHW	CRHR1 rs7209436 rs110402 rs242924	Main effect for child maltreatment on depression in both samples. G×E interaction significant for TAT haplotype and maltreatment on depression significant only for E-Risk sample. Carriers of TAT haplotype who experienced childhood maltreatment had lower risk of depression.
Quinn et al., 2012	Early life stress: ELSQ, self-report	Community sample of MDD and healthy controls	MDD: MINI, clinical interview Depression symptoms: HRSD, self-report; CORE, self-report; DASS, self-report	N = 256 MDD: 128 Control: 128	M range across groups = 37.89–42.07	Australian	5-HTTLPR BDNF Val66Met	Main effect for early life stress on depression. Melancholic > nonmelancholic > controls. G×G×E interaction significant for 5-HTTLPR (s alleles), BDNF (Met allele), and early life stress on nonmelancholic depression. No significant interaction for melancholic depression.
Ressler et al., 2010	Child abuse: CTQ, self-report	Low-income, urban, AA participants recruited from waiting rooms of public hospital	Depression symptoms: BDI, self-report MDD history (subsample of 297): SCID, clinical interview	N = 1,392	Range: 18–65	US: 100% AA	5-HTTLPR rs25531 CRHR1 rs110402 rs7209436 rs4792887	Main effect significant for child abuse on depression symptoms. Main effect not significant for 5-HTTLPR on depression symptoms. G×E interaction not significant for 5-HTTLPR and child abuse on depression symptoms. G×E interaction significant for 5-HTTLPR and child abuse on history of MDD only for s' allele carriers. Main effect not significant for CRHR1. G×E interaction significant for CRHR1, child abuse on current depression symptoms, only for the A allele carriers of rs110402 and protective CRHR1-TCA haplotype. G×G×E interaction significant for CRHR1, 5-HTTLPR, and child abuse on current (adult) depression symptoms.
Ritchie et al., 2009	Childhood stress and trauma: study-made self-report checklist of 25 adverse and 8 protective events and environmental conditions	Random community sample of older adults (65+ yr)	Depression: any 1 of 3: MINI (clinical interview), CES-D (self-report), or on antidepressant medication	N = 942	Median = 72 Range: 65–92	France	5-HTTLPR rs25531	Main effect significant for child trauma and later-life depression and repeated episodes. Risk associated with excessive sharing of parental problems, poverty, mental disorder in parents, excessive punishment, verbal abuse, humiliation, and mistreatment by adult outside family.

Study	Predictor/adversity measure	Outcome measure	N (%)	Age	Country/ethnicity	Gene	Findings
	Adverse events in past year: Gospel Oak, self-report						GxE interaction significant for 5-HTTLPR and child trauma on depression. Carriers of l′ allele raised in poverty and with excessive sharing of parental problems.
Sjöberg et al., 2006	Childhood psychosocial adversity: single- vs. multifamily housing; nuclear family vs. separated parents; interview; traumatic conflict with family (yes/no), composite score of interview	Depression symptoms: DSRS, self-report	N = 200 (40.5%)	16, 19	Sweden	5-HTTLPR	GxE×Sex interaction significant for 5-HTTLPR, adversity, and sex on depression. Boys with l allele had higher risk for depression when living in public housing and with separated parents. Girls with s allele had higher risk for depression when experienced traumatic conflicts with family.
Surtees et al., 2006	Childhood adversity and adult adversity in past 5 yr: HLEQ	MDD, past year: HLEQ, structured self-report	N = 4,175 (53%)	Range: 41–80	UK	5-HTTLPR	Main effects significant for childhood and recent adversity on depression. GxE interaction not significant.
Taylor et al., 2006	Stressful early family environment: RF, self-report Recent stressful events: self-generated list of 10 major life events	Depression symptoms: BDI	N = 118 (43%)	Range: 18–29 M=20.6	US: 38% As 34% AA	5-HTTLPR	Main effect significant for early life stress on depression scores. GxE interaction significant for 5-HTTLPR and early life stress and depression. GxE interaction significant for 5-HTTLPR and recent life stress and depression. Carriers of s/s genotype exhibited higher depression in the face of early or recent life stress. Carriers of s/s genotype had less depression if they reported supportive early environment or recent positive experiences, compared with carriers of s/l or l/l.
Uher et al., 2011	Childhood maltreatment: E-Risk study: CTQ, self-report Dunedin study: composite score of mother-child interactions at age 3 yr, parent report of harsh discipline, multiple changes in primary caregiver, retrospective report of physical and sexual abuse	MDD single or persistent episodes: DIS, clinical interview	N = 2,153 E-Risk: n=930 (0%) Dunedin: n = 847 (52%)	E-Risk: M=40 Dunedin: M=32	E-Risk: UK: 90% NHW Dunedin: New Zealand: 90%+ NHW	5-HTTLPR	Main effect significant for childhood maltreatment on persistent depression. Main effect not significant for 5-HTTLPR on persistent depression. GxE interaction significant for 5-HTTLPR (s/s genotype) and childhood maltreatment on persistent depression, but not single episode of depression.

(continued)

Table 33.2. (continued)

Study	Trauma Types Assessed	Sample Selection	Outcome: Assessments	N (% male)	Age (yr)	Country/ Nationality: Race/Ethnicity	GENE dbSNP	Findings
Veletza et al., 2009	Stressful life experiences in childhood and young adulthood: open questionnaire	University students in medicine and molecular biology	Depression symptoms: ZDRS	N = 181 (66.3%)	Range: 18–33 Median = 22	Greece	5-HTTLPR	G×E interaction significant for 5-HTTLPR and serious adverse life events. Carriers of s allele who experienced serious adverse life event scored high on depression and other measures of psychological distress. Carriers of l/l genotype without adversity scored higher than s allele carriers on measures of depression and other psychological distress.
Wichers et al., 2008	Childhood adversity: CTQ, omitted sexual and physical abuse items	Female participants drawn from longitudinal general population twin study	Depression symptoms: SCL-90	N = 621 (0%)	Range: 18–46	Belgian: NHW	5-HTTLPR BDNF Val66Met rs6265	Main effect of BDNF Met allele on childhood adversity, controlling for age, income, and education. G×G×E interaction significant for BDNF (Met), 5-HTTLPR (s alleles), and childhood adversity on depression. BDNF Met alleles moderated effect of childhood adversity on risk of depression. Effect of BDNF Met allele moderated by 5-HTTLPR s allele.
PTSD								
Binder et al., 2008	Child abuse and non-child abuse trauma: TEI, self-report	Nonpsychiatric hospital / medical health clinic patients	PTSD: CAPS, clinical interview; PSS, self-report	N = 762 (~43%)	M = ~41 (SD = 14)	US: 95% AA 2% NHW 3% Other	FKBP5 rs3800373 rs992105 rs9296158 rs737054 rs1360780 rs1334894 rs9470080 rs4713916	Main effects significant for child abuse and adult trauma predicting adult PTSD symptoms. G×E interaction significant for rs3800373 (risk C), rs9296158 (A), rs1360780 (T), and rs9470080 (T) and severity of child abuse in prediction of adult PTSD symptoms.
Mercer et al., 2012	Child abuse and lifetime trauma: TLEQ, self-report Exposure to mass shooting: self-report	College females participating in longitudinal study, assessed for PTSD following school shooting	Post-shooting PTSD: DEQ, self-report	N = 204 (0%)	M = 20.1	US: 77.5% NHW 13.7% AA	SLC6A4 STin2 5-HTTLPR rs25331	No main effect of child abuse on post-shooting PTSD symptoms. No main effect of lifetime trauma on post-shooting PTSD symptoms. Main effect of degree of mass shooting exposure on post-shooting PTSD symptoms. No main effects for STin2 or 5-HTTLPR on post-shooting PTSD symptoms. Main effect significant for rs25331 on post-shooting PTSD symptoms.

Study	Sample	Measures	N	Age	Ethnicity	Gene/variant	Findings
							GxE interaction significant for *s-HTTLPR* and shooting exposure on post-shooting PTSD symptoms. Low-expressing genotypes *s'/s'* associated with higher post-shooting PTSD.
Nelson et al., 2009	Participants from family twin study	Child abuse: CTI, phone interview; PTSD: SSAGA-II, phone interview	N = 2,594	NR	NR	*GABRA2* rs279836 rs279826 rs279858 rs279871	No main effect of gene/variant on PTSD risk. Significant GxE interaction between composite lifetime history of trauma exposure and 3 out of 4 risk alleles for adult PTSD.
van Zuiden, 2012	Childhood trauma: ETI, self-report; Deployment stressors: 13-item checklist; Dutch Armed Forces assessed pre-deployment and 6 months post-deployment to Afghanistan	PTSD: SRIP, self-report; Depression and anxiety symptoms: SCL-90	N = 448 (100%) PTSD+: 35	M = 29 (SD = 9)	Dutch: 95% NHW	*GR tth111l* rs1002957; *GR ER22/23EK* rs6189/90; *GR N363S* rs6195; *GR BclI* rs41423247; *GR A3669G 9β* rs6198; *FKBP5* rs3800373 rs1360780	Main effect significant for childhood trauma and PTSD symptoms. No significant main effect for GR or *FKBP5* and PTSD diagnosis. Main effect not significant for childhood trauma on pre-deployment GR number (biomarker for PTSD risk). GxE interaction significant between GR haplotype and childhood trauma in predicting pre-deployment GR number.
Xie et al., 2009	Adult trauma: SSADDA (PTSD module); Child adversity (before 13 yr): SSADDA (Environment module); TE subjects recruited from 4 university medical centers 100% TE	PTSD: SSADDA (PTSD modules), clinical interview	N = 1,252 PTSD+: 229 (42%) PTSD−: 1,023 (54%)	Range: 17–79 M = 39 (SD = 11)	US: 47% NHW 53% AA	*5-HTTLPR* rs4795541 rs25531	Significant main effect for childhood adversity and adult trauma on PTSD. No main effect of gene/variant on PTSD risk. GxE interaction significant for adult trauma on PTSD risk. GxE interaction significant for childhood trauma only for NHW. GxE interaction significant for adult trauma and child adversity. *s'* allele associated with risk in exposed participants. Highest-risk group: *s'/s'* and adversity and trauma.
Xie et al., 2010	Adult trauma: SSADDA (PTSD module); Child adversity (before 13 yr): SSADDA (Environment module); Subjects recruited from 4 university medical centers	PTSD and alcohol dependence: SSADDA, clinical interview	N = 2,427 (54.4%)	M = 38.6 (SD = 10.8)	US: 47% NHW 53% AA	*FKBP5* rs3800373 rs9296158 rs1360780 rs9470080	Main effect for childhood adversity on adult PTSD. No main effect for *FKBP5* genotype on PTSD. GxE interaction significant for rs9296158 and childhood adversity on PTSD in AA only. AA with rs9470080 T/T had lowest risk of PTSD compared with other genotypes in the absence of childhood adversity exposure, but had highest risk when exposed.

Table 33.2. (continued)

Study	Trauma Types Assessed	Sample Selection	Outcome: Assessments	N (% male)	Age (yr)	Country/ Nationality: Race/Ethnicity	GENE dbSNP	Findings
								NHW rs3800373 (risk A), rs9296158 (G), rs1360780 (C), and rs9470080 (C) carriers had higher risk of PTSD if also alcohol-dependent, compared with subjects with other genotypes.
Xie et al., 2012	Child adversity (before 13 yr): SSADDA (Environment module)	High prevalence of substance-dependence comorbidity	PTSD: SSADDA (PTSD modules), clinical interview	N = 5,178 (56%)	M = 40.5 (SD = 11.2)	US: 46% AA 54% NHW	5-HTTLPR	Main effect for child adversity and PTSD, with greater number of categories endorsed related to increased risk for PTSD.
								G×E interaction significant for 5-HTTLPR and childhood adversity on PTSD only for NHW. Carriers of one or two copies of the s allele and with childhood adversity had increased risk for PTSD.

Abbreviations. AA, African American; As, Asian; ASPD, antisocial personality disorder; DHS, Department of Human Services; fMRI, functional magnetic resonance imaging; HW, Hispanic white; M, mean; MDD, major depressive disorder; MDE, major depressive episode; NHW, non-Hispanic white; NL, the Netherlands; NR, not reported; ns, not significant; SD, standard deviation; TE, traumatic event; UCLA, University of California, Los Angeles; UK, United Kingdom; US, United States.

Assessment abbreviations. ASSIS, Arizona Social Support Interview Schedule; BDI, Beck Depression Inventory; BDI-II, Beck Depression Inventory I-II; BFI-44, Big Five Inventory; BSI, Brief Symptom Inventory; C-SSAGA, Child Semi-Structured Assessment for Genetics of Alcoholism; CAPS, Clinician Administered Posttraumatic Stress Disorder Scale; CDI, Child Depression Inventory; CES-D, Center for Epidemiological Studies–Depression Scale; CIDI, Composite Interview Diagnostic Instrument; CORE, CORE Assessment of Psychomotor Change; CTI, Christchurch Trauma Inventory; CTQ, Child Trauma Questionnaire; DASS, Depression Anxiety Stress Scale; DEQ, Distressing Event Questionnaire; DIS-III-R, National Institute of Mental Health Diagnostic Interview Schedule for DSM-III-R; DISC, Diagnostic Interview Schedule for Children; DSRS, Depression Self-Rating Scale; ELSQ, Early Life Stress Questionnaire; ETI, Early Trauma Inventory; GDAS, Goldberg Depression and Anxiety Scales; HADS, Hospital Anxiety and Depression Scale; HLEQ, Health and Life Experiences Questionnaire; HRSD, Hamilton Rating Scale for Depression; K-SADS-PL, Schedule for Affective Disorders and Schizophrenia for School-Age Children–Present and Lifetime Version; LEIDS-R, Leiden Index of Depression Sensitivity–Revised; LTE, List of Life-threatening Experiences; LTE-Q, List of Threatening Events Questionnaire; MADRS, Montgomery Asberg Depression Scale; MCS, Maltreatment Classification System; MFQ, Mood and Feelings Questionnaire; MINI, Mini International Neuropsychiatric Interview; NEO-PI, NEO-Five Factor Inventory; NEO-PI-R, NEO-Five Factor Inventory–Revised; PAPA, Preschool Age Psychiatric Assessment; PSS, Posttraumatic Stress Disorder Symptom Scale; RF, Risky Families questionnaire; SCID, Structured Clinical Interview for Diagnostic and Statistical Manual of Mental Disorders; SCL-90, Symptom Checklist 90; SCL-90-R, Symptom Checklist 90 Revised; SPQ, Social Problems Questionnaire; SRIP, Self-Rating Inventory for PTSD; SSADDA, Semi-Structured Assessment for Drug Dependence and Alcoholism; SSAGA-II, Semi-Structured Assessment for the Genetics of Alcoholism; TEI, Trauma Events Inventory; TLEQ, Traumatic Life Events Questionnaire; TRF, Teacher Report Form; YSR, Youth Self Report; ZDRS, Zung Depression Rating Scale.

Molecular G×E and PTSD

In comparison with the large number of G×E studies on depression reviewed above, few studies have examined G×E interactions in relation to PTSD. This is particularly surprising given that a PTSD diagnosis, by definition, requires exposure to an environmental event (i.e., trauma). To date, there have been more than 40 molecular genetic studies of PTSD (Cornelis et al., 2010), with only 12 studies explicitly examining G×E interactions, one-third of which examined 5-HTTLPR (see table 33.2).

Of these 12 G×E studies, only half focused on events experienced during childhood. All of the G×E studies of PTSD and childhood events included retrospective assessments of the childhood environmental events. Significant interactions between variation in numerous candidate genes (e.g., GABRA2, Nelson et al., 2009; 5-HTTLPR, Xie et al., 2009) and childhood trauma were found in predicting adult PTSD symptoms and diagnosis. Particular attention was paid to examination of single nucleotide polymorphisms (SNPs) in the FKBP5 gene (which plays a role in modulating the glucocorticoid stress response) and severity of trauma exposure in relation to adult PTSD symptoms. Interestingly, variation in FKBP5 was found to interact with severity of child abuse but not with severity of other trauma types in predicting adult PTSD symptoms, even after adjusting for the effects of adult depressive symptoms (Binder et al., 2008). Other work found similar interactions between the FKBP5 gene and childhood adversity, more generally defined, in predicting adult PTSD symptoms (Xie et al., 2010). Similarly, van Zuiden and colleagues (2012) assessed a sample of soldiers pre- and post-deployment and found that childhood trauma interacted with a glucocorticoid receptor (GR) haplotype (a cluster of SNPs on a single chromosome) in predicting greater pre-deployment GR number, a presumed biological risk marker for PTSD. Indeed, pre-deployment GR number was associated with greater risk for post-deployment PTSD in this sample. These findings suggest a potentially unique and long-lasting role of child abuse and adversity in the modulation of genetic risk for adult PTSD.

The remaining G×E studies of PTSD focused on adult-onset environmental events. As in the depression literature, the majority of the studies investigated 5-HTTLPR in relation to a range of adult-onset environmental events (e.g., hurricane exposure, level of social support, county-level crime, lifetime traumatic events). Findings are mixed; some studies reported that the s′ variant of the 5-HTTLPR gene was predictive of a greater likelihood of PTSD under these conditions (Kilpatrick et al., 2007; Koenen & Galea, 2009), whereas other studies found that the l′ variant interacts with the "E" variable (Grabe et al., 2009). Finally, Kolassa and colleagues (2010) found that number of lifetime traumatic events predicted lifetime PTSD among those with s′/l′ and l′/l′ (i.e., evidence for a standard dose-response relationship for trauma and PTSD) but not those with s′/s′ gen-

otypes in a sample of Rwandan genocide survivors. Individuals with the s/s genotype were at elevated risk for PTSD regardless of the number of previous traumatic events they had experienced. The remaining adult environment studies investigated other genetic variants (e.g., RGS2, COMT).

Taken together, these studies provide evidence for various trauma and environmental characteristics modifying the relationship between a limited selection of genotypes and risk for PTSD in a range of samples. For example, childhood trauma may have lasting effects that may interact with certain genetic factors in promoting the long-term risk for PTSD. Additionally, as evidenced by some of the adult trauma literature, environmental events (e.g., trauma load) may have differential effects on the basis of genotype, such that individuals with certain genetic variants may be more sensitive to the effects of trauma at any level. However, the small number of studies examining G×E interactions in relation to PTSD, particularly the number assessing environmental events occurring in childhood, makes conclusive statements on any one investigation difficult. In addition, all the assessments of childhood trauma/abuse have been retrospective (i.e., individuals with greater risk for PTSD in adulthood may be more likely to report a history of childhood trauma). Further research, particularly with child and adolescent samples, is greatly needed to further the current literature.

G×E and Treatment

The findings on gene-environment interplay have a number of implications for prevention and intervention studies. As discussed by Beauchaine and colleagues (2008), there is potential for the use of genetic markers to identify populations at greatest risk. In other words, genetic markers either may facilitate targeted treatments by identifying those who, following exposure, are at greatest risk for later problems or may help to inform treatment tailoring. For example, one could postulate that genetic variation in the serotonergic system might inform the likelihood that someone would respond to psychopharmacological intervention that targets serotonin. Indeed, for depression, candidate markers in SLC6A4 have been associated with treatment response to SSRIs, such as citalopram (Mrazek et al., 2009), escitalopram (Huezo-Diaz et al., 2009), paroxetine (Wilkie et al., 2008), and a mix of SSRIs (Illi et al., 2011; Smits et al., 2008). Although this relationship was not consistently found across studies (Gudayol-Ferré et al., 2010), a recent meta-analysis concluded that SLC6A4 is implicated in SSRI response (Porcelli, Fabbri, & Serretti, 2012). HTR2A has also been associated with SSRI depression response (Kishi et al., 2010; Wilkie et al., 2008). One recent investigation identified a significant interaction between stressful life events and SLC6A4 in response to escitalopram (Keers et al., 2011).

If the SSRI benefits can be modified by an interaction between environmental influences and stressful life events, then environmental modification (through additional supports, minimization of stress exposure, and psychosocial intervention) may be especially important for individuals with the *5-HTTLPR s'* allele. Indeed, as some have conceptualized *5-HTTLPR* to be a marker of plasticity and sensitivity to the environment rather than risk for psychopathology, *5-HTTLPR* is one promising marker for "therapygenetics" (Beevers, 2012). *5-HTTLPR* variation was examined in a small sample (n = 42) of patients who underwent exposure-based cognitive behavioral therapy for PTSD (Bryant et al., 2010), with findings suggesting that *s'* carriers were less responsive to treatment than patients with the *l'/l'* genotype. Another investigation of cognitive behavioral therapy for children with anxiety disorders (n = 584; ages 6–13) reported a more positive treatment response among children with the *s/s* genotype than children with the *s/l* or *l/l* genotypes (Eley, 2012). The triallelic *5-HTTLPR* genotype was also tested in a small study (n = 69) of exposure-based cognitive behavioral therapy for panic disorder in adults (Lonsdorf, 2010). Although no effect for *5-HTTLPR* and treatment outcome was observed, the study found a main effect of symptom severity over time, with *s'* carriers showing higher symptoms than participants with the *l'/l'* genotype. Participants with the *COMT Val158Met Met/Met* genotype were less likely to benefit from treatment than those with at least one *Val* allele.

Although no studies have examined genetic factors in maltreatment prevention efforts, prevention research in the arena of risk behaviors has reported interactions between intervention and genotype. In a series of publications, Brody and colleagues described an interaction between *5-HTTLPR* and risk behaviors among youths participating in a family-based prevention program targeting initiation of risk behavior (Brody, Beach, et al., 2009; Brody, Chen, et al., 2009). Specifically, the researchers reported that participants with the *s* allele in the control condition initiated risk behaviors at twice the rate of youths with the *s* allele in the prevention condition (Brody, Beach, et al., 2009). They attributed this difference to the importance of parenting for youths with the *s* allele. This investigation in many ways exemplifies the potential for genetic markers to identify the highest-risk youths and the youths who are likely to benefit from a behavioral intervention, including interventions that influence components of the child's environment (i.e., parenting) in addition to child-directed treatments. These interventions could be adopted at a higher system level through neighborhood or school programming and could be especially influential.

METHODOLOGICAL CONSIDERATIONS

GxE research involves some critical methodological considerations, which, when inadequately addressed, can lead to erroneous conclusions. Although relatively few studies adhere to recommended guidelines for reporting, replication difficulties in this field and increasing evidence for the vulnerability of GxE analyses to statistical artifacts (e.g., Eaves & Silberg, 2003) have led to the development of some guidelines: STROBE (STrengthening the Reporting of OBservational studies in Epidemiology) and STREGA (STrenghtening the REporting of Genetic Association studies; Little et al., 2009). As we briefly review here, it is important for consumers of the GxE literature to be aware of the importance of (1) considering key covariates (i.e., sex, age or developmental period, ancestry), (2) definitions/coding of the target genes, (3) how environment is measured and scaled, (4) how the outcome is measured and scaled, and (5) analytical considerations, including sample size.

The first, critical consideration in GxE research is the need to control for, or stratify on, key covariates such as sex, age or developmental period, and ancestry (race/ethnicity). Although several studies reviewed here found different GxE effects for males and females (e.g., Eley et al., 2004; Uddin et al., 2010), studies that do not explicitly test for sex effects may be ignoring a critical confound that could explain the observed findings. Age and developmental stage are important considerations because the risk of exposure to certain types of maltreatment, such as sexual violence increases, over time and sharply peaks for females around early adolescence (U.S. Department of Health and Human Services, 2008), and neuroscience research suggests that there may be sensitive periods for environmental exposures (Gunnar & Quevedo, 2007; Lupien et al., 2009; Walker, Sabuwalla, & Huot, 2004). Additionally, risk for some internalizing disorders changes over the course of childhood and adolescence, with sex differences in depression, for example, emerging in adolescence (Kessler et al., 2005; Rudolph, 2009; Tambs & Mourn, 1993).

In addition to the key covariate of sex, all genetic research is vulnerable to population stratification, which occurs when a sample includes subpopulations characterized by little mating between them, such that the subsamples show differences in allele frequencies that are unrelated to the phenotype under investigation (Freedman et al., 2004; Hutchison et al., 2004; Pritchard & Rosenberg, 1999). If there are differences in prevalence or genetic mechanism of the phenotype between subpopulations, "discovery" of an allelic difference may be erroneously attributed to the phenotype. These differences in allele frequency generally correspond to ancestry, making it important for GxE research to test for ancestry-related frequency differences in the study sample. Although reliance on self-reports of ancestry (i.e., race/ethnicity) is better than ignoring population stratification, it is preferable to use genetic markers (ancestry informative markers), as individuals may be unaware of the specific mixture of their ancestry. Genetic research should also test for Hardy-Weinberg equilibrium, which is a test of whether genotype frequencies are consistent with random mating in the studied population.

The second key methodological consideration for genetically informative studies pertains to the numerical coding of the genotype for analyses. All coding and subsequent analyses should correspond to the expected mode of inheritance for genetic effects. For example, whereas most studies examining *5-HTTLPR* assume a dose effect of the *s* allele (i.e., test *s/s*, *s/l*, and *l/l*), others combine the *s/s* and *s/l* genotypes, assuming a dominance effect (i.e., that one allele, in this case the *s* allele, masks the phenotypic expression of the other allele, here the *l* allele, at the same locus). In other words, a dominance model of *5-HTTLPR* assumes that the *s/s* and *s/l* genotypes will have the same phenotypic expression. Many candidate genes have been tested for their functional differences in protein levels, which can be used to inform whether analyses should focus on a dose effect or a dominance effect.

Third, the way the environment is measured and the variability of environmental exposures in the sample are another key consideration. Caspi and colleagues (2010) note that for analyses of dichotomous variables, the power to detect G×E interactions declines as the proportion of the sample with the risk allele or risk environment diverges from 50%. Accordingly, if the entire sample is exposed or unexposed to a given risk (or intervention) environment, it quickly becomes impossible to detect a G×E effect. Therefore, a richer characterization of experiences of child maltreatment is warranted, beyond a simple "exposed" and "unexposed" classification.

Fourth, the outcome scaling and coding—such as continuous symptom count versus dichotomous diagnosis—has crucial implications for the resulting analysis plan and interpretation of interactions. Continuous measures are more statistically powerful and have the additional benefit of decreasing statistical error due to miscategorization of "subthreshold" individuals (Caspi et al., 2010; Plomin & Davis, 2009). The choice to use continuous versus dichotomous measures is critical not only for power but also for confidence in the findings, as artifactual interactions can occur secondary to subtle changes in the definition and scaling of the variables (Jinks & Fulker, 1970; Kraft et al., 2007; Mather & Jinks, 1982; Moffit, Caspi, & Rutter, 2006; Neale & Cardon, 1992). In fact, changing the scale of the outcome can create interactions not previously existing or eliminate interactions once present (Kraft & Hunter, 2009). The way the outcome is scaled and whether the G×E effect is tested on the additive scale (i.e., risks sum in their effect, such as linear regression) or the multiplicative scale (i.e., risks multiply in their effects, such as logistic regression) can influence whether a G×E effect is observed (Greenland & Rothman, 1998; Institute of Medicine Board on Health Sciences Policy, 2006). The use of logistic regression techniques to identify interactions in G×E studies is widespread, but it is important to note that this technique can lead to both false-positive and false-negative findings (Caspi et al., 2010; Eaves, 2006; Kraft et al., 2007; Moffit, Caspi, & Rutter, 2006; Munafo et al., 2009).

Finally, the savvy consumer of the G×E literature should be aware of issues regarding statistical power. Interaction effects require larger numbers of subjects for adequate power (Brookes et al., 2001; Luan, Wong, & Wareham, 2001; Uher & McGuffin, 2008), and power depends on allele frequencies in addition to exposure to the "E" event of interest (Munafo et al., 2009). In fact, many of the studies reviewed here are probably underpowered with regard to the estimated number of subjects needed to adequately test for G×E effects (Munafo et al., 2009, 2010).

SUMMARY AND IMPLICATIONS FOR TREATMENT RESEARCH

Beauchaine and colleagues (2008) outline the critical contributions of biological and genetic research to prevention and treatment, providing a "top ten" list. In their list, consistent with the literature reviewed here, they point to evidence that biology moderates the influence of environment on behavioral and psychological outcomes. Both psychosocial and psychopharmacological treatment approaches can be conceptualized as "environmental" influences for examination in G×E studies. Beauchaine et al. expand on the importance of biological moderation of environmental influence, pointing to some evidence that the interaction of biology and environment may explain more variance than the main effects themselves. As they and others (Cisler, Amstadter, & Nugent, 2011) point out, temperament is closely tied to biological and genetic factors and has been shown to predict response to environmental influences ranging from maltreatment to intervention response. Thus, it follows that our understanding of why some individuals respond differently to trauma and to intervention may be enhanced by careful examination of biological factors such as genetics that influence these responses. A biologically informed understanding of treatment effects may be particularly relevant when considering early maltreatment effects, as early neural systems affect the development and functioning of later neural systems (Beauchaine et al., 2008). Accordingly, prevention or intervention efforts aimed early in development may be especially critical for subsequent adjustment. This could partly explain why some of the most robust evidence for G×E has been found for childhood maltreatment rather than adult life experiences.

In sum, the G×E literature on depression and PTSD is growing rapidly and has suffered from many nonreplications. The majority of these studies have examined retrospective accounts of childhood traumatic events, which is not without significant limitations. Very few studies have explored the potential interplay between genes and "environment" as defined by psychopharmacological or psychosocial treatment, and among those studies that have done so, none were conducted using interventions for youths who have been maltreated. Nonetheless, such investigations can inform the fields of both genetics and intervention science because they can help to characterize the mechanisms through which the effects of both inheritance and intervention influence outcomes such as depression and PTSD.

References

Aguilera, M., Arias, B., Wichers, M., Barrantes Vidal, N., Moya Higueras, J., Villa Martín, E., et al. (2009). Early adversity and 5-HTT-BDNF genes: New evidences of gene-environment interactions on depressive symptoms in a general population. *Psychological Medicine, 39*(9), 1425–1432.

Amstadter, A. B., Aggen, S. H., Knudsen, G. P., Reichborn-Kjennerud, T., & Kendler, K. S. (2012). A population-based study of familial and individual-specific environmental contributions to traumatic event exposure and posttraumatic stress disorder symptoms in a Norwegian twin sample. *Twin Research and Human Genetics, 15*(5), 656–662.

Antypa, N., & Van der Does, A. (2010). Serotonin transporter gene, childhood emotional abuse and cognitive vulnerability to depression. *Genes, Brain and Behavior, 9*(6), 615–620.

Åslund, C., Leppert, J., Comasco, E., Nordquist, N., Oreland, L., & Nilsson, K. W. (2009). Impact of the interaction between the 5HTTLPR polymorphism and maltreatment on adolescent depression. A population-based study. *Behavior Genetics, 39*(5), 524–531.

Beach, S. R., Brody, G. H., Gunter, T. D., Packer, H., Wernett, P., & Philibert, R. A. (2010). Child maltreatment moderates the association of MAOA with symptoms of depression and antisocial personality disorder. *Journal of Family Psychology, 24*(1), 12.

Beauchaine, T. P., Neuhaus, E., Brenner, S. L., & Gatzke-Kopp, L. (2008). Ten good reasons to consider biological processes in prevention and intervention research. *Development and Psychopathology, 20*(3), 745–774. doi:10.1017/S0954579408000369

Beevers, C. G. (2012). Therapygenetics: Moving towards personalized psychotherapy treatment. *Trends in Cognitive Sciences, 16*(1), 11. doi:10.1016/j.tics.2011.11.004

Bet, P. M., Penninx, B. W., Bochdanovits, Z., Uitterlinden, A. G., Beekman, A. T., van Schoor, N. M., et al. (2009). Glucocorticoid receptor gene polymorphisms and childhood adversity are associated with depression: New evidence for a gene-environment interaction. *American Journal of Medical Genetics Part B: Neuropsychiatric Genetics, 150*(5), 660–669.

Binder, E. B., Bradley, R. G., Liu, W., Epstein, M. P., Deveau, T. C., Mercer, K. B., et al. (2008). Association of FKBP5 polymorphisms and childhood abuse with risk of posttraumatic stress disorder symptoms in adults. *JAMA, 299*(11), 1291–1305.

Brody, G. H., Beach, R. H., Philibert, R. A., Chen, Y., & McBride Murry, V. (2009). Prevention effects moderate the association of 5-HTTLPR and youth risk behavior initiation: Gene × environment hypotheses tested via randomized prevention design. *Child Development, 80*(3), 645–661.

Brody, G. H., Chen, Y.-F., Beach, S. R. H., Philibert, R. A., & Kogan, S. M. (2009). Participation in a family-centered prevention program decreases genetic risk for adolescents' risky behaviors. *Pediatrics, 124*(3), 911–917. doi:10.1542/peds.2008-3464

Brookes, S. T., Whitley, E., Peters, T. J., Mulheran, P. A., Egger, M., & Davey Smith, G. (2001). Subgroup analyses in randomised controlled trials: Quantifying the risks of false-positives and false-negatives. *Health Technology Assessment, 5*, 1–56.

Brown, G. W., & Harris, T. O. (2008). Depression and the serotonin transporter 5-HTTLPR polymorphism: A review and a hypothesis concerning gene-environment interaction. *Journal of Affective Disorders, 111*, 1–12.

Browne, A., & Finkelhor, D. (1986). Impact of child sexual abuse: A review of the research. *Psychological Bulletin, 99*(1), 66–77.

Bryant, R. A., Felmingham, K. L., Falconer, E. M., Pe Benito, L., Dobson-Stone, C., Pierce, K. D., & Schofield, P. R. (2010). Preliminary evidence of the short allele of the serotonin transporter gene predicting poor response to cognitive behavior therapy in posttraumatic stress disorder. *Biological Psychiatry, 67*(12), 1217–1219. doi:10.1016/j.biopsych.2010.03.016

Carver, C. S., Johnson, S. L., Joormann, J., LeMoult, J., & Cuccaro, M. L. (2011). Childhood adversity interacts separately with 5-HTTLPR and BDNF to predict lifetime depression diagnosis. *Journal of Affective Disorders, 132*(1), 89–93.

Caspi, A., Hariri, A. R., Holmes, A., Uher, R., & Moffit, T. E. (2010). Genetic sensitivity to the environment: The case of the serotonin transporter gene and its implications for studying complex diseases and traits. *American Journal of Psychiatry, 167*, 509–527.

Caspi, A., Sugden, K., Moffitt, T. E., Taylor, A., Craig, I. W., Harrington, H. L., et al. (2003). Influence of life stress on depression: Moderation by a polymorphism in the 5-HTT gene. *Science, 301*, 386–389.

Chipman, P., Jorm, A., Prior, M., Sanson, A., Smart, D., Tan, X., et al. (2007). No interaction between the serotonin transporter polymorphism (5-HTTLPR) and childhood adversity or recent stressful life events on symptoms of depression: Results from two community surveys. *American Journal of Medical Genetics Part B: Neuropsychiatric Genetics, 144*(4), 561–565.

Chipman, P., Jorm, A. F., Tan, X.-Y., & Easteal, S. (2010). No association between the serotonin-1A receptor gene single nucleotide polymorphism rs6295C/G and symptoms of anxiety or depression, and no interaction between the polymorphism and environmental stressors of childhood anxiety or recent stressful life events on anxiety or depression. *Psychiatric Genetics, 20*(1), 8–13.

Chorbov, V. M., Lobos, E. A., Todorov, A. A., Heath, A. C., Botteron, K. N., & Todd, R. D. (2007). Relationship of 5-HTTLPR genotypes and depression risk in the presence of trauma in a female twin sample. *American Journal of Medical Genetics Part B: Neuropsychiatric Genetics, 144*(6), 830–833.

Cicchetti, D., Rogosch, F. A., & Oshri, A. (2011). Interactive effects of corticotropin releasing hormone receptor 1, serotonin transporter linked polymorphic region, and child maltreatment on diurnal cortisol regulation and internalizing symptomatology. *Development and Psychopathology, 23*(4), 1125.

Cicchetti, D., Rogosch, F. A., & Sturge-Apple, M. L. (2007). Interactions of child maltreatment and serotonin transporter and monoamine oxidase A polymorphisms: Depressive symptomatology among adolescents from low socioeconomic status backgrounds. *Development and Psychopathology, 19*(4), 1161.

Cicchetti, D., Rogosch, F. A., Sturge-Apple, M., & Toth, S. L. (2010). Interaction of child maltreatment and 5-HTT polymorphisms: Suicidal ideation among children from low-SES backgrounds. *Journal of Pediatric Psychology, 35*(5), 536–546.

Cisler, J. M., Amstadter, A. B., & Nugent, N. R. (2011). Genetic and environmental influences on post-trauma adjustment in children and adolescents: The role of personality constructs. *Journal of Child and Adolescent Trauma, 4*, 301–317.

Conway, C. C., Hammen, C., Brennan, P. A., Lind, P. A., & Najman, J. M. (2010). Interaction of chronic stress with serotonin transporter and catechol-O-methyltransferase polymorphisms in predicting youth depression. *Depression and Anxiety, 27*(8), 737–745.

Cornelis, M., Nugent, N. R., Amstadter, A. B., & Koenen, K. C. (2010). Genetics of post-traumatic stress disorder: Review and recommendations for genome-wide association studies. *Current Psychiatry Reports, 12*(4), 313–326.

Drury, S. S., Theall, K. P., Smyke, A. T., Keats, B. J., Egger, H. L., Nelson, C. A., et al. (2010). Modification of depression by

COMT val158met polymorphism in children exposed to early severe psychosocial deprivation. *Child Abuse & Neglect, 34*(6), 387–395.

Dunn, E. C., Gilman, S., Slopen, N. B., Willett, J. B., & Monlar, B. E. (2012). The impact of exposure to interpersonal violence on gender differences in adolescent-onset major depression. *Depression and Anxiety, 29*, 392–399.

Dunn, E. C., Uddin, M., Subramanian, S. V., Smoller, J. W., Galea, S., & Koenen, K. C. (2011). Gene-environment interaction (GxE) research in youth depression: A systematic review with recommendations for future research. *Journal of Child Psychology and Psychiatry, 52*(12), 1223–1238.

Eaves, L. J. (2006). Genotype × environment interaction in psychopathology: Fact or artifact? *Twin Research and Human Genetics, 9*(1), 1–8.

Eaves, L. J., & Silberg, J. L. (2003). Modulation of gene expression by genetic and environmental heterogeneity in timing of a developmental milestone. *Behavior Genetics, 33*, 1–6.

Eley, T. C. (2012). Therapygenetics: The 5HTTLPR and response to psychological therapy. *Molecular Psychiatry, 17*(3), 236. doi:10.1038/mp.2011.132

Eley, T. C., Sugden, K., Corsico, A., Gregory, A. M., Sham, P., McGuffin, P., et al. (2004). Gene-environment interaction analysis of serotonin system markers with adolescent depression. *Molecular Psychiatry, 9*, 908–915.

Elzinga, B. M., Molendijk, M. L., Voshaar, R. C. O., Bus, B. A., Prickaerts, J., Spinhoven, P., et al. (2011). The impact of childhood abuse and recent stress on serum brain-derived neurotrophic factor and the moderating role of BDNF Val66Met. *Psychopharmacology, 214*(1), 319–328.

Fergusson, D. M., Horwood, L. J., Miller, A. L., & Kennedy, M. A. (2011). Life stress, 5-HTTLPR and mental disorder: findings from a 30-year longitudinal study. *British Journal of Psychiatry, 198*(2), 129–135.

Freedman, M. L., Reich, D., Penney, K. L., McDonald, G. J., Mignault, A. A., Patterson, N., et al. (2004). Assessing the impact of population stratification on genetic association studies. *Nature Genetics, 36*(4), 388–393.

Fu, Q., Koenen, K. C., Heath, A. C., Bucholz, K. K., Nelson, E., Goldberg, J., et al. (2007). PTSD and major depression: Same genes, different environments? *Biological Psychiatry, 62*(10), 1088–1094.

Gatt, J., Nemeroff, C., Dobson-Stone, C., Paul, R., Bryant, R., Schofield, P., et al. (2009). Interactions between BDNF Val66Met polymorphism and early life stress predict brain and arousal pathways to syndromal depression and anxiety. *Molecular Psychiatry, 14*(7), 681–695.

Gatt, J. M., Williams, L. M., Schofield, P. R., Dobson-Stone, C., Paul, R. H., Grieve, S. M., et al. (2010). Impact of the HTR3A gene with early life trauma on emotional brain networks and depressed mood. *Depression and Anxiety, 27*(8), 752–759.

Goodyer, I. M., Croudace, T., Dudbridge, F., Ban, M., & Herbert, J. (2010). Polymorphisms in BDNF (Val66Met) and 5-HTTLPR, morning cortisol and subsequent depression in at-risk adolescents. *British Journal of Psychiatry, 197*(5), 365–371.

Grabe, H. J., Schwahn, C., Appel, K., Mahler, J., Schulz, A., Spitzer, C., et al. (2010). Childhood maltreatment, the corticotropin-releasing hormone receptor gene and adult depression in the general population. *American Journal of Medical Genetics Part B: Neuropsychiatric Genetics, 153*(8), 1483–1493.

Grabe, H. J., Schwahn, C., Mahler, J., Schulz, A., Spitzer, C., Fenske, K., et al. (2012). Moderation of adult depression by the serotonin transporter promoter variant (5-HTTLPR), childhood abuse and adult traumatic events in a general population sample. *American Journal of Medical Genetics Part B: Neuropsychiatric Genetics, 159*(3), 298–309.

Grabe, H. J., Spitzer, C., Schwahn, C., Marcinek, A., Frahnow, A., Barnow, S., et al. (2009). Serotonin transporter gene (SLC6A4) promoter polymorphisms and susceptibility to posttraumatic stress disorder in the general population. *American Journal of Psychiatry, 166*(8), 926–933.

Greenland, S., & Rothman, K. J. (1998). Concepts of interaction. In K. J. Rothman & S. Greenland (Eds.), *Modern epidemiology* (2nd ed., pp. 349–342). Philadelphia, PA: Lippincott-Raven Publishers.

Gudayol-Ferré, E., Herrera-Guzmán, I., Camarena, B., Cortés-Penagos, C., Herrera-Abarca, J. E., Martínez-Medina, P., et al. (2010). The role of clinical variables, neuropsychological performance and SLC6A4 and COMT gene polymorphisms on the prediction of early response to fluoxetine in major depressive disorder. *Journal of Affective Disorders, 127*(1–3), 343–351. doi:10.1016/j.jad.2010.06.002

Gunnar, M., & Quevedo, K. (2007). The neurobiology of stress and development. *Annual Review of Psychology, 58*, 145–173.

Haeffel, G. J., Getchell, M., Koposov, R. A., Yrigollen, C. M., De Young, C. G., af Klinteberg, B., et al. (2008). Association between polymorphisms in the dopamine transporter gene and depression evidence for a gene-environment interaction in a sample of juvenile detainees. *Psychological Science, 19*(1), 62–69.

Hammen, C., Brennan, P. A., Keenan-Miller, D., Hazel, N. A., & Najman, J. M. (2010). Chronic and acute stress, gender, and serotonin transporter gene-environment interactions predicting depression symptoms in youth. *Journal of Child Psychology and Psychiatry, 51*(2), 180–187.

Hardy, J., & Low, N. C. (2011). Genes and environments in psychiatry: Winner's curse or cure? *Archives of General Psychiatry, 68*(5), 455–456.

Huezo-Diaz, P., Uher, R., Smith, R., Rietschel, M., Henigsberg, N., Marušič, A., et al. (2009). Moderation of antidepressant response by the serotonin transporter gene. *British Journal of Psychiatry, 195*(1), 30–38. doi:10.1192/bjp.bp.108.062521

Hutchison, K. E., Stallings, M., McGeary, J., & Bryan, A. (2004). Population stratification in the candidate gene study: Fatal threat or red herring? *Psychological Bulletin, 130*(1), 66–79.

Illi, A., Poutanen, O., Setälä-Soikkeli, E., Kampman, O., Viikki, M., Huhtala, H., et al. (2011). Is 5-HTTLPR linked to the response of selective serotonin reuptake inhibitors in MDD? *European Archives of Psychiatry and Clinical Neuroscience, 261*(2), 95–102. doi:10.1007/s00406-010-0126-x

Institute of Medicine Board on Health Sciences Policy. (2006). Study design and analysis for assessment of interactions. In *Genes, behavior, and the social environment: Moving beyond the nature/nurture debate* (pp. 161–180). Washington, DC: National Academies Press.

Jinks, J. L., & Fulker, D. W. (1970). Comparison of the biometrical genetical, MAVA, and classical approaches to the analysis of human behavior. *Psychological Bulletin, 73*(5), 311–349.

Juhasz, G., Chase, D., Pegg, E., Downey, D., Toth, Z. G., Stones, K., et al. (2009). CNR1 gene is associated with high neuroticism and low agreeableness and interacts with recent negative life events to predict current depressive symptoms. *Neuropsychopharmacology, 34*(8), 2019–2027.

Juhasz, G., Dunham, J. S., McKie, S., Thomas, E., Downey, D., Chase, D., et al. (2011). The *CREB1-BDNF-NTRK2* pathway in depression: Multiple gene-cognition-environment interactions. *Biological Psychiatry, 69*(8), 762–771.

Karg, K., Burmeister, M., Shedden, K., & Sen, S. (2011). The serotonin transporter promoter variant (5-HTTLPR), stress, and depression meta analysis revisited: Evidence of genetic moderation. *Archives of General Psychiatry, 68*(5), 444–454.

Kaufman, J., Yang, B.-Z., Douglas-Palumberi, H., Grasso, D., Lipschitz, D., Houshyar, S., et al. (2006). Brain-derived neurotrophic factor–5-HTTLPR gene interactions and environmental modifiers of depression in children. *Biological Psychiatry, 59*(8), 673–680.

Kaufman, J., Yang, B.-Z., Douglas-Palumberi, H., Houshyar, S., Lipschitz, D., Krystal, J. H., et al. (2004). Social supports and serotonin transporter gene moderate depression in maltreated children. *Proceedings of the National Academy of Sciences of the United States of America, 101*(49), 17316–17321.

Keers, R., Uher, R., Huezo-Diaz, P., Smith, R., Jaffee, S., Rietschel, M., et al. (2011). Interaction between serotonin transporter gene variants and life events predicts response to antidepressants in the GENDEP project. *Pharmacogenomics Journal, 11*(2), 138–145. www.nature.com/tpj/journal/v11/n2/suppinfo/tpj201014s1.html

Kendler, K. S., & Baker, J. H. (2007). Genetic influences on measures of the environment: A systematic review. *Psychological Medicine, 37*(5), 615–626. doi:10.1017/S0033291706009524

Kendler, K. S., Bulik, C. M., Silberg, J., Hettema, J. M., Myers, J., & Prescott, C. A. (2000). Childhood sexual abuse and adult psychiatric and substance use disorders in women. *Archives of General Psychiatry, 57*, 953–959.

Kessler, R. C., Berglund, P., Demler, O., Jin, R., Merikangas, K. R., & Walters, E. E. (2005). Lifetime prevalence and age-of-onset distributions of DSM-IV disorders in the National Comorbidity Survey Replication. *Archives of General Psychiatry, 62*, 593–602.

Kilpatrick, D. G., Koenen, K. C., Ruggiero, K. J., Acierno, R., Galea, S., Resnick, H. S., et al. (2007). Serotonin transporter genotype and social support and moderation of posttraumatic stress disorder and depression in hurricane-exposed adults. *American Journal of Psychiatry, 164*(11), 1–7.

Kishi, T., Yoshimura, R., Kitajima, T., Okochi, T., Okumura, T., Tsunoka, T., et al. (2010). HTR2A is associated with SSRI response in major depressive disorder in a Japanese cohort. *Neuromolecular Medicine, 12*(3), 237–242. doi:10.1007/s12017-009-8105-y

Koenen, K. C., & Galea, S. (2009). Gene-environment interactions and depression. *JAMA, 302*(17), 1859–1862. doi:10.1001/jama.2009.1575

Kolassa, I., Ertl, V., Eckart, M., Glockner, F., Kolassa, S., Papassotiropoulos, A., et al. (2010). Association study of trauma load and SLC6A4 promoter polymorphism in PTSD: Evidence from survivors of the Rwandan genocide. *Journal of Clinical Psychiatry, 71*(5), 543–547.

Kraft, P., & Hunter, D. J. (2009). The challenge of assessing complex gene-environment and gene-gene interactions. In M. J. Khoury, S. R. Bedrosian, M. Gwinn, J. P. T. Higgins, J. P. A. Ioannidis, & J. Little (Eds.), *Human genome epidemiology: Building the evidence for using genetic information to improve health and prevent disease* (2nd ed., 165–187). New York, NY: Oxford University Press.

Kraft, P., Yen, Y. C., Stram, D. O., Morrison, J., & Gauderman, W. J. (2007). Exploiting gene-environment interaction to detect genetic associations. *Human Heredity, 63*(2), 111–119.

Kranzler, H. R., Feinn, R., Nelson, E. C., Covault, J., Anton, R. F., Farrer, L., et al. (2011). A CRHR1 haplotype moderates the effect of adverse childhood experiences on lifetime risk of major depressive episode in African-American women. *American Journal of Medical Genetics Part B: Neuropsychiatric Genetics, 156*(8), 960–968.

Little, J., Higgins, J. P. T., Ioannidis, J. P. A., Moher, D., Gagnon, F., von Elm, E., et al. (2009). STrengthening the REporting of Genetic Association studies (STREGA): An extension of the STrengthening of Reporting of OBservational studies in Epidemiology (STROBE) statement. *Journal of Clinical Epidemiology, 62*, 597–608.

Lonsdorf, T. B. (2010). The COMTval158met polymorphism is associated with symptom relief during exposure-based cognitive-behavioral treatment in panic disorder. *BMC Psychiatry, 10*(1), 99. doi:10.1186/1471-244x-10-99

Luan, J. A., Wong, M. Y., & Wareham, N. J. (2001). Sample size determination for studies of gene-environment interaction. *International Journal of Epidemiology, 30*, 1035–1040.

Lupien, S. J., McEwen, B. S., Gunnar, M. R., & Heim, C. (2009). Effects of stress throughout the lifespan on the brain, behaviour, and cognition. *Nature Reviews Neuroscience, 10*(6), 434–445.

Lyons, M. J., Goldberg, J., Eisen, S. A., True, W., Tsuang, M. T., & Meyer, J. M. (1993). Do genes influence exposure to trauma? A twin study of combat. *American Journal of Medical Genetics, 48*(1), 22–27.

Mather, L., & Jinks, J. (1982). *Biometrical genetics; the study of continuous variation* (3rd ed.). New York, NY: Chapman and Hall.

Mercer, K. B., Orcutt, H. K., Quinn, J. F., Fitzgerald, C. A., Conneely, K. N., Barfield, R. T., et al. (2012). Acute and posttraumatic stress symptoms in a prospective gene × environment study of a university campus shooting. *Archives of General Psychiatry, 69*(1), 89–97. doi:10.1001/archgenpsychiatry.2011.109

Moffit, T. E., Caspi, A., & Rutter, M. (2006). Measured gene-environment interactions in psychopathology: Concepts, research strategies, and implications for research, intervention and public understanding of genetics. *Perspectives on Psychological Science, 1*, 5–27.

Molnar, B. E., Buka, S. L., & Ronald, C. (2001). Child sexual abuse and subsequent psychopathology: Results from the national comorbidity survey. *American Public Health Association, 91*, 753–760.

Monroe, S. M., & Reid, M. W. (2008). Gene-environment interactions in depression research: Genetic polymorphisms and life-stress polyprocedures. *Psychological Science, 19*(10), 947–956.

Mrazek, D. A., Rush, A. J., Biernacka, J. M., O'Kane, D. J., Cunningham, J. M., Wieben, E. D., et al. (2009). SLC6A4 variation and citalopram response. *American Journal of Medical Genetics Part B: Neuropsychiatric Genetics, 150B*(3), 341–351. doi:10.1002/ajmg.b.30816

Munafo, M. R., Durrant, C., Lewis, G., & Flint, J. (2009). Gene × environment interactions at the serotonin transporter locus. *Biological Psychiatry, 65*, 211–219.

Munafo, M. R., Durrant, C., Lewis, G., & Flint, J. (2010). Defining replication: A response to Kaufman and colleagues. *Biological Psychiatry, 67*, e21–23.

Neale, M. C., & Cardon, L. R. (1992). *Methodology for genetic studies of twins and families*. Dordrecht, Netherlands: Kluwer Academic Publishers.

Nederhof, E., Bouma, E., Oldehinkel, A. J., & Ormel, J. (2010). Interaction between childhood adversity, brain-derived neurotrophic factor *val/met* and serotonin transporter promoter polymorphism on depression: The TRAILS study. *Biological Psychiatry, 68*(2), 209–212.

Nelson, E. C., Agrawal, A., Pergadia, M. L., Lynskey, M. T., Todorov, A. A., Wang, J. C., et al. (2009). Association of childhood trauma exposure and GABRA2 polymorphisms with risk of posttraumatic stress disorder in adults. *Molecular Psychiatry, 14*, 234–238.

Nelson, E. C., Martin, N. G., Heath, A. C., Madden, P. A. F., Bucholz, K. K., Statham, D. J., et al. (2012). Common heritable contributions to low-risk trauma, high-risk trauma, posttraumatic stress disorder, and major depression. *Archives of General Psychiatry, 69*(3), 293–299.

Nierenberg, A. A. (2009). The long tale of the short arm of the promoter region for the gene that encodes the serotonin uptake protein. *CNS Spectrums, 14*(9), 462–463.

Nikulina, V., Widom, C. S., & Brzustowicz, L. M. (2012). Child abuse and neglect, *MAOA*, and mental health outcomes: A prospective examination. *Biological Psychiatry, 71*(4), 350–357.

Nilsson, K. W., Sjöberg, R. L., Leppert, J., Oreland, L., & Damberg, M. (2009). Transcription factor AP-2β genotype and psychosocial adversity in relation to adolescent depressive symptomatology. *Journal of Neural Transmission, 116*(3), 363–370.

Nugent, N. R., Tyrka, A. R., Carpenter, L. L., & Price, L. H. (2011). Gene-environment interactions: Early life stress and risk for depressive and anxiety disorders. *Psychopharmacology, 214*(1), 175–196. doi:10.1007/s00213-010-2151-x

Owens, M. J., & Nemeroff, C. B. (1994). Role of serotonin in the pathophysiology of depression: Focus on the serotonin transporter. *Clinical Chemistry, 40*(2), 288–295.

Plomin, R., & Davis, O. S. P. (2009). The future of genetics in psychology and psychiatry: Microarrays, genome-wide association, and non-coding RNA. *Journal of Child Psychology and Psychiatry, 50*(1–2), 63–71.

Polanczyk, G., Caspi, A., Williams, B., Price, T. S., Danese, A., Sugden, K., et al. (2009). Protective effect of CRHR1 gene variants on the development of adult depression following childhood maltreatment: Replication and extension. *Archives of General Psychiatry, 66*(9), 978.

Porcelli, S., Fabbri, C., & Serretti, A. (2012). Meta-analysis of serotonin transporter gene promoter polymorphism (5-HTTLPR) association with antidepressant efficacy. *European Neuropsychopharmacology, 22*(4), 239–258. doi:10.1016/j.euroneuro.2011.10.003

Pritchard, J. K., & Rosenberg, N. A. (1999). Use of unlinked genetic markers to detect population stratification in association studies. *American Journal of Human Genetics, 65*(1), 220–228.

Quinn, C. R., Dobson-Stone, C., Outhred, T., Harris, A., & Kemp, A. H. (2012). The contribution of BDNF and 5-HTT polymorphisms and early life stress to the heterogeneity of major depressive disorder: A preliminary study. *Australian and New Zealand Journal of Psychiatry, 46*(1), 55–63.

Ressler, K. J., Bradley, B., Mercer, K. B., Deveau, T. C., Smith, A. K., Gillespie, C. F., et al. (2010). Polymorphisms in CRHR1 and the serotonin transporter loci: Gene × gene × environment interactions on depressive symptoms. *American Journal of Medical Genetics Part B: Neuropsychiatric Genetics, 153*(3), 812–824.

Risch, N., Herrell, R., Lehner, T., Kung-Yee, L., Eaves, L., Hoh, J., et al. (2009). Interaction between the serotonin transporter gene (5-HTTLPR), stressful life events, and risk of depression: A meta analysis. *JAMA, 301*(23), 2462–2471.

Ritchie, K., Jaussent, I., Stewart, R., Dupuy, A.-M., Courtet, P., Ancelin, M.-L., et al. (2009). Association of adverse childhood environment and 5-HTTLPR genotype with late-life depression. *Journal of Clinical Psychiatry, 70*(9), 1281.

Rudolph, K. D. (Ed.). (2009). *Adolescent depression* (2nd ed.). New York, NY: Guilford Press.

Rutter, M. (2010). Gene-environment interplay. *Depression and Anxiety, 27*, 1–4.

Sartor, C. E., McCutcheon, V. V., Pommer, N. E., Nelson, E. C., Grant, J. D., Duncan, A. E., et al. (2011). Common genetic and environmental contributions to posttraumatic stress disorder and alcohol dependence in young women. *Psychological Medicine, 41*(7), 1497–1505.

Shanahan, M. J., & Hofer, S. M. (2005). Social context in gene-environment interactions: Retrospect and prospect.

Journals of Gerontology: Series B, Psychological Sciences and Social Sciences, 60(1), 65–76.

Sjöberg, R., Nilsson, K. W., Nordquist, N., Ohrvik, J., Leppert, J., Lindstrom, L., et al. (2006). Development of depression: Sex and the interaction between environment and a promoter polymorphism of the serotonin transporter gene. *International Journal of Neuropsychopharmacology, 9*(4), 443.

Smits, K. M., Smits, L. J. M., Peeters, F. P. M. L., Schouten, J. S. A. G., Janssen, R. G. J. H., Smeets, H. J. M., et al. (2008). The influence of 5-HTTLPR and STin2 polymorphisms in the serotonin transporter gene on treatment effect of selective serotonin reuptake inhibitors in depressive patients. *Psychiatric Genetics, 18*(4), 184–190. doi:110.1097/YPG.1090b1013e3283050aca

Stein, M. B., Jang, K. J., Taylor, S., Vernon, P. A., & Livesley, W. J. (2002). Genetic and environmental influences on trauma exposure and posttraumatic stress disorder: A twin study. *American Journal of Psychiatry, 159*(10), 1675–1681.

Sullivan, P. F., Neale, M. C., & Kendler, K. S. (2000). Genetic epidemiology of major depression: Review and meta-analysis. *American Journal of Psychiatry, 157*, 1552–1562.

Surtees, P. G., Wainwright, N. W., Willis-Owen, S. A., Luben, R., Day, N. E., et al. (2006). Social adversity, the serotonin transporter (5-HTTLPR) polymorphism and major depressive disorder. *Biological Psychiatry, 59*(3), 224–229.

Tambs, K., & Mourn, T. (1993). Low genetic effect and age-specific family effect for symptoms of anxiety and depression in nuclear families, halfsibs and twins. *Journal of Affect Disorders, 27*(3), 183–195.

Taylor, S. E., Way, B. M., Welch, W. T., Hilmert, C. J., Lehman, B. J., & Eisenberger, N. I. (2006). Early family environment, current adversity, the serotonin transporter promoter polymorphism, and depressive symptomatology. *Biological Psychiatry, 60*(7), 671–676.

Thapar, A., Harold, G., Rice, F., Langley, K., & O'Donovan, M. (2007). The contribution of gene-environment interaction to psychopathology. *Development and Psychopathology, 19*, 989–1004.

Thase, M. E. (Ed.). (2009). *Neurobiological aspects of depression* (2nd ed.). New York, NY: Guilford Press.

True, W. J., Rice, J., Eisen, S. A., Heath, A. C., Goldberg, J., Lyons, M. J., & Nowak, J. (1993). A twin study of genetic and environmental contributions to liability for posttraumatic stress symptoms. *Archives of General Psychiatry, 50*(4), 257–264.

Uddin, M., Koenen, K., de los Santos, R., Bakshis, E., Aiello, A., & Galea, S. (2010). Gender differences in the genetic and environmental determinants of adolescent depression. *Depression and Anxiety, 27*(7), 658–666.

Uher, R., Caspi, A., Houts, R., Sugden, K., Williams, B., Poulton, R., et al. (2011). Serotonin transporter gene moderates childhood maltreatment's effects on persistent but not single-episode depression: Replications and implications for resolving inconsistent results. *Journal of Affective Disorders, 135*(1), 56–65.

Uher, R., & McGuffin, P. (2008). The moderation by the serotonin transporter gene of environmental adversity in the aetiology of mental illness: Review and methodological analysis. *Molecular Psychiatry, 13*, 131–146.

Uher, R., & McGuffin, P. (2010). The moderation by the serotonin transporter gene of environmental adversity in the etiology of depression: 2009 update. *Molecular Psychiatry, 15*, 18–22.

U.S. Department of Health and Human Services, Administration for Children and Families, Administration on Children, Youth and Families, Children's Bureau. (2008). *Child maltreatment, 2006.* Washington, DC: U.S. Government Printing Office.

Van Os, J., & Jones, P. B. (1999). Early risk factors and adult person-environment relationships in affective disorder. *Psychological Medicine, 29*, 1055–1067.

van Zuiden, M., Geuze, E., Willemen, H. L. D. M., Vermetten, E., Maas, M., Amarouchi, K., et al. (2012). Glucocorticoid receptor pathway components predict posttraumatic stress disorder symptom development: A prospective study. *Biological Psychiatry, 71*(4), 309–316. doi:10.1016/j.biopsych.2011.10.026

Veletza, S., Samakouri, M., Emmanouil, G., Trypsianis, G., Kourmouli, N., & Livaditis, M. (2009). Psychological vulnerability differences in students—Carriers or not of the serotonin transporter promoter allele *S*: effect of adverse experiences. *Synapse, 63*(3), 193–200.

Vergne, D. E., & Nemeroff, C. B. (2006). The interaction of serotonin transporter gene polymorphisms and early adverse life events on vulnerability for major depression. *Current Psychiatry Reports, 8*, 452–457.

Walker, E. F., Sabuwalla, Z., & Huot, R. (2004). Pubertal neuromaturation, stress sensitivity, and psychopathology. *Development and Psychopathology, 16*, 807–824.

Wankerl, M., Wust, S., & Otte, C. (2010). Current developments and controversies: Does the serotonin transporter gene–linked polymorphic region (5-HTTLPR) modulate the association between stress and depression? *Current Opinion in Psychiatry, 23*(6), 582–587.

Wichers, M., Kenis, G., Jacobs, N., Mengelers, R., Derom, C., Vlietinck, R., et al. (2008). The BDNF Val-66Met × 5-HTTLPR × child adversity interaction and depressive symptoms: An attempt at replication. *American Journal of Medical Genetics Part B: Neuropsychiatric Genetics, 147*(1), 120–123.

Wilkie, M. J. V., Smith, G., Day, R. K., Matthews, K., Smith, D., Blackwood, D., et al. (2008). Polymorphisms in the SLC6A4 and HTR2A genes influence treatment outcome following antidepressant therapy. *Pharmacogenomics Journal, 9*(1), 61–70. www.nature.com/tpj/journal/v9/n1/suppinfo/6500491s1.html

Xie, P., Kranzler, H. R., Farrer, L., & Gelernter, J. (2012). Serotonin transporter 5-HTTLPR genotype moderates the effects of childhood adversity on posttraumatic stress disorder risk: A replication study. *American Journal of Medical Genetics Part B: Neuropsychiatric Genetics, 159*(6), 644–652.

Xie, P., Kranzler, H. R., Poling, J., Stein, M. B., Anton, R. F., Bradley, B., et al. (2009). Interactive effect of stressful life events and the serotonin transporter 5-HTTLPR genotype on posttraumatic stress disorder diagnosis in 2 independent populations. *Archives of General Psychiatry, 66*(11), 1201–1209.

Xie, P., Kranzler, H. R., Poling, J., Stein, M. B., Anton, R. F., Farrer, L. A., & Gelernter, J. (2010). Interaction of FKBP5 with childhood adversity on risk for post-traumatic stress disorder. *Neuropsychopharmacology, 35*(8), 1684–1692. doi:10.1038/npp.2010.37

Zammit, S., & Owen, M. J. (2006). Stressful life events, 5-HTT genotype and risk of depression. *British Journal of Psychiatry, 188*, 199–201. doi:10.1192/bjp.bp.105.020644

34

Resilience and Posttraumatic Growth in Abused and Neglected Children

GENERAL CONSIDERATIONS

Maltreated children experience resilience when provided with the resources they need to cope effectively. Though individual factors associated with resilience are most often studied, the ease with which a child's environment facilitates the conditions children need to recover and grow after abuse and neglect is just as important to the child's positive outcomes. This chapter reviews the protective factors that both nurture and maintain resilience among children who have experienced maltreatment, exploring a set of principles that explain which factors are most likely to influence developmental outcomes in which contexts. A social ecological understanding of resilience (Ungar, 2011a, 2011b) is used to show that interventions that help children are most effective when they closely match the child's needs. Interventions exert more or less influence (a differential impact) depending on the amount of exposure to maltreatment the child has experienced. The focus of the chapter then shifts to the efficacy of interventions by social service providers. It concludes with a discussion of how social policy can shape children's resilience after abuse and neglect.

Studies of internalizing and externalizing problems among children and adults with histories of abuse and neglect identify a heightened risk for disorder, but an interest in resilience is focusing the attention of researchers and clinicians on the estimated 20% of children who seem to avoid problems—demonstrating a capacity either to maintain normative functioning or to recover from temporary declines in functioning or, on rare occasions, reporting functioning better than they did prior to the abuse (Haskett et al., 2006). These patterns are described as *resilience* or *posttraumatic growth* and are indicative of interactions between individuals and adverse environments that facilitate adaptation that sustains well-being. These interactions,

however, are dependent as much (or more) on the capacity of children's families, schools, and communities to make resources available and accessible to maltreated children as on the individual coping capacities of the children themselves (Jaffee et al., 2007; Ungar, 2011b). This social ecological understanding of resilience deemphasizes the individual child's personal resources and instead emphasizes qualities of the child's environment as the most important protective factors that predict resistance to the effects of abuse, recovery after declines in functioning, and occasionally, better than expected growth. Those who report better than expected functioning are thought to experience posttraumatic growth (PTG), a concept closely related to resilience. PTG describes one pathway through adversity that results in new patterns of thinking, feeling, and behaving that integrate lessons learned from exposure to adversity.

While the relationship between resilience and child maltreatment is becoming better understood, much of the resilience research with maltreated children has focused more on the child's characteristics and characteristics related to the child's attachments to caregivers than on the quality of the complex systems of care developed to meet children's needs or other aspects of children's meso- and macro-systemic interactions. Interventions by those mandated to protect children, by providers of voluntary treatment, and by social policies that make services available and accessible have a great deal of influence on whether children can use their capacities under stress (Pancer et al., 2012). A successful foster care placement, continuity in engagement with their families of origin for older youths in care, the accessibility of trauma counseling, safety in the child's community or family, the coordination of multidisciplinary services, child protection legislation—these and many other systemic factors make it more or less likely that a child will recover from abuse. Individual-level factors such as the child's attribution of blame for the abuse, locus of control, personality factors such as persistence, and relational characteristics such as the ability to attach to others are also important to resilience, but these interact in complex patterns with the environment and the risks that are present.

THE RELATIONSHIP BETWEEN MALTREATMENT AND RESILIENCE

Bonanno and Mancini (2012), in their look at developmental trajectories after potentially traumatizing events (PTEs), show that individuals cope in multiple ways and that resilience (or resistance) is relatively common. Most people show a remarkably common capacity to recover from trauma, though a great deal of that recovery and resistance to a decline in functioning is related to our ability to find the resources that support our well-being. This understanding of resilience focuses as much attention on the environment around the abused child as on the child herself. In this respect, the study of resilience is showing a pattern of changing conceptualization similar to that occurring in the study of trauma. Early trauma work related to deficits in the individual (the war veteran who malingers) rather than the psychological burden imposed on the individual by contextual factors (such as war). Trauma is now understood to be the reaction to PTEs resulting from an environment stressing an individual and exhausting her resources to cope. Individual factors such as a predisposition to depression and a history of other trauma may shape the person's response to a specific traumatic event. In other words, as Bonanno and Mancini explain, trauma (such as that resulting from abuse and neglect) is not a quality of the individual but a result of interactional processes and environmental factors that shape the way individuals cope with the PTE.

Resilience is very similar, with our ability to cope with adversity being a function of the severity and duration of the risk factors endured and the capacity of both the individual and his environment to facilitate adaptation that contributes to an experience of well-being. If most of us recover, and if resilience is, as it has been described, a common everyday capacity for most people, then we might rightly assert that it is our ability as humans to create facilitative environments (e.g., attachments to caregivers, safe communities) and cognitions (e.g., an internal locus of control) that is protective when we are exposed to maltreatment. This ability to create resilience is only partially an individual's exercise of personal agency; it is just as much a reflection of the social policies of governments that result in resources such as child welfare workers and trauma counseling being made available to children so that PTEs do not have long-term consequences.

This relationship between context and resilience can be shown in studies of the combination of individual, family, and neighborhood factors that distinguish resilient from nonresilient maltreated children. For example, in a national longitudinal study of 1,116 twin pairs and their families, Jaffee and colleagues (2007) showed that individual strengths predicted resilience for children only in contexts where a maltreated child was exposed to low amounts of stress in the environment. In more highly stressed family and neighborhood settings, it was the quality of the environment rather than individual characteristics of the child that predicted well-being When approached this way, and children were matched for the level of abuse and neglect they had experienced, the nonresilient children (in this study, those that showed above-average levels of problem behaviors at ages 5 and 7) exhibited a positive relationship between the child's exposure to higher levels of stress and more problem behaviors. The environmental stressors included parents with antisocial personality traits and lower intelligence and neighborhoods with higher crime, lower levels of social cohesion, and little informal social control. In such contexts, even if a child had a better than average number of strengths, his or her experience of maltreatment was still predictive of higher than average levels of problem behaviors at school.

If we understand resilience as a set of factors and processes that mitigate the impact of exposure to risk, change developmental trajectories so that children are helped to adapt in positive ways, improve self-esteem, and open opportunities to experience social support and other determinants of well-being (Rutter, 1987), then there is abundant evidence that children who have been maltreated can develop resilience when their environments are responsive to their needs. *The challenge, however, is to know which protective factor is best suited to which type of abuse experience for which child in which context.* Specifically, to know how resilience will appear in the life of a child who is maltreated, we need to assess:

- The type of maltreatment
- The severity of the maltreatment
- The duration of the maltreatment
- The individual's response to the maltreatment (attribution of causality; meaning ascribed to the PTE)
- The culturally held values related to the maltreatment
- The contextual factors that influence which resources are available and accessible
- The likely symptoms that will result from the maltreatment

Considering all these factors complicates the understanding of processes that facilitate resilience. For example, internalizing problems such as depression have been shown to be moderated by aspects of resilience for a population of urban, low-income, highly traumatized, predominantly African American adults (Wingo et al., 2010). Furthermore, these same factors associated with resilience also interact with other trauma experiences frequently present in the lives of adults who have experienced adverse childhood events related to maltreatment, such as witnessing violence in their homes and harsh discipline. In this case, aspects of people's marginalization because of race and class are critical to how abuse is experienced, the psychological symptoms that follow, and which factors are most likely to protect individuals from problems later on.

In general, however, maltreated children tend to show less resilience than children exposed to other types of developmental risk such as poverty or a parent with a substance abuse problem (Haskett et al., 2006). Children are also likely to show resilience in one functional domain, such as academics or peer interactions, but lack strengths in others or show less positive functioning over time. Therefore, if we are to understand resilience, we need to first understand the nature of the individual's exposure to risk and how that exposure is either mitigated or accentuated by the child's environment. Different types of maltreatment are strongly associated with different forms of psychopathology later in life, with aspects of resilience likely to be most effective when they interrupt environment-individual interactions. For example, Powers et al. (2011) found that emotional abuse, but not physical or sexual abuse, was related to later development of schizotypal personality disorder. Other personality disorders in adults are also strongly related to childhood abuse, though these relationships may be mediated by the development of PTSD. Likewise, a study of 84 high-functioning women who had previously been in foster care and had received scholarships for postsecondary education showed differences in their placement histories depending on whether they had been sexually or physically abused (Breno & Galupo, 2007). Sexual abuse victims were more likely to have histories of restrictive housing, and they had changed foster placements twice as often. These differences in patterns of risk and the responses by service providers (e.g., stability of placement) affected both life trajectories and trauma-related beliefs after maltreatment. Trauma-related beliefs and sense of powerlessness were both negatively correlated with resilience. In this case, as others, it is the nature of the adversity the child experiences, the quality of the response by caregivers to mitigate the impact of that adversity, and individual factors such as cognition that combine to create a complicated explanation for resilience.

Neither individual nor environmental factors alone can account for the reason some children do well and others do not. Collin-Vezina et al. (2011), for example, showed that multiple forms of trauma are related to sexual concerns and posttraumatic stress and depression and dissociation, as well as lower levels of resilience as measured by the Child and Youth Resilience Measure-28 (Ungar & Liebenberg, 2011). The youths with the highest levels of trauma showed a steady decline in the resources they had available to protect themselves, including concurrent decreases in individual, relational, community, and cultural resources.

Further adding to this complexity, posttraumatic stress disorder (PTSD) may result from childhood maltreatment itself or from other life events that are not directly related to maltreatment. The combination of a history of abuse and PTSD makes it more likely that an individual will develop a personality disorder (Powers et al., 2011). With regard to resilience, interventions that address the aftereffects of emotional abuse, such as a secure attachment to a foster parent following removal from an abusive family of origin, would be expected to decrease the likelihood of both PTSD and the development of a personality disorder later in life.

Our understanding of the processes associated with resilience as they relate to child abuse is moving toward this level of specificity in its identification of the impact of protective factors. We know, for example, that it is childhood trauma, not childhood life events themselves, that is a risk factor for adult depressive and anxiety disorders and the comorbidity between the two (Hovens et al., 2010). However, a specific type of childhood trauma may not be strongly associated with a specific psychiatric disorder later in life. Unlike the research by Powers et al. (2011) that found emotional abuse produced distinct outcomes, childhood trauma may produce a number of possible mental health challenges during adulthood. A different risk factor, though, such as placement in care during childhood has been found to be associated with later anxiety and depression in a sample of nearly 2,000 adults in the Netherlands, none of whom had a lifetime diagnosis of either depression or anxiety at the time of their interview (Hovens et al., 2010).

Just as it is now commonplace to conduct detailed diagnoses of the risk factors confronting an abused child, the same care needs to be taken when assessing resilience. For example, with regard to resilience, results from the Netherlands study suggest that by not removing children from their homes whenever possible, alternative interventions such as in-home support and ecological models of intervention such as family group conferencing (Burford & Hudson, 2000) that maintain the child's contact with his biological parents may be protective against two types of internalizing behaviors—depression and anxiety—during adulthood.

Even as we see the need for greater specificity in understanding which protective factors are most helpful for which children in which contexts, studies of resilience among populations exposed to adversity continue to identify generic sets of protective processes that are likely to mitigate the impact of abuse and prevent the development of trauma. These aspects of resilience vary by study. For example, Rutter (1987) named four processes: (1) reduction of risk impact, (2) reduction of negative chain reactions, (3) establishment and maintenance of self-esteem and self-efficacy, and (4) opening up of opportunities. In a more ecologically sensitive approach to the study of resilience, and one that takes into account cultural variations, Ungar et al. (2007) identified seven factors that are associated with resilience: (1) nurturing relationships, (2) a positive identity, (3) experiences of control (efficacy), (4) social justice, (5) access to material resources, (6) a sense of cohesion and belonging in one's family, school, and community, and (7) cultural adherence. Each of these seven factors is experienced by a young person as codependent on the others, such that improvement in one can facilitate increases in another.

DIFFERENTIAL IMPACT

One way to reconcile the tension between the need to identify specific protective factors in a child's life and generic processes that are likely to protect all maltreated children is to study the differential impact of protective factors. A single factor can have different influences depending on the child's level of risk exposure and the nature of the risk. In general, the greater an individual's risk exposure and vulnerability, the more the protective factors exert a positive influence on the individual's psychosocial development. This principle of differential impact helps to explain why some protective factors promote well-being across an entire population, some are effective only for individuals who have been exposed to lower levels of adversity, and some are most predictive of good outcomes for individuals who experience the most severe PTEs.

A factor that is relatively commonplace among nonmaltreated children, such as a prosocial peer group or an adult mentor, can have a profound impact on the maltreated child's life course (Cyrulnik, 2008). The protective factor compensates for a child's lack of supports and offers a differential response to the child's need for help in dealing with the risk factors he faces. For example, whereas a child exposed to minimal risk has lots of access to peers and mentors, the deprived child may experience both (peer group and/or mentor) as his only source of support. The difference is akin to that between the child who comes home after school to a well-resourced, stable home where he is monitored and expected to succeed academically and the neglected child who has none of these supports at home but has one adult at school (a coach, teacher, counselor, or school administrator) who helps him see his potential to overcome his disadvantage. The resulting paradox is that many maltreated and socially excluded children experience higher rates of self-reported school engagement than their less disadvantaged peers (Shernoff & Schmidt, 2008). For the maltreated child, school may offer the only source of social support available. Therefore, in contexts where there is higher exposure to risk, environmental factors that change risk impact and open new opportunities for personal development are likely to be more strongly associated with resilience than are individual factors (Jaffee et al., 2007).

This relative influence of individual and environmental factors has implications for intervention. Whereas at lower levels of risk, more individualized treatment is likely to be effective, children exposed to severe abuse and neglect will require structural supports such as a stable living situation, physical safety, education tailored to their needs, and accessible treatment with a provider who remains constant. More individually focused interventions such as those that address cognitions and the psychological symptoms related to PTSD may not be as effective until these systemic factors are addressed.

If we have previously imagined that resilience is a quality of the individual or have assumed that resilience is the result of environment-person interactions in which both sides of the equation are equal, it is because we have not included in the psychological research a sociopolitical perspective. At higher levels of risk, structural changes related to social policy, service accessibility, and sociocultural factors such as stigma and racism all shape the opportunities that maltreated children have to thrive. Individual factors are less likely to influence these complex macro-systemic factors that determine whether children are provided with what they need in contexts where they experience social exclusion (Bottrell & Armstrong, 2012).

This same differential impact appears in studies of gene-environment interactions and epigenetics as they relate to maltreatment. According to Heim and Binder (2012), early experiences that stress neurobiological systems are implicated in later emotional regulation and increase vulnerability to stress and risk for depression later in life: "However, not all cases with early adverse experiences develop depression later in life and there is substantial variability in the outcomes of early life stress, including resilience" (p. 103). Therefore, a range of responses are expected, depending on multiple factors associated with early adverse events, such as the severity, duration, and developmental period during which abuse and neglect occur. The potential impact on a child is further confounded by differences in stress reactivity, though the precise models to explain these patterns are still developing. In general, abuse before and after puberty help to predict differences between a predisposition toward depression (resulting from earlier exposure to adversity) and PTSD (later exposure). As Heim and Binder suggest in their review of the literature, "it is conceivable that early life stress at different developmental stages can lead to differential neurobiological phenotypes with differential vulnerability to depression, as a function of the relative plasticity of different brain regions and the effects of sex hormones" (p. 105). Furthermore, studies of epigenetics are suggesting that there are gene-environment interactions that include both individual-level and community-level factors that influence gene expression (social support, crime, poverty). The specificity of one or more protective mechanisms is particularly important when predicting which factor is most likely to enhance which child's capacity to cope under which types of stress.

For example, cultural transmission across generations and preservation of identity through the revitalization of a culture have been shown to protect Aboriginal populations in Canada that experienced the cultural genocide resulting from more than a hundred years of forced placement of children into residential schools. The high levels of both mental illness and addictions among indigenous populations are associated with their firsthand experience of maltreatment at the schools, as well as the vicarious trauma of growing up in the care of a parent or grandparent who had attended a residential school (Elias et al., 2012). In this case, where the exposure is high and the resources within a child's family and community are depleted, there is a need for structural supports—including kinship care, family group conferencing, and other forms of community response that match the children's need for a culturally sensitive intervention. Examples such as these show there are temporal, social, and contextual characteristics to the way we adapt and how the impact of stressors is moderated (Bonanno & Mancini, 2012).

POSTTRAUMATIC GROWTH

A concept related to resilience is posttraumatic growth, defined by Kilmer (2006) as a perceived beneficial change to individuals following an experience of trauma. The concept was first used by Tedeschi and Calhoun (1996, 2004), who identified five domains of growth following exposure to trauma-inducing events such as disability or loss of a spouse: adults experience "greater appreciation of life and changed sense of priorities; warmer, more intimate relationships with others; a greater sense of personal strength; recognition of new possibilities or paths for one's life; and spiritual development" (Tedeschi and Calhoun, 2004, p. 6). In much the same way that resilience depends on the quality of the environment that children experience and the nature of their maltreatment, McElheran and colleagues (2012) suggest that "traumatic events that are unexpected, longer-lasting, and of severe intensity impede the recovery process" (pp. 74–75). These qualities of the experience will greatly influence children's outcomes, even where there has been a history of good functioning before the traumatic event and children have had access to social support. The variability in outcomes results from a complex pattern of cognitions and experiences that influence the development of PTG. Access to social support, rumination on life-changing events, development of cognitive schema to explain the events, and development of narratives that provide acceptable explanations for the tragedy can all result in PTG despite enduring distress (McAdams, 1993; Tedeschi & Calhoun, 2004). In other words, there is the possibility that PTG can exist even while the risks associated with disorder remain.

In the case of children, however, PTG may be less likely among younger children, largely due to their less mature cognitive abilities and spiritual development. If children show the capacity to heal from exposure to trauma, it may be more a function of their closer relationships with social supports that are, by necessity, present in a child's life. Likewise, as Kilmer (2006) suggests, "a child's assumptive world is less firmly entrenched or embedded than an adult's" (p. 267) and therefore is more likely to be flexible enough to accommodate the experience of trauma into a new narrative about the world.

HIDDEN ASPECTS OF CHILDREN'S COPING WITH ABUSE AND NEGLECT

Whereas *posttraumatic growth* results in children with narratives of survival and of growth that looks very positive, *hidden resilience* is another pattern of coping that is also effective but far less welcome. Both terms refer to a child's use of coping strategies that are adaptive but beyond normal expectations. Ungar (2004) observed hidden resilience among a population of mental health clients who had resorted to delinquency and other problem behaviors when their pathways to resilience were poorly resourced. A child with a history of severe neglect, for example, may purposefully commit a crime to secure the safety of incarceration and the predictable support of professional helpers.

To illustrate this pattern further, we can look at children's perception of control over controllable and uncontrollable events. Wyman (2003) showed that children who were more stress-resilient and lived in difficult situations (such as with a parent with an addiction or where there was family violence) did best because they could properly assess their opportunities to change their situation and the resources that were available. Where they had control over such things as conflict with other children, the children did best when they exercised control. To outsiders, this realistic appraisal may appear to disadvantage a child who does not conform with the expectations of professional helpers or behave in a particular way that they consider appropriate (i.e., avoiding conflict in all circumstances). In practice this means there will always be an element of negotiation between children and their caregivers when it comes to determining which strategies are most effective in contexts with few resources or with culture-based value systems that violate a child's right to equal participation. Returning to the study by Wyman, his findings showed the following pattern of hidden resilience:

> The group of children who demonstrated enhanced adjustment in high-adversity families reported low levels of affective responsiveness to others' feelings and low acceptance of others' affect expressiveness compared to competent youths in more favorable settings. They also reported minimal engagement and emotional involvement with their primary caregivers. In contrast, they reported positive beliefs in their own competence and had positive expectations for their futures. Those findings were consistent with the hypothesis that more restrictive affective management strategies would help children to reduce distress associated with family turmoil and disappointment over unmet emotional needs. Firm psychological boundaries in relationships with adult family members (e.g., limited expectations) may have enabled them to experience competence in other avenues. In contrast, positive adaptation for children in more favorable family climates was associated with emotional

responsiveness and with skills for promoting and maintaining close emotional connections with family. (Wyman, 2003, p. 310)

As the example shows, atypical behavior may produce positive outcomes for a maltreated child in specific contexts. Therefore, in some cases, an inflated perception of one's self can lead to this protective avoidant style (Wyman, 2003). Wyman concludes that "processes that are beneficial to children in one context may be neutral, or even deleterious, in another" (p. 314).

This pattern is not an anomaly. A study by Seidman and Pedersen (2003) of ethnically diverse students in New York City found that a detaching profile, one in which the young person was less involved with parents, was actually far more adaptive and protected children when caregivers were dysfunctional, hassling, or enmeshing. Likewise, Kolar, Erickson, and Stewart (2012) found in their qualitative study of street-involved youths that participants showed differences in self-rated health that might not indicate mental health but that these assessments often overlooked important coping strategies. Employing a stance of critical realism in which "researchers account for participants' experiences as both agentic and embedded in structural and social contexts that exist independently from experience but that are always socially mediated" (p. 748), they found that the youths they interviewed (many of whom had experienced maltreatment) used the dual strategies of violence and social distancing, which were "(1) the active attempts of [street-involved youths] in our study to remove themselves from certain social groups or persons, and (2) their development of anti-social coping mechanisms in the form of attitudes and outlooks on life, such as a non-discriminating and intense distrust of others due to hurtful experiences" (p. 749).

INTERVENTIONS

Remarkably, there is little in the resilience literature that has investigated patterns of service use by maltreated children and youths after abuse. This is particularly odd because a child or youth who experiences maltreatment is, over time, likely to be identified to professionals by members of his community. Where services exist, many of these children will go on to receive help from multiple mandated and voluntary providers (Ungar et al., in press).

The problem, however, is not with the quantity of services but with their lack of coordination. In Simmel's (2012) review of the state of child welfare needs and services, she notes that there are still many children in the child welfare system who have untreated mental health needs. Her review traces the history of child abuse interventions from the publication of Jane Knitzer's (1982) *Unclaimed Children*, which identified the needs of children with serious emotional disturbances and led to the establishment of legislation to provide systems of care (Stroul & Friedman, 1986). Echoing the need for complexity in how we intervene to

promote resilience, Simmel (2012) shows that in many cases, the child welfare system becomes the mental health care provider when children are unable to navigate to services before placement.

While these patterns of service provision do get services to children and youths, there are no evidence-based treatments that are specific to building resilience among maltreated children—although, as this volume shows, a great number of programs promote processes that are associated with resilience among children who have experienced violence and neglect. The evidence that specific interventions help maltreated children become more resilient, however, is a patchwork of competing results.

For example, Anctil and colleagues (2007) showed that for graduates from an intensive foster placement service, services were related to positive mental health outcomes: "When evaluating the long-term effect of specific risk factors associated with foster care (e.g., child abuse and neglect and placement experiences), alongside services designed to enhance and develop protective factors, the risk factors' effect was negligible on adult psychological outcomes" (p. 1021). For youths taken into care because of abuse, the factors that promote resilience are specific to the context in which they are being raised. Placement decisions, however, are not necessarily benign when the risk is moderate or low or when the placement itself exposes children to other risks, including disengagement from their family of origin (Frensch & Cameron, 2002).

Matching intervention to child also means matching the child's developmental age to the type of intervention provided. A survey of interventions by Benoit, Coolbear, and Crawford (2008) identified age-appropriate interventions (in this case, for children under the age of 3) that addressed the child's need for a sense of safety, engagement of the caregivers in treatment, and resolution of the problems caregivers face in getting to treatment. These interventions also helped the nonmaltreating caregiver (when present) to be emotionally available to the child and helped in resolving conflicts and negative sequelae of behavior between caregiver and child. As expected, most of these interventions focused on creating facilitative social ecologies for children by helping their caregivers become better navigators and negotiators for the resources that protect children from risk exposure, opening opportunities for growth, and reducing the impact of maltreatment when it does occur. There is evidence that early interventions that change environments in these ways can result from large-scale prevention efforts. In their look at 15-year outcomes among parents who participated in the Better Beginnings, Better Futures Project, Pancer and colleagues (2012) showed that parents in the intervention group had better outcomes than parents in a control community with regard to their engaging in fewer risky behaviors and having lower rates of depression and more community involvement. In this case, it was the resilience of the caregiver to change, the ability of the child's extended support network to respond, and the flexibility of service providers in ensuring available and accessible treatment that improved outcomes and prevented the trauma that follows abuse.

The factors that make an intervention resilience-promoting are necessarily linked to the nature of the child's abuse history. The relationship is somewhat complicated, with different patterns evident. For example, while a history of sexual or physical abuse among opiate users is associated with worse medical status, worse family relationships, less engagement with psychiatric care, and lower quality of life than for substance-using peers without a history of abuse, substitution drug treatments appear to be equally effective for both groups (Oviedo-Joekes et al., 2010). As the example illustrates, processes that bolster resilience are most likely to result when interventions are matched to a maltreated individual's needs.

SOCIAL POLICY

When considering social policy and resilience for maltreated children and youths, we need to anticipate the protective factors that can be influenced by policy, such as placement decisions for children who are removed from their parents. In Kernan and Lansford's (2004) review of the impact of the U.S. Adoption and Safe Families Act of 1997, they show that overall, children in foster care do better than children who are reunited with their families of origin. Therefore, it appears that reunification is a risk factor and placement is protective for children who are maltreated. The evidence, however, also strongly suggests that because reunification tends to be a higher risk for families that are ethnic and racial minorities and are therefore likely to be economically and socially marginalized, the real protective factor against developmental problems is children's placement in financially better-off or financially stable and less marginalized homes. A more comprehensive effort to foster resilience (when understood as dependent on the child's social ecology) might be to address the poverty of the child's biological parents and provide resources for family support.

Interestingly, when older youths are studied separately, they show patterns of resisting placement when their needs are not negotiated, in particular with regard to foster placement. Once again, social policy that emphasizes youths' participation in their case planning and placement decisions, as well as a more nuanced implementation of policy that is sensitive to the psychosocial needs of children who are maltreated, is likely to facilitate children's and youths' ease of access to the resources needed to maintain their well-being despite maltreatment. In this regard, a social ecological model of resilience focuses attention on both the individual and the environment, suggesting that changes to the environment will profoundly affect the developmental path of maltreated children just as much as, and probably more than, the changes that individuals make themselves.

CONCLUSIONS

The abused and neglected child shows patterns of coping that reflect successful navigations towards resources and negotiations for resources to be provided in ways that are meaningful for the child. In some instances, children show posttraumatic growth and exceed expectations; in others, children show hidden resilience and appear to function poorly, though they may in fact be making the best use possible of whatever resources are available and accessible. Therefore, while individual factors are very important, the adversity experienced by the maltreated child makes it more likely that environmental factors will have a differential impact on the child's recovery and growth. In this regard, services for these children are one of the most important aspects of their social ecologies that make resilience more likely. Services and the social policies that shape them work best when they help create conditions for abused and neglected children to navigate and negotiate in ways that they and their caregivers value.

References

Anctil, T. M., McCubbin, L. D., O'Brien, K., & Pecora, P. (2007). An evaluation of recovery factors for foster care alumni with physical or psychiatric impairments: Predictors of psychological outcomes. *Children and Youth Services Review, 29,* 1021–1034.

Benoit, D., Coolbear, J., & Crawford, A. (2008). Abuse, neglect, and maltreatment of infants. *Encyclopedia of Infant and Early Childhood Development, 1–3,* 1–11.

Bonanno, G. A., & Mancini, A. D. (2012). Beyond resilience and PTSD: Mapping the heterogeneity of responses to potential trauma. *Psychological Trauma, 4*(1), 74–83.

Bottrell, D., & Armstrong, D. (2012). Local resources and distal decisions: The political ecology of resilience. In M. Ungar (Ed.), *The social ecology of resilience: A handbook of theory and practice* (pp. 247–264). New York, NY: Springer Publishing.

Breno, A. L., & Galupo, M. P. (2007). Sexual abuse histories of young women in the U.S. child welfare system: A focus on trauma-related beliefs and resilience. *Journal of Child Sexual Abuse, 16*(2), 97–113.

Burford, G., & Hudson J. (Eds.). (2000) *Family group conferencing: New directions in community-centered child and family practice.* New York, NY: Aldine de Gruyter.

Collin-Vezina, D., Coleman, K., Milne, L., Sell, J., & Daigneault, I. (2011). Trauma experiences, maltreatment-related impairments, and resilience among child welfare youth in residential care. *International Journal of Mental Health and Addictions, 9,* 577–589.

Cyrulnik, B. (2008). Children in war and their resilience. In H. Parens, H. P. Blum, & S. Akhtar (Eds.), *The unbroken soul: Tragedy, trauma, and resilience* (pp. 23–36). Lanham, MD: Jason Aronson.

Elias, B., Mignone, J., Hall, M., Hong, S. P., Hart, L., & Sareen, J. (2012). Trauma and suicide behaviour histories among a Canadian indigenous population: An empirical exploration of the potential role of Canada's residential school system. *Social Science & Medicine, 74,* 1560–1569.

Frensch, K. M., & Cameron, G. (2002). Treatment of choice or a last resort? A review of residential mental health placements for children and youth. *Child and Youth Care Forum, 31*(5), 313–345.

Haskett, M. E., Nears, K., Ward, C. S., & McPherson, A. V. (2006). Diversity in adjustment of maltreated children: Factors associated with resilient functioning. *Clinical Psychology Review, 26*, 796–812.

Heim, C., & Binder, E. B. (2012). Current research trends in early life stress and depression: Review of human studies on sensitive periods, gene-environment interactions, and epigenetics. *Experimental Neurology, 233*, 102–111.

Hovens, J. G. F. M., Wiersma, J. E., Giltay, E. J., van Oppen, P., Spinhoven, P., Penninx, B. W. J. H., & Zitman, F. G. (2010). Childhood life events and childhood trauma in adult patients with depressive, anxiety and comorbid disorders vs. controls. *Acta Psychiatrica Scandinavica, 122*, 66–74.

Jaffee, S. R., Caspi, A., Moffitt, T. E., Polo-Tomas, M., & Taylor, A. (2007). Individual, family, and neighborhood factors distinguish resilient from non-resilient maltreated children: A cumulative stressors model. *Child Abuse & Neglect, 31*, 231–253.

Kernan, E., & Lansford, J. E. (2004). Providing for the best interests of the child? The Adoption and Safe Families Act of 1997. *Applied Developmental Psychology, 25*, 523–539.

Kilmer, R. P. (2006). Resilience and posttraumatic growth in children. In L. G. Calhoun & R. G. Tedeschi (Eds.), *Handbook of posttraumatic growth: Research and practice* (pp. 264–288). New York, NY: Psychology Press.

Knitzer, J. (1982). *Unclaimed children: The failure of public responsibility to children and adolescents in need of mental health service.* Washington, DC: Children's Defense Fund.

Kolar, K., Erickson, P. G., & Stewart, D. (2012). Coping strategies of street-involved youth: Exploring contexts of resilience. *Journal of Youth Studies 15*(6), 744–760. doi:10.1080/13676261.2012.677814

McAdams, D. (1993). *The stories we live by.* New York, NY: William Morrow.

McElheran, M., Briscoe-Smith, A., Khaylis, A., Westrup, D., Hayward, C., & Gore-Felton, C. (2012). A conceptual model of post-traumatic growth among children and adolescents in the aftermath of sexual abuse. *Counselling Psychology Quarterly, 25*(1), 73–82.

Oviedo-Joekes, E., Marchand, E., Guh, K., Marsh, D., Brissette, D., Krausz, S., et al. (2010). History of reported sexual or physical abuse among long-term heroin users and their response to substitution treatment. *Addictive Behaviors, 36*, 55–60.

Pancer, S. M., Nelson, G., Hasford, J., & Loomis, C. (2012). The Better Beginnings, Better Futures Project: Long-term parent, family, and community outcomes of a universal, comprehensive, community-based prevention approach for primary school children and their families. *Journal of Community & Applied Social Psychology, 23*(3), 187–205. doi:10.1003/casp/2110

Powers, A. D., Thomas, K. M., Ressler, K. J., & Bradley, B. (2011). The differential effects of child abuse and posttraumatic stress disorder on schizotypal personality disorder. *Comprehensive Psychiatry, 52*, 438–445.

Rutter, M. (1987). Psychosocial resilience and protective mechanisms. *American Journal of Orthopsychiatry, 57*, 316–331.

Seidman, E., & Pedersen, S. (2003). Holistic contextual perspectives on risk, protection and competence among low-income urban adolescents. In S. S. Luthar (Ed.), *Resilience and vulnerability: Adaptation in the context of childhood adversities* (pp. 318–342). Cambridge, UK: Cambridge University Press.

Shernoff, D. J., & Schmidt, J. A. (2008). Further evidence of an engagement-achievement paradox among U.S. high school students. *Journal of Youth and Adolescence, 37*, 564–580.

Simmel, C. (2012). Highlighting adolescents' involvement with the child welfare system: A review of recent trends, policy developments, and related research. *Children and Youth Services Review, 34*, 1197–1207.

Stroul, B., & Friedman, R. (1986). *A system of care for children and youth with severe emotional disturbances* (Revised ed.). Washington, DC: Georgetown University Child Development Center.

Tedeschi, R. G., & Calhoun, L. G. (1996). The Posttraumatic Growth Inventory: Measuring the positive legacy of trauma. *Journal of Traumatic Stress, 9*, 455–471.

Tedeschi, R. G., & Calhoun, L. G. (2004). Posttraumatic growth: Conceptual foundations and empirical evidence. *Psychological Inquiry, 15*(1), 1–18.

Ungar, M. (2004). *Nurturing hidden resilience in troubled youth.* Toronto, ON: University of Toronto Press.

Ungar, M. (2011a). *Counselling in challenging contexts.* Belmont, CA: Brooks/Cole.

Ungar, M. (2011b). The social ecology of resilience: Addressing contextual and cultural ambiguity of a nascent construct. *American Journal of Orthopsychiatry, 81*, 1–17.

Ungar, M., Brown, M., Liebenberg, L., Othman, R., Kwong, W. M., Armstrong, M., & Gilgun, J. (2007). Unique pathways to resilience across cultures. *Adolescence, 42*(166), 287–310.

Ungar, M., & Liebenberg, L. (2011). Assessing resilience across cultures using mixed methods: Construction of the Child and Youth Resilience Measure. *Journal of Multiple Methods in Research, 5*(2), 126–149.

Ungar, M., Liebenberg, L., Landry, N., & Ikeda, J. (in press). Caregivers, young people with complex needs, and multiple service providers: A study of triangulated relationships and their impact on resilience. *Family Process.*

Wingo, A. P., Wrenn, G., Pelletier, T., Gutman, A. R., Bradley, B., & Ressler, K. J. (2010). Moderating effects of resilience on depression in individuals with a history of childhood abuse or trauma exposure. *Journal of Affective Disorders, 126*, 411–414.

Wyman, P. A. (2003). Emerging perspectives on context specificity of children's adaptation and resilience: Evidence from a decade of research with urban children in adversity. In S. S. Luthar (Ed.), *Resilience and vulnerability: Adaptation in the context of childhood adversities* (pp. 293–317). Cambridge, UK: Cambridge University Press.

PART VII Legal Issues

35

DONALD C. BROSS, PH.D., J.D.

Legal Issues Related to Child Maltreatment and Its Therapy

GENERAL CONSIDERATIONS

The topics of this chapter are the reporting and treatment of child abuse, information related to court reports and testimony, the contrast between civil and criminal proceedings, and a few of the special legal topics of child maltreatment. Since any of these topics might lend themselves individually to extensive legal analysis, the purpose here is to list and briefly describe the issues and direct the reader, when appropriate, to more extensive sources or examples.

MANDATED CHILD ABUSE REPORTING AND HIPAA CONSIDERATIONS

Against a limited backdrop of intellectual controversy on the value and consequences of mandatory reporting of child maltreatment (Mathews & Bross, 2008), reporting of suspected child abuse and neglect is the legally enforced practice in all U.S. states and many districts, territories, and possessions. Originally, all 50 states independently enacted child abuse reporting laws that focused on severe physical abuse (Paulsen, 1967). The original state laws were, to a degree, standardized by Pub. L. No. 93-247, which applied the federal spending power, using small grants to states as incentives to achieve relative compliance with national standards for reporting. Changes encouraged by federal granting authority included expansion of the reporting requirement to virtually every form of maltreatment, including neglect, as well as requirements for the appointment of legal representatives for maltreated children whose cases came to court. The inclusion of neglect as a requirement of reporting laws resulted in a vastly increased number of child maltreatment reports. The reporting system has been the basis for analyzing how important child maltreatment is to the United States, to what degree child maltreatment is being addressed, and the extent to which public investment should be made to address the problem.

Since the landmark decision of *Landeros v. Flood* (1976), remarkably few cases of liability for failure to report have been litigated, and of those known, most resulted in settlements out of court, which do not lead to appeals and thus have not been documented in places easily accessible to non-lawyers (Bross, 1987). Cases for not reporting have been documented more often than cases of malicious reporting, and a legislative grant of "good faith immunity" from civil or criminal liability for child abuse reporting is universal in the United States (Child Welfare Information Gateway, 2010). The exception to this effective shield from liability is found in litigation related to divorce, child custody, and visitation proceedings. "The American Psychological Association's Presidential Task Force on Violence and the Family found that batterers are twice as likely to seek custody as non-batterers" (Haralambie, 2010, citing the taskforce's report of 1996). However, "When a parent attempts to obtain the protection of the child welfare and judicial system, but the courts do not believe that abuse has occurred, the would-be protector has no place else to turn. Each subsequent attempt to get help may be viewed as vindictiveness, paranoia, hypervigilance, or attempts to 'alienate' the child from the other parent. Parents may actually be ordered not to make further CPS [child protective services] reports or to first have a report screened by some other professional, even if such orders put parents who are mandated reporters at risk of violating mandatory reporting laws" (p. 408). Even in this contentious area, however, any lawsuits against professional participants tend to be filed under various claims of negligence—for example, related to evaluation or treatment—and are commonly filed against a professional reporter for the mere act of reporting.

A significant form of tort suit liability is being imposed with respect to child abuse and neglect. Lawsuits against churches (Berry, 1992) and youth organizations that have employees or volunteers who molested children (Boyle, 1994) are usually brought on the grounds of failure to select, screen, train, and supervise adults who work with children. This liability is particularly visible in the scandal involving Penn State University and its football program, and in fact, one of the grounds for the lawsuits being brought is the failure to report the abuse. However, colleges and universities in the United States have not had specific statutory duties to report, except to the extent that the state law encompasses everyone in the state and requires a report. At least one state enacted a specific law requiring reports from colleges as a result of the Penn State scandal.*

The threshold for reporting in most jurisdictions is reasonable suspicion. "Reasonable suspicion" is a legal standard that depends on what a reasonable person in the same or similar circumstance would believe is a reasonable suspicion. Since, for physicians only, suspicion is a medical "term of art," it is possible that a physician might not reach the conclusion that there is a statutory "suspicion" of child maltreatment pending completion of necessary tests or scans. However, reporters are not required to "prove" child abuse but rather, once a reasonable level of concern is reached, are required by reporting laws to enlist protective services or police to complete the overall evaluation or investigation. On the other hand, notwithstanding the law, I am aware of at least one case in which a psychologist thought he was following a statutory mandate to report suspected sexual abuse and, through what appears to be a series of failed investigation and inadequate representation, ended up losing his livelihood.

State reporting laws address confidentiality issues that include testimonial privilege and duties of nondisclosure. HIPAA (the Health Insurance Portability and Accountability Act) and federal laws on substance abuse address confidentiality through laws against nondisclosure, but with modifications that address state child abuse reporting laws. Two distinct applications of the law of confidentiality can be defined. "Testimonial privileges" refer to the right of a patient or client not to have information from confidential professional-client communications become testimony in court. In contrast, "duties of nondisclosure" refer to laws and custom related to divulging or sharing personal, confidential information related to business records, therapeutic files and communications, and personal data, including income, taxes, or health status, whenever such events occur without the permission of the person to whom the information applies. Federal laws have recognized and addressed conflicts between state reporting laws and federal protections for privacy with respect to child maltreatment.

HIPAA is a modern example of highly developed laws on nondisclosure. HIPAA addresses PHI, or protected health information, and prescribes who may and may not have access to PHI without the patient's express permission. Written into HIPAA is an exception to the prohibition of disclosure of PHI when a state law requires reporting of child abuse and neglect. As noted already, child maltreatment reporting is legislated as a legal duty in all 50 states. However, it is also true that states can vary as to disclosure or reporting of information to agencies other than child protective services. A committee of the American Academy of Pediatrics analyzed these statutes as follows (see also Davidson, 2003):

> All states have laws that mandate reporting of suspected child abuse or neglect, and HIPAA rules allow disclosure of protected health information without legal guardian authorization under these circumstances. In general, if a pediatrician suspects abuse or neglect, as defined within state statutes, then he or she is obligated to disclose information to the appropriate investigative agencies, which in most states includes CPS and law enforcement agencies.
>
> Section 164.512(f) places limitations on the information released to law enforcement but not to CPS agencies. However, if a law enforcement agency is a designated authority by the state to receive and investigate child abuse reports, the pediatrician may disclose all protected health information important to the investigation without legal guardian authorization. In other circumstances, the physician may disclose protected health information to law enforcement without authorization if there is a probability of imminent physical injury to the patient, physician, or another person or if the child is missing and a law enforcement agency confirms it is investigating a missing person. (Committee on Child Abuse and Neglect, 2010)

In a related area, federal law regulates confidentiality of substance abuse records (42 C.F.R. Part 2). However, with respect to reports of child abuse and neglect, "The restrictions on disclosure do not apply to the reporting under State law of incidents of suspected child abuse and neglect to the appropriate State or local authorities" (U.S. Department of Health and Human Services, 2011, p. 4).

LEGAL ARGUMENTS ABOUT INTERVIEWS AND THERAPY

Statements made during interviews or during therapy are variable in terms of their legal implications. Outside specifically protected relationships or settings, such as when in police custody or a therapeutic setting, what a person states can be used against him or her in court as an "admission against interest" or confession. Not every such situation can be enumerated here because there are too many possible scenarios, such as participation in legal, business, hu-

---

*Protection of Vulnerable Persons (HB 1355) was signed into law in Florida by Governor Rick Scott in 2012 and is asserted to be the first such law enacted in the United States (Palm Beach Post, 2012).

man resources, investment, or other confidential meetings at which statements made must be kept confidential by all participating, unless some overriding principle permits breaching the confidentiality of the meeting. The focus here, therefore, is specifically on questions as to when a statement to a therapist will or will not fall under a duty of disclosure or perhaps a courtroom abrogation of the usual testimonial privilege.

Initial reporting of child maltreatment by therapists, as addressed above, is generally mandated in the United States, notwithstanding a therapeutic, substance abuse, or medical duty of nondisclosure. Less clear is the degree to which additional information can or must be provided as the investigation of a report proceeds. In some states, the law is clear that participation in the investigation by providing information is authorized. Since the specifics of state law and details of the relationship can vary greatly, advice from a lawyer competent to offer advice on such issues should be sought unless the therapist is certain of his or her duties and responsibilities. Examples, with extensive analysis of the duties of psychologists and how these duties vary with circumstances, can be found in Melton et al.'s (2007) *Psychological Evaluations for the Courts* (third edition). When there is doubt, recourse to a lawyer for one's agency or to one's own lawyer can lead to a court motion to restrict the professional's testimony from being required, as in the instance of a court order "quashing a subpoena."

Many professionals understand that courtroom testimony for children can be traumatic to the children, even if the prosecutor sometimes decides the testimony is unavoidable. The question of whether a caseworker, therapist, or physician who is evaluating a child client or patient may testify as to what is said by the child—that is, testify as to what the child said to the therapist (hearsay) in lieu of the child's testimony—depends on a legal analysis of the facts of the setting, the relationship to the person who heard the child's words, and the extent to which the information received by the professional would be perceived as something that reasonable persons would expect to be used in court. When the statement of a victim to a professional is to be used for criminal prosecution, the facts surrounding the statement are likely to be scrutinized with particular care, focusing particularly on whether the statement can be considered "testimonial" (*Crawford v. Washington*, 2004). For the physician or therapist in the regular practice of diagnosis and therapy, taking a "history" of why the adult brought a child for care or why the child is seeking care is standard practice and should not be considered "testimonial." However, if the interview takes place in an investigative location, such as in a child protective services office or in the presence of a police officer, then it is more likely that the child victim will have to be made available at trial for cross-examination, if the statement is crucial to the trial (e.g., *Maryland v. Snowden*, 2005). Forensic interviews are generally more likely to lead to cross-examination of the victim whenever she or he is competent and "available" to testify.

Evidence that the child is "unavailable" for medical or psychological reasons must be reviewed by the court on a case-by-case basis.

DOCUMENTATION AS IT RELATES TO TESTIMONY OR INTRODUCTION AS EVIDENCE

Physicians are taught to practice "evidence-based medicine," meaning that their diagnosis and treatment of patients is to be guided by the best available science whenever possible. Other treating professionals involved in child maltreatment cases should follow this example when they can. At the same time, not all important evidence is scientific in nature. Non-opinion, factual information is powerful and important in all court proceedings. What a witness has heard, seen, or even felt, tasted, or smelled can be crucial evidence. Keeping a chronological, "business-like" record of evaluation and treatment of a client increases the likelihood that if the professional is called to testify on behalf of a child or parent, her or his memory can be refreshed with the record, and if the record comes into court, the record will be found more credible or accorded greater "dignity" because of the way in which it has been maintained. However, in criminal trials, if the information is only about treatment and if release of the therapeutic record or testimony will hurt the child, the court can be asked to prevent the testimony. The court can restrict admission of therapeutic records following a review "in chambers" (by the judge only) that determines that the therapeutic record is not relevant to the criminal trial (*Pennsylvania v. Ritchie*, 1987). While some lawyers advise their professional clients not to keep detailed records due to concerns that something in the record will be used to make the professional seem careless, there is an important counter consideration: that the competent professional's best response to criticism or even a lawsuit is a written record of competent, careful, thoughtful, and thorough practice.

The purpose of keeping contemporaneous and business-like records is to undermine criticism that the professional's memory is flawed or that the professional is sloppy and hence "unprofessional," or, in other words, not to be trusted. Testimony that might be offered as to the many ways that memory can fail any person is made harmless to the extent that the information is recorded in a careful manner as close as possible to the time of the actual encounter.

For physicians and others responsible for obtaining and guarding physical evidence, the term "chain of evidence" is well appreciated. The concept is clear: it is unjust to convict or even hold accountable any person based on evidence that might have been mixed up or contaminated with physical evidence not gathered at the time or in the manner asserted by the prosecuting attorney. In other words, evidence must be exactly as it is purported to be, connected directly and indisputably with a defendant. Thus, creating a chain of evidence means making a record of the sequence of individuals taking successive custody of physical material that has been gathered and preserved at every step before it is presented in court. The process must assure the judge and jury that the evidence in question was gathered, guarded, preserved, and brought before the court in exactly the way that the witness being used to offer the evidence and to confirm its authenticity swears to be true.

Physicians need no reminders about the tradeoffs between "specificity" and "sensitivity' in biological tests. For example, there are a number of tests for the more than 30 sexually transmitted infections (STIs), or sexually transmitted diseases (STDs) (on laboratory diagnosis of STDs, see sources cited in Holmes et al., 2008, pp. 2139–2140). No forensically relevant test is both perfectly sensitive and perfectly specific. A most sensitive test for chlamydia inevitably produces a percentage of "false positives," indicating that a tested individual has or did have the disease when in fact the individual does not and did not. A more specific test risks a smaller percentage of false positives, meaning that if the test produces a positive result it is more likely (as compared with the sensitive test) that the person has or did have chlamydia. However, using the more specific test increases the likelihood that a person who is infected will not be diagnosed as being infected, because the more specific the test, the less sensitive it will be compared with other tests for the same condition. And, even the most specific test can still produce false positives. One remedy—which is still imperfect, for practical and scientific reasons—is to screen a patient with a very sensitive test for an STD and, if it is positive, to retest with a more specific test that is not as likely to produce a "false-positive" result.

The value of visual images of physical harm to children can be taken for granted, perhaps in part because many would view taking photos as something ordinary. Health professionals don't have time allocated for photography courses during their graduate and postgraduate training. Nor are social workers trained or, as a general rule, experienced professionally in taking photos as part of their evaluations. Before a judge or jury, who of course did not see firsthand the visible injuries to a child, noting that all of the child's injuries, at the opening of a case, could be largely invisible due to healing, the question can easily arise: "What was the harm?" The more obvious and more visible the injury, the more it is likely to be true that a picture is worth a thousand words.

TESTIMONY AS TO FACTS OR OPINIONS

Factual information is the necessary basis for any opinion accepted by a court, and until experience teaches a witness otherwise, the necessity of understanding how to present factual testimony well can be overlooked or undervalued. The direct experience with a patient or client of a professional called to testify in a child protection matter provides the essential source for the most important factual testimony. Without a factual foundation, opinion evidence has virtually no value. Good factual testimony is the strongest form of testimony. Good factual testimony provides a judge or jury with information that, whenever possible, "speaks for itself" and minimizes any features of opinion or possible bias from the witness. Professionals can learn to better observe and document the behaviors, including interactions of children and caregivers, that inform us about the quality of parenting, safety, and relationships.

It is true that different professionals to some extent gather different types of factual information. While physicians (Dubowitz & Bross, 1992) and caseworkers (Bross, 2000) gather different types of information in some areas, much of what they are told about by children or parents and what they observe is often the same—the same or closely related behaviors and indications of parenting capacity or incapacity, child trauma or child well-being. All professionals working with child abuse and neglect must be able to manage their own tendency to practice "gaze aversion"—the tendency of every person to look away from disquieting information. In a different but related way, any professional can practice "self-protection" from secondary trauma by oversimplifying many family situations in a stereotyped response that overestimates a child's safety or underestimates protective factors present. Factual information that can be observed and documented is extensive: What issue of harm or safety brings a child to attention? What is the parent's perception of the child? How well does the parent describe the child? How has the child grown and developed? Are these descriptions at all detailed, consistent with what others observe, and sensitive to the abilities of children as they develop? Does the parent reasonably attribute good and bad traits in the child as well as trends of progress or delay? How much does the parent express an insistence that the child does what the parent needs, and how well can the parent recognize any way in which the parent is contributing to the child's lack of safety or positive growth? As observed through either a proper interactional study or other competent clinical assessment, how do child and parent interact with each other, and to what extent are they interacting with positive or negative behaviors? Judges and jurors, like professionals, make attributions of behaviors and do so when given a factual basis for their attributions (Jones & Davis, 1965). Most people prefer to have facts given to them so that they can make up their own minds, and observations of the behaviors of people about whom decisions are to be made will be received with more confidence if the observations occur over time and with different observers, and if the individuals in question are seen in different settings (Kelley, 1967).

Because no professional is expert in everything, one way to approach the problem of opinion testimony is to anticipate what factual information might be needed in court that the professional can recognize early and to find a way to involve others with more expertise. Thus, screening for developmental disability, substance abuse disorders, alcohol use disorder, mental illness, and domestic violence can lead to requests for additional information by the court without the caseworker or physician having to make a concluding opinion or diagnosis.

Questions about who can offer opinion testimony can be sufficiently complicated that a potential witness might make a study of this issue by referring to treatises (the best general treatise on evidence with respect to child witness law and practice is Myers, 2011), or more efficiently, the witness can rely on the summoning attorney to explain what opinions will be sought and in what manner on the witness stand. Moreover, without being qualified as an expert witness, it is often possible for a witness to make statements of great value in answer to questions on whether the behaviors of a particular child or parent are especially unusual or typical in the experience of the witness who has worked with many similar individuals. A comprehensive guide for psychologists, also useful for nonpsychologists who must testify about behavioral matters, is Melton et al.'s (2007) *Psychological Evaluations for the Courts*.

THE "LEGAL APPARATUS" IN CIVIL VERSUS CRIMINAL CASES

Sufficiently experienced non-lawyer witnesses can eventually acquire not only a working knowledge but a highly nuanced understanding of the different types of courts and legal processes. Simplistically, criminal courts exist to punish individuals who have acted wrongfully to a criminal extent and, through criminal prosecution, to deter others from similar bad acts in the future. Retribution, rehabilitation, and conciliation can be factors in the criminal justice system and frequently are not. With respect to child maltreatment, one published study suggested that a very small percentage of "confirmed" cases of child maltreatment result in criminal prosecution (Tjaden & Thoennes, 1992), and the particular cases filed depend on such factors as the background and characteristics of the perpetrator and victim, severity of abuse, and nature of the available evidence, along with maternal support of the victim (Cross, De Vos, & Whitcomb, 1994). The Bill of Rights of the U.S. Constitution, to a degree, incorporates a criminal code into the nation's fundamental law, thus affording special protections for defendants in all American criminal proceedings. Therefore, criminal proceedings have a highly rigorous set of procedures and rules of evidence intended to provide due process and fairness. What a witness says and what evidence will be permitted into the trial are much more limited than what is permitted in noncriminal proceedings.

The simplest way to describe civil proceedings is that all "actions in law" that are noncriminal proceedings are civil in nature. Because the United States is a nation of law, there is virtually no form of conflict for which redress cannot be sought in the civil courts. Terms for these legal proceedings include torts (negligence law suits), contracts, administrative law, wills, trusts, commercial code, zoning, divorce and child custody, admiralty law, and the list goes on. One subset of civil law should be of particular interest to anyone concerned with child maltreatment: public health, mental health, chemical dependency, and child dependency and protection. While these latter forms of law are noncriminal in their intent—that is, they are intended to be ameliorative rather than punitive in character—they are actions that must be brought by involving state agencies or state-licensed agencies. All of these proceedings, in one way or another, determine the "status" of an individual or (in the instance of public health and restaurants or other businesses affecting public health) business entities. A neglected area of social science, law, and therapy is recognition that law is "an intervention variable." Even though most research currently informing the practices of child protection is based on work with "involuntary" interventions (i.e., with populations of children and parents who came to attention due to reporting), few have bothered to carefully examine when and why such interventions are necessary or unnecessary or what trade-offs exist in managing cases through legal involvement—or at least, the possibility of legal involvement (Bross, 2009).

One area in which little has been done to study "best practices" is the coordination of criminal and civil approaches to child maltreatment. While conflict between different professions is not unknown, and opinions about the harm induced by criminal, civil, or no legal interventions are debated, only rarely have researchers tried to examine the comparative outcomes for civil and criminal proceedings (Runyan et al., 1988; Whitcomb et al., 1994). Similarly, there are few studies that carefully compare reunification and termination of the child-parent legal relationship. As an example of a situation in which only the criminal law is likely to be effective, prosecution of the online exploitation of children relies on law enforcement officers to investigate and hold individuals accountable, including those who go so far as to try to meet their child victims. On the other hand, if maltreatment is very severe, the criminal law can place a parent in prison, but only a child protection agency can pursue a decision to free a child for adoption due to extreme and "untreatable" issues of parenting. Moreover, while termination of the parent-child legal relationship has been addressed in many legal decisions and state statutes, the process has almost never been addressed in terms of how professionals manage the issue with respect to their own emotions and background. Termination of the child-parent legal relationship is a fundamentally psychological process for all involved, even if it can only occur within a legal framework, and rarely has this area of law been addressed explicitly in terms of how law must respond for the psychological well-being of both the families and the professionals involved (for an example of a termination law that responds with all these measures to demands for fairness in terminations, see Bross, 1978; see also Bross, 1995).

POSSIBLE LEGAL CONSEQUENCES FOR THERAPISTS AND CASEWORKERS RESPONDING TO CHILD MALTREATMENT

Obvious violations of duties due to clients, including professional boundary violations or even sexual transgressions (Bouhoutsos et al., 1993), have potential remedies through state professional grievance committees and lawsuits. A review of any state's log of professional grievances is likely to reveal instances of professional impropriety with clients. Already mentioned is the difficulty of all therapists in working with divorce custody matters. In general, liability for working as a therapist for children and parents raises the same risks of claims that arise for any behavioral health therapist, such as not identifying a suicidal patient and preventing self-injury, failure to obtain informed consent, or negligent misdiagnosis (Melton et al., 2007, pp. 81–85).

The role of caseworkers involved in placement decisions exposes them to one of the oldest recorded forms of liability for failures in child protection in the United States—that is, failing to properly select, train, and monitor placements, including foster placements (Bross, 1983). A newer but not yet fully appreciated potential source of liability, a risk that should not be overstated at this time, is the possibility of a lawsuit being filed for interviewing a child without a search warrant. Such a case was filed on the West Coast and was eventually reviewed by the U.S. Supreme Court. Both a caseworker and a law enforcement officer interviewed, at her school, a 9-year-old student who was reported to be a victim of child sexual abuse. Notwithstanding the subsequent conviction of the child's father for abuse, both professionals were sued by the mother on behalf of the victim for a violation of the child's rights against an unlawful search under the Fourth Amendment to the U.S. Constitution. In *Camreta v. Greene* (2011, p. 4), the U.S. Supreme Court reviewed the decision of the 9th Circuit Court of Appeals, in which the Federal Appellate Court ruled that the interview was a violation of the Fourth Amendment. Writing for the majority, Justice Sotomayor summarized what the 9th Circuit Court of Appeals was saying. "Government officials investigating allegations of child abuse," the court warned, "should cease operating on the assumption that a 'special need' automatically justifies dispensing with traditional Fourth Amendment protections in this context." The Court of Appeals ruling found that the child was interviewed in the absence of a warrant, a court order, exigent circumstances, or parental consent. While the decision most clearly applies to states covered by the 9th Circuit Court of Appeals, it serves as a general warning that courts in the future can look carefully at whether child protection evaluations, especially if a criminal case might result, must be done as if they were being conducted as a criminal investigation. While the two professionals in *Camreta v. Greene* did not end up having to pay damages, workers might need advice on the meaning of "exigent circumstances" from their legal counsel when their inves-

tigation may include the likelihood of a crime having been committed.

LEGAL DECISIONS INVOLVING EMOTIONALLY DIFFICULT TOPICS

The psychological nature of many situations in which law is called upon for a remedy is not always considered, by many of those involved in the case, from a psychological perspective. Law properly applied reflects and accurately recognizes and incorporates human experience, intelligence, and emotion, to the extent possible. For example, it is not always possible to avoid the criminal ramifications of child abuse. If a child has been mortally injured but lingers, and questions of brain death or other questions of end-of-life decision making arise, agencies and courts must respond to the circumstances created by the injury. Whereas parents normally must make end-of-life decisions for their children, the possibility that a parent is responsible criminally for the child's death can end up taking the decision out of the parent's control. For example, the first time the Harvard Criteria for Brain Death were applied by a court order in the United States was in a child abuse death in which a guardian ad litem was appointed to agree to a child's removal from life support because the parent, facing criminal charges that would be more severe once the child died, refused to consent to the removal of life support (*Lovato v. Dist. Court*, 1979).

When termination of the child-parent legal relationship becomes a necessary consideration, it is not surprising if some involved in the case feel that involuntary "divorce" between child and parent is like a death in the family or, at the very least, represents a professional failure. Most children wish to be with a parent no matter how abusive, although there are exceptions. The problem is that, in the words of Dr. C. Henry Kempe, there are some parents who love their children very, very much, but not at all well. Physicians and nurses cannot continue to work with the most difficult medical cases unless they can accept that all of us eventually die and that the measure of success is preventing avoidable illness and death and providing all possible comfort to patients who cannot survive. Notwithstanding these perhaps obvious observations, Elizabeth Kübler-Ross (1969) revealed in her book on death and dying how many physicians and nurses wouldn't openly speak of a patient's impending death with the patient, justifying their behavior as a protection for the patient, while the patient felt isolated and alone, often in full knowledge of his or her condition. If there is something in a caregiver's behavior or condition that might be akin to "cancer of the soul," then not being able to find or provide treatment or support sufficient to enable a particular parent of a specific child to safely care for that child might describe such a situation.

A sense of "due process" enacted or codified into law providing the basis for termination of the parent-child legal relationship should meet or exceed the legal requirements for termination, as well as persuade most people who care about child maltreatment of the fundamental fairness of the entire process. A first step would be a statute that provides parents with clear notification from the first filing and service of process related to an allegation of child maltreatment, as well as a statutory scheme that provides for a civil trial by jury or judge resulting in an adjudication of child abuse or neglect and provides free legal counsel for indigent parents. Next, the parent should have a right to a treatment plan, a plan approved by the judge as appropriate to address the conduct or condition that led to the child abuse or neglect. Any termination decision must be made by clear and convincing evidence that the plan was refused by the parent or failed to correct the conduct or condition, and, indeed, the U.S. Supreme Court has ruled that all aspects of the termination decision must meet a "clear and convincing" standard of proof (*Santosky v. Kramer*, 1982). Added to these due process requirements for a possible termination should be a finding of specific parental unfitness and, finally, but not before meeting the first steps in the process, a ruling that termination of the parent-child legal relationship would be in the child's best interests. If the case proceeds to a termination hearing, not only should the parent and the child be represented independently, but the parent should be able to present a professional witness to testify as to the parent's capacity to parent the child in question, paid for by the state, subject only to court review of the reasonableness of costs. The parent should be provided with free transcripts on appeal if termination is ordered, and there should be a requirement for post-termination review with the added requirement of a post-termination report filed independently by the child's guardian ad litem or attorney. The purpose of the post-termination report would be to decrease delays in the child's adoption and to increase the likelihood that the adoption will succeed. Such a statute should not only meet U.S. Constitutional requirements but provide a conscientious balance for the rights of all involved (for an example of a statute containing all of these provisions, see *Colorado Revised Statutes* § 19-3-601 et seq.).

LEGAL AUTHORIZATION FOR CARE OF CHILDREN IN SPECIFIED CIRCUMSTANCES

In general, parents, or those in a parental capacity, are the lawful custodians and only decision-makers in all matters related to the care of their children, including medical care. In some specific circumstances, this general rule will not be enforced due to overriding considerations of child safety. For example, if a child is being seen by a physician who suspects child abuse, some state laws authorize the physician to undertake a few enumerated steps to document or diagnose the abuse. For example, in the State of Colorado:

> C.R.S. §19-3-306. Evidence of abuse—color photographs and X-rays. (1) Any child health associate, person licensed to practice medicine in this state, registered nurse or licensed practical nurse, hospital personnel engaged in the admission, examination, care, or treatment of patients, medical examiner, coroner, social worker, psychologist, or local law enforcement officer who has before him a child he reasonably believes has been abused or neglected may take or cause to be taken color photographs of the areas of trauma visible on the child. If medically indicated, such person may take or cause to be taken X rays of the child.

Many states have laws providing for physicians to call a judge, child protection agency, or law enforcement officer to report that a child is being taken from a hospital against medical advice, as in the example of a child suspected to be maltreated and taken before the diagnostic workup can be completed. When a child is in the custody of a child protection agency, a judge can be asked to order treatment necessary for the child's health. More broadly, in instances of medical care neglect, a court order or court adjudication can be sought for care to save the life of the child or to prevent serious bodily injury. There are at least 10 or 11 factors that courts will consider and weigh before ordering treatment over the objections of the parents, such as whether denial of treatment will lead to death or serious bodily injury, and with what probability; whether the treatment can be delayed until the child is older; whether the treatment is standard and widely accepted; the probability that the treatment will succeed; and for a child who is old enough to be consulted or to consent, the wishes of the child (Bross, 1982; Bross & DeHerrera, 2005).

CHANGING PRACTICES AND LEGAL IMPLICATIONS

Child protection can be evidence-based or slogan-driven, and susceptible to swings of public opinion that affect funding and practices. Without a legal framework, even voluntary child protection would become unpredictable in terms of duties, liabilities, powers, and limitations. With the advent of family-group decision making and differential response, priorities of prevention, treatment, and record keeping are changing. Intended and unintended consequences of each change will inevitably be reflected in the law. This is an important reason for "law as an intervention variable" to become part of research, training, practice, and policy in child protection.

CONCLUSIONS

There are many legal issues associated with child maltreatment and its therapy, and the professionals who do the diagnosing and treating, as well as children and parents drawn into the child protection system, need and deserve to have access to legal advice. Caseworkers who are part of or have access to multidisciplinary teams view their communications with medical and legal colleagues favorably, when compared with those who do not have such access (Fryer et al., 1988). Over 470 lawyers in the United States are certified child welfare law specialists, and they are practicing in 33 states (D. Trujillo, Administrator, Child Welfare Law Certification Program, National Association of Counsel for Children, personal communication, November 11, 2012). While specialists are not available everywhere, agencies responsible for working with more than a few cases of child maltreatment annually should have ready access to expert legal resources. Law is an essential foundation for child protection, as surely as law forms the basis for other government activities clearly intended to ameliorate unacceptable human health problems, as illustrated by the examples of public health and mental health. The law enumerates the authority, procedures, and limitations for those acting within the child protection environment. If at all possible, experienced child protection lawyers should always be available to those working to protect children.

References

Berry, J. (1992). *Lead us not into temptation: Catholic priests and the sexual abuse of children.* New York, NY: Doubleday.

Bouhoutsos, J., Holroyd, J., Lerman, H., Forer, B. R., & Greenberg, M. (1993). Sexual intimacy between psychotherapists and patients. *Professional Psychology: Research and Practice, 14*(2), 185–196.

Boyle, P. (1994). *Scouts honor: Sexual abuse in America's most trusted institution.* Rocklin, CA: Prima Publishing.

Bross, D. C. (1978). Termination of the parent-child legal relationship in Colorado. *Colorado Lawyer, 7*(3), 362–376.

Bross, D. C. (1982). Medical care neglect. *Child Abuse & Neglect, 5*(4), 375–382.

Bross, D. C. (1983). Professional and agency liability for child protection negligence. *Law, Medicine, and Society, 11*(2), 71–75.

Bross, D. C. (1987). Professional and agency liability for negligence in child protection. In D. C. Bross & L. F. Michaels (Eds.), *Foundations of child advocacy* (pp. 181–196). Denver, CO: National Association of Counsel for Children.

Bross, D. C. (1995). Terminating the parent-child legal relationship as a response to child sexual abuse. *Loyola Law Review, 26*(2), 287–319. [Excerpted and republished in D. E. Abrams & S. H. Ramsey, *Children and the law: Doctrine, policy and practice* (pp. 543–546), St. Paul, MN: West, 2000.]

Bross, D. C. (2000). Witness preparation for trials related to child abuse or neglect. In L. King & M. R. Ventrell (Eds.), *Improving the professional response to children in the legal system* (pp. 143–152). Denver, CO: National Association of Counsel for Children.

Bross, D. C. (2009). Involuntary therapy: A good idea? In A. Kellogg (Ed.), *Standing at the forefront: Effective advocacy in today's world* (pp. 229–250). Denver, CO: National Association of Counsel for Children.

Bross, D. C., & DeHerrera, N. (2005). Refusal of therapy for children: Factors affecting judicial decisions to override parental decisions. In A. G. Donnelly (Ed.), *State of the art advocacy for children, youth, and families* (pp. 147–158). Denver, CO: National Association of Counsel for Children.

Camreta v. Greene, 131 S. Ct. 2020, 179 L. Ed. 2d 1118 (2011).

Child Welfare Information Gateway. (2010). *Mandatory reporters of child abuse and neglect: summary of state laws.* Washington, DC: U.S. Department of Health and Human Services, Children's Bureau. www.childwelfare.gov/systemwide/laws _policies/statutes/manda.cfm

Committee on Child Abuse and Neglect. (2010) Child abuse, confidentiality, and the Health Insurance Portability and Accountability Act. *Pediatrics, 125*(1), 197–201.

Crawford v. Washington, 541 U.S. 36 (2004).

Cross, T., De Vos, E., & Whitcomb, D. (1994). Prosecution of child sexual abuse: Which cases are accepted? *Child Abuse & Neglect, 18*(8), 663–677.

Davidson, H. (2003). *The impact of HIPAA on child abuse and neglect cases.* Washington, DC: American Bar Association.

Dubowitz, H., & Bross, D. C. (1992). The pediatrician's documentation of child maltreatment. *American Journal of the Diseases of Childhood, 146,* 596–599.

Fryer, G. E., Jr., Poland, J. E., Bross, D. C., & Krugman, R. D. (1988). The child protective service worker: A profile of needs, attitudes, and utilization of professional resources. *Child Abuse & Neglect, 12*(4), 481–490.

Haralambie, A. M. (2010). Collateral proceedings. In D. N. Duquette and A. M. Haralambie (Eds.), *Child welfare law and practice* (2nd ed., pp. 399–414). Denver, CO: National Association of Counsel for Children.

Holmes, K. K., Sparling, P. F., Stamm, W. E., Piot, P., Wasserheit, J. N., Corey, L., et al. (2008). *Sexually transmitted diseases* (4th ed.). New York, NY: McGraw Hill Medical.

Jones, E. E., & Davis, K. E. (1965). From acts to dispositions: The attribution process in person perception. In L. Berkowitz (Ed.), *Advances in experimental social psychology* (Vol. II, pp. 219–266). New York, NY: Academic Press.

Kelley, H. H. (1967). Attribution theory in social psychology. In D. Levine (Ed.), *Nebraska symposium on motivation* (Vol. 15, pp. 192–240). Lincoln, NE: University of Nebraska Press.

Kübler-Ross, E. (1969). *On death and dying.* London, UK: Routledge.

Landeros v. Flood, 131 Cal. Rptr. 69, 551 P.2d 389 (1976).

Lovato v. Dist. Court, 198 Colo. 419, 601 P.2d 1072 (1979).

Maryland v. Snowden, 867 A.2d 314 385 Md. 64 (Md. Ct. App., 2005).

Mathews, B., & Bross, D. C. (2008). Mandated reporting is still a policy with reason: Empirical evidence and philosophical grounds. *Child Abuse & Neglect, 32*(5), 511–516.

Melton, G. B., Petrila, J., Poythress, N. G., & Slobogin, C. (2007). *Psychological evaluations for the courts: A handbook for mental health professionals and lawyers* (3rd ed.). New York, NY: Guilford Press.

Myers, J. E. B. (2011). *Myers on evidence of interpersonal violence: Child maltreatment, intimate partner violence, rape, stalking, and elder abuses* (5th ed.). New York, NY: Aspen Publishers.

Palm Beach Post. (2012, April 27). "Penn State" child abuse reporting law signed into law by Gov. Scott. www.palm beachpost.com/news/news/state-regional/penn-state-child -abuse-reporting-law-signed-into-l/nN3S7

Paulsen, M. (1967). Child abuse reporting laws: The shape of legislation. *Columbia Law Review, 67*(1), 1–49.

Pennsylvania v. Ritchie, 480 U.S. 39 (1987).

Runyan, D. K., Everson, M., Edelsohn, G., Hunter, W., & Coulter, M. (1988). Impact of legal intervention on sexually abused children. *Journal of Pediatrics, 113*(4), 647–653.

Santosky v. Kramer, 455 U.S. 745 (1982).

Tjaden, P., & Thoennes, N. (1992). Legal intervention in child maltreatment cases. *Child Abuse & Neglect, 16,* 807–821.

U.S. Department of Health and Human Services, Substance Abuse and Mental Health Services Administration. (2011). *Applying the substance abuse confidentiality regulations 42 CFR Part 2 (revised).* www.samhsa.gov/about/laws/SAMHSA _42CFRPART2FAQII_Revised.pdf

Whitcomb, D., DeVos, E., Cross, T., Peeler, N., Runyan, D. K., Hunter, W., et al. (1994). *The child victim as witness: Research report.* Washington, DC: Office of Juvenile Justice and Delinquency Prevention.

INDEX